DICTIONARY OF MEDICAL BIOGRAPHY

DICTIONARY OF MEDICAL BIOGRAPHY

Volume 4, M–R

Edited by

W. F. Bynum *and* Helen Bynum

GREENWOOD PRESS
Westport, Connecticut • London

Library of Congress Cataloging-in-Publication Data

Dictonary of medical biography / edited by W. F. Bynum and Helen Bynum.
     p.   cm.
     Includes bibliographical references and index.
     ISBN 0–313–32877–3 (set : alk. paper) — ISBN 0–313–32878–1 (v. 1 : alk. paper) —
     ISBN 0–313–32879–X (v. 2 : alk. paper) — ISBN 0–313–32880–3 (v. 3 : alk. paper) —
     ISBN 0–313–32881–1 (v. 4 : alk. paper) — ISBN 0–313–32882–X (v. 5 : alk. paper)
     1. Medicine—Biography. 2. Healers—Biography. I. Bynum, W. F. (William F.), 1943– . II. Bynum, Helen.
    R134.D57 2007
    610—dc22   2006022953

British Library Cataloguing in Publication Data is available.

Library of Congress Catalog Card Number: 2006022953
ISBN: 0–313–32877–3 (set)
        0–313–32878–1 (vol. 1)
        0–313–32879–X (vol. 2)
        0–313–32880–3 (vol. 3)
        0–313–32881–1 (vol. 4)
        0–313–32882–X (vol. 5)

First published in 2007

Greenwood Press, 88 Post Road West, Westport, CT 06881
An imprint of Greenwood Publishing Group, Inc.
www.greenwood.com

Printed in the United States of America

The paper used in this book complies with the
Permanent Paper Standard issued by the National
Information Standards Organization (Z39.48–1984).

10   9   8   7   6   5   4   3   2   1

CONTENTS

CONTRIBUTORS

Göran Åkerström
Academic Hospital, Uppsala, Sweden
Sandström

Seema Alavi
Jamia Millia University, New Delhi, India
Aziz

Angelo Albrizio
Institut d'Histoire de la Médecine et de la Santé,
Geneva, Switzerland
De Giovanni

W. R. Albury
University of New South Wales, Sydney,
Australia
Bichat, Broussais, Corvisart des Marets, Magendie

Marta de Almeida
Museu de Astronomia e Ciências Afins,
Rio de Janeiro, Brazil
Ribas

Cristina Álvarez Millán
UNED, Madrid, Spain
Ibn Buṭlān, Al-Majūsī, Ibn al-Nafīs, Al-Rāzī, Ibn Rushd,
Ibn Zuhr

Stuart Anderson
LSHTM, London, England
Beecham, Holloway, Squibb

Warwick Anderson
University of Wisconsin–Madison, Madison, WI,
USA
Burnet, Cleland

Jon Arrizabalaga
CSIC, Barcelona, Spain
Laguna, Sanches, Torrella

S. N. Arseculeratne
University of Peradeniya, Peradeniya,
Sri Lanka
M. Paul, Wickramarachchi

Mikel Astrain
Universidad de Granada, Granada, Spain
Lardizábal Dubois

Guy Attewell
Wellcome Trust Centre for the History of Medicine
at UCL, London, England
Medical Traditions in South Asia, Abd ul-Hamīd,
M. Ajmal Khān, M. A'zam Khān, Saīd

Nara Azevedo
Casa de Oswaldo Cruz, Fundação Oswaldo Cruz,
Rio de Janeiro, Brazil
Cruz

Søren Bak-Jensen
Medical Museion, Copenhagen, Denmark
Fibiger, Friderichsen, Gram, Hagedorn,
Pindborg, Salomonsen

Martha Baldwin
Stonehill College, Easton, MA, USA
Dionis

Marta Aleksandra Balinska
Institut national du cancer, Paris, France
Hirszfeld, Rajchman, Śniadecki

Rosa Ballester
Universidad Miguel Hernández, Alicante-Valencia, Spain
Martínez Vargas

Scott Bamber
UNICEF, Bangkok, Thailand
Jivaka

Richard Barnett
Wellcome Trust Centre for the History of Medicine
at UCL, London, England
Godlee, Knox, Long, W. Morton, Read, Simpson, Wakley

Josep Lluís Barona
Universidad de Valencia Blasco, Valencia, Spain
Ramón y Cajal, Trueta i Raspall

Penelope Barrett
Wellcome Trust Centre for the History of Medicine
at UCL, London, England
Li Shizhen

Alexander R. Bay
Chapman University, Orange Campus, CA, USA
Takaki

Elaine Beale
Cherhill, Wiltshire, England
Ingen Housz

Norman Beale
Cherhill, Wiltshire, England
Ingen Housz

Denise Best
California State University, Fresno, CA, USA
Pokrovskaia

Anne-Emanuelle Birn
University of Toronto, Toronto, ON, Canada
Morquio

Carla Bittel
Loyola Marymount University, Los Angeles, CA, USA
Baker, A. Jacobi, M. P. Jacobi, Van Hoosen

Johanna Bleker
ZHGB, Institut für Geschichte der Medizin,
Berlin, Germany
Henle, Schoenlein

Michael Bliss
University of Toronto, Toronto, ON, Canada
Cushing, Dandy

Hans Blom
Erasmus Universiteit, Rotterdam, the Netherlands
Mandeville

Michel Bonduelle
University of Paris, Paris, France
Duchenne de Boulogne, Guillain

Christopher Booth
Wellcome Trust Centre for the History of Medicine
at UCL, London, England
Haygarth, Hurst, Lettsom, Sherlock

Cornelius Borck
McGill University, Montreal, QC, Canada
Berger

Mineke Bosch
Universiteit Maastricht, Maastricht,
the Netherlands
Jacobs

David Bradley
LSHTM, London, England
Macdonald

Gunnar Broberg
University of Lund, Lund, Sweden
Linnaeus

Alejandra Bronfman
University of British Columbia, Vancouver,
BC, Canada
Finlay y Barres, Guiteras Gener

Linda Bryder
University of Auckland, Auckland, New Zealand
Gordon, King, Liley

Chris Burton
University of Lethbridge, Lethbridge, AB,
Canada
Burdenko, Fedorov, Semashko, Solev'ev

Helen Bynum
Shadingfield, Suffolk, England
Halsted, Harinasuta, Rogers, Snow, Steptoe

Ricardo Campos
CSIC, Madrid, Spain
Rubio Gali

Franco Carnevale
Azienda Sanitaria di Firenze, Florence, Italy
Devoto, Ramazzini

Ana María Carrillo
UNAM, Mexico City, Mexico
Montoya Lafragua

Ian Carter
University of Auckland, Auckland, New Zealand
M. Bell

Ramón Castejón-Bolea
Universidad Miguel Hernández, Alicante, Spain
Azúa y Suárez

Rafael Chabrán
Whittier College, Whittier, CA, USA
Hernández

Iain Chalmers
The James Lind Initiative, Oxford, England
Cochrane

Joël Chandelier
Ecole française de Rome, Rome, Italy
Gentile da Foligno

Rethy Chhem
University of Western Ontario, London, ON,
Canada
Yajnavaraha

Indira Chowdhury
Tata Institute of Fundamental Research,
Mumbai, India
*Chopra, Dharmendra, Mukerji, Pandit,
Ramalingaswami, P. Sen, Vakil*

Charlotte Christensen-Nugues
University of Lund, Lund, Sweden
Harpestreng

Amy Eisen Cislo
Washington University, St Louis, MO, USA
Gilbert the Englishman

Catherine S. Coleborne
Waikato University, Hamilton, New Zealand
Manning

Andrea Contini
University of Paris XII, Paris, France
Basaglia

Roger Cooter
Wellcome Trust Centre for the History of Medicine
at UCL, London, England
Braid, Charnley, Gall, R. Jones, Treves, Wells

Anne Cottebrune
Ruprecht-Karls-Universität Heidelberg,
Heidelberg, Germany
Fischer, Wagner

Christopher Crenner
KUMC, Kansas City, KS, USA
*Bowditch, Codman, Edsall, J. Jackson, Jarvis,
Minot*

Anna Crozier
University of Edinburgh, Edinburgh, Scotland
Atiman, Cook, Kasili, Spoerry, C. Williams

Ivan Crozier
University of Edinburgh, Edinburgh, Scotland
*Dickinson, Ellis, Haire, Hirschfeld, C. Mosher,
E. Mosher, Reich, Sanger, Stopes*

Marcos Cueto
Universidad Peruana Cayetano Heredia,
Lima, Peru
*Balmis, Candau, Horwitz Barak, Houssay,
Monge Medrano, Núñez Butrón, Paz Soldán,
Soper*

Michael Z. David
University of Chicago, Chicago, IL, USA
Pavlovskii, Sklifosovskii

Rosalie David
University of Manchester, Manchester,
England
Imhotep

Annemarie de Knecht-van Eekelen
CITO International, Arnhem, the Netherlands
De Lange

Ana Cecilia Rodríguez de Romo
Universidad Nacional Autónoma de México,
Mexico City, Mexico
*Arias de Benavides, Bernard, Bustamante
Vasconcelos, Chávez Sánchez, Izquierdo
Raudón, Liceaga, Martínez Báez, Montaña
Carranco*

Michelle DenBeste
California State University, Fresno, CA, USA
Pokrovskaia

Michael Denham
Wellcome Trust Centre for the History of Medicine
at UCL, London, England
M. Warren

Sven Dierig
Max-Planck-Institut, Berlin, Germany
Brücke, Ludwig

Derek A. Dow
University of Auckland, Auckland, New
Zealand
Buck, Gillies, Hercus, G. Robb, Scott

Alex Dracobly
University of Oregon, Eugene, OR, USA
Fournier, Ricord

Jean-Jacques Dreifuss
Centre Médical Universitaire, Geneva,
Switzerland
Coindet, Prevost

Ariane Dröscher
University of Bologna, Bologna, Italy
*Bassini, Bizzozero, Cotugno, Lombroso, Perroncito,
Rasori, Rizzoli*

Jacalyn Duffin
Queen's University, Kingston, ON, Canada
Laennec

Marguerite Dupree
University of Glasgow, Glasgow, Scotland
Anderson, Blackwell, Jex-Blake

Achintya Kumar Dutta
University of Burdwan, West Bengal, India
Brahmachari

William Eamon
New Mexico State University, Las Cruces, NM, USA
Nicholas of Poland

Myron Echenberg
McGill University, Montreal, QC, Canada
Brazil, Girard, A. Gregory, Jamot, Simond, Yersin

Wolfgang U. Eckart
Ruprecht-Karls-Universität Heidelberg,
Heidelberg, Germany
*Büchner, Dietl, Domagk, Sachs, Sauerbruch, Schwalbe,
Sennert, Skoda, Wundt, Zeiss*

Flávio Coelho Edler
Casa de Oswaldo Cruz, Fundação Oswaldo Cruz,
Rio de Janeiro, Brazil
Wucherer

Martin Edwards
Wellcome Trust Centre for the History of Medicine
at UCL, London, England
Balint

Kristen Ann Ehrenberger
University of Illinois, Urbana-Champaign, IL, USA
Drake

Antoinette Emch-Dériaz
University of Florida, Gainsville, FL, USA
Tissot

Eric J. Engstrom
ZHGB, Berlin, Germany
Kraepelin

Gunnar Eriksson
Uppsala Universitet, Uppsala, Sweden
Rudbeck

Bernardino Fantini
Institut d'Histoire de la Médecine et de la Santé,
Geneva, Switzerland
*Baglivi, Bovet, Celli, Dubini, Fabrizi da Acquapendente,
Golgi, Grassi, Lancisi, Pacini, Puccinotti, Redi, Sanarelli*

F. N. Fastier
University of Otago, Dunedin, New Zealand
Smirk

Morten Fink-Jensen
University of Copenhagen, Copenhagen, Denmark
Bartholin

Michael A. Flannery
University of Alabama at Birmingham,
Maylene, AL, USA
*J. Jones, Lloyd, McDowell, Newton, Nott, E. Warren,
D. Williams*

Yajaira Freites
IVIC, Caracas, Venezuela
Balmis, Beauperthuy, Gabaldón, Razetti

Charlotte Furth
University of Southern California, Los Angeles,
CA, USA
Zhu Zhenheng

Namrata R. Ganneri
Independent scholar, Mumbai, India
Joshi, Rakhmabai, Scudder

Michelle Garceau
Princeton University, Princeton, NJ, USA
Chauliac, William of Saliceto

Amy Gardiner
LSHTM, London, England
Burkitt

Nina Rattner Gelbart
Occidental College, Los Angeles, CA, USA
Du Coudray

Toby Gelfand
University of Ottawa, Ottowa, ON, Canada
Bayle, Bernheim, Bourneville, Charcot, Desault, Hayem,
Lapeyronie, Lasègeu, Péan, Petit, Sée

Jacques Gélis
University of Paris, Paris, France
Baudelocque

Dario Generali
Edizione Nazionale delle Opere di Antonio Vallisneri,
Milan, Italy
Vallisneri

Norman Gevitz
Ohio University, Athens, OH, USA
A. Still

James Gillespie
University of Sydney, Sydney, Australia
Argyle, Cilento

Florence Eliza Glaze
Coastal Carolina University, Conway, SC, USA
Constantine the African, Gariopontus

Christopher Goetz
Rush University Medical Center, Chicago, IL,
USA
Déjerine, Marie

Asaf Goldschmidt
Tel Aviv University, Tel Aviv, Israel
Li Gao, Liu Wansu, Qian Yi, Wang Weiyi,
Xu Shuwei

Christoph Gradmann
University of Oslo, Oslo, Norway
Klebs, Koch, Pettenkofer, Rabinowitsch-Kempner

John L. Graner
Mayo Clinic, Rochester, MN, USA
C. Mayo, W. Mayo

Joanna Grant
London, England
Wang Ji

Monica H. Green
Arizona State University, Tempe, AZ, USA
Trota

Samuel H. Greenblatt
Brown University, Pawtucket, RI, USA
Broca

David Greenwood
University of Nottingham, Nottingham,
England
Florey

Alberto Alonso Guardo
Universidad de Vallodolid, Vallodolid, Spain
Bernard of Gordon

Patrizia Guarnieri
Università degli Studi de Firenze, Florence, Italy
Bufalini, Cerletti, Chiarugi, Concetti, De Sanctis,
Morselli, Mya

Annick Guénel
LASEMA, Villejuif, France
Tùng Tôn Thất

Anita Guerrini
University of California, Santa Barbara, CA,
USA
G. Cheyne

Anne Y. Guillou
L'Université de Haute-Bretagne, Rennes, France
Pen

Bert Hall
University of Toronto, Toronto, ON, Canada
Guido da Vigevano

June Hannam
University of the West of England, Bristol, England
R. Paget

Caroline Hannaway
NIH History, Bethesda, MD, USA
Alibert, Cruveilhier, Dunglison, Dupuytren, Louis, Parran

Signe Lindskov Hansen
Copenhagen, Denmark
Finsen

Marta E. Hanson
Johns Hopkins University, Baltimore, MD, USA
Wu Youxing, Ye Gui, Zhang Jiebin

Susan Hardy
University of New South Wales, Sydney, Australia
Gillbee

Mark Harrison
Wellcome Unit for the History of Medicine, University of Oxford, Oxford, England
Carter, Christophers, Fayrer, Martin, Parkes, Ross

Joy Harvey
Independent scholar, Somerville, MA, USA
Bert, Bertillon, Brès, Edwards-Pilliet, Littré, Rayer, Tardieu, Trousseau, Vulpian

Mike Hawkins
Wellcome Trust Centre for the History of Medicine at UCL/Imperial College, London, England
Willis

E. A. Heaman
McGill University, Montreal, QC, Canada
Fleming, Sanderson, Wright

R. van Hee
Universiteit Antwerpen, Antwerp, Belgium
Depage, Vesalius

Jürgen Helm
Martin Luther Universität, Halle-Wittenberg, Halle, Germany
Brunfels, Erxleben, Frank, Gersdorff, Hoffmann, Stahl

John Henry
University of Edinburgh, Edinburgh, Scotland
Caius, Dubois, Fernel, Harvey, Linacre, Lower, Turquet, Winsløw

Volker Hess
ZHGB, Berlin, Germany
Behring, Frerichs, Kraus, Leyden, Traube, Wunderlich

Martha Hildreth
University of Nevada, Reno, NV, USA
Brouardel, Grancher

Caroline Hillard
Washington University, St Louis, MO, USA
Del Garbo, Mondino de' Liuzzi

Gilberto Hochman
Casa de Oswaldo Cruz, Fundação Oswaldo Cruz, Rio de Janeiro, Brazil
Barros Barreto, Chagas, Cruz, Fraga, Penna, Pinotti, Ribas, Wucherer

Hans-Georg Hofer
University of Manchester, Manchester, England
Krafft-Ebing, Wagner-Jauregg

Eddy Houwaart
Vrije Universiteit Medisch Centrum, Amsterdam, the Netherlands
Ali Cohen

Joel D. Howell
University of Michigan, Ann Arbor, MI, USA
Elliotson, Flick, Gerhard, Heberden, Herrick, Lewis

Elisabeth Hsu
University of Oxford, Oxford, England
Chunyu Yi

Christian Huber
Sigmund Freud-Privatstiftung, Vienna, Austria
Breuer, Jung

Rafael Huertas
CSIC, Madrid, Spain
Orfila i Rotger, Rodríguez Lafora

Teresa Huguet-Termes
Universitat Autònoma de Barcelona, Barcelona, Spain
Cardenal Fernández

Frank Huisman
University Medical Center, Utrecht/Universiteit Maastricht, Maastricht, the Netherlands
Einthoven, Hijmans van den Bergh, Loghem, Sylvius

Marion Hulverscheidt
Ruprecht-Karls-Universität Heidelberg,
Heidelberg, Germany
Basedow, Hegar

J. Willis Hurst
Emory University, Atlanta, GA, USA
White

Erik Ingebrigsten
Norwegian University of Science and Technology,
Trondheim, Norway
Holst

Lorentz M. Irgens
University of Bergen, Bergen, Norway
Hansen

Mark Jackson
University of Exeter, Exeter, England
Blackley, Down, Floyer, Freeman, Seguin, Tredgold

Bengt Jangfeldt
Center for the History of Science, Royal Academy of
Science, Stockholm, Sweden
Munthe

Mark Jenner
University of York, York, England
*Chamberlen, Clowes, Glisson, D. Turner, Wiseman,
Woodall*

William Johnston
Wesleyan University, Middletown, CT, USA
*Gotō Konzan, Hanaoka, Manse, Sugita, Yamawaki,
Yoshimasu*

Peter Jones
King's College Library, Cambridge, England
Arderne, Yperman

Eric Jorink
Constantijn Huygens Instituut, the Hague,
the Netherlands
*J. Heurnius, O. Heurnius, Lemnius, Piso,
Swammerdam*

Robert Jütte
Robert Bosch Stiftung, Stuttgart, Germany
*Auenbrugger, Hahnemann, Hirsch, Hufeland, Kaposi,
Rolfink, Rubner*

Oliver Kahl
University of Manchester, Manchester, England
Ibn at-Tilmīdh

Harmke Kamminga
University of Cambridge, Cambridge, England
Eijkman

Amalie M. Kass
Harvard Medical School, Boston, MA, USA
Cabot, Channing, Churchill, Dameshek, Kelly, Sims

Matthew Howard Kaufman
University of Edinburgh, Edinburgh, Scotland
Ballingall, C. Bell, Brodie, Guthrie, Liston, McGrigor

Amy Kemp
Indiana University, Bloomington, IN, USA
Souza

Helen King
University of Reading, Reading, England
*Agnodice, Archagathus, Hippocrates, Machaon,
Podalirius*

Stephanie Kirby
University of the West of England, Bristol, England
Nightingale

Rina Knoeff
Universiteit Maastricht, Maastricht,
the Netherlands
G. Bidloo, Boerhaave

Carl Henrik Koch
University of Copenhagen, Copenhagen,
Denmark
Stensen

Peter Koehler
Wever Hospital, Heerlen, the Netherlands
Babinski, Brown-Séquard, Winkler

Luuc Kooijmans
Universiteit van Amsterdam, Amsterdam,
the Netherlands
Ruysch

Maria Korasidou
Panteion University of Athens, Athens, Greece
Geroulanos, Goudas, Papanicolaou, Vouros, Zinnis

Jan K. van der Korst
Loosdrecht, the Netherlands
Camper, Swieten

Samuel Kottek
Hebrew University, Jerusalem, Israel
Astruc

Simone Petraglia Kropf
Casa de Oswaldo Cruz, Fundação Oswaldo
Cruz, Rio de Janeiro, Brazil
Chagas

Howard I. Kushner
Emory University, Atlanta, GA, USA
Gilles de la Tourette

Ann F. La Berge
Virginia Tech, Blacksburg, VA, USA
Parent-Duchâtelet, Villermé

Paul A. L. Lancaster
University of Sydney, New South Wales, Australia
Gregg

Øivind Larsen
University of Oslo, Oslo, Norway
Schiøtz

Christopher Lawrence
Wellcome Trust Centre for the History of
Medicine at UCL, London, England
*Cheselden, Culpeper, Lind, Mead, Pott, Pringle,
Salk, Sydenham, Trotter*

Sean Hsiang-lin Lei
National Tsing-hua University, Hsinchu, Taiwan
Yu Yan

Efraim Lev
University of Haifa, Haifa, Israel
Asaph

Milton James Lewis
University of Sydney, Sydney,
Australia
Cumpston

Shang-Jen Li
Institute of History and Philology, Academia
Sinica, Taipei, Taiwan
*Bruce, Hobson, Leishman, Lockhart, Manson,
Parker*

Kai Khiun Liew
Wellcome Trust Centre for the History of Medicine
at UCL, London, England
Chen Su Lan

Vivienne Lo
Wellcome Trust Centre for the History of Medicine
at UCL, London, England
Medicine in China

Stephen Lock
Aldeburgh, Suffolk, England
*The Western Medical Tradition, Beecher, Cooper,
Crile, Dale, Doll, Ferrier, Fishbein, Gull, Hart,
Hastings, G. Holmes, Keynes, Mitchell,
Pappworth, Pickles, Ryle, Saunders, Trudeau*

Winifred Logan
Glasgow, Scotland
Stephenson

Brigitte Lohff
Medizinische Hochschule Hannover,
Hannover, Germany
Autenrieth, Baer, Blumenbach, Müller, Oken, Reil

Jorge Lossio
University of Manchester, Manchester, England
Carrión, Espejo, Unanue

Ilana Löwy
CERMES, Villejuif, France
Aleksandrowicz, Bieganski, Biernacki, Korczak

Kenneth M. Ludmerer
Washington University, St Louis, MO, USA
Flexner

Joan E. Lynaugh
University of Pennsylvania Nursing School,
Philadelphia, PA, USA
L. Dock, L. Richards, I. Robb

Kan-Wen Ma
Wellcome Trust Centre for the History of Medicine
at UCL, London, England
Bian Que

Helen MacDonald
University of Melbourne, Carlton, Victoria,
Australia
W. MacKenzie

Andreas-Holger Maehle
University of Durham, Durham/Wolfson Research
Institute, Stockton, England
Moll

Susanne Malchau
Aarhus Universitet, Aarhus, Denmark
Mannerheim, Reimann

John Manton
University of Oxford, Oxford, England
Johnson, Lambo, Schweitzer

Predrag J. Markovic
Institute for Contemporary History, Belgrade, Serbia
Batut, Djordjević, Lazarević, Kostić, Nešić, Štampar, Subbotić

Shula Marks
SOAS, London, England
Gale, Gear, Gillman, Gluckman, Kark, Waterston

José Martínez-Pérez
Universidad de Castilla-La Mancha, Albacete, Spain
Calandre Ibáñez, Jiménez Díaz, Marañón Posadillo

Àlvar Martínez-Vidal
Universidad Autónoma de Barcelona, Barcelona, Spain
Gimbernat i Arbós, Giovannini

Romana Martorelli Vico
Università di Pisa, Pisa, Italy
Lanfranc, Ugo Benzi

J. Rosser Matthews
Williamsburg, VA, USA
Biggs, Bouchard, Bouchardat, Chapin, Greenwood, Hill

Janet McCalman
University of Melbourne, Melbourne, Australia
Balls-Headley, Bryce, Campbell, Macnamara, Scantlebury Brown

Louella McCarthy
University of Sydney, Sydney, New South Wales, Australia
D'Arcy

Laurence B. McCullough
Baylor College of Medicine, Houston, TX, USA
Hooker, Rush

Susan McGann
RCN Archives, Edinburgh, Scotland
Fenwick

James McGeachie
University of Ulster, Newtownabbey, Northern Ireland
Corrigan, Graves, W. Jenner, M. Mackenzie, Stokes, Wilde

Alessandro Medico
Washington University, St Louis, MO, USA
Peter of Abano

Rosa María Medina-Doménech
Universidad de Granada, Granada, Spain
Goyanes Capdevilla, Guilera Molas

Alfredo Menéndez
Universidad de Granada, Granada, Spain
Casal Julián

Sharon Messenger
Wellcome Trust Centre for the History of Medicine at UCL, London, England
Livingstone

Alexandre Métraux
Dossenheim, Germany
S. Freud, Goldstein

Dmitry Mikhel
Saratov State University, Saratov, Russia
Botkin, Erisman, Manassein, Molleson, Ostroumov, Zakhar'in

Bridie Andrews Minehan
Bentley College, Waltham, MA, USA
Ding Fubao, Yen

Consuelo Miqueo
Universidad de Zaragoza, Zaragoza, Spain
Piquer Arrufat

Néstor Miranda Canal
Universidad El Bosque y de la Universidad de Los Andes, Bogotá, Colombia
Vargas Reyes

Jorge Molero-Mesa
Universidad Autònoma de Barcelona, Barcelona, Spain
Sayé i Sempere

Laurence Monnais
Université de Montréal, Montreal, QC, Canada
Medical Traditions in Southeast Asia: From Syncretism to Pluralism

Maria Teresa Monti
CSPF-CNR, Milan, Italy
Spallanzani

Francisco Moreno de Carvalho
Independent scholar, São Paulo, Brazil
Amatus Lusitanus, Orta

Edward T. Morman
Baltimore, MD, USA
Bartlett, H. Bigelow, J. Bigelow, Billings, Da Costa, Pepper, Thayer, Welch

Barbara Mortimer
Edinburgh, Scotland
Sharp

Anne Marie Moulin
CNRS-CEDEJ, Cairo, Egypt
Bordet, Davaine, Laveran, Netter, Roux, Widal

Wolf-Dieter Müller-Jahncke
Hermann-Schelenz-Institut für Pharmazie und
Kulturgeschichte, Heidelberg, Germany
Paracelsus

Jock Murray
Dalhousie University, Halifax, Nova Scotia, Canada
*Abbott, Banting, Bethune, Gowers, Grenfell, Huggins,
J. H. Jackson, Macphail, Osler, Parkinson, Penfield, Selye*

Takeshi Nagashima
Keio University, Tokyo, Japan
Gotō Shinpei, Kitasato, Miyairi, Nagayo, Noguchi, Shiga

Michael J. Neuss
Columbia University, New York, NY, USA
Al-Anṭākī

Michael Neve
Wellcome Trust Centre for the History of Medicine
at UCL, London, England
Beddoes, Gully, Head, Prichard, Rivers, Winslow

Malcolm Nicolson
University of Glasgow, Glasgow, Scotland
Alison, Baillie, Donald, J. Hunter, W. Hunter, Lister, Smellie

Ingemar Nilsson
University of Gothenburg, Gothenburg, Sweden
Acrel

Sherwin Nuland
Yale University, New Haven, CT, USA
Beaumont, Bloodgood, Kubler-Ross, McBurney, Mott, Murphy

Eva Nyström
University of Uppsala, Uppsala, Sweden
Rosén von Rosenstein

Ynez Violé O'Neill
UCLA, Los Angeles, CA, USA
Paré

Diana Obregón
Universidad Nacional de Colombia Edificio Manuel
Ancizar, Bogotá, Colombia
Carrasquilla, García-Medina

Ambeth R. Ocampo
National Historical Institute, Manila, Philippines
Rizal

Guillermo Olagüe de Ros
Universidad de Granada, Granada, Spain
García Solá, Nóvoa Santos, Urrutia Guerezta

Jan Eric Olsén
University of Lund, Lund, Sweden
Gullstrand, Holmgren

Todd M. Olszewski
Yale University, New Haven, CT, USA
Cannon, D. Dock

Willie T. Ong
Makati Medical Center, Makati, Philippines
Acosta-Sison

Giuseppe Ongaro
Ospedale di Padova, Padova, Italy
*Aranzio, Aselli, Bellini, Benivieni, Berengario da Carpi,
Borelli, Cardano, Cesalpino, Colombo, Cornaro,
Da Monte, Eustachi, Falloppia, Malpighi, Mattioli,
Mercuriale, Morgagni, Santorio, Scarpa, Severino,
Tagliacozzi, Valsalva, Zacchia*

Ooi Keat Gin
Universiti Sains Malaysia, Penang, Malaysia
Danaraj, Lim Boon Keng, Wu Lien-Teh

Teresa Ortiz-Gómez
Universidad de Granada, Granada, Spain
Arroyo Villaverde, Soriano Fischer

Abena Dove Osseo-Asare
University of California, Berkeley, CA, USA
Ampofo, Barnor, De Graft-Johnson, C. Easmon

Nelly Oudshoorn
Universiteit Twente, Enschede,
the Netherlands
Laqueur

Caroline Overy
Wellcome Trust Centre for the History of
Medicine at UCL, London, England
Livingstone

Steven Palmer
University of Windsor, Windsor, Ontario,
Canada
*Calderón Guardia, Durán Cartín,
Fernández y Hernández*

José Pardo-Tomás
CSIC, Barcelona, Spain
Monardes

Lawrence Charles Parish
Jefferson Medical College, Philadelphia, PA, USA
Bateman, Duhring, Gross, Hutchinson, Shippen, Willan

Eldryd Parry
Tropical Health and Education Trust, London, England
Burkitt

Adell Patton Jr.
University of Missouri, St Louis, MO, USA
Boyle, J. Easmon, Odeku, Togba

Harry W. Paul
University of Florida, Gainesville, FL, USA
Pasteur, Rothschild

John Pearn
University of Queensland, Brisbane, Australia
Bancroft, Beaney, Coppleson, Fairley, Halford, MacGregor

Steven J. Peitzman
Drexel University College of Medicine, Philadelphia, PA, USA
Addis, Bright, A. Richards, Scribner

Kim Pelis
National Institutes of Health, Bethesda, MD, USA
Barker, Councilman, Gorgas, Hammond, Nicolle, Reed, T. Smith

Concetta Pennuto
Université de Genève, Geneva, Switzerland
Ficino, Fracastoro

José Morgado Pereira
Universidade de Coimbra, Coimbra, Portugal
Egas Moniz

Jacques Philippon
Salpêtrière-Pitié Hospital, Paris, France
Mondor

Howard Phillips
University of Cape Town, Rondebosch, South Africa
Abdurahman, Barnard, Barry, Naidoo, Orenstein, Xuma

Jean-François Picard
CNRS, Paris, France
Debré, Delay, Hamburger, Leriche, Roussy, Vincent

Mikhail Poddubnyi
Voenno-meditsinskii Zhurnal, Moscow, Russia
N. Bidloo, Buial'skii, Dobroslavin, Gaaz, Inozemtsev, Pirogov, Pletnev

Hans Pols
University of Sydney, Sydney, Australia
Beard, Beers, Bowlby, Burton-Bradley, Grinker, Klein, Laing, Stillé

María-Isabel Porras-Gallo
University of Castilla-La Mancha, Madrid, Spain
Obrador Alcalde

Patricia E. Prestwich
University of Alberta, Edmonton, AB, Canada
Magnan, Moreau de Tours, Morel

Lawrence M. Principe
Johns Hopkins University, Baltimore, MD, USA
Helmont

Armin Prinz
Medizinische Universität Wien, Vienna, Austria
Wenckebach

Cay-Ruediger Pruell
Albert-Ludwigs-Universität, Freiburg, Germany
Aschoff, Cohnheim, Conti, Ehrlich, Rokitansky, Virchow

Constance Putnam
Independent scholar, Concord, MA, USA
Balassa, Bene, Duka, O. W. Holmes, Korányi, Markusovszky, Meigs, Morgan, Semmelweis, G. Shattuck, N. Smith, J. Warren

Emilio Quevedo
Universidad Nacional de Colombia, Bogotá, Colombia
Franco

Sean Quinlan
University of Idaho, Moscow, ID, USA
A. Louis, Quesnay

Camilo Quintero
University of Wisconsin–Madison, Madison, WI, USA
Mutis y Bosio

Roger Qvarsell
University of Linköping, Linköping, Sweden
Huss

Karina Ramacciotti
Universidad de Buenos Aires, Buenos Aires, Argentina
Carrillo, Mazza, Rawson

Mridula Ramanna
SIES College, University of Mumbai, Mumbai, India
Bentley, Choksy, Jhirad, Khanolkar, Lad, Morehead, J. Turner

Matthew Ramsey
Vanderbilt University, Nashville, TN, USA
*Civiale, Desgenettes, Fourcroy, Portal, Richerand, Velpeau,
Vicq d'Azyr*

Ismail Rashid
Vassar College, Poughkeepsie, NY, USA
Fanon, Horton

Carole Reeves
Wellcome Trust Centre for the History of Medicine
at UCL, London, England
*Abt, Battey, Buchan, Budd, Cole, Darwin, Holt, Keen,
Lane, S. Morton, Prout, Rock, Sabin, Scharlieb, Seacole,
Spock, Tait*

C. Joan Richardson
University of Texas Medical Branch, Galveston, TX,
USA
Barton

Philip Rieder
Université de Genève, Geneva, Switzerland
Bonet, De La Rive, Le Clerc, Odier, Reverdin, Tronchin

Ortrun Riha
Universität Leipzig, Leipzig, Germany
Isaac Israeli

Julius Rocca
University of Birmingham, Birmingham, England
*Aëtius, Aretaeus, Aristotle, Asclepiades, Caelius Aurelianus,
Celsus, Dioscorides, Empedocles, Erasistratus, Herophilos,
Pliny, Scribonius Largus, Soranus, Whytt*

Julia Rodriguez
University of New Hampshire, Durham, NH, USA
Aráoz Alfaro, Coni, Grierson, Ingenieros

Esteban Rodríguez-Ocaña
Universidad de Granada, Granada, Spain
Ferrán y Clúa, Pittaluga Fattorini

Volker Roelcke
Justus-Liebig Universität, Giessen, Germany
Alzheimer, Bleuler, Kretschmer, Mitscherlich, Rüdin

Hugo Röling
Universiteit van Amsterdam, Amsterdam,
the Netherlands
Rutgers

Naomi Rogers
Yale University, New Haven, CT, USA
Kenny

Anastasio Rojo
University of Valladolid, Valladolid, Spain
Bravo de Sobremonte, Mercado, Valles

Nils Rosdahl
Medical Museion, Copenhagen Denmark
Madsen

Barbara Gutmann Rosenkrantz
Harvard University, Cambridge, MA, USA
Hardy, L. Shattuck

Leonard D. Rosenman
UCSF, San Francisco, CA, USA
Frugard

Fred Rosner
Mount Sinai School of Medicine, New York,
NY, USA
Maimonides

Lisa Rosner
Richard Stockton College, Pomona, NJ, USA
*Bennett, Brown, Christison, Cullen, Ferriar, J. Gregory,
Laycock, Monro, Percival, Withering*

Frederic Roy
Université de Montréal, Montreal, QC,
Canada
Suvannavong

Marion Maria Ruisinger
Friedrich-Alexander-Universität,
Erlangen-Nuremberg, Germany
Heister

Han van Ruler
Erasmus Universiteit, Rotterdam,
the Netherlands
Blankaart, Bontekoe, Graaf

Andrea Rusnock
University of Rhode Island, Kingston,
RI, USA
*Arbuthnot, Bond, Boylston, E. Jenner, Jurin, Sutton,
Waterhouse*

Fernando Salmón
Universidad de Cantabria, Santander, Spain
Arnald, López Albo

Lutz D. H. Sauerteig
University of Durham, Durham/Wolfson
Research Institute, Stockton, England
Blaschko

Walton O. Schalick III
Washington University, St Louis, MO, USA
*Gilles de Corbeil, Henry of Mondeville, John of
Gaddesden, John of Saint-Amand, Peter of Abano, Peter
of Spain, Richard the Englishman, Taddeo, William of
Brescia*

Volker Scheid
University of Westminster, London, England
Ding Ganren, Fei Boxiong, Yun Tieqiao

Aina Schiøtz
Universitetet i Bergen, Bergen, Norway
Evang

William Schneider
Indiana University, Indianapolis, IN, USA
Hirszfeld, Pinard, Richet, Tzanck

Heinz Schott
Rheinische Friedrich-Wilhelms-Universität,
Bonn, Germany
Mesmer

Andrew Scull
University of California San Diego, San Diego, CA,
USA
*Brigham, Cotton, Dix, Earle, Haslam, Meyer, Ray,
Tuke*

Nikolaj Serikoff
The Wellcome Library, London, England
*The Islamic Medical Tradition, Aḥmad, Ibn al-Bayṭār,
Al-Bīrūnī, Clot Bey, Foley, Ḥaddād, Ibn al-Haytham,
Mahfouz, Ibn al-Māsawayh, Meyerhof, Ibn Sīnā, Sournia,
Van Dyck, Waldmeier, Al-Zahrāwī*

Jole Shackelford
University of Minnesota, Minneapolis, MN, USA
Severinus

Sonu Shamdasani
Wellcome Trust Centre for the History of Medicine
at UCL, London, England
*Adler, Forel, A. Freud, Gesell, Janet, Menninger, Putnam,
Sullivan*

Patrick Henry Shea
Rockefeller Archive Center, Sleepy Hollow, NY, USA
Carrel

Sally Sheard
University of Liverpool, Liverpool, England
*Bevan, Beveridge, Chadwick, Farr, Newman, Newsholme,
Shuttleworth, T. S. Smith*

Dongwon Shin
Korean Advanced Institute of Science and
Technology, Taejon, Korea
Choe Han'gi, Heo, Sejong, Yi Jema

Barry David Silverman
Northside Hospital, Atlanta, GA, USA
Taussig

Mark E. Silverman
Emory University, Atlanta, GA, USA
Flint, Hope, J. Mackenzie

Jelena Jovanovic Simic
Zemun, Serbia
*Batut, Djordjević, Lazarević, Kostić, Nešić, Štampar,
Subbotić*

P. N. Singer
London, England
Galen

Kavita Sivaramakrishnan
Public Health Foundation of India, New Delhi,
India
G. Sen, P. Sharma, T. Sharma, Shukla, Vaid, Varier

Morten A. Skydsgaard
University of Aarhus, Aarhus, Denmark
Panum

Jean Louis De Sloover
Erpent (Namur), Belgium
Dodonaeus

David F. Smith
University of Aberdeen, Aberdeen, Scotland
Orr

F. B. Smith
Australian National University, Canberra, Australia
W. Thomson

Thomas Söderqvist
Medical Museion, Copenhagen, Denmark
Jerne

Marina Sorokina
Russian Academy of Sciences, Moscow, Russia
*Al'tshuller, Briukhonenko, Haffkine, Ilizarov, Iudin,
Negovskii, Semenovskii*

David Sowell
Juniata College, Huntingdon, PA, USA
Perdomo Neira

Eduard A. van Staeyen
Leiden, the Netherlands
Guislain

Frank W. Stahnisch
Johannes Gutenberg-Universität, Mainz, Germany
*Graefe, Griesinger, His, C. Vogt, O. Vogt, Warburg,
Wassermann*

Ida H. Stamhuis
Vrije Universiteit Amsterdam, Amsterdam,
the Netherlands
Quetelet

Darwin H. Stapleton
Rockefeller Archive Center, Sleepy Hollow, NY, USA
Hackett

Jane Starfield
University of Johannesburg, Bertsham, South Africa
Molema, Moroka

Martin S. Staum
University of Calgary, Calgary, AB, Canada
Cabanis

Hubert Steinke
University of Bern, Bern, Switzerland
Haller

Oddvar Stokke
National Hospital, Oslo, Norway
Følling, Refsum

Michael Stolberg
Universität Würzburg, Würzburg, Germany
Bartisch, Fabricius, Fuchs, Platter, Rösslin, Scultetus

Marvin J. Stone
Baylor University Medical Center, Dallas, TX, USA
Coley, Ewing, Farber, E. Graham, Hodgkin, Wintrobe

Hindrik Strandberg
Helsinki, Finland
Willebrand, Ylppö

Karin Stukenbrock
Martin-Luther-Universität Halle-Wittenberg,
Halle, Germany
*Brunfels, Erxleben, Frank, Gersdorff, Hoffmann,
Stahl*

Charles Suradji
Jakarta, Indonesia
Soedarmo

Akihito Suzuki
Keio University, Yokohama, Japan
*Medicine, State, and Society in Japan, 500–2000,
Asada, Baelz, Conolly, Hata, Mori, Ogata, Pompe van
Meerdervoort, Siebold, Yamagiwa*

Mika Suzuki
Shizuoka University, Shizuoka, Japan
Ogino, Yoshioka

Victoria Sweet
UCSF, San Francisco, CA, USA
Hildegard of Bingen

Simon Szreter
University of Cambridge, Cambridge,
England
McKeown

Cecilia Taiana
Carleton University, Ottawa, ON, Canada
Lacan

Ian Tait
Aldeburgh, Suffolk, England
Browne

Jennifer Tappan
Columbia University, New York, NY, USA
Trowell

Robert Tattersall
University of Nottingham, Nottingham,
England
*Abel, Addison, Albright, Doniach, Hench, Horsley,
Joslin, Minkowski, Starling*

Kim Taylor
Kaimu Productions, Shanghai, China
Hatem, Zhu Lian

Manuela Tecusan
University of Cambridge, Cambridge, England
*Alcmaeon, Anaximander, Andreas, Democedes,
Democritus, Diocles, Diogenes, Oribasius, Paul
of Aegina, Philistion, Plato, Praxagoras, Rufus*

Bert Theunissen
Universiteit Utrecht, Utrecht, the Netherlands
Donders

Michel Thiery
Stichting Jan Palfyn en Museum voor
Geschiedenis van de Geneeskunde, Ghent, Belgium
Palfyn

C. Michele Thompson
Southern Connecticut State University,
New Haven, CT, USA
Lán Ông, Tuệ Tĩnh

Carsten Timmermann
University of Manchester, Manchester, England
Bauer, Grotjahn, McMichael, Pickering, D. Richards,
Rosenbach

Tom Treasure
St George's Hospital Medical School, London,
England
Beck, Blalock, C. E. Drew, C. R. Drew, Favaloro, Gibbon,
Hufnagel

Ulrich Tröhler
University of Bern, Bern, Switzerland
Bergmann, Billroth, Kocher, Langenbeck,
Mikulicz-Radecki, Nissen, Quervain

Arleen Marcia Tuchman
Vanderbilt University, Nashville, TN, USA
Zakrzewska

Marius Turda
Oxford Brookes University, Oxford, England
Babeş, Cantacuzino, Ciucă, Marinescu

Trevor Turner
Homerton University Hospital, London, England
Maudsley

Peter J. Tyler
Edgecliffe, New South Wales, Australia
W. Armstrong, Bland, Fiaschi, Mackellar, Skirving,
Stuart, Thompson

Michael Tyquin
Making History, Darlington, New South Wales,
Australia
Dunlop

Tatiana Ul'iankina
Institute of the History of Science and Technology,
Moscow, Russia
Mechnikov, Sechenov

G. van der Waa
Rotterdam, the Netherlands
Gaubius

Lia van Gemert
Universiteit Utrecht, Utrecht, the Netherlands
Beverwijck

Maria Vassiliou
University of Oxford, Oxford, England
Belios, Livadas

Jan Peter Verhave
UMCN, Nijmegen, the Netherlands
Swellengrebel

Joost Vijselaar
Trimbos-Instituut, Utrecht, the Netherlands
Schroeder van der Kolk

Jurjen Vis
Amsterdam, the Netherlands
Foreest

An Vleugels
National University of Singapore, Singapore
Kerr

Hans de Waardt
Vrije Universiteit Amsterdam, Amsterdam,
the Netherlands
Wier

Keir Waddington
Cardiff University, Cardiff, Wales
Abernethy, Brunton, Garrod, Gee, Lawrence,
J. Paget

Lisa K. Walker
University of California, Berkeley, CA, USA
Khlopin, Teziakov

John Walker-Smith
Wellcome Trust Centre for the History of
Medicine at UCL, London, England
G. Armstrong, G. Still, Underwood, West

Paul Weindling
Oxford Brookes University, Oxford, England
Verschuer

Dora B. Weiner
UCLA, Los Angeles, CA, USA
Esquirol, Larrey, Percy, Pinel, Tenon

Kathleen Wellman
Southern Methodist University, Dallas, TX, USA
La Mettrie, Patin, Renaudot

Ann Westmore
The University of Melbourne, Parkville, Victoria,
Australia
Cade

James Whorton
University of Washington, Tacoma, WA, USA
Eddy, S. Graham, Kellogg, Lust, B. Palmer, D. Palmer, S. Thomson, Trall

Ann Wickham
Dublin City University, Dublin, Ireland
A. Jones

Elizabeth A. Williams
Oklahoma State University, Stillwater, OK, USA
Boissier de la Croix de Sauvages, Bordeu

Sabine Wilms
Paradigm Publications, Taos, NM, USA
Ge Hong, Sun Simiao, Tao Hongjing

Warren Winkelstein, Jr.
University of California, Berkeley, CA, USA
Emerson, Frost, Goldberger, Hamilton, Kinyoun, Lane-Claypon, Park, Paul, Wynder

Michael Worboys
University of Manchester, Manchester, England
Allbutt, Bristowe, W. W. Cheyne, Moynihan, Simon, Syme

Jill Wrapson
University of Auckland, Auckland, New Zealand
Barnett

Marcia Wright
Columbia University, New York, NY, USA
Park Ross

Rex Wright-St Clair (deceased)
Huntingdon, Hamilton, New Zealand
A. Thomson

Henrik R. Wulff
Medical Museion, Copenhagen, Denmark
Hirschsprung

Ronit Yoeli-Tlalim
Warburg Institute, London, England
Sangye Gyatso, Yuthog Yontan

William H. York
Portland State University, Portland, OR, USA
Despars, Valesco of Tarenta

Benjamin Zajicek
University of Chicago, Chicago, IL, USA
Bekhterev, Korsakov, Pavlov

Soledad Zárate
Universidad de Chile, Santiago, Chile
Cruz-Coke Lassabe

Alfons Zarzoso
Museu d'Història de la Medicina de Catalunya, Barcelona, Spain
Pedro-Pons, Puigvert Gorro

Franz Zehentmayr
Salzburg, Austria
Zhang Yuansu

Barbara Zipser
Wellcome Trust Centre for the History of Medicine at UCL, London, England
Al-Mawṣilī

Patrick Zylberman
CERMES, Villejuif, France
Sand

ABBREVIATIONS

AMA	American Medical Association
ANB	*American National Biography*
BA	Bachelor of Arts
BCE	Before Common Era
BCG	Bacillus Calmette-Guérin (tuberculosis vaccination)
BM	Bachelor of Medicine
BMA	British Medical Association
BMJ	*British Medical Journal*
CBE	Commander, The Most Excellent Order of the British Empire
CE	Common Era
ChB	Bachelor of Surgery
ChD	Doctor of Surgery
ChM	Master of Surgery
CIE	Companion, The Most Eminent Order of the Indian Empire
KCIE	Knight Commander, The Most Eminent Order of the Indian Empire
CM	Master of Surgery
CMB	Combat Medical Badge (U.S. Army)
CMG	Companion, The Most Distinguished Order of St Michael and St George
CMO	Chief Medical Officer
CMS	Church Missionary Society
CSI	Companion, The Most Exalted Order of the Star of India
CSIRO	Commonwealth Scientific and Industrial Research Organization (Australia)
DAMB	*Dictionary of American Medical Biography*
DAuB	*Dictionary of Australian Biography* (available online)
DBE	Dame of the British Empire
DBI	*Dizionario Biografico degli Italiani*
DGMS	Director General Medical Service (military)

DMed	Doctor of Medicine
DNZB	*Dictionary of New Zealand Biography* (available online)
DPM	Diploma of Psychological Medicine
DSB	*Dictionary of Scientific Biography*
DSO	Distinguished Service Order (military British)
ECT	Electo-convulsive Therapy
EEG	Electroencephalogram
FAO	Food and Agriculture Organization (United Nations)
FRCP	Fellow Royal College of Physicians
FRCPEdin/FRCPEd	Fellow Royal College of Physicians Edinburgh
FRCS	Fellow of the Royal College of Surgeons
FRCSEdin/FRCSEd	Fellow Royal College of Surgeons Edinburgh
FRS	Fellow of the Royal Society
FRSEdin/FRSEd	Fellow of the Royal Society of Edinburgh
GBH	General Board of Health (England and Wales)
GMC	General Medical Council (UK)
GP	General Practitioner
ICN	International Council of Nursing
ICS	Indian Civil Service
IHB	International Health Board (Rockefeller Foundation)
IMS	Indian Medical Service
IOC	Institute Oswaldo Cruz
JAMA	*Journal of the American Medical Association*
KCSI	Knight Commander, The Most Exalted Order of the Star of India
LLD	Doctor of Laws
LMS	Licentiate in Medicine and Surgery
LRCP	Licentiate of the Royal College of Physicians
LRCPEdin/LRCPEd	Licentiate of the Royal College of Physicians Edinburgh
LRCSEdin/LRCSEd	Licentiate of the Royal College of Surgeons Edinburgh
LRFPS	Licentiate of the Royal Faculty of Physicians and Surgeons of Glasgow
LSA	Licentiate of the Society of Apothecaries
LSHTM	London School of Hygiene and Tropical Medicine
LSMW	London School of Medicine for Women
MA	Master of Arts
MB	Bachelor of Medicine
MBCM	Bachelor of Medicine Master of Surgery
MC	Military Cross
MD	Doctor of Medicine
mg	milligram
MMed	Master of Medicine
MO	Medical Officer
MoH	Medical Officer of Health
MRC	Medical Research Council
MRCNZ	Medical Research Council of New Zealand
MRCOG	Member of the Royal College of Gynaecologists
MRCP	Member of the Royal College of Physicians
MRCS	Member of the Royal College of Surgeons
MS	Multiple Sclerosis
NHMRC	National Health and Medical Research Council (Australia)
NSDAP	National Socialist Party (Nazi Germany)
NSW	New South Wales (Australia)
OAS	Organization of American States
OBE	Officer, The Most Excellent Order of the British Empire
Oxford DNB	*Oxford Dictionary of National Biography* (UK)
PASB	Pan American Sanitary Bureau

PhD	Doctor of Philosophy
QVJIN	Queen Victoria Jubilee Institute of Nursing
RACP	Royal Australasian College of Physicians
RACS	Royal Australasian College of Surgeons
RAMC	Royal Army Medical Corps (UK)
RBNA	Royal British Nurses Association
RCP	Royal College of Physicians
RCPEdin	Royal College of Physicians of Edinburgh
RCS	Royal College of Surgeons
RCSEdin	Royal College of Surgeons of Edinburgh
RMO	Resident Medical Officer
RSTMH	Royal Society of Tropical Medicine and Hygiene
SA	Sturm Abteilung [Storm Section] (Nazi Germany)
SLSAA	Surf Lifesaving Association of Australia
SS	Schutzstaffel [Protective Squadron] (Nazi Germany)
STD	Sexually Transmitted Diseases
UCH	University College Hospital (London, England)
UCL	University College London (England)
UNICEF	United Nations Children's Fund
UNRRA	United Nations Relief and Rehabilitation Administration
WHO	World Health Organization
YMCA	Young Men's Christian Association

LIST OF ENTRIES

Kark, Sidney
Kasili, Edward G.
Keen, William W.
Kellogg, John H.
Kelly, Howard A.
Kenny, Elizabeth
Kerr, Norman S.
Keynes, Geoffrey L.
Khān, Muhammad Ajmal
Khān, Muhammad A'zam
Khanolkar, Vasant R.
Khlopin, Grigorii V.
King, Frederic Truby
Kinyoun, Joseph James
Kitasato Shibasaburō
Klebs, Edwin
Klein, Melanie
Knox, Robert
Koch, H. H. Robert
Kocher, Emil T.
Korányi, Frigyes
Korczak, Janusz
Korsakov, Sergei S.
Kostić, Aleksandar Đ.
Kraepelin, Emil W. M. G.
Krafft-Ebing, Richard von
Kraus, Friedrich
Kretschmer, Ernst
Kubler-Ross, Elisabeth
La Mettrie, Julien Offroy de
Lacan, Jacques-Marie É.
Lad, Bhau D.
Laennec, René T. H.
Laguna, Andrés
Laing, Ronald D.
Lambo, Thomas A.
Lán Ông
Lancisi, Giovanni M.
Lane, William Arbuthnot
Lane-Claypon, Janet E.
Lanfranc of Milan
Langenbeck, Bernhard
Lapeyronie, François de
Laqueur, Ernst
Lardizábal Dubois, Vicente de
Larrey, Jean D.
Lasègue, Charles
Laveran, Charles L. A.
Lawrence, William
Laycock, Thomas
Lazarević, Laza K.
Le Clerc, Daniel
Leishman, William B.
Lemnius, Levinus
Leriche, René

Lettsom, John C.
Lewis, Thomas
Leyden, Ernst von
Li Gao
Li Shizhen
Liceaga, Eduardo
Liley, Albert W.
Lim Boon Keng
Linacre, Thomas
Lind, James
Linnaeus, Carl
Lister, Joseph
Liston, Robert
Littré, Émile
Liu Wansu
Livadas, Gregory A.
Livingstone, David
Lloyd, John Uri
Lockhart, William
Loghem, Johannes J. van
Lombroso, Cesare
Long, Crawford W.
López Albo, Wenceslao
Louis, Antoine
Louis, Pierre-C.-A.
Lower, Richard
Ludwig, Carl F. W.
Lust, Benedict
Macdonald, George
MacGregor, William
Machaon
Mackellar, Charles K.
Mackenzie, James
Mackenzie, Morell
MacKenzie, William C.
Macnamara, Annie J.
Macphail, John A.
Madsen, Thorvald J. M.
Magendie, François
Magnan, J. J. Valentin
Mahfouz, Naguib M. P.
Maimonides
Al-Majūsī
Malpighi, Marcello
Manase Dōsan
Manassein, Viacheslav A.
Mandeville, Bernard de
Mannerheim, Eva C. L. S.
Manning, Frederick Norton
Manson, Patrick
Marañón Posadillo, Gregorio
Marie, Pierre
Marinescu, Gheorghe
Markusovszky, Lajos
Martin, James Ranald

Martínez Báez, Manuel
Martínez Vargas, Andrés
Ibn Māsawayh
Mattioli, Pietro A.
Maudsley, Henry
Al-Mawṣilī
Mayo, William J.
Mayo, Charles H.
Mazza, Salvador
McBurney, Charles
McDowell, Ephraim
McGrigor, James
McKeown, Thomas
McMichael, John
Mead, Richard
Mechnikov, Elie
Meigs, Charles D.
Menninger, Karl
Mercado, Luis de
Mercuriale, Girolamo
Mesmer, Franz A.
Meyer, Adolf
Meyerhof, Max
Mikulicz-Radecki, Johannes von
Minkowski, Oskar
Minot, George R.
Mitchell, Silas Weir
Mitscherlich, Alexander
Miyairi Keinosuke
Molema, Seetsele M.
Moll, Albert
Molleson, Ivan I.
Monardes, Nicolás B.
Mondino de' Liuzzi
Mondor, Henri
Monge Medrano, Carlos
Monro, Alexander, *secundus*
Montaña Carranco, Luis J.
Montoya Lafragua, Matilde P.
Moreau de Tours, Jacques-Joseph
Morehead, Charles
Morel, Bénédict-Augustin
Morgagni, Giovanni B.
Morgan, John
Mori Rintarō
Moroka, James S.
Morquio, Luis
Morselli, Enrico
Morton, Samuel G.
Morton, William T. G.
Mosher, Clelia D.
Mosher, Eliza M.
Mott, Valentine
Moynihan, Berkeley G. A.
Müller, Johannes Peter

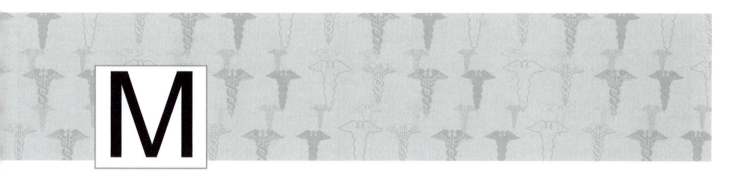

M

MACDONALD, GEORGE (b. Sheffield, England, 22 June 1903; d. London, England, 10 December 1967), *malariology, tropical hygiene.*

Macdonald, the son of J. S. Macdonald FRS, professor of physiology in the universities of Sheffield and then Liverpool, was educated at King Edward VII School in Sheffield and at Liverpool University, where in 1924 he graduated in medicine and also obtained his Diploma in Tropical Medicine and Hygiene. The posts he then held from 1925 to 1945 gave him a unique experience with malaria and its control. He first went to Sierra Leone as research assistant at the Sir Alfred Lewis Jones Laboratories in Freetown, there beginning work on malaria epidemiology, the subject to which he devoted his life. In 1929 he moved to the malaria survey of India for two years as a research officer, so gaining experience with both African and Asian malaria by the age of twenty-eight, when he returned to the UK to obtain his MD at Liverpool University and his Diploma of Public Health (London).

From 1932 to 1937, Macdonald was principal medical officer at the Mariani Medical Association's tea estates in Assam. There he studied Ronald Ross's (1857–1932) epidemiological model of malaria transmission (rescuing it from two decades of oblivion because of the mathematics) and tested it against observed incidence of malaria. He became assistant director of the Ross Institute (1937), spending eighteen months in Ceylon (now Sri Lanka) before being drawn into

the RAMC during World War II, during which he formed and commanded the First Malaria Field Laboratory for the War Office in 1940, working in the Mediterranean. He was appointed Brigadier and Consultant Malariologist (1942) to the armies that fought in North Africa and then advanced through Italy. This was when the residual insecticide DDT first became available for malaria control.

In 1947 he succeeded Sir Malcolm Watson (1873–1955) as director of the Ross Institute, which by then was based in the building of the London School of Hygiene and Tropical Medicine, and he also became the first professor of tropical hygiene in the University of London, posts that he held until his death. In his first few years in the chair, he brought to fruition his prolonged reflection on malaria transmission, in a series of papers that re-examined each stage of the cycle. Macdonald felt that his key advance on Ross was inclusion of the process of superinfection (those already having malaria could acquire further infections with malaria whilst still infected), but more important was his lucid analysis of mosquito biology affecting transmission, development of an analytical formula for the basic case-reproduction number, and his exposition of this in terms comprehensible to epidemiologists (as distinct from mathematicians). This gave powerful insight into two key issues of the time: the stability of transmission—whether viewed as the excess of transmission over what was needed to maintain the infection or as the relative difficulty of malaria control under different vectors—and the relative efficacy of residual insecticides (such as the recently introduced DDT) as compared with larviciding. He thus created a rational quantitative epidemiology of malaria and a rational basis for malaria control at the time when it was most needed.

The heroic age of malaria control was about to begin. Residual insecticides held the promise of breaking transmission, and Macdonald was one of the small group who drove the concept of global malaria eradication as a flagship endeavor of the young WHO. At the Kampala malaria conference of 1950, he pressed the case, driven by his experience with the damage done by malaria (and in spite of being the one person with analytical understanding of its extreme difficulty in Africa).

Macdonald played a key role in the WHO committees driving the eradication program, and he used the Ross Institute insectaries to pioneer the genetics of insecticide resistance. His own research turned to schistosomiasis (in the hope that more malaria research would be unnecessary), for which he used computer models to tackle its epidemiology and control, and his presidential address to the Royal Society of Tropical Medicine and Hygiene (RSTMH) presented the case for tropical hygiene as a discipline, only two years before his premature death.

George Macdonald greatly influenced UK tropical medicine policy in the colonial transition era and was immensely respected worldwide for his scientifically rigorous approach to the practical control of disease in developing countries.

Bibliography

Primary: 1973. (Bruce-Chwatt, L. J., and V. J. Glanville, eds.) *Dynamics of Tropical Disease* (Oxford); 1957. *Epidemiology and Control of Malaria* (Oxford).

Secondary: Bruce-Chwatt, L. J., 1973. 'Professor George Macdonald, 1903–1967' in Bruce-Chwatt, L. J., and V. J. Glanville, eds., *Dynamics of Tropical Disease* (Oxford) pp. 3–4; *Munk's Roll*; *Oxford DNB*.

David Bradley

MACGREGOR, WILLIAM   (b. Hillockhead, Aberdeenshire, Scotland, 20 October 1846; d. Aberdeen, Scotland, 3 July 1919), *colonial administration, public health, medicine, botany, anthropology.*

MacGregor, the son of Agnes Smith and her crofter husband John MacGregor, worked initially as a farm laborer and then attended Tillyduke village school, where his ability soon attracted attention. Partly through self-education and partly with the help of friends, he was able to attend Aberdeen Grammar School in 1865, at the age of nineteen. He then studied medicine at Anderson's Medical College in Glasgow and at the Universities of Aberdeen and Edinburgh. After receiving his MD (1874) he commenced practice at the relatively senior age of twenty-eight years, at the Royal Lunatic Asylum, Aberdeen.

In 1873 he was appointed assistant medical officer in the Seychelles, thus following in the long tradition of Scottish doctors who went to the limits of the known world to promote the health of their fellows on colonial outposts, on expeditions, and on missions of mapping and exploration. In 1874 he was appointed resident surgeon at Port Louis in Mauritius and in the following year went to Fiji as chief medical officer. He remained in Fiji for thirteen years, receiving successive appointments as receiver general and as colonial secretary. During his time as medical officer, a measles epidemic killed 40,000 Fijians out of an estimated population of 150,000. His wife died from dysentery there in 1877. While in Fiji, he was decorated for gallantry with the Clarke Gold Medal, for his personal heroism in saving three people from a shipwreck near Suva in 1884.

MacGregor's most challenging post was his appointment as the first administrator of the Territory of Papua (then British New Guinea), for which he was given the formal title of lieutenant governor in 1895. In what was then an unexplored and unknown country, in which fierce tribal warfare was the norm, he organized an efficient police service, tackled the difficult problems of land tenure and labor, and conducted important explorations. He also contributed considerably to scientific knowledge in ethnography and botany. For his research, scholarship, and administrative skills, he received the Founder's Medal of the Royal Geographical Society.

From 1898 until 1902 he was governor of Lagos, where he assisted Sir Ronald Ross's research on the transmission of malaria by mosquitoes. In 1904 he was appointed governor of Newfoundland and there took a major role in campaigns to reduce tuberculosis. He explored extensively in Labrador, and his knowledge of mathematics, natural science, and medicine led to significant advances in meteorology and anthropology.

From 1909 to 1914 he was governor of Queensland, his last colonial posting. On 10 December 1909, he gave his assent to the University of Queensland Bill and dedicated Government House to be the center of Queensland's first university. He was appointed the foundation chancellor and took a vigorous and very influential role in University Senate deliberations. He instituted a fund for the establishment of the Faculty of Medicine, a goal that was not realized until 1936. MacGregor's personal insistence ensured high matriculation standards for University entry, a policy that meant that Queensland graduates enjoyed equal status with those of other British universities. He criticized the ill treatment of the Australian Aborigines, was a strong advocate for greater resources for medical research, and officially opened the Institute of Tropical Medicine in Townsville.

Sir William MacGregor was the most successful and accomplished of all the medically qualified civil administrators in the British Colonial Service. Many honors were showered upon him in his lifetime. He was created KCMG, made a Privy Councillor, and was awarded many honorary degrees, including a Cambridge DSc for his contributions to natural history. His personal herbarium and ethnographic collections are to be found in many repositories, including those of the Queensland Museum. His most durable memorials are the numerous species of plants, mosses, and grasses in many parts of the world that bear his name.

Bibliography

Secondary: Pearn, J. H., 1990. 'Doctor Governor, Sir William MacGregor—and the Queensland Medical School.' *Medical Journal of Australia*, 153: 708–711; *Oxford DNB*.

John Pearn

MACHAON AND PODALIRIUS (apocryphal), *surgery, general medicine.*

According to Paracelsus, the four men through whom God revealed medicine were Apollo, Machaon, Podalirius, and Hippocrates. Machaon and Podalirius appear in several brief passages of the *Iliad* as the sons of Asclepius, who in Homer's time was not yet regarded as a god, but rather as a physician who had been taught by the centaur Chiron. Their mother is later named as Epione, daughter of Heracles. That both sons were medical practitioners suggests that medicine was taught within the family in Greece in the mid–eighth century BCE. According to Homer, both served as soldiers in the Greek army under Agamemnon in the campaign against Troy, as well as acting as its doctors; Machaon treated the prince Menelaus before himself being wounded.

Of Machaon it was said that 'A healer is worth many other men/in cutting out arrows and spreading soothing drugs'; Alexandrian commentators later ignored the second line, with its specifically military reference, to increase their praise of physicians in general. Besides removing arrows and applying ointments, Machaon is also represented as removing bad blood by sucking it out. Homeric medicine also included the use of prayer, above all to Apollo, father of Asclepius, and incantations were used to staunch blood loss. Homer's detailed description of wounds and the range of vocabulary he used to describe them have led some modern scholars to believe that, like Machaon, he too was a doctor in the Greek army; however, this could also simply indicate that doctors and their patients shared knowledge of what would have been common experiences.

More detail on both men is given in Greek epic, as well as in the biographies of Hippocrates, who was a descendant of Podalirius. Machaon is supposed to have been one of the soldiers inside the Trojan Horse, and to have died of the wounds he received in combat with the sons of Telephus, although later tradition attributed sons to him as well. His grave in Messenia was visited by those seeking cures. Podalirius, according to Stephanus of Byzantium, settled on the coast of Asia Minor, where he treated the daughter of the king of Caria, who had fallen from a roof. He successfully bled her, and her delighted father rewarded him with a small kingdom, in which Podalirius founded two cities.

From the time of Alexandrian medicine onward, the two men have often been portrayed as representing different aspects or branches of medicine, with Machaon as the patron of surgery and Podalirius the patron of medicine— two of the three branches of medicine in ancient thought, the third being the use of diet. There is some evidence of this difference between them in the primary sources; for example, when Machaon treated the wounded Ajax, Podalirius noted that the patient was suicidal. However, differences between the two have been overemphasized. The brothers appear together on the arms of the Royal College of Surgeons, England, Machaon carrying an arrow and Podalirius the staff of Asclepius, complete with snake.

Bibliography

Primary: Homer, *Iliad* 2.729–733; 11.832–835; 11.514–515.

Secondary: Saunders, Kenneth B., 1999. 'The Wounds in *Iliad* 13–16.' *Classical Quarterly* 49: 345–363; Smith, Wesley D., 1979. *The Hippocratic Tradition* (Ithaca, NY); Lorenz, R., 1976. *Beiträge zur Hygiene bei Homer* (Munich).

Helen King

MACKELLAR, CHARLES KINNAIRD (b. Sydney, Australia, 5 December 1844; d. Woollahra, Australia, 14 July 1926), *public health, eugenics.*

Mackellar was the son of Scottish parents—Isabella McGarvie, the widow of a well-known journalist and pastoralist, and Frederick Mackellar, a physician who became the first salaried medical officer at the Sydney Infirmary (renamed Sydney Hospital in 1881). Charles was educated at Sydney Grammar School before moving to Port Macquarie with his family, where he spent several years farming. He then went to Scotland, graduating MB ChM from the University of Glasgow in 1871.

Upon returning to Sydney, Mackellar took an appointment as honorary surgeon at Sydney Infirmary (1873–77) to complement his nearby private medical practice. Starting from 1882 he was a physician at Sydney Hospital, and soon became a director (1884–1903). He also became a director of the (Royal) Prince Alfred Hospital (1886–1917).

In September 1881 the first serious smallpox epidemic struck New South Wales. Mackellar was appointed to the advisory body that later evolved into the Board of Health. He subsequently took up a staff position as government health officer, with control over port quarantine. In August 1883 he was appointed inaugural president of the Board of Health, as well as becoming a member of the Pharmacy Board and the Medical Board, which accredited practitioners in those disciplines. He was active in various medical organizations, including a term as president of the New South Wales Branch of the British Medical Association (1883–84).

One of his private patients was the attorney general, who persuaded Mackellar to relinquish his official appointments in order to enter politics. He was nominated to the Legislative Council (1885), where he introduced some public health legislation, and also served briefly as Minister for Mines. After federation of the Australian colonies, he was elected to a vacancy in the Commonwealth Senate in 1903, but served only a short term before resuming his place on the State Legislative Council, where he remained until 1925.

Mackellar had long been interested in the welfare of neglected children, initially convinced that environmental factors determined the development of the young, although he modified these views later. He was president of the State Children's Relief Board (1902–14), where he became embroiled in disputes with the bureaucracy over their preference for institutional care. In 1903 Mackellar was reappointed to a vacancy on the Board of Health, almost immediately thereafter becoming chairman of a Royal Commission inquiring into the reasons for the decline in the birthrate.

He took a dominant position in the proceedings, with the comprehensive report published in 1904 largely reflecting his own conservative values. The report regarded birth control as a selfish indulgence that would lead to 'racial suicide'. Mackellar advocated a ban on publication of information about this practice, plus prohibitions on the sale of contraceptives. An underlying concern was that national efficiency would be reduced if healthy British stock were diluted with 'foreign' races. It was only a short step from here to supporting the sterilization of 'unfit' people, such as the mentally defective. By now Mackellar placed more emphasis on the role of heredity, at a time when eugenicist ideology was widely accepted in Australian medical and intellectual circles.

When he married Marion Buckland in 1877, Mackellar acquired extensive pastoral interests. He succeeded his father-in-law as a director of the Bank of New South Wales, the largest in Australia, eventually becoming its chairman. His business affairs took precedence over his medical career after he became a director of some of Australia's leading companies, but his influence on the profession remained strong.

Bibliography

Primary: 1912. 'The Neglected Child in New South Wales.' *Nineteenth Century* 72: 953–963.

Secondary: Garton, S., 1986. 'Sir Charles Mackellar: Psychiatry, Eugenics, and Child Welfare in New South Wales, 1900–1914.' *Historical Studies* 22: 21–34; Dickey, B., 1977. 'Care for Deprived, Neglected and Delinquent Children.' *Journal of the Royal Australian Historical Society*, 63: 167–183; AuDB.

Peter J. Tyler

MACKENZIE, JAMES (b. Scone, Perthshire, Scotland, 4 April 1853; d. London, England, 26 January 1925), *medicine, cardiology.*

Mackenzie, a general practitioner whose determination to fathom the symptoms and prognosis of his patients led to the beginning of modern cardiology, was born on a farm near Scone, Scotland. An undistinguished pupil, he left school at fifteen to apprentice to a pharmacist in Perth and later in Glasgow. Turning from pharmacy to medicine, he schooled at Edinburgh University (1874–78) and then trained at the Edinburgh Infirmary for a year. Mackenzie, at age twenty-six, was invited to join a practice in Burnley, an industrial town in northern England. He soon discovered that his patients rarely fit the textbook description of disease—'I couldn't tell the nature of a single symptom from which my patients' suffered, such as pain and irregular heart'—and was frustrated because he could not predict outcome (Smith, 1975, p. 215). Inspired by the example of his partner's remarkable powers of deduction gained from long experience, Mackenzie decided to study the natural history of symptoms. Over a twenty-eight–year period, he conducted laborious clinical research within the confines of a very busy practice. He later stated, 'One special function of a consultant is to foretell what is going to happen to a patient if treated, or if left untreated. To obtain this knowledge it is necessary to see patients through the various stages of disease. And this can only be done by the individual who has the opportunity' (Smith, 1975, p. 217).

After a woman under his care died of a rhythm disturbance, he also resolved to record venous and arterial pulses to decipher rhythm disturbances. Using a modified kymograph, he was able to interpret and name the jugular 'a, c, and v waves' and various rhythm disturbances. These original studies, correlated with symptoms and prognosis, first published in 1891–92, provided an important early understanding of arrhythmias and conduction disturbances and established the value of the graphic method. His book *The Study of the Pulse* (1902), was published a year before Willem Einthoven's (1860–1927) first clinical paper on the electrocardiogram. When his book received little attention, Mackenzie moved to London in 1907, age fifty-four, to convince the medical community of the significance of his research. Armed with data and possessing a vigorous personality, Mackenzie achieved respect and stature after a cool initial reception. His subsequent book, *Diseases of the Heart* (1908), established Mackenzie as an authority, and he was appointed to the Mount Vernon Hospital and later to the London Hospital, where he started cardiac research departments. In addition to arrhythmias, he published original work on referred pain, angina pectoris, digitalis, heart failure, and pregnancy. His teaching 'a heart is what a heart can do' was instrumental in turning attention toward cardiac function and away from excessive concern about murmurs and arrhythmia. During World War I he helped establish a military hospital to study the important problem of 'soldier's heart'. After the war, in 1918, he moved to St Andrews to start an Institute for Clinical Research devoted to long-term investigation of symptoms. He suffered from angina pectoris and died from a myocardial infarction at age seventy-one. Mackenzie's clinical investigations, textbooks, and influence on others, especially Thomas Lewis (1881–1945) and John Parkinson (1885–1976), nurtured the rise of cardiology as a specialty. For his many contributions, he was knighted (1915) and eulogized as one of the greats in British medicine.

Bibliography

Primary: 1902. *The Study of the Pulse* (Edinburgh); 1908. *Diseases of the Heart* (London).

Secondary: Silverman, Mark E., 1994. 'From Rebellious Palpitations to the Discovery of Auricular Fibrillation: Contributions of Mackenzie, Lewis, and Einthoven.' *American Journal of Cardiology* 73: 384–389; Mair, Alex, 1986. *Sir James Mackenzie MD: General Practitioner* (Edinburgh); Smith, Carter, Sr., and Mark E. Silverman, 1975. 'A Letter from Sir James Mackenzie to Dr. Carter Smith, Sr.' *Circulation* 51: 212–217; *Oxford DNB.*

Mark E. Silverman

MACKENZIE, MORELL (b. Leytonstone, Essex, England, 7 July 1837; d. London, England, 3 February 1892), *surgery, laryngology.*

Mackenzie was the son and nephew of general practitioners in Leytonstone and Tiverton, respectively, and was also related to the Bristol physician J. Addington Symonds. His father, Stephen Mackenzie, fractured his skull and was instantly killed after being thrown from his carriage in 1851. Subsequently, Mackenzie abandoned his studies at Dr Greig's school, Walthamstow, and worked as a clerk in the Union Insurance Office, studying in the evenings to prepare for matriculation at London University. A maternal aunt subsequently paid for his training at the London Hospital, where he distinguished himself. After he was admitted MRCS (1858), his aunt supported two further years of study in Paris and Vienna as well as his establishment of a practice in London.

The formative moment of Mackenzie's career came during a visit to Budapest when he met the Hungarian physiologist Johann Czermak (1828–73) who was starting to investigate the laryngoscope's (recently invented by the renowned Parisian singing master Manuel Garcia) potential for diagnosis and treatment of diseases of the throat. As a result of this fortuitous encounter, Mackenzie introduced the instrument to England, where, shortly after his return, he was appointed resident medical officer to the London Hospital. After eighteen months, he became the hospital's first medical registrar and also passed the London University MB with honors in three subjects (1861) and took his MD (1862). Briefly practicing in George Street, Hanover Square, he was awarded the Jacksonian prize of the RCS (1863) for his essay 'On the pathology and treatment of diseases of the larynx'. In the same year Mackenzie opened the dispensary for diseases of the throat, later the Throat

Hospital, Golden Square. Appointed assistant physician to the London Hospital (1866), he became full physician (1873), sharing the lectureship in physiology at the hospital with John Hughlings Jackson (1835–1911). In 1874 Mackenzie resigned from all his commitments at the London Hospital save for the course of summer lectures he continued to give until 1885.

Mackenzie had wanted to devote himself to diseases of the throat since the early 1860s, and by 1874 the Throat Hospital was attracting huge numbers of both patients and students, many of the latter from abroad. His private practice was extensive and lucrative although Mackenzie was renowned for the number of poor patients he treated and without taking a fee. His prominence as a practitioner stemmed from his surgical dexterity in removing laryngeal growths through the mouth. His prowess in this surgical method made him dismissive of other ways of treating such growths, and this intolerance earned him numerous enemies within the profession. Mackenzie was also a technical innovator, inventing various instruments and appliances for treating the throat; he tended to downplay these innovations as mere 'mechanical ingenuity'.

One obituarist observed, 'Like all men who have come into extensive practice at the outset of their professional life, his knowledge of disease was founded rather on clinical observation than pathological research' (*British Medical Journal*, 1892, i, p. 363). He firmly believed in specialism as the main means of medical advance. Prominently involved in establishing special departments at the London Hospital and 'a conspicuous figure amongst contemporary laryngologists', he captured a degree of public attention through the forceful tone of his 1888 articles on specialism in the *Fortnightly Review* (reprinted in *Essays*, 1893). Mackenzie's assertiveness was primarily determined by his awareness of continuing resistance to specialism within the London medical establishment. Even with a Harley Street address, he noted, 'we are just a little doubtful as to our position in the social scale' (cited in Roy Porter, *The Greatest Benefit*, 1999, p. 385). Despite Mackenzie's international renown for surgical dexterity, the London Throat Hospital enjoyed what *Lancet* (1892, i, p. 394) described as a 'somewhat chequered' history. Dissension between Mackenzie and his staff (1877) resulted in an inquiry into the hospital's administration and the publicly and professionally damaging withdrawal of the patronage of the Prince of Wales. This negative publicity notwithstanding, Mackenzie was invited to be president of the Section of Laryngology at the 1884 International Medical Congress at Copenhagen, and at its foundation (1888) the British Laryngological Society elected him its first president.

Mackenzie's international renown led to his involvement in the case of Crown Prince Frederick of Germany's cancerous laryngeal growth. Hope for the Prince's survival engendered by Mackenzie's reputation, and the initial success of his ministrations brought a knighthood from Queen

Victoria and the Grand Cross and Star of the Royal Order of Hohenzollern from Frederick, after he had succeeded to the imperial throne. But Frederick's reliance on and preference for Mackenzie over his German counterparts generated profound resentment, feeding into the anti-English sentiments of Bismarck and his faction at the Hohenzollern court. What had appeared to be remission turned into relapse during Mackenzie's involvement from his arrival in Berlin in May 1887, through Rudolf Virchow's (1821–1902) inconclusive microscopical examinations, and through the tracheotomy Mackenzie performed in February 1888, and Frederick died that June. The disquiet and resentments of the German doctors progressively grew, and in the immediate aftermath of the death, a public controversy erupted, threatening a wider crisis in Anglo-German relations. Mackenzie's published response to German accusations of malpractice brought censure from the RCP and RCS. Never having enjoyed good health and being a long-term asthmatic, his brief stint as the most controversial medical man of the day undoubtedly hastened Mackenzie to an early grave, at age fifty-five.

Bibliography

Primary: 1865. *The use of the laryngoscope* (London); 1880–84. *Manual of diseases of the throat and nose* 2 vols. (London); 1888. *The fatal illness of Frederick the Noble* (London); 1893. *Essays* (London).

Secondary: Stevenson, Robert Scott, 1946. *Morell Mackenzie* (London); Anon., 1892. 'Sir Morell Mackenzie.' *British Medical Journal* i: 394–395; Anon., 1892. 'Sir Morell Mackenzie.' *Lancet* i: 362–363; *Oxford DNB.*

James McGeachie

MACKENZIE, WILLIAM COLIN (b. Kilmore, Victoria, Australia, 9 March 1877; d. Kew, Victoria, 29 June 1938), *orthopedic surgery, comparative anatomy.*

MacKenzie, the son of Ann McKay and her husband John MacKenzie, a Scottish-born draper, was educated at the University of Melbourne, graduating MB (1898), MD (1901), BS (1902). He served as resident medical officer at the (Royal) Melbourne Hospital and the (Royal) Children's Hospital (1899–1901) before traveling to Europe for further study at the orthopedic clinics of Oskar Vulpius in Heidelberg and Robert Jones in Liverpool and developing his interest in the treatment of infantile paralysis (poliomyelitis). He became FRCSEdin in 1903.

Returning to Melbourne the following year, MacKenzie established an orthopedic practice and lectured at the university, where he shared Richard Berry's interest in distinguishing between criminal and racial 'types'. In 1908, during a polio epidemic, MacKenzie developed a distinctive method of treatment, integrating elements from the work of Thomas, Jones, and Vulpius. He promoted the early re-education of patients' muscles within their capa-

bilities, once the acute phase of the disease had been resolved, dismissing the use of massage and electricity as worse than useless and arguing that muscle fiber should be 'coaxed, but not driven . . . conserved, and not indiscriminately torn or cut through at surgical operations'. His thinking was also influenced by broader debates: MacKenzie saw the important psychological benefit to a patient in being able to quickly regain erect posture, which he also promoted because he viewed erect posture as being associated with human evolution.

In 1915 MacKenzie returned to London to work with (Sir) Arthur Keith, Conservator of the Hunterian Museum at the Royal College of Surgeons, who later recalled MacKenzie's arrival with 'a precious cargo of dead Australian animals'. MacKenzie wrote his *Action of Muscles: Including Muscle Rest and Muscle Re-education*, worked with Keith to catalogue war wound specimens, and became a council member of the Anatomical Society of Great Britain and Ireland. In 1917, at the request of Robert Jones (who was then Inspector of Military Orthopaedics), he established a rehabilitation unit at the Military Orthopaedic Hospital, Shepherd's Bush.

On returning to Australia after the war, MacKenzie's main work became the study of comparative anatomy. He lectured at the university, where he met Winifred Smith, his future wife. MacKenzie collected, dissected, and published on Australian fauna, which he viewed as living fossils whose structure and function required urgent study before they became extinct. He also debated the antiquity of unearthed human remains with fellow anatomists Frederick Wood Jones and Grafton Elliot Smith.

MacKenzie offered his valuable collection of comparative anatomical specimens to the Australian government, and from 1930 it formed the basis of the Australian Institute of Anatomy in Canberra. Knighted in 1929 for his services to Australian zoology and medicine, MacKenzie was the Institute's first director and professor of comparative anatomy. He boasted that the Institute housed 'the greatest collection of dissections of our animals and histological preparations in the world today'. The Institute subsequently attracted many donations, including Aboriginal skeletal remains.

In 1937 MacKenzie was elected the first honorary member of the Australian Orthopaedic Association. He died in Melbourne a year later; his best-known ongoing contributions to Australian science are the Sir Colin MacKenzie Fauna Sanctuary (established 1934) and the concept of rehabilitation.

Bibliography

Primary: 1919. *The Action of Muscles; Including Muscle Rest and Muscle Re-education* (London); 1924. 'The Australian Fauna and the Medical Student.' *The Speculum: The Journal of the Melbourne Medical Students' Society* 114: 9–11; 1924. *Intellectual Development and the Erect Posture* (Melbourne).

Secondary: Hart, John A. L., 2003. 'Sir Colin Mackenzie: A Remarkable Legacy.' *Australian and New Zealand Journal of Surgery* 73: 443–448; Robin, Libby, 2003. 'Collections and the Nation: Science, History and the National Museum of Australia.' *Historical Records of Australian Science* 14: 251–289; Keith, Arthur, 1950. *An Autobiography* (London); *AuDB*.

Helen MacDonald

MACNAMARA, ANNIE JEAN   (b. Beechworth, Victoria, Australia, 1 April 1899; d. Victoria, 13 October 1968), *poliomyelitis, rehabilitation.*

Macnamara was the second daughter of Victorian-born parents John Macnamara, clerk of courts, and his wife Annie, née Fraser. Scholarships took her to the Presbyterian Ladies' College and the University of Melbourne where she graduated MB, BS in 1922 with exhibitions in surgery and anatomy and the Beaney scholarship in surgery. She became a resident medical officer at the (Royal) Melbourne Hospital.

In May 1923 Macnamara was appointed resident at the (Royal) Children's Hospital. She remained until 1925 when, having graduated MD, she became clinical assistant to the Children's outpatients' physician and entered private practice with a special emphasis on poliomyelitis. From 1925 to 1931 she was consultant and medical officer responsible to the Poliomyelitis Committee of Victoria led by Dr John Dale and in 1930–31 was honorary adviser on polio to official authorities in New South Wales, South Australia, and Tasmania. From 1928 to 1951 she was honorary medical officer to the Yooralla Hospital School for Crippled Children.

The 1925 polio epidemic prompted Macnamara to test the use of immune serum in the treatment of patients at the preparalytic stage. Convinced of the value of the method, she published and defended her results in Australian and British journals in 1927–35, notably with F. G. Morgan in *Lancet* of 27 February 1932. The therapy, difficult to administer properly, was damned by the discouraging findings of W. H. Park in New York in 1931, even though Macnamara was quick to pinpoint vital weaknesses in his procedures. The efficacy of the treatment has in fact never been disproved, and although its general adoption was 'wrecked', she believed, 'on the rocks of carelessness' in America, she continued to use it privately. Her discovery, in collaboration with Macfarlane Burnet, of the existence of more than one strain of polio virus (reported in 1931 in the *British Journal of Experimental Pathology*) has, however, been acknowledged as an early step toward the development of the Salk vaccine. Although research still appealed to her, and she worked part-time at the Walter and Eliza Hall Institute in Melbourne in 1933–37 on serum and psittacosis, her special field remained conservative orthopedics.

While overseas on a Rockefeller fellowship (1931–33), she preached the necessity for adequate aftercare of disabled persons, met President Roosevelt, ordered Australia's first artificial respirator, and armed herself with new ideas for splinting and rehabilitation. She also wrote to health departments around the world canvassing the possibility that the polio virus was transmitted through milk.

On 19 November 1934 Macnamara married Joseph Ivan Connor, a dermatologist. They were to have two daughters. She won great renown for her orthopedic work, being appointed DBE in 1935. During the 1937–38 polio epidemic she supervised patient care at both the Children's and Fairfield hospitals. Her method was to splint the paralyzed part of the body until the damaged nerve had recovered and then patiently re-educate the muscles. She spent much time not only with her patients but also with her splintmaker, devising ingenious restraining devices. She belonged to the Consultative Council for Polio from 1937–42 and 1946–47 and served on the 1935 Queensland royal commission investigating Sister Elizabeth Kenny's treatment. Wisely, she supported the establishment of an experimental Kenny treatment centre at Brighton (Hampton), at the same time acquiring improved hospital facilities for herself. Her work extended to victims of lead poisoning and cerebral palsy and to healthy people with poor posture. The first center for spastic children in Australia was opened, on her recommendation, at the Children's Hospital in 1940.

From girlhood Macnamara had an affinity with the land, and from 1933 her advocacy was instrumental in the introduction of myxomatosis to combat the rabbit plague. In 1952–53 'myxo' was reputed to have augmented the wool check by at least £30 million, and woolgrowers gave her £800 and a clock. In 1964 the CSIRO's animal house at the Keith Turnbull Research Station, Frankston, was named in her honor. The University of Melbourne awarded her an honorary LLD in 1966. Neglectful of her own health and a chain smoker, Dame Jean died from heart disease on 13 October 1968.

Bibliography

Secondary: Yule, Peter, 1999. *The Royal Children's Hospital* (Rushcutters Bay); Zwar, D., 1984. *The Dame* (Melbourne); *AuDB*.

Janet McCalman

MACPHAIL, JOHN ANDREW   (b. Orwell, Prince Edward Island, Canada, 24 November 1864; d. Montreal, Canada, 23 September 1938), *medical journalism, literature.*

Born in the rural Prince Edward Island, son of William Macphail and Catherine Moore Smith, Macphail regarded his life and his community as idyllic, and they would inform his views and his writing throughout his life. His father became Inspector of Schools and later supervisor for the Public Hospital for the Insane in Charlottetown and encouraged his education. He was educated at Uigg School and Prince of Wales College and became the 'principal' of the one-room school. After three years, he had enough money to enter McGill University in Montreal, working as a reporter to further support himself. He obtained his BA in 1888 and MD, CM in 1891.

After a period abroad, he became the professor of pathology at Bishop's College during the brief period it had a medical school, and when that faculty was absorbed into McGill in 1907, he was given the position as professor of the history of medicine, a position created for him because of his interests. Macphail was a prolific writer and became recognized as a prominent literary figure in Canada, and although his professorship and most of his stimulating lectures were on medical history, little of his writing was on this topic. He was made a Fellow of the Royal Society of Canada in 1910.

He was more committed to his academic pursuits than clinical practice, but did occasional work for insurance companies. He was not a skilled researcher but did become involved in chemical investigation for the lobster industry of Prince Edward Island. He was editor of the highly respected *University Magazine* from 1907 to 1920 and editor of the *Montreal Medical Journal*. He convinced the delegates at the annual meeting of the Canadian Medical Association that they must have a journal and was instrumental in joining this journal with the *Maritime Medical News* to form the *Canadian Medical Association Journal*, becoming its founding editor. He gave a personal financial guarantee for the journal, and the first issue appeared on 1 January 1911.

Although he was fifty years old and had lost sight in one eye in an accident, he tried to enlist at the outbreak of war in 1914; he was refused until he made a personal appeal to the Prime Minister. He joined the Canadian Field Ambulance Service and spent over twenty months at the front. In 1917 he was invited to give the Cavendish Lecture in London, speaking on 'A Day's Work', referring to the work of the Canadian medical corps at the battle of Vimy. In 1918 Macphail was knighted for his wartime services and his literary career. In 1922, while working on the history of the Canadian medical corps, he was awarded an honorary LLD from McGill University. The official history of the Canadian forces in World War I was published in 1925 to acclaim by many and protest from others because of the personal views expressed and his criticism of leadership, particularly of Sir Sam Hughes, Canadian Minister of Militia.

He had a close brush with death by a bullet from a mentally deranged man in 1921. In his later years, he became a 'man of means' and encouraged music, literature, and drama in the community of Orwell, returning to his birthplace for rest and writing each year. He and his brother experimented with agricultural methods and were responsible for and began experiments in agriculture on his family farm.

Although professor of medical history for thirty years, he was best known as a writer and social critic, one of the most distinguished men of letters in Canada. His favorite writing was the essay, but he also wrote ten books and wrote on subjects as varied as military history, education, the Bible, evolution, feminism, agriculture, family values, biography, and poetry. In his essays he put forward strong views based in his rural Scottish Presbyterian roots. He had a traditional and romantic view of rural life and of family and the place of women in society. His lasting work, still in print and popular, is his semiautobiographical novel *The Master's Wife* (the master is William, his father), which reveals life in rural Prince Edward Island and which was written in the 1930s and published after his death by his children. The 140-acre Macphail Homestead in Orwell is maintained by a foundation in his name and is open to the public.

Bibliography

Primary: 1911. 'Style in Medical Writing.' *Can. Med. Assoc. J.* 146: 2197–2198; 1925. *Official History of the Canadian Forces in the Great War 1914–1919, The Medical Services* (Ottawa); 1929. 'Evolution of Life.' *Annals of Medical History* (n.s.) 1: 533–561; 1939. *The Master's Wife* (Montreal).

Secondary: Campbell, D., 2002. '"I Would Not Have Missed It for the World": Sir Andrew Macphail's War.' *Island Magazine* 51: 2–10, 52: 2–9; Shortt, S. E., 1978. 'Sir Andrew Macphail: Physician, Philosopher, Founding Editor of CMAJ.' *Can. Med. Assoc. J.* 118: 323–326; Robertson, I. R., 1974. 'Sir Andrew Macphail as a Social Critic.' PhD thesis, University of Toronto; Stuart, H. A., 1944–45. 'Sir Andrew Macphail.' *Hist. Bull.* (Calgary Associate Clinic) 9: 61–67; Francis, W. W., 1939. 'Sir Andrew Macphail.' *Bulletin of the History of Medicine* 7: 799–800.

Jock Murray

MADSEN, THORVALD JOHANNES MARIUS

(b. Copenhagen, Denmark, 18 February 1870; d. Gjorslev Manor, St Heddinge, Denmark, 14 April 1957), *microbiology, public health, international health.*

Madsen was son of Wilhelm Hermann Oluf Madsen (1844–1917) and Albertine Henriette (née Petersen). His father was an artillery officer, internationally known as the inventor of the Madsen machine gun and Minister of War from 1901 to 1904. Madsen graduated from school at the age of sixteen and consequently needed special permission to start studies in medicine at Copenhagen University. During his studies he attended the first voluntary course in bacteriology at the University's recently established Laboratory of Medical Bacteriology, organized by Professor C. J. Salomonsen. The same year he suffered from diphtheria. His lifelong interest in the disease was based on this personal experience.

Madsen graduated in 1893 and worked one year as a locum for a rural general practitioner. He then commenced research at a new laboratory for serotherapeutics established by Salomonsen, who had promised Madsen a position as assistant during his attendance at the bacteriology course. During the next two years Madsen worked on problems related to the diphtheria toxin and antitoxin. The results were presented in his thesis on experimental investigations on the diphtheria toxin (1896). The laboratory had

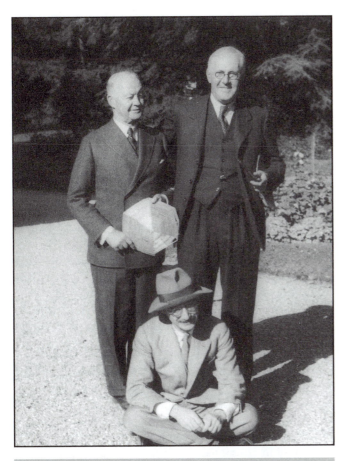

Thorvald Madsen (standing left) with Sir Henry Dale (right, see biographical entry) and Ludwik Rajchman (seated, see biographical entry) in the park of the League of Nations, 1937. Photograph, Library of the Statens Serum Institut, Copenhagen.

the task of developing methods for the production of serum for treatment of diphtheria, and Madsen's work established basic scientific knowledge on toxin and antitoxin. At the same time it gave him insight into the difficulties of comparing results from different laboratories. Based on his experiments he considered the methods of Paul Ehrlich to measure the activity of antitoxin to be superior to those favored by the Institut Pasteur.

After defending his thesis, Madsen continued to do research at the laboratory. At the same time, he was attached to clinical hospital departments in Copenhagen, among them the epidemic hospital, Blegdamshospitalet. Here Johannes Fibiger conducted a major study on the efficiency of Danish diphtheria serum, which had been available since 1895. The study revealed an apparent beneficial effect of serum treatment. However, in his last scientific publication (1956), Madsen stated that he had at the time of the study felt uncertain about that interpretation. His continued research with Salomonsen was primarily on aspects related to immunology, both in general and that of diphtheria. He further studied the binding of toxin and

antitoxin with the Swedish chemist Svante Arrhenius (1859–1927), who became a Nobel laureate in 1903. They showed the differences in binding capacity as well as binding velocity of various sera.

His early work and his relation to Salomonsen gave Madsen, in the last years of the century, access to leading microbiologists, most notably including Paul Ehrlich in Germany but also others in France. In 1901 Madsen visited the United States, where he met many leading American microbiologists. He also contracted typhoid fever and was admitted to Johns Hopkins Hospital.

Madsen's travels gave him important inspiration in his scientific work. They further brought him onto friendly terms with leading scientists and refined his skills in English, French, and German. He also obtained knowledge about the organization of institutions that combined research and production of sera, like the Robert Koch Institute and the Institut Pasteur. This made him an obvious ally for Salomonsen, who finally obtained government and parliamentary backing to establish a proper state-financed institution to take over the production of diphtheria antitoxin. The Statens Serum Institute was inaugurated in 1902 with Salomonsen as director and Madsen as head of laboratory. The opening was attended by leading scientists from many European countries, and a number of Madsen's scientific results were presented in a Festschrift.

In the following years Madsen extended the activities of the institute beyond serum production, taking up Widal and Wasserman testing. A proposal to extend an old state institution producing smallpox vaccine was submitted to a standing medical reform committee. As a consequence, the committee presented a draft bill for the enlargement of Statens Serum Institute, making it the national institute for diagnostic, preventive, and therapeutic microbiology. The change came into force in 1910 and Madsen became the sole director. Over the next thirty years he developed the institute, taking up new methods of diagnosis, and developed BCG and diphtheria vaccines. The institute established an epidemiological service, which enabled rapid disclosure in outbreaks and which conducted studies on diseases like tuberculosis. The Rockefeller Foundation supported such studies and also assisted in the physical extension of the institute in the interwar years. Starting from a handful of persons at its opening in 1902, the institute's staff totaled 379 when Madsen retired in 1940.

Alongside his administrative duties as a director, Madsen continued his scientific work with the many researchers he was able to attach to the institute. This ran in parallel with an increasing engagement in international affairs, which, however, had a significant domestic dimension as well. For example, in 1908 Madsen went to St Petersburg during a cholera epidemic. As a consequence he was able to obtain funds to establish a cholera laboratory at the institute.

During World War I Madsen traveled in Russia on behalf of the Danish Red Cross and with backing by the

Danish government, to bring relief to the prisoners of war from the Central Powers, and he was also on reverse missions to Germany. He was received in both countries by the empresses, who held honorary Red Cross positions.

Following the war, the League of Nations' Covenant came into force, as the first part of the Treaty of Versailles. It contained a mandate for the League to take action on international health. The first steps were taken at meetings in 1919 and 1920. Other interested and active bodies were the League of Red Cross Societies and the Office International d'Hygiène Publique (OIHP). This organization was established in 1907 and was particularly concerned with international control of contagious diseases, and Madsen became the Danish member after the war. The intention of the founding fathers of the League of Nations' Health Organization (LNHO) had been to incorporate OIPH into the new body. This was, however, blocked by the OIHP and some of its member countries, notably France and the United States.

A compromise was reached whereby the LNHO was governed by a Health Committee with members appointed both from the Council of the League of Nations and from OIHP, which remained unchanged. This arrangement had the inherent benefit that the American delegate to the OIHP, normally the U.S. Surgeon General, was a member. The LNHO's operative wing was the Health Section, which formed part of the League's secretariat, and Ludwik Rajchman was appointed director. At the first meeting of the Health Committee in August 1921, the French member, Léon Bernard, proposed Madsen as president, and was seconded by his British counterpart. The reasons given for the nomination were that Madsen was a man of science, with skills in the two official languages of the League, English and French, and that he was a member of the OIPH.

The immediate health concerns in postwar Europe were famine and epidemics in the eastern parts, with the partial breakdown of the infrastructure, including health services, as a secondary issue. Rajchman had been engaged in American-supported relief work, e.g., in Poland, and that effort continued under the auspices of LNHO, though funds were scarce. Attention to other disaster-stricken areas followed suit, for example in the aftermath of the Greek-Turkish war. The LNHO never obtained regular funds of a magnitude to run their own relief programs. However, it developed an epidemiological surveillance system, which eventually included the colonies of the European countries. Later a special bureau was established in Singapore for the Far East.

In the course of the 1920s the LNHO started work on a broad range of activities in the field of public health, through the establishment of standing commissions. Madsen became chairman of the commission of biological standardization, an issue that had been close to his heart for decades. It was formally established in 1924, though work had begun earlier. Sir Henry Dale became the commission's vice-chairman. The bulk of work on standardization of microbiological products was carried out at Statens Serum Institute, while most work on other products, such as vitamins and insulin, was done at Dale's institute in London. However, international experts oversaw all of the work and the final approval rested with the Health Committee upon recommendation from the appropriate standing commission.

At an early stage Madsen tried to extend the work of LNHO beyond the founding countries of the League of Nations. He succeeded in including German scientists in early work on standardization, even though Germany only became a member of the League in 1926. That was accomplished against French *and* German opposition. Both he and Rajchman obtained good working relations with public health authorities in the USSR as well. In addition, Madsen kept close contacts with American scientists and funding bodies, such as the Rockefeller Foundation.

Madsen was president of the Health Committee for five successive three-year terms. During his years in office, he traveled extensively to all corners of the world, initially mostly in trouble areas. From 1937 onward he was honorary president after the Committee's structure was changed. Although acknowledging the need for him in Denmark, the Secretary General of the League pleaded with the Danish government to allow Madsen to continue as president. In articles, interviews, and lectures, Madsen promoted the concept of international health and the role of LNHO, and he had an eye for the possibility of promoting Danish medical science in parallel with his work for LNHO. This is illustrated by his Flexner lectures on infectious disease in Denmark and in Baltimore in March 1937 and in his Harvey Lecture on the LNHO the previous month, in which he carefully emphasized the role of American physicians and scientists in the international work.

In the latter part of the 1930s, international work became difficult. Madsen assisted in getting some Jewish scientists out of Germany, including Fritz Kauffmann (1899–1978), who received a position at Statens Serum Institute. Rajchman, also a Jew, was forced out of the League of Nations in early 1939, and Madsen attended the last meeting of the Health Committee in November of that year.

Madsen retired from his post as director of Statens Serum Institute just after the German occupation of Denmark (1940–45). During that period Madsen was engaged in activities primarily related to the combat of tuberculosis, which had been a lifelong interest. That paved the way for a countrywide tuberculosis screening and BCG vaccination program after the war. In 1947 Madsen chaired the international microbiology congress in Copenhagen, which allowed him to re-establish many personal contacts. Rajchman had become head of UNICEF and used Madsen as an advisor. He further appointed him head of relief operations in Italy, a post which lasted until Madsen turned eighty.

Madsen started his career with important scientific achievements. He continued research activities until late in life and was able to attract many researchers to his institute. He had a reputation for underlining the scientific significance of the work of his collaborators at the institute in his many international presentations, and he had great pleasure in seeing members of his staff promoted and honored. He was described as an extremely helpful superior and a person who was able to delegate. He developed the Statens Serum Institute into one of the leading microbiological institutions in Europe. Through his humanitarian work from the World War I years through 1950, Madsen played in significant role in making health a responsibility of the international community. In the interwar years he developed international, technical cooperation and supported, with diplomatic caution, most of Rajchman's ambitions of creating a broad public health policy for the LNHO.

Madsen consequently received numerous scientific honors and decorations from many countries. He married Emilie (Misse) Gad (1884–1957) in 1906. They had four children and they showed grand hospitality in Copenhagen, where Madsen's wife became a most admired hostess. Madsen died at a family reunion at the estate of his daughter and son-in-law.

Bibliography

Primary: 1896. *Experimentelle Undersøgelser over Difterigiften.* thesis, Copenhagen University; 1937. 'The Scientific Work of the Health Organization of the League of Nations.' *Harvey Lectures 1936–1937,* pp. 145–168; 1937. *Lectures on the Epidemiology and Control of Syphilis, Tuberculosis and Whooping Cough, and Other Aspects of Infectious Disease* (Baltimore); 1940. *Statens Seruminstitut; Instituttets Udvikling 1902–1940.* (Copenhagen); 1956. (with Madsen, S.). 'Diphtheria in Denmark; from 23,695 to 1 Case—Post or Propter?' *Danish Medical Bulletin* 3: 112–121.

Secondary: Parnas, Joseph, 1980. *Thorvald Madsen; Leader in International Health* (Copenhagen); Schelde-Møller, E., 1970. *Thorvald Madsen; I Videnskabens og Menneskehedens Tjeneste* (Copenhagen); Jensen, K. A., 1957. 'Thorvald Johannes Marius Madsen 18. februar 1870–14. april 1957.' *Oversigt over Det kgl. Danske Videnskabernes Selskabs. Virksomhed.* 1957–58: 99–107.

Nils Rosdahl

MAGENDIE, FRANÇOIS (b. Bordeaux, France, 6 October 1783; d. Sannois, France, 7 October 1855), *physiology, pharmacology.*

Magendie was the elder son of Antoine Magendie, a Bordeaux surgeon originally from the Pyrenees region of France, and Marie Nicole de Perey de Launay, a native of Paris. Notwithstanding the aristocratic flavor of Mme Magendie's maiden name, Antoine Magendie was a follower of the egalitarian social philosophy of Jean-Jacques Rousseau (1712–78), in honor of whom the couple's second son was named Jean-Jacques. There were no other

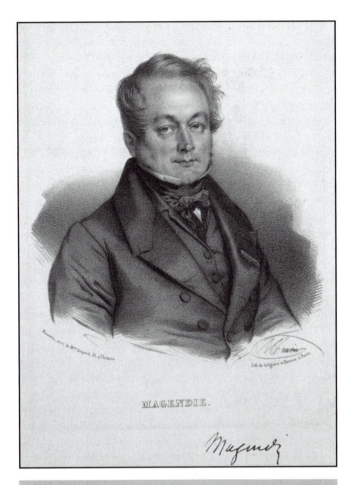

François Magendie. Lithograph by Nicolas-Eustache Maurin. Iconographic Collection, Wellcome Library, London.

children, and in May 1792, after a prolonged illness, Mme Magendie died in Paris, where the family had relocated during the previous year.

With the advent of the Republic some months after his wife's death, Antoine became politically active in the municipal government of Paris. As a youth, François shared his father's republican sympathies, and throughout his life he retained a liberal political outlook combined with a philosophical disposition toward skepticism and materialism.

In accordance with Rousseau's educational principles, Antoine kept his sons away from formal schooling during their childhood years, with the result that at the age of ten François could still neither read nor write. He soon afterward entered primary school, however, and quickly made up lost time.

In 1799 he became an apprentice to the surgeon Alexis Boyer (1757–1833), who was then associate professor of operative medicine at the School of Medicine, the successor institution to the Faculty of Medicine, which had been abolished during the revolution in 1793. Magendie, although too young at the time to be enrolled in the medical school, was soon selected as Boyer's anatomical assistant and began teaching informal anatomy classes to other students.

In addition to human anatomy, he also took an interest in comparative anatomy and dissected animal specimens obtained from Georges Cuvier (1769–1832) at the Museum of Natural History. He later entered formal medical study and in 1803 passed his first competitive examination, enabling him to obtain a hospital placement as a medical student. After progressing through the required examinations, he graduated in 1808 as a doctor of medicine.

In 1809 Magendie launched his career as a medical scientist by publishing a theoretical critique of the prevailing approach to physiological explanation and a series of experimental reports. In all these papers Magendie drew upon the legacy of Xavier Bichat (1771–1802), but in varying ways: negatively in the case of theory and positively in the case of experimentation.

Bichat's explanatory approach, like that of many physiologists at the time, sought to identify the normal phenomena of life by means of careful observation and then to classify these phenomena in meaningful categories. Groups of related phenomena were explained by positing an underlying vital principle or property that was said to give rise to them. In his paper entitled 'Some General Ideas on the Phenomena Peculiar to Living Bodies', Magendie criticized this approach, arguing that experimentation was needed—both to provide a more accurate account of what the phenomena of life actually were and to reveal the processes by which these phenomena occurred.

To give an initial orientation to this proposal, he recommended that the existing lists of vital properties be abandoned and that physiologists treat all the phenomena of life as arising from processes of two kinds: micro-level processes that resulted in growth and nutrition, and macro-level processes that resulted in functional actions. The many differences in these functional actions were to be accounted for by the organization of the anatomical parts involved and thus were amenable to experimental study. In giving this theoretical priority to nutrition and function, Magendie was reflecting within physiology the priority that Cuvier had given these phenomena in his comparative anatomy.

Cuvier, however, was not an experimenter, whereas Bichat had used experiments extensively in his researches on accidental death. So despite his rejection of Bichat's theories, it was probably not coincidental that the young Magendie designed his experiments in ways that parallel those of Bichat. Using procedures that Bichat had employed to study asphyxiation, Magendie and his collaborator, the botanist and physician A. Raffeneau-Delile, investigated the effects of newly-discovered vegetable poisons on mammals, showing that the poison (later identified as strychnine) first entered the bloodstream and then acted on the animal's spinal cord.

The experiments of 1809 left some questions unresolved, as was often the case with Magendie's investigations throughout his career. Whenever he obtained conflicting experimental results he typically preferred to report what he had found without attempting to reconcile discrepancies—a practice for which he was later criticized by his student and successor, Claude Bernard (1813–78). Nevertheless, it is generally agreed that Magendie's 1809 collaboration with Raffeneau-Delile represents the beginning of systematic experimental pharmacology.

In 1811 Magendie became a demonstrator in anatomy at the School of Medicine, but in 1813 he resigned from this position, possibly because his brusque and often rude manner had brought him into conflict with his colleagues. He registered his medical diploma at the local prefecture at this time, so that he could enter private practice, and he also rented an amphitheatre where he began offering a private course in experimental physiology. His demonstrations of experimental techniques on live animals attracted both medical students and medical graduates, and the success of this course prompted him to write a textbook in two volumes entitled *An Elementary Precis of Physiology* (1816–17).

Unlike previous physiology textbooks, Magendie's *Precis* was oriented toward experimentation rather than systematic theory. In the introduction he extended the attack on the prevailing approaches to physiological explanation that he had begun in 1809. Even if the laws of living phenomena should have some unique features, he argued, they must always act in concert with the laws of physics and chemistry, and therefore it is the relationship between living phenomena and physicochemical phenomena that physiology must experimentally investigate. In support of this position the *Precis* included extensive reports of Magendie's own experiments as well as those of colleagues and collaborators. The textbook was translated into a number of other languages, and it went through three substantive French editions by 1834 (and an unaltered 'fourth edition' in 1836), with each of the revisions making the work's orientation more empirical and less speculative.

To further his medical practice and obtain a clinical setting in which to study the therapeutic effects of new medications, Magendie sought a hospital post in 1818. He was successful in the competitive examination but did not obtain a formal position until 1826, when he was appointed to the Salpêtrière hospital in Paris. In the meantime, he was able to make ward rounds at the principal Parisian hospital, the Hôtel Dieu, in collaboration with physicians who were located there.

The year 1821 saw a number of major events in Magendie's life. He was elected to the Academy of Sciences and the Royal Academy of Medicine, which provided recognition of his achievements to date, and he launched two innovative publications. Building on his continuing interest in pharmacological research and the therapeutic potential of chemical substances, he brought out a *Formulary for the Preparation and Use of Many New Remedies*. This compilation was based in large part on Magendie's own studies and came to be in great demand, going through many successive editions. He also founded a new periodical in 1821, the *Journal of Experimental Physiology and Pathology* (the last two words of the title were added in 1822). Magendie's journal was the first to be devoted exclusively to physiology, and it served to further disseminate his view that physiological science was necessarily experimental.

Magendie was no stranger to controversy throughout his career. His most elaborate dispute was with the British anatomist and surgeon Charles Bell (1774–1842). In the course of his experiments on the nervous system, Magendie demonstrated in 1822 that the dorsal and ventral roots of the spinal nerves have different functions, relating to sensation and motion respectively. Magendie was accused of plagiarism by Bell, on the basis of work the latter had done in 1821, and many protracted and unpleasant exchanges followed. Most commentators now agree first, that Magendie was unaware of the details of Bell's work in 1822, although he may have learned something of its general features from the Bell's collaborator, John Shaw; second, that Bell in 1821 correctly proposed that the dorsal and ventral roots have different functions, but did not correctly identify these functions; and third, that Magendie in 1822 provided the first experimental demonstration of these different functions, now summarized as the Bell-Magendie Law.

The controversy with Bell, together with Magendie's 1824 visit to London and the experimental demonstrations he publicly gave there, brought him to the attention of British antivivisectionists, and in 1825 he was denounced in parliamentary debates on the prevention of cruelty to animals. Although he was relatively indifferent to the suffering of his experimental animals, Magendie's reputation in nineteenth-century Britain and America as a monster who delighted in torturing animals was a fiction concocted for political purposes.

Magendie's position in France was also affected by political currents. Twice during the period of the Bourbon Restoration (1815–30), in 1822 and 1827, he had been recommended to the king by the Academy of Sciences for appointment to the chair of medicine at the College of France. On each occasion another candidate, more acceptable to the government and the Church, had received royal approval. But after the fall of the Bourbons in the July Revolution of 1830, Magendie's political liberalism was no longer an obstacle to his career. In December 1830 he received an appointment to the Hôtel Dieu, the pinnacle of the Parisian hospital system, and in March 1831 he was appointed, after another recommendation from the Academy of Sciences, to the chair of medicine at the College of France.

In his lectures at the College, Magendie continued to stress the importance of physics and chemistry for physiology and medicine, despite general resistance to this position from the French medical establishment. His most significant series of lectures were those on the physical phenomena of life (1832–38) and on the nervous system (1838–39). Both series led to important publications. The last four semesters of lectures from the first series appeared as separate volumes after each course and were later reprinted in four volumes as *The Physical Phenomena of Life* (1842). In the interval, the course on the nervous system was published in two volumes as *Lectures on the Functions and Maladies of the Nervous System* (1839-41).

Magendie's collaboration with Claude Bernard began in 1839, when the young Bernard began to prepare specimens for Magendie's demonstrations at the College. From then until the latter's death the association continued in various forms, with Bernard taking on some of Magendie's lecturing duties at the College from 1847, and then all of them from 1853. Magendie's marriage in 1830 to Henriette Bastienne de Puisaye, a prosperous widow, had provided him with financial security and a country property at Sannois, where he increasingly spent his time as he grew older. In his last years he suffered from shortness of breath, probably caused by a heart condition, and from rheumatism. He died at Sannois on the day following his seventy-second birthday.

Bibliography

Primary: 1816–17. *Précis élémentaire de physiologie* (Paris); 1821. *Formulaire pour l'emploi et la préparation de plusieurs nouveaux médicaments, tel que la noix vomique, la morphine, l'acide prussique, la strychnine, la vératrine, les alcalis des quinquinas, l'iodide, etc.* (Paris); 1839–41. *Leçons sur les fonctions et les maladies du système nerveux, professées au Collège de France* (Paris); 1842. *Phénomènes physiques de la vie: Leçons professées au Collège de France* (Paris).

Secondary: Lesch, John E., 1984. *Science and Medicine in France: The Emergence of Experimental Physiology, 1790–1855* (Cambridge, MA); Albury, William Randall, 1977. 'Experiment and Explanation in the Physiology of Bichat and Magendie.' *Studies in History of Biology* 1: 47–131; Olmsted, J. M. D., 1945. *François Magendie: Pioneer in Experimental Physiology and Scientific Medicine in XIX Century France* (New York, 1981 reprint); DSB.

W. R. Albury

MAGNAN, (JACQUES JOSEPH) VALENTIN (b. Perpignan, France, 16 March 1835; d. Paris, France, 27 September 1916), *psychiatry.*

Magnan was born to a family of modest means. After completing his secondary schooling in Perpignan, he studied medicine in Montpellier and later in Lyons, where he became interested in psychiatry. In 1863 Magnan continued his studies in Paris, as a psychiatric intern at Bicêtre and the Salpêtrière. He defended his medical thesis in 1866, and in 1867 he was appointed to the Admissions Office at the new Parisian public asylum of Sainte-Anne, where patients were examined, certified, and quickly dispatched to the various public asylums around Paris. Magnan remained at the Admissions Office until his retirement in 1912. By 1879 he was the sole admitting physician and examined over 3,000 patients annually.

Magnan quickly recognized that the Admissions Office offered unparalleled opportunities for clinical observation and statistical analysis. He had already become interested in alcoholism, particularly the toxic effects of the popular apéritif absinthe. In 1874 he published his book *De l'alcoolisme*, in which he drew on his extensive clinical experience at the Admissions Office to describe and classify a wide range of alcoholic disorders. Magnan also warned that alcoholism was a major cause of degeneration and that it threatened to destroy French society. The novelist Émile Zola based his dramatic account of alcoholic delirium on Magnan's clinical description. The book was translated into English, Russian, and Portuguese, and brought him international recognition. Magnan's research was also used extensively by the French temperance movement.

In the 1880s and 1890s Magnan focused his research on developing Morel's theory of degeneration. He defined degeneration as a deterioration of the organism from the state of its immediate forebears, rather than from Morel's primal norm, and he delineated two large categories of mental illness, hereditary degeneration and *délire chronique,* or chronic delusional insanity. He also expanded the descriptions of the mental and emotional signs of degeneration. Magnan's work reflected the increasing importance of degeneration theory for French psychiatry, but his system of classifications provoked three years of intense debate among his colleagues and was never adopted by the *Société médico-psychologique,* the professional society of French psychiatrists.

Magnan was also an influential teacher and a leader in the reform of psychiatric care. In 1868 he began his clinical lessons at the Admissions Office and, by his retirement, it was estimated that he had trained half the psychiatrists practicing in Parisian asylums. By the 1880s he had transformed his service from a triage and emergency center to a 120-bed clinic with a high staff-patient ratio, where he could institute reforms that were not always feasible in the average asylum service. In 1874 he abolished the use of straitjackets at the Admissions Office and substituted a less-confining garment. By 1878, however, he had adopted a policy of complete nonrestraint. He abandoned the use of cells in 1897 and instituted the practice of *clinothérapie,* or prolonged bed rest, arguing that mental patients had to be treated as ordinary hospital patients. In the 1890s Magnan and his former student Paul-Maurice Legrain began a campaign to establish special treatment centers for alcoholics, at a time when medical and popular opinion held that alcoholics were incurable. At his death and later in 1935, at celebrations marking the centenary of his birth, Magnan was praised as a great clinician in the nineteenth-century French tradition of clinical medicine and as a worthy successor to Pinel in his devotion to his patients.

Bibliography

Primary: 1874. *De l'alcoolisme: des diverses formes du délire alcoolique et de leur traitement* (Paris); 1891. *Leçons cliniques sur les maladies mentales* (Paris); 1892. *Le délire chroniqiue à évolution systématique* (Paris and Montreal).

Secondary: Dowbiggin, Ian, 1996. 'Back to the Future: Valentin Magnan, French Psychiatry, and the Classification of Mental Diseases, 1885–1925.' *Social History of Medicine* 9: 383–408; Prestwich, Patricia E., 1988. *Drink and the Politics of Social Reform: Antialcoholism in France since 1870* (Palo Alto); Sérieux, Dr Paul, 1921. *V. Magnan. Sa vie et son oeuvre* (Paris).

Patricia E. Prestwich

MAHFOUZ, NAGUIB MIKHĀ'IL PĀSHĀ (b. Mansoura, Egypt, 5 January 1882; d. Cairo, Egypt, 25 July 1974), *gynecology, obstetrics.*

Mahfouz, an Egyptian Christian, was the son of a cotton and cereal merchant. He attended the American Mission School, then the Government Primary School. In 1898 he entered Kasr El-Aini Medical School, where European professors predominantly held the teaching posts. Mahfouz started his medical career by combating outbreaks of cholera in Upper Egypt and was very successful in finding contaminated wells.

Kasr El-Aini School at that time did not have a department for obstetrics and gynecology. Mahfouz decided to become an obstetrician after he attended a labor that ended fatally for both mother and child. After graduating in 1902, Mahfouz was appointed as anesthetist to the Kasr El-Aini hospital, where he started a weekly gynecological outpatients' clinic. The great success of this clinic resulted in the dedication of two whole wards soon after to obstetric and gynecological patients. During the subsequent fifteen years, Mahfouz attended about 2,000 women.

In 1929 Mahfouz was appointed as professor of obstetrics and gynecology at Kasr El-Aini medical school. He also served as obstetrician and gynecologist to the Egyptian royal family. His pioneering work on the surgical repair of urinary and rectal fistulae brought him international acclaim. Moreover, a maternity unit, long absent from Kasr El-Aini hospital, was finally established thanks to his efforts. Mahfouz taught in this department for more than thirty years. In 1919 he started a pioneering scheme whereby the midwives, whom he trained to highest standards, were allowed to deliver women in their homes. Also in the same year he introduced Egypt's first antenatal clinic. By 1930 Mahfouz had collected three thousand rare specimens in obstetrics and gynecology, obtained from his operations, and in that year he offered the museum that housed them as a gift to the Kasr El-Aini hospital.

Mahfouz was a prolific writer. He authored a number of books and articles, including his autobiography, *The Life of an Egyptian Doctor*, an important source for the modern history of medicine in Egypt. His medical writings include *Atlas of Mahfouz's Obstetric and Gynaecological Museum* (1949).

Mahfouz received a number of honors, including the Order of Nile and an Honorary Fellowship of the Royal College of Obstetricians and Gynaecologists of England, among many others. He was a devout Christian and a man of strict principles. He successfully opposed Egyptian bureaucracy and won great acclaim for himself and his department. In 1911 Mahfouz helped to deliver a baby. In appreciation of his competence, compassion, and dedication, the baby was named after him. This baby grew up to become the Nobel laureate, Naguib Mahfouz.

Bibliography

Primary: 1938. 'Ectopic Pregnancy.' *The Journal of Gynaecology and Obstetrics of the British Empire* 45: 209–230; 1949. *Atlas of Mahfouz's Obstetric and Gynaecological Museum (Altrincham)*; 1966. *The Life of an Egyptian Doctor* (Edinburgh and London).

Secondary: Simaika, Samir Mahfouz, and Youssef Simaika, 2004. 'Naguib Mahfouz: The Man Who Dedicated His Life to the Betterment of Women's Health.' *Watani International* 25 July, p. 2; Ebeid, Makram, Amin 2004. 'Naguib Pasha Mahfouz: A Grandson Remembers.' *Watani International* 25 July, p. 2.

Nikolaj Serikoff

MAIMONIDES, RABBI MOSES BEN MAIMON (aka MOSHE BEN MAIMON, MUSSA BIN MAIMUN IBN ABDALLAH AL-KURTUBI AL-ISRAILI) (b. Córdoba (Cordova), Spain, 30 March 1138; d. ?, buried Tiberias, Palestine, 13 December 1204), *medicine, ethics.*

Maimonides was born on Passover eve in the Hebrew year 4898 to a mother who died in childbirth; he was then raised by his father, Maimon. Following persecution by the Almohades in Córdoba, the family was forced into a peripatetic existence in southern Spain and northern Africa for the next decade, finally settling in Fes, Morocco. Thereafter they traveled to Palestine and Egypt.

As with many medieval figures, Maimonides' youth remains largely unknown. He probably benefited from a semiprivate course of education, judging from his reference in *Medical Aphorisms* to 'the elders before whom I have read', and he knew the son of the great physician Ibn Zuhr (known as Avenzoar in the Latin West). It is clear that he had a wide exposure to Arabic translations of Greek authors, including Hippocrates, Aristotle, and Galen, as well as to original Arabic writers, such as Rhazes, Alfarabius, and, of course, Ibn Zuhr. From these beginnings, and after the death of his father and brother around 1166, Maimonides turned to medicine for a living. He rapidly rose to court physician under the Vizier (government official) and Egyptian Regent al Fahil, and under Saladin the Great. While Saladin and Richard the Lionheart were fighting in the Crusades, King Richard reputedly invited Maimonides to be his own court physician; the latter declined. Maimonides then served Saladin's son, whose demands were a burden on the physician, as suggested in a letter of 1199. By this point, his fame as both physician and theologian-philosopher was widespread.

In the latter role, Maimonides headed the Jewish community in Egypt. His wide learning and religious convictions inspired his first significant work, *Commentary on the Mishnah* (1168), which includes the distilled thirteen central beliefs of Judaism, as well as his greatest text, the *Mishneh Torah* (1178), a fourteen-volume synthesis of Talmudic and biblical law. Twelve years later, he finished his greatest philosophical work, *Guide for the Perplexed*, which arbitrated between Jewish theological doctrine and Aristotelian philosophical principles. These three texts form his 'trilogy.' Nevertheless, this polymath also wrote books on logic, the commandments, resurrection, commentaries on the Talmud, several epistles, and over six hundred responsa. Given his fame, a number of pseudo-Maimonidean texts were written, some as late as 1783.

His medical work exists in ten texts, all of which were written in Arabic, and frequently translated into Hebrew during the Middle Ages. The first, *Extracts from Galen* [The Art of Cure], was directed at students of medicine, being a selection of quotations verbatim from Galen.

The second, *Commentary on the Aphorisms of Hippocrates*, was generated from a translation of Hippocrates by Hunayn ibn Ishaq (Johannitius, ninth century). It displays some of Maimonides' independence, as he was critical of both Hippocrates and Galen when his own experience led to a different conclusion.

The third text is the fifteen-hundred aphorism collection, *Medical Aphorisms of Moses*. While the sources are all Greek and late Roman, the organization is dizzyingly comprehensive, ranging from anatomy to pathology and diagnosis, systemic diseases and therapies, regimen and medical curiosities. The *Aphorisms* was also translated into Latin during the thirteenth century, and printed in a variety of fifteenth-century and later editions.

The fourth text, *Treatise on Hemorrhoids*, was probably written for a young member of the Sultan's family. The format is that of a regimen directed at an individual with a specific condition; the regimenal recommendations include foods to be sought or avoided as well as viable pharmaceutical and physical therapies. As a good medieval physician, Maimonides endorsed interventions in lifestyle; surgery and phlebotomy were a last resort.

The fifth is *Treatise on Sexual Intercourse*, a text also written for one of Saladin's promiscuous young relatives, Sultan al-Muzaffar Omar Ibn Nur ad-Din. The recommendations include diets and drugs with both aphrodisiac and antiaphrodisiac effects. A spurious longer version of this comparatively short text developed a life of its own some years later. In the original regimen as in others, Maimonides recommended moderation.

The sixth is *Treatise on Asthma*, which discusses in thirteen chapters how a patient with severe respiratory complaints can mitigate their effects through diet, drugs, and climatic sensitivity. This particular patient's symptoms were so severe as to provoke headaches, which impaired his ability to wear a turban. Nevertheless, the last chapter's recommendations were intentionally very general for the promotion of health in any patient.

The seventh is *Treatise on Poisons and Their Antidotes*. Given its subject, *Poisons* was popular among both medieval readers and modern ones; the latter extol its 'scientific and modern' approach toward the subject. Written at the behest of Vizier al-Fadil for the poisoned layman wishing assistance before a physician is available, Maimonides used the text as a vehicle to praise its patron's accomplishments, while endorsing two general antidotes, theriac and the electuary of Mithridates.

The eighth is a *Regimen of Health* (written in 1198). This text represents a four-chapter response to the mood swings of Saladin's son and successor. The third chapter in particular highlights Maimonides' 'healthy mind in a healthy body' philosophy. Later authors have found in its precepts a harbinger of psychosomatic medicine. The regimenal prescriptions are largely Hippocratic and Galenic and concentrate on the six nonnaturals for intervention. Given its generalizability, the text was popular in both the medieval and modern eras.

The ninth is *Discourse on the Explanation of Fits*, written about 1200 for Sultan al-Malik al-Afdal. Some later interpreters have considered it the so-called 'fifth chapter' of the *Regimen of Health*. The text confirms the recommendations of the Sultan's other physicians and closes with an hourly list of regimenal prescriptions.

The tenth is *Glossary of Drug Names*, consisting of a 405-paragraph long pharmacopoeia with drugs listed in Arabic, Berber, Greek, Persian, Spanish, and Syrian. The text was rediscovered in the early twentieth century and does not have as extensive a premodern influence.

The *Medical Aphorisms* are indicative of Maimonides' range of medical thought, which was accompanied by an acute clinical eye as well. His descriptions of diabetes suggest a thoughtful geographic epidemiology, based on his own observations; Maimonides concluded that the condition is more common in the warmer climes. He accurately described the signs and symptoms of pneumonia, hepatitis, digital clubbing in pulmonary disease, stroke, and the signs of emphysema. While he cogently cited previous authors, he was not shy to advance his own experience, both diagnostically and therapeutically. His *Treatise on Hemorrhoids* endorsed medical intervention over surgical because of the etiologic consequences of treating a medical condition with surgery. His affinity for medical regimen induced him to include some of his broader lifestyle rules in *Mishneh Torah* and *Code of Jewish Law*.

Overall, despite some modern critics who find his theological/philosophical works more original, Maimonides' medical texts are distinctive for their synthesis, concision, and systematic structure and lucidity. During the Middle Ages, *Medical Aphorisms*, *Poisons*, and *Regimen of Health* were particularly influential. Many medieval and modern authors have agreed with Sir William Osler's identification of Maimonides as the 'Prince of Physicians'.

Bibliography

Primary: Rosner, Fred, 1963–1995. *Maimonides' Medical Writings* vols. 1–7 (Haifa); Rosner, Fred, and Süssman Muntner, 1969. *The Medical Writings of Moses Maimonides. Treatise on Hemorrhoids and Maimonides' Answers to Queries* (Philadelphia); Bos, Gerrit, 2002. *Maimonides On Asthma: A Parallel Arabic-English Edition* (Provo, UT).

Secondary: Rosner, Fred, and Samuel S. Kottek, eds., 1993. *Moses Maimonides. Physician, Scientist and Philosopher* (Northvale, NJ); Rosner, Fred, 1980. 'Maimonides, the Physician: A Bibliography.' *Clio Medica* 15: 75–79.

Fred Rosner

AL-MAJŪSĪ, ʿALĪ B. AL-ʿABBĀS (aka HALY ABBAS)

(b. al-Ahwāz, Iran, first quarter of the tenth century; d. Shiraz, Iran?, *c.* 994), *medicine*.

ʿAlī ibn al-ʿAbbās al-Majūsī was probably born in Ahwāz, near the Persian city of Shiraz, to which he is supposed to have moved at an early date. He studied medicine under the physician of that city Abū Māhir Mūsa b. Yūsuf b. Sayyār, of whom he kept a respectful memory. No more details of his life have come down to us, and even the place and date of his death are unknown. Al-Majūsī was an influential medical author in the Western tradition, in which he was known as Haly Abbas. The nickname 'al-Majūsī', meaning 'the Magician', has always been understood as a reference to the Zoroastrian religion of his ancestors. Although the family's conversion to Islam must have taken place at least in the generation of the author's grandfather, the fact that he does not mention the prophet Muḥammad in the introduction of his work, and that his argument for the excellence of medicine does not refer to the Koran, suggests that he lacked Muslim zeal.

As a physician, he called himself *al-mutaṭabbib*, which may indicate that he was not only a medical author, but also a practitioner. He is said to have been particularly successful in the treatment of fevers. He left just one work, entitled *Kitāb Kāmil al-ṣināʿa al-ṭibbiya* [The Complete Book of the Medical Art], also known as *Kitāb al-Malikī* [The Royal Book] because it was dedicated to the Buwayhid king ʿAḍūḍ al-Dawla (d. 983). In the introduction of this manual, he gave a detailed account of medical works available in his time. Being particularly critical toward his predecessor al-Rāzī for the lack of organization of the voluminous *Kitāb al-Hāwī* as much as for the conciseness of the *K. al-Manṣūrī*, al-Majūsī's aim was to produce an improved medical compendium presenting comprehensive coverage of the topic. According to the author's intention, the work contains everything a physician should know, from the four elements to anatomy and physiology, pathology, diagnosis, therapy by medicines, and surgery. This work, then, constituted the best synthesis of medical science of its time because of its careful organization and its reasonable proportions. Its balanced division of theory and practice was a feature that established a common format in later medieval medical texts. Recognized as a masterpiece, it was adopted as the chief textbook of medicine for students until, some hundreds of years later, it was overshadowed by Ibn Sīnā's *Qānūn*. Under the title *Pantegni*, its translation became highly regarded in Europe less than one century after, through the free adaptation made by the physician and translator Constantine the African (*c.* 1010–87), who had been born in Carthage and settled in Italy as a monk of the abbey of Monte Cassino, and who did not credit the actual author. Stephanus of Antioch made a second, more faithful translation in 1127 under the title *Liber Regius* (Venice, 1492), which acknowledged the true authorship. Along with other medieval Islamic medical treatises such as Avicenna's *Canon* (Ibn Sīnā's *Qānūn*), al-Majūsī's medical treatise was incorporated into the medical curriculum of European universities.

Bibliography

Primary: Koning, P. de, 1903. *Trois traités d'anatomie arabe* (Leiden) pp. 90–427 (French translation of the anatomical section of the *Kāmil al-ṣinā*); 1996. *Kitāb Kāmil al-ṣinā 'a al-ṭibbiya* 2 vols. (Frankfurt am Main).

Secondary: 1996. *'Ali ibn al-'Abbās al-Majūsī (4th/10th cent.): Texts and Studies*, collected and reprinted by Sezgin, F. (Frankfurt am Main); Burnett, C., and D. Jacquart, eds. 1994. *Constantine the African and 'Alī ibn al-'Abbās al-Magūsī: The Pantegni and Related Texts* (Leiden); Richter-Bernburg, L., 1982–2003. [*s.v.* 'Ali b. 'Abbās al-Majūsī] in Yarshater, Ehsan, ed. *Encyclopaedia Iranica* 11 vols. (London and Costa Mesa) vol. I, pp. 837–838; *DSB*.

Cristina Álvarez Millán

MALPIGHI, MARCELLO (b. Crevalcore, Bologna, Italy, baptized 10 March 1628; d. Rome, Italy, 29 November 1694), *medicine, microscopy, comparative anatomy, embryology.*

Malpighi was the son of Marcantonio Malpighi and Maria Cremonini. He enrolled at the University of Bologna in 1646, where he was taught by the Peripatetic philosopher Francesco Natali, attending in particular the lessons on Aristotle's *De generatione et corruptione*. He also attended courses on astronomy and mathematics. Natali, whom Malpighi always held in great esteem and affection, persuaded him to study medicine. At first he was pupil of Bartolomeo Massari, and then of Andrea Mariani (d. 1661). He was among the nine students including Carlo Fracassati (*c.* 1630–72) allowed to attend the dissections and vivisections Massari conducted in his own house. His active participation in this group, which was decidedly modern and antitraditionalist, placed him somewhat at odds with the more conservative members of the University, and was one of the reasons for his conflict with the Sbaraglia family, which was later exacerbated by other events.

On 26 April 1653 Malpighi graduated in medicine and philosophy. Just three years later, in February 1656, the senate of Bologna nominated him lecturer in logic at the university, a post he had been denied in previous years because he was not a native of Bologna. However, towards the end of the same year the Grand Duke of Tuscany, Ferdinand II, called him to the chair of theoretical medicine at the University of Pisa. The three years he spent in Pisa were fundamental to the formation of Malpighi's science. Influenced by Giovanni Alfonso Borelli (1608–79), professor of mathematics in the same university, Malpighi turned from Peripateticism to a 'free and Democritean philosophy'. He also participated, together with Claude Aubry (Claudius Auberius), the Lorraine anatomist who had also been invited to Pisa, in animal dissections in Borelli's home laboratory and, through Borelli, entered the scientific orbit of Galileo Galilei's school, which was at that time best represented in Tuscany, at the Accademia del Cimento (1657–67). It was in Borelli's home laboratory at Pisa, in 1657, that Malpighi and Aubry discovered two mechanically significant anatomic structures, without the help of a microscope, by employing 'artful and subtle' anatomy, e.g., boiling, soaking, and laceration to separate the parts and aid their examination. Malpighi discovered the spiral fibers of the heart by cooking and maceration, whereas Aubry revealed the seminiferous tubules in the testicle of a wild boar by cooking it and by studying the organ in the mating season, when it is at the peak of its performance and therefore of greater turgidity. In this case Aubry appealed to the so-called 'microscope of nature', claiming that the boar's large testicle corresponded to a magnified human testicle: Malpighi often used this 'method' himself. 'Artful and subtle' anatomy enjoyed its full development after the introduction of optical magnification—i.e., of the microscope—into biological research, and Malpighi is considered the founder of microscopic anatomy because of his systematic association of the microscope with anatomical techniques.

In 1659, however, at the termination of his three-year contract for teaching theoretical medicine, Malpighi, who abhorred Pisa's climate, chose to return to Bologna as extraordinary lecturer in theoretical medicine. Toward the end of 1660 he assumed the ordinary lectureship at the university in practical medicine. Meanwhile, with Carlo Fracassati, he continued dissecting and vivisecting and using the microscope, made some fundamental discoveries about the lungs, which he immediately communicated to Borelli in his two letters *De pulmonibus observationes anatomicae* and *De pulmonibus epistola altera* (1661). Unfortunately the hostility of the Bolognese academic environment, with its particularly influential and pugnacious Galenists, affected Malpighi. His situation deteriorated further after his brother Bartolomeo killed Tommaso Sbaraglia during a street brawl. Malpighi sought a position away from Bologna, and thanks to the help of Borelli managed to obtain a chair in Messina (where Borelli had also taught).

In 1662 Malpighi became the first professor of ordinary medicine at the University of Messina and began teaching on 14 November 1662. In the four years he spent at Messina (1662–66), Malpighi continued his research on fundamental structures, sometimes using marine animals from the Strait of Messina.

Four years later he returned once more to Bologna to lecture in practical medicine. On 21 February 1667 he married Francesca Massari, the sister of his former teacher. At the end of 1667 Malpighi began his association with the Royal Society of London, which requested a scientific correspondence with him in a letter dated 28 December 1667; the Society subsequently supervised the printing of all his later works. The Royal Society showed interest in his studies on silkworms and the anatomy of plants, and as early as 1669 Malpighi was able to send his manuscript *De bombyce* to the Royal Society, which immediately had it printed and made him an honorary member. After dealing ingeniously with embryological questions in his *De formatione pulli in ovo* (1673), between 1673 and 1678 Malpighi turned his interests to the anatomy and histology of plants. Between 1667 and 1668 Malpighi broke off his epistolary relationship with his old friend and teacher Borelli. The motives for this are not clear; he may have been upset because Borelli disagreed with him over certain scientific questions. Borelli, however, greatly regretted this and did everything he could to restore their friendship, but in vain.

In 1691 Antonio Pignatelli was elected Pope Innocent XII. Malpighi had cured him while he had been a cardinal legate in Bologna, and now when the new pope summoned him to Rome as papal archiater and personal physician, Malpighi accepted immediately. He transferred to the papal court where was able to continue his research, assisted by his pupil Giorgio Baglivi (1668–1707). He died there, in his apartments in the Quirinal Palace.

De pulmonibus

Malpighi's first—and fundamental—work was the *De pulmonibus*, two short letters that were sent to Borelli in Pisa and published in Bologna in 1661. Traditionally the lungs were considered as fleshy viscera, endowed with a sanguine nature and hot-humid temperament. When Malpighi examined them under a microscope, he found instead an aggregate of membranous alveoli (Malpighi's vesicles) opening into the ultimate tracheobronchial ramifications and surrounded by a capillary network. He had discovered the communication, until then sought for in vain, between arteries and veins. These observations were of fundamental importance, both because for the first time the pulmonary parenchyma (and subsequently other parenchymas) could be seen to have a structure, and because the observation of the capillaries confirmed the theory of the circulation of the blood and ensured its general acceptance.

In *De pulmonibus* Malpighi demonstrated his complete mastery of the methods of microscopic anatomy. He used instruments of different magnifying powers and made observations with both reflected and transmitted light. In the preparation of specimens he employed various anatomical techniques, such as drying, boiling, and insufflation of the tracheobronchial tree or of systems of blood vessels; vascular perfusion; and deaeration by crushing, corrosion, or a combination of these methods. He also used the 'microscope of nature' and chose to examine the frog, believing that in that way he could visualize, with a relatively small magnification, a feature as minute as the capillary: in fact, the capillary network itself is so fine in mammals that Malpighi was never able to observe it with the microscopes available to him. He acutely remarked that nature was accustomed 'to undertake its great works only after a series of attempts at lower levels, and to outline in imperfect animals the plan of perfect animals' (*De pulmonibus*, 1661).

Malpighi saw the structure of the lung as air cells surrounded by a network of blood vessels. He interpreted this structure as a well-devised mechanism to ensure the mixing of chyle particles with blood particles, i.e., for the conversion of chyle to blood (then called hematosis), a function that the Galenists attributed to the liver. In 1647 Jean Pecquet (1622–74) had shown that the chyle, instead of being conveyed to the liver, was introduced into the blood in the superior vena cava, at a point shortly before that vessel reached the heart, and was then distributed to the lungs through the pulmonary artery.

Neurology

The results of the research Malpighi conducted during the four years at Messina were published in a series of works in 1665–66, for the main part dedicated to three important topics: neurology (nerves), adenology (glands), and hematology (blood). With his two closely related booklets *De lingua* (1665) and *De externo tactus organo* (1665), Malpighi also provided an anatomic basis for mechanistic esthesiology. In his anatomical letter *De lingua* he reported the separation of two layers from the surface of the tongue, the horny layer and the reticular (or mucous) layer now named after him, thus revealing the papillary body in which he distinguished the three orders of papillae, functioning as gustatory receptors. He supposed that these papillae were reached through pores in the reticular layer and thereby stimulated by sapid particles dissolved in the saliva, the organic liquid whose significance had been recognized a few years earlier by Niels Stensen (aka Nicholas Steno, 1638–86). One can clearly recognize the influence of Galileo, who suggested in *Il saggiatore* (1623) that the very small taste particles, when 'placed on the upper surface of the tongue and, mixed with its moisture, penetrate it and carry the tastes, pleasant or otherwise, according to the differences in the touching of the different shapes of these tiny corpuscles, and according to whether they are few or many, faster or slower'. Malpighi discovered analogous structures in the skin. In *De externo tactus organo* he described the cutaneous (or tactile) papillae, i.e., the tactile receptors, which he understood to be—like the lingual papillae—the peripheral endings of nerves.

Malpighi's discovery of sensory receptors formed part of his wider neuroanatomical research. The treatise *De cerebro*, published in 1665 with *De lingua*, was mainly concerned with the white substance of the central nervous system, which he found to be composed of the same fibers forming nerves. Malpighi conceived these fibers as long, fine channels filled with a liquid—the nervous fluid—which was secreted by the cortical gray matter, or, more precisely, by the cortical glands. In the later treatise *De cerebri cortice* (1666) he believed he had managed to demonstrate these glands, but his results were in fact an artifact. However, with his findings, whether correct or incorrect, Malpighi managed to construct a nervous mechanism comprising the entire neural course from the brain's cortex to the nerves' peripheral endings: a sort of 'neuron', in which transmission of the nervous impulse could be compared to transmission of a mechanical impulse through a liquid mass in accordance with Pascal's principle.

Glands, or 'Secretion Machines'

During his time in Messina, Malpighi also conducted research on the structure of another mechanism fundamental to iatromechanical atomism: the gland, or 'secretion machine'. The function of the secretion machine was to select specific particles of blood brought by an afferent artery, to separate them from others flowing back through an efferent vein, and to introduce them, as an independent liquid, into an excretory duct. The model of the secretion machine was a sieve, which offered an *a priori* explanation of the operation of the secreting mechanism by postulating a proportionality of form and dimension between the pores and the particles to be separated.

In *De externo tactus organo* Malpighi presented his scheme of the elementary gland. His secreting mechanism was based on a follicle at the center that on the one hand was continued into the secretary tubule, and on the other hand was surrounded by the ultimate ramifications of the arteries, veins, and nerves. He attributed this elementary glandular structure to the four organs (liver, cerebral cortex, kidneys, and spleen) described in the four treatises (*De hepate, De cerebri cortice, De renibus,* and *De liene*) constituting his *De viscerum structura* (1666). Of the four treatises, the one most important for the subtlety of its research and the importance of its findings was the *De renibus*, in which he described the renal corpuscles (Malpighi's corpuscles) and the renal pyramids constituting the kidney's medullary substance (Malpighi's pyramids). The splenic follicles, i.e., the Malpighian nodules visible to the naked eye inside the spleen, were described in the *De liene*.

More than twenty years later Malpighi further developed his theory of glandular structure in the epistolary dissertation *De structura glandularum conglobatarum consimiliumque partium*, dated June 1688 and published in London the following year. The distinction between 'conglobate' glands (e.g., lymph nodes) and 'conglomerate' glands (whose structure is manifestly globular, such as the salivary glands and the pancreas) was made in 1663 by Franciscus dele Boë (or Sylvius, 1614–72). Less than half of the treatise was devoted to 'conglobate' glands; for the rest, Malpighi reported additional observations on glands that were already known and considerably expanded his earlier work on the secretory mechanism.

Hematology

Malpighi's *De polypo cordis* concerned hematology and appeared in 1666 as an appendix to *De viscerum structura*. So-called 'heart polyps' had been observed with a certain frequency in the cardiac cavities and large blood vessels, especially in patients who had died from severe cardiorespiratory insufficiency. Previous authors had explained such polyps in various ways, even invoking traditional humoral theory. Malpighi instead claimed that the polyps resulted from an intravital process of coagulation, which had as its model the coagulation of blood extracted from the organism. The study of coagulum allowed Malpighi to demonstrate that the 'phlogistic crust' was, despite its whitish color, derived from the whole blood. He found that the coagulum, after repeated washings, 'from being intensely red and black becomes white, while the water is reddened by the extracted particles of color'. Microscopical examination of a clot of coagulum also enabled Malpighi to observe, as separate components, the interlacing white fibers arising from the conglutination of much smaller but similarly shaped filaments (analogous to what occurs in the crystallization of salts) and the red fluid that filled the interstices of these fiber meshes. Seen under the microscope, this red fluid was composed of a host of red 'atoms', thus confirming the discovery of the red corpuscles, which he had already observed in Messina and reported in *De omento* (1665). In fact, in 1663, while studying the hedgehog's mesentery under the microscope, he had noticed some *globuli rubescentes* flowing through a blood vessel, which he initially interpreted as globules of fat, but in 1664, upon repeating the observation on a newborn kitten's mesentery, he realized that these globules were part of the blood.

Embryology and Development

In *De polypo cordis* Malpighi also stressed the methodological importance of studying simple animals in order to understand more complex ones. *De bombyce* (1669), on the silkworm, and later embryological and botanical works edited by the Royal Society in the 1670s were part of this program. In *De bombyce* Malpighi carefully described each of the three stages—larva, chrysalis, and moth—through which the silkworm passed during development; moreover, he dealt with some of the specific structures of silkworms, including air ducts (tracheae) and the blood duct, which has a number of pulsating centers (corcula).

Malpighi brought a fine structural content to embryology—ultimately a valuable aid to illustrating the morphology of the adult—in *De formatione pulli in ovo* (1673) and *Appendix repetitas auctasque de ovo incubato observationes continens* (1675). After a careful re-examination of his embryological texts and the original plates Malpighi drew to illustrate his works on chick development, Howard Adelmann (1966) defended Malpighi against the charge of preformationism—the view of Cole and Needham. According to Malpighi, the fetus and its rudiments were not pre-existing at fecundation, but formed after fecundation. Malpighi's chief embryological discoveries in this work were the vascular area embraced by the terminal sinus, the cardiac tube and its segmentation, aortic arches, somites, neural folds and tube, cerebral and optic vesicles, protoliver, glands of the prestomach, and feather follicles.

Plant Anatomy and Pathology

Malpighi also studied plants with extraordinary success. *Anatome plantarum*, which appeared in London in two parts (1675 and 1679), earned him acclaim (along with Nehemiah Grew) for founding the microscopic study of plant anatomy. He found that plants also have a mechanical structure: he described their ducts (some of which he compared to the tracheae of insects) and their basic 'cellular' structure (an aggregate of 'utricles'), which Hooke had already described (as 'cellulae') in the *Micrographia* of 1665.

Malpighi also made considerable contributions to vegetable pathology, particularly in his study of plant galls, which he described as a morbid alteration of the structure of the infested plant. Antonio Vallisneri (1661–1730) later showed (1700) that the insect larvae in galls, whose presence had been demonstrated by Malpighi, emerged from eggs deposited by insects on the plants, refuting the claims for spontaneous generation.

Legacy

In *De polypo cordis* and subsequent treatises Malpighi made explicit reference to pathological material obtained during autopsies, recognizing the importance of local lesions. He gathered an extensive collection of anatomico-medical histories, the result of autopsies carried out 'to investigate the causes and effects of the disease'. In his medical anatomy (or practical anatomy, as it was then called), in his emphasis on those aspects of anatomy proper to medical practice, and above all, in his use of anatomico-clinical parallelism, Malpighi shaped the work of at least two generations of researchers. His pupils included Ippolito Francesco Albertini (1662–1738) and Antonio Valsalva (1666–1723), and the *De sedibus et causis morborum per anatomen indagatis* of their pupil, Giovanni Battista

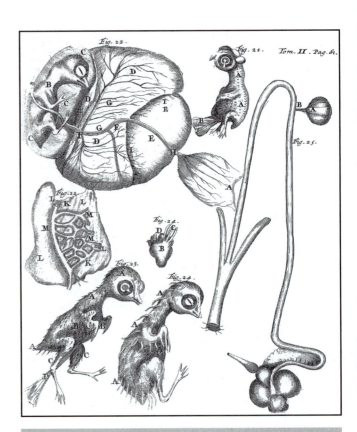

Development of the chick embryo. Engraving from *De formatione pulli in ovo* (*Opera omnia*), London, 1687. Rare Books, Wellcome Library, London.

Morgagni (1682–1771), represents one of the most important developments of Malpighi's work.

Finally, Malpighi wrote an important methodological work, his *Risposta* to *De recentiorum medicorum studio* (1689) of Giovanni Girolamo Sbaraglia (1641–1710), in which he supported rational medicine against the empiricists. Rational medicine was also the basis for his many *Consultationes*, which attest to the medical practice that he carried out concurrently with his biological researches.

Bibliography

Primary: 1686–87. *Opera omnia* 2 vols. (London) (repr. Leiden, 1687); 1661. *De pulmonibus observationes anatomicae* (Bologna) and *De pulmonibus epistola altera* (Bologna) (English trans. Young, James, 1929–30. *Proceedings of the Royal Society of Medicine Section of the History of Medicine* 23: 1–11); 1665. *Epistolae anatomicae de cerebro, ac lingua . . . quibus anonymi accessit exercitatio de omento, pinguedine, et adiposis ductibus* (Bologna); 1665. *De externo tactus organo anatomica observatio* (Naples); 1666. *De viscerum structura exercitatio anatomica . . . accedit dissertatio . . . de polypo cordis* (Bologna); 1669. *Dissertatio epistolica de bombyce* (London); 1673. *Dissertatio epistolica de formatione pulli in ovo* (London); 1675. *Anatomes plantarum pars prima. Cui subjungitur appendix iteratas et auctas de ovo incubato observationes continens* (London); 1679. *Anatomes plantarum pars altera* (London); 1684. 'Dissertatio epistolica varii argumenti' [addressed to Jacob Spon]. *Philosophical Transactions of the Royal Society of London* 14: 601–608, 630–636; 1689. *De structura glandularum conglobatarum consimiliumque partium epistola* (London); 1697. *Opera posthuma* (London) (repr. Amsterdam, 1698); 1713. *Consultationum medicinalium centuria prima* (Padua); 1747. *Consultationum medicarum nonnullarumque dissertationum collectio* (Venice); 1967. (Belloni, Luigi, ed.) *Opere scelte* (Turin).

Secondary: Adelmann, Howard B., 1966. *Marcello Malpighi and the Evolution of Embryology* 5 vols. (Ithaca, NY); *DSB*.

Giuseppe Ongaro

MANASE, DŌSAN

(b. Kyoto, Japan, 23 October 1507; d. Kyoto, 23 February 1594), *Chinese-Japanese medicine, Li-Zhu (Jp. Ri-Shu) medicine, diagnostics, pulse.*

Manase Dōsan was born in Kyoto at a time when the city was the capital for both the Ashikaga shogun and the emperor. His father belonged to the Hattori clan and his mother to the Megata, but his father died the day after he was born and his mother died while he was still a small child. He then lived with his aunt and older sister until, at age ten, he entered a Buddhist temple near Kyoto. Three years later, he entered Shōkokuji, the renowned Rinzai Zen temple in Kyoto. However he later decided not to become a Buddhist priest and instead started the serious pursuit of poetry, and at age twenty-two he journeyed to eastern Japan to study at the Ashikaga School, contemporary Japan's leading center for the study of Confucian thought.

Medical Studies

While there, two years later in 1531, he met Tashiro Sanki (1465-1544?), a physician who had studied for twelve years in China and returned to Japan to profess the ideas of the Li-Zhu (Jp. Ri-Shu) school of medicine. Tashiro had originally been from the region of eastern Japan close to the Ashikaga school, and he returned there after finishing his studies in China. Although he was one of the first in Japan to practice the Li-Zhu school, Tashiro would have remained an obscure rural physician if Manase had not become his student.

The Li-Zhu school was based on the ideas of Li Gao (aka Li Dongyuan) (Jp., Ri Tōen; 1180–1251) and Zhu Zhen-heng (aka Zhu Danxi) (Jp. Shu Tankei; 1282–1358). Li had been active during the late Chin and early Yuan dynasties, and Zhu had built on his ideas while developing new ideas and practices of his own. Both Li and Zhu had emphasized the balance of Yin and Yang energies in their theories of pathology and therapy, and based many of their ideas on their interpretations of the early Chinese classics, the *Suwen* and *Nanjing*.

Li believed that all diseases were caused by an excess of delight (a Yang energy) or anger (a Yin energy), a loss of moderation in food or drink, inappropriate cold or humidity, or an excess of work. By focusing on these causes, he established an etiological theory that distinguished internal and external causes. External causes included exposure to cold, winds, heat, and humidity; internal conditions included imbalances of food and drink. Among the internal organs, Li considered the spleen to be the center of Yin and the stomach to be the center of Yang; when the qi (Jp. ki, 'vital energy') in these two organs fell out of balance, pathological symptoms then manifested themselves in other parts of the body. Li's therapeutic methods emphasized medicinal and dietary supplements with the aim of re-establishing the balance between the Yin and Yang forms of qi.

Zhu Danxi studied medicine with a physician who had studied under Li Gao. Zhu extended Li's medical ideas with a theory that interpreted disease as the excess of Yang and an insufficiency of Yin. With this, he combined previous ideas of external and internal harms to establish what became the Chinese medical mainstream for centuries. Indeed, it was approximately one-hundred and fifty years after Zhu's death that Tashiro Sanki studied medicine in China, but what he learned there was based on the original texts of Li and Zhu, as well as later interpretations.

Kyoto

Manase studied under Tashiro until the death of the latter, after which he returned to Kyoto. Manase started his own practice there in 1545 and achieved great fame after successfully treating the ruling shogun, Ashikaga Yoshiteru (1536–65). During the following years he treated a large number of the most important warlords of the time, and for over twenty years ran his own school of medicine, which was called the Keitekiin.

At this time, medical practice in Japan was socially divided in ways similar to contemporary European practices. Practitioners of internal medicine were held in the highest prestige. The most highly regarded were members of a small number of families who, through their inherited positions as court physicians, attended the emperor and other members of the imperial court in Kyoto. Just below them in status were physicians who attended the shogun and other powerful warlords. Other internists could be found in urban areas, and could be hired by anybody with sufficient funds. However, even those who held high-ranking inherited positions faced competition. In premodern Japan, medicine was one of the few professions whereby a person with sufficient intelligence and means could become socially mobile: physicians who could cure difficult cases were always in demand. From the sixteenth century onward, it was expected that a trained internist would be fluent in the Confucian classics and in the Song dynasty (960–1279) interpretations of those classics; possession of intellectual abilities reinforced the possibility of social mobility through medicine. Before this time, Buddhist priests often acted as physicians, and as a consequence medical ideas before the sixteenth century tended to be based on a combination of Buddhist thought and Chinese medical texts.

In addition to practitioners of internal medicine, there were specialists in surgery, gynecology and obstetrics, ophthalmology, and dentistry. While many practitioners of these specializations received some degree of training, generally they were not expected to be grounded in Confucianism in the way that was expected of an internist. In addition, the higher social standing of well-trained internists was based on the fact that they were familiar with the theory and, to some degree, the practices of other specializations.

At the Keitekiin, where Manase is said to have taught over 800 students, the training of internists in a broad range of Chinese Confucian and medical texts became institutionalized. Although no clear record of the program of study remains, it was necessary to have a broad intellectual foundation in order to be conversant with the medical texts that Manase himself wrote. In addition to emphasizing the theories and practices of the Li-Zhu school, he also used an eclectic selection of Chinese works that included the *Shanghanlun* (Jp. *Shōkanron*) by Zhang Zhongjing (Jp. Chō Chūkei; 196–220), a work that became central to later schools of Japanese medicine.

Manase's Approach to Medical Practice

Manase's approach to medical practice was most clearly outlined in a list of fifty-seven rules for practitioners. While many of these rules clearly focused on diagnostic and therapeutic criteria, others dealt with ethical concerns. First on the list was a simple statement of 'compassion and benevolence', two of the guiding principles of Confucian ethics that the physician should keep in mind. The second clearly established his diagnostic procedure, which started with pulse diagnosis and the establishment of the disease name. Pulse diagnosis was a highly developed tactile analysis of the qualities of the pulse; it allowed the physician to assess the patient's condition and whether the case was critical. However, the third rule required the physician to discern whether the patient was indeed ready to put complete faith in the physician or, as a later rule stated, whether the patient also would be putting their faith in prognosticators. Unless the patient placed complete faith in the physician, there was no reason to attempt proper treatment.

One key for reaching a diagnosis, devising a therapeutic regimen, and establishing a prognosis was a four-step procedure of questioning the patient and making visual, aural, and tactile observations. Other important criteria that the physician had to keep in mind included the course of the illness to that point; the patient's sex, age, weight, and diet; and if the patient were a woman, it was necessary to consider the possibility of pregnancy, which was important in determining the illness, its causes, and treatment. All of these observations were vital to understanding the balance of positive and negative qi in the patient, which then determined the course of therapy. Treatments included infusions, powders, and pills, as well as acupuncture and moxibustion. During the course of treatment, it was important for the physician to monitor for efficacy. These rules were spelled out on a piece of paper that a physician trained in the Manase school could use as a checklist when visiting patients.

Manase was important to Japanese medical history not only as a medical educator, but also as an author of medical texts. His most important text, one that remained central to internal medicine in Japan for over two centuries, was the *Keitekishū*, a work in eight volumes that borrowed heavily from various Chinese medical works. It examined topics in nomenclature and nosology, etiology, pulse diagnosis, differential diagnosis, prognosis, and therapy for a broad range of illnesses. Manase also wrote important texts on gynecology and obstetrics, pharmaceuticals, acupuncture and moxibustion, and regimens for health maintenance (Ch. *yangsheng*, Jp. *yōjō*).

Manase's Legacy

Manase's patients included not only the leading warlords of the day, but also some of the Jesuit priests who were proselytizing Catholicism in Japan during the late sixteenth century. According to the Portuguese Jesuit Louis Frois (1532–97), Manase himself converted to Catholicism and in doing so became more influential than the ruling military hegemon, Toyotomi Hideyoshi (1537–98). Frois described Manase as a polymath, conversant not only in the Chinese classics but also in the main works of Buddhism. And like many other leading intellectuals as well as the politically important of his day, he also was renowned as a master of the tea ceremony.

Manase had only one son, who died at an early age. In order to continue the Manase line, he then adopted his nephew and named him Manase Gensaku (1549–1631). He proved highly able and received permission to attend the emperor in 1581. The list of Gensaku's patients is even more illustrious than that of his adoptive father, and included two emperors, Ōgimachi (1517–93) and Goyōzei (1571–1617), the hegemon Toyotomi Hideyoshi and his son, Toyotomi Hidetsugu (1568–95), and the second Tokugawa shogun, Tokugawa Hidetada (1579–1632). At the order of the emperor, Gensaku assumed his father's name and became the second-generation Dōsan. Gensaku also had an unintended but pervasive influence on Japanese culture by reviving the custom of drinking sake laced with medicinal herbs (*otoso*) on New Year's Day; it was said to prevent illness throughout the year. By urging the Tokugawa shogun to do this, the custom quickly became popular throughout the country.

Gensaku built on his adoptive father's successes in education and medical theory. He continued operation of Keitekiin, the school that Dōsan had established, and wrote widely used texts on internal medicine, pharmaceuticals, and health maintenance. The style of medicine that he practiced, called the Goseiha (literally the 'Later Generation School') remained influential until the nineteenth century, and continues to influence Chinese-style medicine (Kanpō) in Japan to the present.

Although the medical ideas and practices advocated by the Goseiha were highly influential, they did not monopolize contemporary medicine. One competing set of ideas was advanced by the extraordinarily long-lived Nagata Tokuhon (1513–1630). Nagata was renowned for the relative simplicity of his medical thought as well as for his eccentric behavior. He believed that illness arose when food and drink stagnated in the body and created poisons; this occurred because wind and cold entered the body and caused internal maladies. The theoretical basis for Nagata's ideas depended solely on the *Shanghanlun*, and he derided Goseiha ideas and practices. Nagata's method of practicing medicine was also in marked contrast to that of Goseiha physicians. Where the Manase family had achieved fame and fortune in the capital city of Kyoto and its imperial court, Nagata was based in what is now Yamanashi prefecture and rode around the country on the back of an ox, selling his medicine for eighteen copper pieces.

The Manase school systematized Japanese medicine and became a foil against which later medical theorists would react. In this way Manase Dōsan was the father of early modern medical practice in Japan and an intellectual giant of his day. During the second half of the sixteenth century, the same years during which a unified, early modern Japanese state started to replace the previous network of autonomous feudal domains, Manase Dōsan did more than any previous physician to create a systematic Japanese approach to medical thought and practice. Manase based his approach on Chinese ideas and practices, which offset the generally empirical methods that had dominated Japanese medicine until then.

Bibliography

Primary: 1995. *Manase Dōsan zenshū* [Collected Works of Manase Dōsan] (Osaka); 1995. *Keitekishū* (Kyoto).

Secondary: Yakazu, Dōmei, 1982. *Kinsei Kanpō igakushi* [Kanpō Medicine in Early Modern Japan] (Kyoto); Fujikawa, Yū, 1972. *Nihon igaku shi* [Medical History of Japan] (Tokyo).

William Johnston

MANASSEIN, VIACHESLAV AVKSENT'EVICH (b. Verkhnie Devlezeri, Kazan province, Russia, 3 March 1841; d. St Petersburg, Russia, 13 February 1901), *therapeutics*.

Manassein was the ninth son of former officer Avksenti Petrovich Manassein and Maria Petrovna Dronova. After finishing at the gymnasium in Kazan, Manassein studied law in St Petersburg (1853–56) under pressure of his father, but eventually left as he wanted to be a physician. His brother Nikolai Manassein would later become Minister of Justice (1887–93). Manassein attended Moscow University (1857–60), Kazan University (1860), and Derpt (now Tartu) University (1861). All of his transfers from one university to another were caused by his persecution for participation in student political activities. He finished his

medical education at the Medical-Surgical Academy, St Petersburg (1864–66). Afterward, he specialized in the clinic of Sergey Petrovich Botkin (1866–69). From 1870–72 he lived in Germany and Austria.

In 1869 Manassein defended his dissertation on the theme 'Materialy dlia voprosa o golodanii' [Materials on the question of starvation]. He then spent time in Vienna, along with his wife, Maria Mikhailovna Korkunova, one of the first Russian women physicians. There he dealt with the problem of fever and researched *Penicillium glaucum* in professor Julius von Wiesner's mycological laboratory at the Vienna Polytechnic Institute, in which he discovered the antibiotic properties of green mold.

As a researcher Manassein was influenced by Botkin's ideas. He proved that the nervous system renders paramount influence on thermoregulation. He also confirmed that the development of illness depends on both physiological and psychic influences. He discovered that the glycogen of the liver sharply diminishes during fever, and sometimes disappears completely. He also demonstrated that organisms develop artificially high temperatures when rotting substances are introduced into them.

From 1872 he worked as a sessional lecturer in the Medical-Surgical Academy, and from 1875 as adjunct professor in the department of diagnostics, general therapy, and pathology, headed by professor Victor Vilibal'dovich Besser. From 1876 to 1892 he was a professor of the department of partial pathology and internal medicine. During this period Manassein's students completed ninety-one dissertations. In 1874 he established a clinical laboratory, and in 1885 bacteriological examinations began to be performed there. He was also a librarian of the Academy (1872–79).

In his therapeutic practice Manassein recommended gymnastics, massage, and treatment by water and electricity. He was very cautious about medication, and considered koumiss (fermented mare's milk) as a means for treating tuberculosis. As a physician Manassein was an ascetic who avoided private practice and criticized money-grubbing physicians. He helped physicians, students, and writers for free and visited prisoners at the Petropavlovsk fortress.

Manassein was the author of twenty-three scholarly works. He translated and published some works of German medical men and wrote scientific reviews in *Voenno-meditsinskii zhurnal* (1874–76). For twenty years (1880–1901) he edited the weekly magazine *Vrach*, which was the most widely-distributed medical periodical in Russia (the circulation was 6,200 in 1900). His second marriage was childless, but his wife Ekaterina Mikhailovna Dostoevskaia, a niece of writer Fyodor Dostoevsky, helped him in his editorial work. He analyzed the development of medical science in Russia and the West in his magazine and discussed moral and everyday aspects of the life of the physician. He popularized the ideas of social medicine and hygiene and harshly criticized medical unorthodoxies, in particular various forms of popular healing and homeopathy, which were popular among the Russian elite. This activity stimulated the development of the medical profession in Russia.

His social activity was very extensive. He directed the Poor Students' Aid Society (1885–99), worked in the Literary Fund (from 1867) and the St Petersburg Writers Union (1897–1901), and often took part in legal processes. He was one of the organizers of the Pirogov Society and an active participant in early meetings; he organized the aid foundations for physicians and their families ('the Manassein ruble'). Manassein popularized the idea of medical education for women and was a supporter of the diffusion of natural sciences among the people. He left 30,000 volumes of his personal library to Tomsk University. Manassein was one of the famous Russians of his time. Some people hated him, whereas others adored him and named him the 'medical conscience' of Russia.

Bibliography

Primary: 1877. *O znachenii psikhicheskikh vlianii* [About the Significance of Psychical Influences] (St Petersburg); 1879. *Lektsii po obshchei terapii* [Lectures of General Therapy] Part 1 (St Petersburg).

Secondary: Arsen'ev, Georgy Il'ich, 1951. *V. A. Manassein* (Moscow); Zhbankov, Dmitry Nikolaevich, 1926. 'Pamiati Viacheslav Avksent'evich Manasseina' *Vrachebnoe delo* 1: 5–12; Berenstam, Bladimir Vil'iamovich, 1911. 'Iz vospominanii o V.A. Manasseine' [From Reminiscences about V. A. Manassein] *Russkii vrach* 7: 217–231.

Dmitry Mikhel

MANDEVILLE, BERNARD (DE)

MANDEVILLE, BERNARD (DE) (b. [baptized] 20 November 1670 in or near Rotterdam, the Netherlands; d. London, England, 19 January 1733), *psychiatry, medical philosophy, political philosophy.*

Bernard was born in Rotterdam as the son of Michael (de) Mandeville, who was a medical doctor, like his own father and grandfather. Bernard first was a student at the Rotterdam Erasmianum and then matriculated at Leiden University in 1685. In Leiden, he presented two disputations: one on animals as Cartesian machines, the other on human metabolism and its disorders. He earned his MD degree in 1691 with the latter. At the age of twenty-five, he was forced to leave his native city because of his political pamphlets. After completing a grand tour through Europe, he settled in London, where he set up medical practice.

Although Mandeville has been considered notoriously difficult to classify, his writings show a remarkable consistency. It is striking to see how his medical training served to connect the philosophical, political, and economic dimensions of his oeuvre. On leaving the Erasmianum, he delivered an oration on the study of medicine. Mandeville stressed the importance of medicine as a discipline, coming directly after philosophy. According to him, it should be based on empirical observation rather than on hypotheses.

Although satirists and comedians may make fun of the profession, he contended that we should think of the practical effects of medicine instead. In his first Leiden disputation—dedicated to, among others, Burchardus de Volder, the Cartesian professor of medicine and mathematics—Mandeville subtly criticized the Cartesian tenet that animals are automatons. In his second Leiden disputation, he developed a critique of the classical theory of digestion as a process driven by heat. Fish constituted a counterexample to that theory, as did the fact that fever reduces the digestive process. Mandeville's alternative theory made digestion dependent on fermentation: during digestion, chyle and the animal spirits penetrate and dissolve the food. Disorders he considered to be the consequence of either too rich or too much food, and excessive drinking would dissolve the ferment.

Mandeville showed a great interest in hypochondria and hysteria. Sources suggest that he was well prepared to study and treat hysterical fixations on the basis of his theories, working with the basic mechanisms of self-deceit and self-love. In *A Treatise on the Hypochondriack and Hysterick Passions*, Mandeville questioned the nature of medical discourse and the authority of the physician, connecting fermentation and digestion theories to mental and social well-being. The book is structured as a dialogue between a patient and his doctor, and is a commentary partly on the medical profession, partly on hypochondria and hysteria. The logic of this work is twofold: on the one hand, it seeks to demonstrate how doctors and pharmacists make their patients ill and on the other hand, it argues that understanding this process may be part of the cure. The patient in the dialogue—the hypochondriac Misomedon—is dissatisfied with the treatment of his doctors. He decides to study medicine himself, whence he loses all faith in the discipline. His opponent—the physician Philopirio, a lover of commonsensical empiricism, modeled on Mandeville himself—agrees that the modern fashion of book writing among physicians was only reproducing the ill-founded hypotheses then floating around. Instead, it would be better if doctors studied men and their social world.

Mandeville firmly believed that a good satire contained more truth than a learned treatise. It was the medium he used to practice both social criticism and medicine. By exposing the conceit of his time, he tried to point the way to a medicine that was both more modest and more effective. In his book on hypochondria and hysteria, Mandeville pronounced the stomach to be the conscience of the body and diet to be the ultimate cure: 'Let your Diet be Nutritious and inoffensive, and your Cookery be simple, natural.'

Bibliography:

Primary: 1685. *De medicina oratio scholastica* (Rotterdam); 1689. *Disputatio philosophica de Brutorum operationibus* (Leiden); 1691. *Disputatio medica inauguralis de chylosi vitiata* (Leiden); 1711. *A*

Treatise of the Hypochondriack and Hysterick Passions (London) (reprinted 1715, and republished with emendations in 1730); 1714. *The Fable of the Bees, or, Private Vices, Publick Benefits* (London).

Secondary: McKee, Francis, 1995. 'Honeyed Words: Bernard Mandeville and Medical Discourse' in Porter, Roy, ed., *Medicine in the Enlightenment* (Amsterdam and Atlanta) pp. 223–254; Clark, George, 1971. 'Bernard Mandeville, MD, and Eighteenth-Century Ethics.' *Bulletin of the History of Medicine* 45: 430–443.

Hans Blom

MANNERHEIM, EVA CHARLOTTA LOVISA SOFIA (b. Helsinki, Finland, 21 December 1863; d. Helsinki, 9 January 1928), *nursing.*

Baroness Sofia (called Sophia) Mannerheim was the firstborn of Count Carl Robert Mannerheim and Hedvig Charlotta Helena von Julin. She was raised on the family estate with six brothers and sisters, one of whom, Carl Gustaf, was president of Finland from 1944–46. In 1881 Mannerheim moved to Stockholm to be trained as a teacher, and afterward she worked as a governess. In 1885 she returned to Finland, where she worked as a bank employee until she married Baron Hjalmar Constantin Linder in 1896. Their ill-fated marriage ended in 1899 and she decided to take up nursing.

Mannerheim made this decision at a time when professional nursing was still in its early stages and worldwide nursing modeled itself on the Nightingale Training School at St Thomas's Hospital in London. In 1899 Mannerheim was admitted to this prestigious school as a probationer. Three years later she returned to Finland, and in 1904 she was appointed matron of Helsinki Surgical Hospital and thereby as leader of the hospital's school of nursing, which offered a program comprising a one-year period of practical training. Within a few years Mannerheim improved the curriculum, and in 1920 she achieved her objective: a preliminary training school followed by a three-year program of education.

Mannerheim's overriding objective was to develop nursing into an autonomous and recognized professional discipline. She advocated this standpoint on a national level as president of the Finnish nurses' association (1905–25), on a Nordic level as cofounder of the Northern Nurses' Federation 1920, and on an international level as president of the International Council of Nurses (ICN) from 1922–25.

The ICN was founded in 1899 by the British suffragist and nurse Ethel Gordon Fenwick, who stated, 'The nursing profession above all things requires organization; nurses, above all other things, require to be united' (Brush, et al., 1999, p. 1). The vision was that the ICN should be a union of national nursing organizations that was led by and represented nurses only, independent of governmental control.

In 1922 Henny Tscherning from Denmark passed on the presidency of ICN to Mannerheim, and at the same meeting an important collaborator, the Danish woman Christiane Reimann, was elected secretary. World War I had caused the ICN to be at a very low point. It was time to pick up the pieces, and that meant reuniting the existing fourteen memberships and recruiting new ones. Mannerheim's policy was to use inclusion rather than exclusion. With this policy she tactfully handled and solved conflicts concerning countries not able to meet ICNs three-year training standard, associations disagreeing with ICN's eligibility criteria and wanting to admit 'less than professional' nurses' associations, and countries with more than one national association. During her presidency eight memberships were added and many countries established educational programs for nurses and created national nursing associations.

An important issue during Mannerheim's presidency was the handling of conflicts between ICN and the League of Red Cross Societies. The two parties differed about who should speak for nursing in the international community, and they disagreed about who could be called a nurse and the standards for schools of nursing. Mannerheim vigorously defended the value of trained over untrained nurses, and she opposed that many countries used the quickly trained Red Cross 'nurses' as qualified nurses. Consequently the League in 1924 appointed an Advisory Board of Nursing Matters, chaired by Mannerheim. On the board's recommendation the League stopped titling women 'Red Cross Nurses' after brief courses of instruction, and they desisted creating nursing associations that were unable to affiliate with the ICN. Due to Mannerheim's competent handling of this dilemma, she ensured the ICN's position in setting worldwide nursing standards.

Mannerheim proved to be the right person to re-establish the ICN after World War I, and managed to strengthen the organization's position as nursing's international voice for standards of education and practice. She was awarded the Florence Nightingale Medal in 1925.

Bibliography

Secondary: Tallberg, Marianne, 2001. 'Sophie Mannerheim' in Birkelund, Regner, ed., *Omsorg, kald og kamp* (Copenhagen) pp. 357–378; Brush, Barbara L., et al., 1999. *Nurses of All Nations* (Philadelphia); Tuulio, Tyyni, 1948. *Friherrinnan Sophie Mannerheim* (Helsingfors); Edelfelt, Berta, 1932. *Sophie Mannerheim. En levnedsteckning* (Stockholm).

Susanne Malchau

MANNING, FREDERICK NORTON (b. Rothersthorpe, Northamptonshire, England, 25 February 1839; d. Sydney, New South Wales, Australia, 18 June 1903), *psychiatry.*

Born into a farming family, the son of John and Eliza (née Norton), Frederick went on to study at St George's Hospital in London (MRCS LSA 1860), then obtained the MD from the University of St Andrews in 1862. He also spent time in the Royal Navy, acting as a ship's surgeon. Although little is known about his early life, much has been written about Manning's personal qualities and his considerable achievements in the field of mental health until his death.

Like other medical men trained in Britain, Manning sought experience as a physician in the colonies. Carrying letters of introduction to important colonists, he arrived in New South Wales in 1864. Appointed as the medical superintendent of Tarban Creek Lunatic Asylum (later Gladesville Asylum) in 1867 by then Attorney General Henry Parkes, Manning had already garnered knowledge about asylums in different parts of the world, including Britain, Europe, and America. His *Report on Lunatic Asylums* (1868) was a detailed account of asylum administration, patient care, buildings and plans, and different perceptions of insanity and the insane in their social and cultural contexts.

Manning's oversight of the state of asylums for the insane continued after 1879, when, after having spent time as an official asylum inspector for three years, he was appointed inspector general of the insane in the colony. His tenure as inspector general lasted until 1898 and included his significant part in official inquiries into three institutions in different colonies of Australia, as well as several roles in medical administration. Manning not only introduced reforms in asylums, including more efficient admission and discharge procedures, and agitated for better public funding of institutions; he also introduced the training of asylum attendants and nurses, and his status and the respect he earned helped to ensure that public debate around issues of mental health was open and progressive. He spoke warmly about the staff in his institutions when he resigned as medical superintendent. His influence on relevant lunacy legislation in New South Wales, such as the Lunacy Act (1878) and the Lunacy Amendment Act (1881), has been noted by historians. Manning also wrote an important report on insanity among Australian Aborigines, delivered at the 1889 Inter-Colonial Medical Congress in Melbourne.

Manning's achievements included his role as honorary secretary to the Prince Alfred Hospital, his presidency of the New South Wales Board of Health, and his contribution as medical adviser to the colonial government, in particular, his role as the health and emigration officer (1889–92). He was also examiner in psychological medicine at the University of Sydney in the late 1880s. Late in his career, and until his death, he worked as a consultant in mental health from private rooms in Phillip Street, Sydney.

Manning's medical career was illustrious, but never removed from the experiences of the sick and insane. After his death from stomach ulcer in 1903, more than one obituary commented upon the way his life was 'given to the amelioration of a class of suffering which needs special sympathy and insight'. As a final gesture of his sympathy towards the sick and insane he was buried, at his request, in the Gladesville Hospital cemetery.

Bibliography

Primary: Manning, F. N., 1879. *Address delivered on resigning charge as Medical Superintendent of the Hospitals for the Insane at Gladesville and Callan Park* (Sydney); Manning, F. N., 1889. 'Insanity in Australian Aborigines with a brief analysis of 32 cases' in *Inter-Colonial Medical Congress Transactions, 2nd Session* (Melbourne); McDonald, D. I., n.d. 'Frederick Norton Manning.' MS 5147, D. I. McDonald Collection, National Library of Australia.

Secondary: Garton, Stephen, 1988. *Medicine and Madness: A Social History of Insanity in New South Wales, 1880–1940* (Sydney); 1903. 'Death of Dr. Norton Manning.' *The Town and Country Journal* 24 June, p. 37; *AuDB*.

Catharine S. Coleborne

MANSON, PATRICK (b. Oldmeldrum, Scotland, 3 October 1844; d. London, England, 9 April 1922), *tropical medicine.*

Manson was the second son of John Manson, the laird of Fingask and a bank manager, and his wife, Elizabeth Livingston Blaikie. In 1857 the family moved to Aberdeen, where Manson attended the Gymnasium and subsequently the West End Academy. He took to natural history and began his lifelong enthusiasm for fishing and hunting. At the age of fifteen, Manson was apprenticed to a local firm of ironmasters with the intention of becoming an engineer. However, his spine suffered from a curvature, probably caused by heavy workloads, which led to weakness in one arm. He was forced to quit the apprenticeship as a result. Taking five months off, Manson spent the two hours of daily activity allowed by his physicians attending the course in natural history at Aberdeen University. He then entered the University to study medicine after learning that the course would be accepted as part of the medical curriculum (1860). The teaching at Aberdeen Medical School emphasized the importance of natural history and microscopy, and the training turned out to be useful for Manson's parasitological research. Manson served as medical officer to a lunatic asylum in Durham after graduating MB CM with distinction (1865). He gained his MD from Aberdeen University for his dissertation, entitled 'On a Peculiar Affection of the Internal Carotid Artery in Connection with Diseases of the Brain' (1866).

Filariasis

Along with many of his contemporary Scottish medical men, Manson sought professional opportunities overseas. By then his elder brother John was working in Shanghai for the Chinese Imperial Maritimes Customs, an institution controlled by the British after 1858. Through the family connection Manson obtained a position as a medical officer for Customs and was posted to the treaty port Takow in southern Taiwan (1866). His duties included inspecting the incoming ships, taking medical care of their

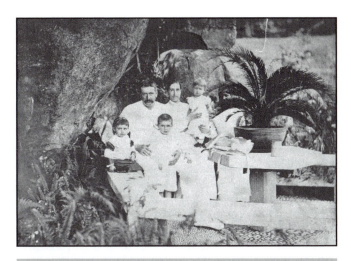

Patrick Manson with his family at Amoy, Fuh-kien, China (now Xiamen, Taiwan), 1881. Photograph, Archives and Manuscripts, Wellcome Library, London.

crews, and performing health examinations and smallpox inoculations on Chinese immigrants.

Manson was transferred to Amoy (now Xiamen), a much busier treaty port than Takow, in 1871. In addition to his duties for Customs, he also worked for a charity hospital funded by foreign merchants and missionaries. At the hospital he encountered many Chinese patients suffering from elephantiasis, a disease that resulted in disfiguring enlargement of the lower limbs or scrotum. Manson, who was a competent clinician, mostly focused on improving the surgical treatment of the disease. His successful operations on many patients increased the hospital's popularity among the Chinese. At the time, Manson considered the disease to be caused by malarial infection, not knowing that some European medical men had attributed it to parasitic infection. The French surgeon Jean-Nicholas Demarquay (1814–75) had discovered the embryonic form of the filarial worm in the fluid aspirated from the swollen scrotum of an elephantiasis patient (1863). Timothy Richard Lewis (1841–86), a British medical officer in India, had detected the worms in the urine and the blood of patients (1871), and he named the parasite *Filaria hominis sanguinis* (now *Filaria bancrofti*).

Manson was granted a furlough and returned to England, where he married the daughter of Captain James Ptolemy Thurburn, Henrietta Isabella (1875), with whom he went on to have five children. He spent time in the British Library consulting medical literature on elephantiasis. The articles by British medical men in India, such as Lewis, Vincent Richards, and Henry Vandyke Carter (1831–97), convinced him that the disease was caused by filarial infection and that there was probably a second host involved in its transmission. Because the worm was present in the blood, Manson suspected that the host was a bloodsucking insect.

Back in Amoy, Manson set out to investigate the disease. He reasoned that the geographical distribution of the second host must coincide with areas where elephantiasis was endemic. Hence, he ruled out fleas, lice, bugs, and leeches, which were distributed much more widely than the disease, and identified a species of mosquito common in Amoy as the most likely candidate. Manson collected mosquitoes that had bitten a Chinese patient suffering from filariasis. He kept the mosquitoes in bottles and dissected a few of them every day to observe the filarial embryos they contained. Manson discovered that, instead of being digested by the mosquitoes, the filarial embryos grew significantly. The experiment was the first to demonstrate insect-borne transmission of disease. Most of Manson's research on filariasis was published in the *Half-Yearly Medical Reports of the Chinese Imperial Maritime Customs*. Thanks to the mediation of the authoritative parasitologist Thomas Spencer Cobbold (1828–86), with whom Manson had been in correspondence, the article announcing this discovery also appeared in the prestigious *Journal of the Linnean Society of London* (1878). Manson, however, fell short of working out the complete life cycle of the filarial worm. He was misled by the contemporary idea that a mosquito fed on human blood only once in its lifetime and speculated that the mosquito died after laying eggs in water. The filarial worms, claimed Manson, escaped into the water afterward and could infect humans who drank the water.

In December 1883, Manson left the Chinese Maritime Customs for Hong Kong to pursue more lucrative private practice. He soon cultivated a successful practice and recruited James Cantlie (1851–1926), another Aberdeen alumnus, from London to join his practice (1887). With Cantlie's proposal and Manson's support, the College of Medicine for the Chinese was founded in October 1887. It was the first Western-style medical school in Hong Kong and eventually became the Medical School of Hong Kong and Victoria University. Manson served as its first dean, and among its earliest students was Sun Yat-sen (1866–1925), who later led the revolution that overthrew the Qing dynasty and became a founder of the Republic of China.

Malaria

Manson retired to Scotland in 1889, but a year later, he was obliged to resume medical practice because depreciation of the Chinese currency had greatly reduced his pension. He went to London to set up a private practice as a consultant in tropical diseases. He was appointed physician to the Seamen's Hospital Society, taking charge of a ward of about fifteen beds at the Albert Dock Hospital (1892). He also visited the Dreadnought Hospital at Greenwich regularly. The post and his contacts with various missionary societies provided him with opportunities to continue his research on tropical diseases and to consolidate his reputation as a leader in the field. Manson began to give public lectures on tropical medicine (1894), first at the Livingstone College in Leytonstone, east London for the missionaries and later at St George's Hospital at Charing Cross. His *Tropical Diseases: A Manual of the Diseases of Warm Climates* (1898) soon became a standard reference work that went through many editions.

Alphonse Lavaren's (1849–1922) discovery of the malarial parasite (1880) galvanized the research and debates on malaria, and once in London, Manson soon immersed himself in this field. He published, in the *British Medical Journal*, a malaria chart to facilitate the microscopic diagnosis of the disease (1894). In an article entitled 'On the nature and significance of the crescentic and flagellated bodies in malarial blood' that appeared in the same journal (1894), he speculated on the biological meaning of the plasmodium's morphological change after its extraction from a human blood vessel. Motile 'flagella' appeared on the surface of the parasites, some of which broke away and moved about in the blood. Manson speculated that these 'flagellated spores' were part of a phenomenon of adaptation that enabled the parasite to continue its existence outside the human body. Analogizing with the life cycle of the filarial worm, Manson conjectured that a bloodsucking insect, most likely the mosquito, was the other host of the malarial parasite. Manson planned to conduct research in India to verify his hypothesis, but lack of funding and the fact that he was suffering from gout prevented him from doing so. In April 1894, Ronald Ross (1857–1932), an officer in the Indian Medical Service who was on furlough in England, came to visit Manson. Ross had been studying malaria in India without being able to observe the parasite in patients' blood. Manson enthusiastically taught Ross the microscopic techniques of observing the plasmodium and expounded to Ross his 'mosquito-malaria theory'. Ross set out to prove Manson's 'Grand Induction' after he returned to India, and Manson continued to provide him with advice and support and used his connections to publicize Ross's findings both at professional meetings and by providing help with publishing in medical journals. Their cooperation via correspondence led to the discovery of the transmission of malaria through the bite of the mosquito when Ross experimentally induced malaria in birds (1898).

School of Tropical Medicine

Manson was appointed Medical Advisor to the Colonial Office, a post that he held for some fifteen years (1897–1912). The health measures that Manson advised for the tropical colonies focused on preventing contact between humans and the insect-vectors of parasitic diseases. He did not, however, favor large-scale sanitary works. Such a view was congenial to the cost-conscious colonial authorities. Manson also put forward a proposal to establish a school of tropical medicine (1897). He argued that most tropical diseases were parasitic diseases in which transmission depended on insects. The prevention and treatment of tropical diseases, argued Manson, required training in helminthology, parasitology, and entomology. Such courses, however, were woefully lacking in the British medical schools. Manson claimed that a school that provided compulsory postgraduate training for medical men who were going to practice medicine in the tropical colonies could greatly improve health conditions in those areas. The proposal won the strong support of Herbert J. Read (1863–1949), who was serving as private secretary to Joseph Chamberlain (1836–1914), the Secretary of State for the Colonies. It also appealed to Chamberlain, who had been arguing that Britain must exploit the resources of her tropical colonies more efficiently in order to retain her leading position in the international competition between European powers. Effective prevention of tropical diseases would facilitate Chamberlain's project of 'constructive imperialism'. There were dissenting voices, however, within the British medical profession. Some medical schools resented the requirement that their graduates must attend another institution before practicing in the colonies and argued that they could provide the training themselves. Manson was able to overcome the resistance thanks to his social skills and, more importantly, the support of the Colonial Office. The London School of Tropical Medicine, one of Manson's lasting legacies, was opened in 1899 and became a key teaching and research institute of the new specialty. After the Rockefeller endowment (1923) it became the London School of Hygiene and Tropical Medicine.

Manson was elected FRS (1900) and became the first president of the Royal Society of Tropical Medicine and Hygiene (1907–09). He was made KCMG in 1903 and was promoted to GCMG upon his retirement from the Colonial Office (1912).

Bibliography

Primary: 1883. *The Filaria Sanguinis Hominis and Certain New Forms of Parasitic Disease in India, China and Warm Climate Countries* (London); 1898. *Tropical Diseases: A Manual of the Diseases of Warm Climates* (London); *1905. Lectures on Tropical Diseases* (London).

Secondary: Li, Shang-Jen, 2002. 'Natural History of Parasitic Disease: Patrick Manson's Philosophical Method.' *Isis* 93: 206–228; Haynes, Douglas M., 2001. *Imperial Medicine: Patrick Manson and the Conquest of Tropical Disease* (Philadelphia); Bynum, W. F., and Caroline Overy, eds., 1998. *The Beast in the Mosquito: The Correspondence of Ronald Ross & Patrick Manson* (Amsterdam); Chernin, Eli, 1983. 'Sir Patrick Manson: An Annotated Bibliography and a Note on a Collected Set of His Writings.' *Reviews of Infectious Diseases* 5: 353–385; Manson-Bahr, Philip, and A. Alcock, 1927. *The Life and Work of Sir Patrick Manson* (London); *DSB; Oxford DNB.*

Shang-Jen Li

MARAÑÓN POSADILLO, GREGORIO (b. Madrid, Spain, 19 May 1887; d. Madrid, 27 March 1960), *medicine, endocrinology, medical humanities.*

Marañón, son of a prominent lawyer, had a culturally privileged upbringing. His father had a great library, which Marañón took advantage of, and among his father's friends were some of the most renowned men of letters in Spain at the turn of the nineteenth century, including Menéndez Pelayo, Pereda, and Galdós. He studied medicine at the Faculty of Madrid (1902–09), where some of his teachers—Olóriz, Cajal, San Martín, Madinaveitia, and Sañudo—influenced the way he saw and understood the profession. After obtaining his PhD with a thesis on the blood in thyroid pathology (1910), he traveled to Frankfurt to study and improve his knowledge of the techniques of chemical biology with Edinger. It was in Germany that he also worked with Paul Ehrlich.

On returning to Spain he was appointed staff physician at the Madrid General Hospital (1911), and carried out numerous clinical and experimental works on infectious diseases and endocrinology. These were followed by other works illustrating the relationship between hormonal activity and various conditions: the climacteric (1919), the sexual nature (1926), and the sexual tendencies (1929). All this research, and other works on thyroid diseases and Addison's disease (1929), resulted in Marañón being considered an authority on endocrinology and a pioneer in making this field of study a medical specialty. As a result of these contributions he became the principal exponent of a generation of doctors dedicated to remodeling and updating medicine in Spain. The successful *Manual de medicina interna* [Handbook on Internal Medicine] (1916–20), which Marañón supervised with Teófilo Hernando and which included the collaboration of the best Spanish clinicians of the time, testifies to this.

In 1922 he was commissioned by the government to study the state of health in a backward area, Las Hurdes. The report gave a desolating picture and attracted the attention of King Alfonso XIII, who visited the area to see the situation firsthand. This trip offered Marañón a chance to see whether or not the monarchy would be able to rise to much-needed modernization in Spain. Marañón was not to find out, due to the coup that led to the dictatorship of 1923–30, but from then on he was to play an active role in political life. A liberal, he disagreed with the dictatorship and supported the establishment of the Republic (1931).

In the meantime his scientific work, which he undertook in part at his own 'Instituto de Patología Médica', was to increase at an amazing rate. Between 1922 and 1936 he published 400 articles and sixteen books, mainly on endocrinology, of which those on the study of sexuality are particularly worth highlighting. Moreover, he produced numerous writings as a historian and essayist. Some notable examples are *Ensayo biológico sobre Enrique IV de Castilla y su tiempo* (1930), *Las ideas biológicas del Padre Feijoo* (1934), and *Vocación y ética* (1936).

He continued to develop both aspects of his work after the Civil War (1936–39). On returning to Spain after a self-imposed exile in Paris (1937–43), where he wrote a celebrated textbook on diagnosis, he moved away from political life and continued his monumental work. His membership as an academic of the five Royal Academies—Medicine, Science, Fine Arts, Spanish Language, and History—illustrate how Marañón's prestige went far beyond the bounds of medicine, making him one of the most representative figures of Spanish culture of the time.

Bibliography

Primary: 1966–77. *Obras completas* 10 vols. (Madrid); 1931. *Estudios de fisiopatología sexual* (Barcelona); 1943. *Manual de diagnóstico etiológico* (Madrid).

Secondary: Botella, José, et al., 2003. *Revisión de la obra médica de Marañón* (Puertollano); Laín, Pedro, 1969. *Gregorio Marañón. Vida, obra y persona* (Madrid); Sánchez Granjel, Luis, 1960. *Gregorio Marañón, su vida y su obra* (Madrid).

José Martínez-Pérez

MARIE, PIERRE (b. Paris, France, 9 September 1853, d. Pradel (Var), France, 3 April 1940), *neurology.*

Marie grew up in the comfortable ambience of the established bourgeoisie. As a hospital intern (1878), he worked under Jean-Martin Charcot at the Salpêtrière hospital. After receiving the MD degree (1885), he continued to be a member of Charcot's inner circle of students, serving as the latter's *chef de clinique* (1886). Marie was a devoted follower of Charcot's clinical-anatomical approach to the study of neurological disease and would remain so throughout his long career. He also contributed to the Salpêtrière project on hysteria during these early years. Marie's main accomplishments, however, were to elucidate an organic neuropathology at all levels: cortical, subcortical, spinal, and peripheral.

In 1886 he published an important study of acromegaly and, that same year, together with Charcot, he described a familial neuropathy with progressive muscular atrophy (which at first was called Charcot-Marie myopathy in France, but is now known as Charcot-Marie-Tooth disease, after A. H. Tooth, who reported the same entity in the same year). Marie's publications on hereditary cerebellar ataxia opened up this field. His work on inherited diseases of the nervous system conformed with the Salpêtrière paradigm of hereditary disease etiology. But Marie also pointed to infections as the likely cause of multiple sclerosis and, breaking with Charcot's emphasis on hereditary causes, implicated syphilis as the necessary precondition for tabes dorsalis.

Following Charcot's death, the prestige of the Salpêtrière school declined. In 1897 Marie, by then an associate professor, went to the Bicêtre hospital, an outlying institution that did not have a significant neurological service at the time. Over the subsequent twenty-five years, Marie made Bicêtre a center for research and instruction. He published a seminal account of spondylitis, and his work on cerebrovascular disease established the modern concept of cerebral lacunes. In 1907 Marie was promoted to the professorship of pathological anatomy.

Marie's midcareer was marked by controversy and debate. He engaged in particularly virulent disagreement with the rival neurologist Jules Déjerine. This culminated in a debate over the cerebral localization of language disorders. Contrary to the generally accepted view, Marie held that these disorders (aphasias) could not be localized to a specific cerebral area (Broca's lobe). His views placed Marie in direct opposition to Déjerine's primary field of research. An emotional exchange followed, after which Marie ceased to write on aphasia. In 1910, the chair of clinical neurology at the Salpêtrière became vacant. Marie and Déjerine were the two obvious candidates. Déjerine, who already led a small unit at the hospital, prevailed. The defeated Marie returned to Bicêtre with little prospect of ever gaining the one available Faculty professorship of neurology, since he was nearly the same age as his rival.

As it turned out, Marie finally did succeed to the Salpêtrière chair when Déjerine died in 1919. Having reached the pinnacle of his profession, he exacted a spiteful revenge on the widow of his deceased rival. Marie gave Mme Déjerine-Klumpke, an accomplished research neurologist in her own right and a frequent collaborator with her husband, just fourteen days to leave the Salpêtrière, together with her laboratory personnel and material.

At age sixty-six, in a France devastated by World War I, Marie's energy had diminished. He endeavored to restore the Salpêtrière to the days when he had served as Charcot's chief resident. Although he managed to preside over an efficient service for teaching and research modeled after Charcot's, it lacked the old dynamism. In 1925, having reached obligatory retirement age, Marie left Paris for the south of France. He returned for professional society meetings but remained detached from advances in neurology during the remaining fifteen years of his life. Weakened by the deaths of his wife and two children, Marie also outlived most of his friends and colleagues. He died at the advanced age of eighty-seven.

Bibliography

Primary: 1926–28. *Travaux et mémoires* 2 vols. (Paris).

Secondary: Goetz, C. G., 2003. 'Pierre Marie: Gifted Intellect, Poor Timing and Unchecked Emotionality.' *J. Hist. Neurosciences* 12: 154–166; Goetz, Christopher G., Michel Bonduelle, and Toby Gelfand, 1995. *Charcot. Constructing Neurology* (New York); Brais, Bernard, 1992. 'The Third Left Frontal Convolution Plays No Role in Language: Pierre Marie and the Paris Debate on Aphasia (1906–1908).' *Neurology* 42: 690–696; Bailey P, 1970. 'Pierre Marie' in Haymaker, W., and F. Schiller, eds., *The Founders of Neurology* (Springfield, IL) pp. 476–479.

Christopher G. Goetz

MARINESCU, GHEORGHE (b. Bucharest, Romania, 28 February 1863; d. Bucharest, 15 May 1938), *neurology.*

Marinescu was born in Bucharest. In 1882, after graduating from the 'Central Seminary' Lyceum, he enrolled at the Faculty of Medicine in Bucharest. In 1889, with the support of Victor Babeş (1854–1926), in whose laboratory of pathological anatomy and bacteriology he worked as an assistant, Marinescu went to Paris to study with Jean-Martin Charcot (1825–93) at his clinic of diseases of the nervous system. He was an innovative student. In 1889, for example, he made the first x-ray photographs in acromegaly. In Paris Marinescu met Pierre Marie (1853–1940), Joseph Babinski (1857–1932), and Fulgence Raymond (1844–98), with whom he cultivated a long friendship. It was Pierre Marie who assigned Marinescu to lecture on the pathological anatomy of acromegaly at the Internal Congress of Medicine in Berlin in 1890. Between 1890 and 1896, Marinescu traveled to Germany on several occasions and studied with Carl Weigert (1845–1904) and Emil Du Bois-Raymond (1872–1929). In 1892, together with Victor Babeş and Paul Oscar Blocq (1860–96), Marinescu published *Atlas der pathologischen Histologie des Nervensystems*, an atlas of the anatomo-pathological aspects of the diseases of the nervous system. Marinescu's collaboration with Paul Blocq continued, and in 1892 they were the first to describe the senile plaques.

In 1897 Marinescu obtained his doctorate in medicine at the Faculty of Medicine in Paris and returned to Romania, where he became the director of the section of nervous diseases at the Pantelimon Hospital in Bucharest. In 1898 he was appointed professor at the clinic of nervous diseases of the Faculty of Medicine and, in the following year, elected a corresponding member of the Romanian Academy. In 1909 he published *La cellule nerveuse*, with a preface by Santiago Ramón y Cajal (1852–1934). In 1912 he was elected a correspondent member of the French Academy of Medicine. In 1913, together with another Romanian neurologist, Ion Minea, Marinescu determined the existence of the syphilitic microorganism *Treponema pallidum*, a discovery later confirmed by the Japanese bacteriologist Hideyo Noguchi (1876–1928).

Marinescu was the founder of the Romanian School of Neurology. He was among the first medical doctors to apply methods from histology and histopathology to neurology. One of Marinescu's original methods consisted of applying the newest experiments in physics and chemistry to the exploration of the nerve cell. For example, he applied ultramicroscopic techniques used in the colloidal theory to study the neuron structure and made daring medical experiments, such as transplants and cultures of nervous tissue. Through the use of the backward degeneration method he also discovered the locations of nerve formations, such as the nucleus of pneumogastric and facial nerve.

The study of the pathological anatomy of the nervous system (especially the regeneration phenomena occurring in the spinal marrow of those suffering from tabes dorsalis and the injuries of the motor neurons in the victims of amyotrophic lateral sclerosis) represents one of Marinescu's main medical achievements. He primarily investigated infections of the nervous system, such as the propagation of the poliomyelitis and the herpetic viruses. Marinescu was also preoccupied with the oxidative ferments in dendrites and the evolution of reflexive tropism. Furthermore, he was among the first in medical history to use the encephalographic method and the conditioned reflexes method in diagnosing hysteria, epilepsy, aphasia, and neurosis. Certain neurological lesions ('Marinescu's hand') and congenital disorders ('Marinescu's syndrome') were named after him. During the last years of his life, he began to write a monograph on the biology of the nerve cell, which he never completed. His international recognition reached its peak in 1925 when Marinescu was invited to evoke the personality of Jean-Martin Charcot at the celebration of the centennial of his birth.

Bibliography

Primary: 1892. (with Babeş, Victor, and Paul Oscar Blocq) *Atlas der pathologischen Histologie des Nervensystems* (Berlin); 1895. *Théorie des neurones* (Berlin); 1909. *La cellule nerveuse* 2 vols. (Paris); 1910. *Maladies des muscles* (Paris).

Secondary: 1955. *Pagini alese din opera lui Gh. Marinescu* (Bucharest).

Marius Turda

MARKUSOVSZKY, LAJOS (b. Csorba, Hungary, 25 April 1815; d. Abbazia, Austro-Hungary [now Opatija, Croatia], 21 April 1893), *surgery, medical publishing, medical education.*

Perhaps best known outside Hungary as a footnote to the story of Ignác Semmelweis, whose close and loyal friend he became, Markusovszky was a towering figure in Hungarian medicine during the second half of the nineteenth century. Next to his mentor, the surgeon János Balassa, Markusovszky was arguably the most outstanding physician at the Pest medical school. He was an active member of Balassa's progressive circle.

Initially, Markusovszky studied law in Pozsony (Pressburg; now Bratislava). As a teacher in Pest, he mingled with doctors, including Balassa, who—recognizing his talent—soon arranged a scholarship enabling Markusovszky to study medicine. When he received his degree in Pest (1844), he was promptly made an assistant in Balassa's surgical clinic. That winter, Markusovszky spent time in Paris hospitals; he then received one of the scholarships for Hungarian surgical trainees in Joseph Wattmann's clinic and attended lectures in Vienna for two years. There he met Semmelweis, with whom he roomed and whom he vigorously supported (not least in encouraging Semmelweis to publish his findings on childbed fever).

Back in Budapest, Markusovszky worked again with Balassa until József Eötvös, the Minister of Education during the 1848 revolution, asked him to establish theoretical and practical courses on military surgery. At the university clinic, Markusovszky also cared for soldiers wounded in the 1848–49 war of independence. Among his patients was the Hungarian patriot, General Arthur Görgey, who subsequently invited Markusovszky to serve as his staff physician. This hardly endeared him to the Austrian authorities; when the revolution failed, he was suspended from the medical faculty.

When Markusovszky sought professional advancement, his promotion was blocked (his Protestantism was used as the justification). But Balassa, recently released from prison himself, once more made Markusovszky his private assistant. Denied a Docent position, Markusovszky in 1857 founded *Orvosi Hetilap* [Medical Weekly], aiming to give Hungarian physicians what the Viennese medical world had in the *Wiener medizinische Wochenschrift*. When *Orvosi Hetilap* celebrated its twenty-fifth anniversary, medical people within and outside Hungary acknowledged Markusovszky's achievement. He edited the paper for thirty-two years (with Imre Poór as co-editor) before stepping down. (The paper still exists, and is Hungary's oldest medical journal.)

Once more collaborating with Balassa, Markusovszky in 1863 founded the *Magyar Orvosi Könyvkiadó Társaság* [Hungarian Medical Book Publishing Society]—an organization modeled on the New Sydenham Society in London—to publish medical works in Hungarian, both translations and original works. At the time of Markusovszky's death, forty-seven volumes had been published, contributing immensely to the continuing education of Hungarian physicians.

In 1867 Eötvös, again Minister of Education, asked Markusovszky to head the section on medical education. Credit goes to him for the raised standards and modernization that resulted. He established model educational institutions and worked diligently to recruit and train truly qualified teachers. He introduced the teaching of hygiene in schools and in 1876 established a National Public Health Council (comprising physicians and educated laypersons) to improve the health of Hungary's citizens.

Markusovszky became a corresponding member of the Hungarian Academy of Sciences in 1863; he was made an 'honored member' in 1890. A medallion was later struck in his memory at the hospital in Szombathely (which bears Markusovszky's name). He was included in Endre Réti's 1954 *Nagy magyar orvosok* [Great Hungarian Physicians] (Budapest); the medical historians György Gortvay (1964) and József Antall (1965) have also written about him and the importance of his activities in medical education, hygiene, public health, and preventive medicine.

Bibliography

Primary: 1905. (Marikovszky, György, ed.) *Markusovszky Lajos Válogatott Munkái* [The Collected Works of Lajos Markusovszky] (Budapest).

Secondary: Albert, E. et al., eds., 1929–34. *Biographisches Lexikon der hervorragenden Ärzte aller Zeiten und Völker* vol. 4 (Berlin) p. 85; Korányi, Frigyes, 1902. *Emlékbeszéd Markusovszky Lajos fölött* [Eulogy of Markusovszky] (Budapest); [Obit.], 1893. 'Ludwig Markusovszky.' *Wiener med. Presse* 18: 708–709.

Constance Putnam

MARTIN, JAMES RANALD (b. Kilmure, Isle of Skye, Scotland, 12 May 1793; d. London, England, 27 November 1874), *surgery, tropical hygiene.*

Martin was born into a clerical family on the Isle of Skye. After the death of his mother, the family left for Inverness, where Martin attended the Royal Academy. He showed an interest in medicine from an early age and received tuition in pharmacy from two local doctors while still at school. After studying at St George's Hospital, London, and becoming MRCS, Martin joined the medical service of the East India Company. In 1817 he began work at the Presidency General Hospital in Calcutta but in 1818 was attached to the Company's army in Fort William, Calcutta. After being promoted to the rank of assistant-surgeon, Martin was dispatched with the army to Orissa, eastern India, to subdue an insurrection.

In 1819 Martin returned to the Presidency Hospital, now promoted to first assistant surgeon. The following year, he was reassigned to military duties and took part in operations against rebellious hill tribes in northern Bengal. While on active service, Martin contracted a fever that rendered him invalid for the next ten months, but through his personal experience of sickness, he became an ardent proponent of preventive medicine. Like most of the other surgeons in the Company's army, Martin believed there was a close association between climate and disease, and this led to him to recommend that troops be garrisoned only in salubrious areas. After returning to Calcutta in 1821, he also pressed for better sanitation in regimental barracks and hospitals, and the governor-general, Lord Hastings, adopted his recommendations.

In 1823 Martin again found himself on active service, in the Burmese War of 1824–26. The war in Burma resulted in heavy casualties from disease, and Martin had little difficulty in persuading the reforming governor-general, William Bentinck, that the army should pay more attention to this problem. He gained Bentinck's support for a system of medical reporting, whereby medical officers wrote on the medical topography of their stations. Martin's own *Medical Topography of Calcutta* (1837) became one of the best known.

The years immediately after the Burma War saw Martin rise rapidly in his chosen profession. After marrying the daughter of Colonel Patton, the quarter-master-general of the Bengal army, he established a successful private practice in Calcutta and in 1828 was appointed to the prestigious post of presidency surgeon and head surgeon of the Native Hospital. It was here that he developed a radical treatment for hydrocephalus using injections of diluted tincture of iodine.

Martin continued to practice in Calcutta until 1840, when poor health forced his return to England. In London he established a thriving practice among friends and acquaintances from India. However, he continued to take an active interest in the health of soldiers and was appointed inspector-general of army hospitals and president of the East India Company's medical board. He also published a number of articles on this subject in *Lancet* and, in 1856, edited the sixth and posthumous edition of James Johnson's classic text on *The Influence of Tropical Climates on European Constitutions.* His interest in soldiers' health also led to Martin's appointment to the royal commission on the sanitary state of the British Army following the Crimean war and, in 1859, to a similar body that examined the army in India.

Martin was elected FRCS in 1845 and was knighted in 1860. He became somewhat deaf in old age but appears to have been in relatively good health until succumbing to pneumonia at his home in Upper Brook Street at the age of seventy-seven.

Bibliography

Primary: 1837. *Notes on the Medical Topography of Calcutta* (Calcutta); 1856. *The Influence of Tropical Climates on European Constitutions* (London).

Secondary: Harrison, Mark, 1994. *Public Health in British India* (Cambridge); 1874. Obituary. *Medical Times and Gazette*, 5 December; *Plarr's Lives*; *Oxford DNB*.

Mark Harrison

MARTÍNEZ BÁEZ, MANUEL (b. Morelia, Michoacán, Mexico, 26 September 1894; d. Mexico City, Mexico, 19 January 1987), *public health, parasitology.*

Martínez Báez was born into a family with a long scientific, cultural, and political tradition in Michoacán. He studied at the Colegio de San Nicolás de Hidalgo, an institution founded on the precepts of Thomas More that provided a solid education, high moral values, group sentiments, and profound pride. He conserved the friendships cultivated at the Colegio throughout his life, and many of the men in his group later formed part of Mexico's political, scientific, and cultural elite between the 1930s and 60s. He studied medicine in Morelia and served as a doctor in the army and in the Cruz Blanca Neutral during the tumultuous years of the Mexican Revolution (1910–17). He worked for two years in the poorest areas of the state, where he came into direct contact with the poverty and human misery that cause disease. In 1925 he settled in Mexico City, where his friends from the Colegio helped him gain access to health-related institutions.

In 1933–34 he worked in the laboratory of the parasitologist Emile Brumpt, studied malaria at the Institute of Tropical Diseases in Hamburg, and won a scholarship from the Rockefeller Foundation to Navalmoral de la Mata, Spain, and the Experimental Station for the Study of Malaria in Rome. This background helps to explain Martínez Báez's later contributions to public health, especially in the area of tropical diseases.

Sensitive to the incongruity between what was studied in foreign books and what he saw in his own country, Martínez Báez systematized the concepts of what was called 'exotic pathology' in a fundamental book that is still required reading today. According to him, 'exotic pathology' or 'tropical medicine' referred to illnesses that needed to be understood, although they were largely unknown in colonizing nations. Climate was not the cause of such maladies, but rather poverty, inadequate social organization, ignorance, and the unequal distribution of wealth. Even today, historians and sociologists of science speak of tropical diseases in the terms that Martínez Báez proposed thirty years ago. For the scientific study of infectious and parasitic diseases in Mexico, he created the National Institute of Tropical Diseases, which bears his name. His research there improved knowledge of the parasite that causes onchocerciasis.

Martínez Báez occupied important positions at universities in Michoacán and Mexico City and participated in the formation and organization of the current National Council of Science and Technology. He led the principal institutions in the field of health in Mexico and served as Sub-Secretary of the Department of Health and Assistance. Internationally, he represented Mexico at several Pan-American expositions and conferences on hygiene. His fluent French and English allowed him to serve as a delegate to meetings of sanitary leaders in Washington, in conferences on alimentation and agriculture in Hot Springs and Quebec, and on the Interim Commission of the Technical Council of the WHO, of which he was a Vice-President. Also, he was a permanent delegate to the United Nations Organization for Education, Science and Culture and presided over that group's Council. In 1946 the Economic and Social Council of the United Nations named him a member of its Committee of Experts. In addition, he served as president of the National Academy of Medicine, was a member of the Colegio Nacional, and earned many national and international honors.

Martínez Báez belonged to a select group of people at a special time. He was interested in culture, science, and human beings. His forceful personality and excellent training as a scientist-diplomat brought prestige to Mexico.

Bibliography

Primary: 1953. *Manual de parasitología médica* (Mexico); 1969. *Factores económicos, culturales y sociales en la génesis de las llamadas enfermedades tropicales* (Mexico).

Secondary: Rodríguez de Romo, A. C., 1997. 'Manuel Martínez Báez' in Magner, Lois, ed., *Doctors, Nurses and Medical Practitioners* (Westport, CT) pp. 177–182; Rodríguez de Romo, A. C. 1993. 'Manuel Martínez Báez: una visión muy personal de las enfermedades tropicales.' *Gaceta Médica de México* 129(1): 81–86.

Ana Cecilia Rodríguez de Romo

MARTÍNEZ VARGAS, ANDRÉS   (b. Barbastro, Lérida, Spain, 27 October 1861; d. Barcelona, Spain, 26 July 1948), *pediatrics.*

Martínez Vargas is one of the central figures of the institutionalization of pediatrics in Spain. Raised in a middle-class family, in a medium-sized town, where new small industries were developing alongside traditional agriculture, he attended a private religious school. He received his degree in medicine from the University of Saragossa in 1882. After obtaining his PhD, he took up his first post in the Princess Hospital in Madrid. Very soon he became interested in child medicine, under the influence of pioneering pediatrics literature in French and German. Another important influence in the early days of his career was Abraham Jacobi (1830–1919), who offered him a job in his pediatric clinic in New York. During his American stage (1883–86), Martínez Vargas also visited Mexico.

As in all European countries, in Spain the domain of a 'medicine for children' was segregated from both obstetrics and internal medicine during the nineteenth century. The first professorship of the specialty was set up by the Medical Syllabus of 1886. Martínez Vargas was one of the pioneers, obtaining, in 1888, the chair of diseases of children at the University of Granada. However, most of his professional activity took place in the University of Barcelona (1891–1931) as a teacher and a head clinician on a special ward and dispensary for children at the University Hospital. He took a very active part in university life as dean of the Faculty of Medicine and, later, as vice-chancellor of the University. There he found the most suitable environment for his scientific and professional interest in the advance of pediatrics.

He showed a great capacity for work and an open-mindedness towards the scientific innovations that were developing in the international arena. His most important contribution toward the diffusion of the main pediatric international texts was as coordinator of the Spanish version (1919) of the *Handbuch der Kinderheilkunde* (Leipzig, 1910–12) by Meihard von Pfaundler (1872–1947) and Arthur Schlossmann (1867–1932).

The birth of pediatrics as a specialty in Spain was promoted by the appearance of specific journals, the constitution of a scientific society, and the organization of congresses. This process cannot be studied without reference to Martínez Vargas's work.

Martínez Vargas attended all the congresses and scientific meetings related to pediatrics. He personally organized, and was the president of, the First Spanish Congress of Pediatrics (Palma de Mallorca, 1914). The Spanish Society of Pediatrics was set up in 1912 with his participation. Years earlier, in 1900, he had founded the first specialized journal, *The Medicine of Children*.

Martínez Vargas belonged to that group of doctors who sought a global solution to the problems of infancy and who strove to reduce the high rates of infant mortality through all possible means. In his view the great task of the twentieth century was the recovery of infancy as a positive value for the family, for society, and for the nation. Besides the demographic and eugenic arguments for the movement, he added economic reasons. The medical-social ideology of Martínez Vargas was akin to the concept of *Nipiology* promoted by the Italian pediatrician Ernesto Cacace (1872–1956), which was a different label for the French *Puériculture*. In 1916 he set up at his birth town a Nipiologic Institute, within the context of the expanding movement to provide healthy milk and medical counseling to newborn infants of working-class mothers.

Finally, one of Martínez Vargas's main concerns was the search for a specific model for the scientific study of children, based on knowledge of the processes of growth and development in these stages of life.

Bibliography

Primary: 1915. *Tratado de Pediatría* (Barcelona); 1927. *La salud en el niño* (Barcelona).

Secondary: Rodriguez-Ocaña, Esteban, 1996. 'Una medicina para la infancia' in Borrás, José, ed., *Historia de la infancia en la España Contemporánea, 1834–1936* (Madrid) pp. 149–192; Ballester, Rosa, and Emilio Balaguer, 1995. 'La infancia como valor y como problema en las luchas sanitarias de principios de siglo en España.' *Dynamis* 15: 177–192.

Rosa Ballester

IBN MĀSAWAYH ABŪ ZAKĀRIYĀ YŪḤANNĀ (aka MESUE) (b. Jundishapur, Iran, *c.* 777; d. Baghdad, Iraq, *c.* 857), *medicine*.

Ibn Māsawayh came from a medical family and studied medicine in Baghdad. His career began under Caliph al-Ma'mūn (r. 813–33) and continued under his successors al-Mu'tasim (r. 833–42), al-Wāthiq (r. 842–47) and al-Mutawakkil (r. 847–61). Like many intellectuals of Iranian origin, he was a Nestorian Christian. He had good command of Syriac and Greek and was representative of Eastern syncretism, which united the practical prescriptions of the East with the mystical speculation of ancient Greek paganism.

Ibn Māsawayh married a daughter of his colleague 'Abdallāh aṭ-Ṭayfūri. We possess descriptions of husband and wife. Ibn Māsawayh described himself as having an oblong face and blue eyes and as being very intelligent. He said his wife was very beautiful but not exactly clever. He had a brother, Michael, who married a daughter of their joint patron, Jibriīl Bakhtīshū'. The Bakhtīshū' family produced a number of medical practitioners, and the Arabic name Bakhtīshū' was applied to skillful practitioners.

Ibn Māsawayh's wit and sayings were widely known. He is said to have had a son whom Ibn Māsawayh believed had not inherited his parents' talents. He apparently said that if it were not for the authorities he would like to dissect his son, as Galen dissected monkeys. By this dissection, he would have learned the cause of his son's stupidity, and also would have provided necessary medical knowledge for others. His son died very young.

Ibn Māsawayh enjoyed a long and fruitful life and lacked neither patrons nor wealth. He contributed to the translation of Greek scientific works. He became the friend and counselor of the Caliphs as well as their physician. His science was a mixture of fantasy, empiricism, and practical observation, of which Ibn Māsawayh became the acknowledged representative. In his period, pharmacy tended to take precedence over medical research, and according to Ibn Māsawayh the remedy, like the malady, was ordained by providence, in the very order of nature. The knowledge of the four qualities (hot, dry, cold, wet), added to knowledge of the properties and the natures as well as the procedures prescribed by the art, enabled the physician to penetrate the secret of universal harmony. This harmony acted on the human body through the four humors (blood, bile, black bile, and phlegm). Pharmacy took into account not only the temperaments but also the seasons, which, thanks to the qualities, have a clearly perceptible affinity with the humors.

Arab authors quoted about thirty-five works composed by Ibn Māsawayh. His Latin works are much longer, which shows that Mesue (the Latin version of this name) was held in high esteem in the West. As late as the fifteenth century, one Petrus Gulosius, a physician of Amalfi, stated (1474) that to read him was as instructive as it was pleasant.

Bibliography

Primary: 1913. *Canones universales divi Mesue de consolatione medicinarum et correctione operationum earundem/Grabadin ejusdem Mesue medicinarum universalium quod antidotarium nuncupatur. Liber ejusdem medicinarum particularium. Additio Petri Apponi medici clarissimi in librum Joannis Mesue. Antidotarium Domini Nicolai* (Venice).

Secondary: Sournia, J. C., and G. Troupeau, 1968. 'Medecine Arabe: Biographies Critiques de Jean Mésué (VIII Siècle) et du Prétendu "Mésué le Jeune" (X Siècle).' *Clio Medica* 3: 109–117; Ullmann, Manfred, 1978. *Islamic Medicine* (trans. Jean Watt) (Edinburgh); *Encyclopaedia of Islam*.

Nikolaj Serikoff

MATTIOLI, PIETRO ANDREA   (b. Siena, Italy, 23 March 1500; d. Trento, Italy, January or February 1577), *medicine, botany.*

The son of Francesco Mattioli and Lucrezia Buoninsegni, Mattioli received his education at Padua when the family (originally from Siena) moved to Venice, where his father practiced medicine. In 1523 he graduated in philosophy and medicine at the University of Padua. After the death of his father he returned to Siena, going thence to Perugia and Rome, but after the sack of the city he went north to Trento. During his stay there, Mattioli continued his research on the simples (medicinal plants), particularly vegetables; he also practiced medicine with great success and became the close friend, adviser, and physician to Cardinal Bernard Clesio, bishop of Trento. While in Trentino, he wrote his first book, *De morbi gallici curandi ratione* (1530), recommending the use of mercury as the cure for syphilis. In 1540, after the death of Cardinal Clesio, the inhabitants of Gorizia invited Mattioli to practice medicine there.

In 1544 he published an Italian translation of the first five books of Dioscorides' *De materia medica*, accompanied by his *Discorsi et commenti*, which, through revisions and additions, made him famous. It was his intention to make available to physicians and pharmacists a practical manual, written in Italian, with a commentary, which would help them to identify the medicinal plants mentioned by Dioscorides. The first edition had no illustrations, but the following edition (1548), also in Italian, was illustrated with a new commentary, and was highly successful. This probably induced Mattioli to publish his Latin translation of Dioscorides' *De materia medica*, including also the sixth book, *De venenis et eorum curatione.* The work was enriched by synonyms in various languages and accompanied by his *Commentarii* and numerous illustrations of plants and animals valuable for the identification of Dioscorides' simples. This Latin edition—known by its abbreviated title of *Commentarii*—went through many editions and was translated into German, French, and Bohemian.

The success of this work was due to its format: it was a practical manual, useful as an everyday source of information for physicians, herbalists, pharmacists, and others, making it possible to identify and compare its plants with those mentioned by Dioscorides and found in nature. This work was totally different from the previous translations of Dioscorides, which usually dwelt more upon the philological critique of the text, rather than its medical and botanical aspects. Mattioli introduced much new information, partly derived from his direct observation of plants and partly obtained from other authors. Many of the illustrations were his own, or were derived from original drawings made available by other scholars. His work gathered together and coordinated all that was known of medical botany at that time. Mattioli's study of the medicinal effects of plants gave priority to the observation of their morphological characteristics, and therefore his work is less valid from the point of view of descriptive botany, even though

he did describe many new species. The species *Matthiola* was named in his honor.

The enormous fame that Mattioli had won resulted in him being summoned to Prague as court physician, first to Ferdinand I (1503–64), and then to Maximilian II (1527–76). In 1570 he left Prague, retiring to Innsbruck and Trentino. He had relations with the leading botanists of his time, including some—notably Melchiorre Guilandino (c. 1520-89), Luigi Anguillara (1512-70), and Amato Lusitano (1511-68)—with whom he had violent arguments.

Bibliography

Primary: 1598. (Bauhin, Caspar, ed.) *Opera quae extant omnia* (Frankfurt); 1530. *De morbi gallici curandi ratione* (Bologna); 1544. *Di Pedacio Dioscoride Anazarbeo libri cinque della historia et materia medicinale* (Venice); 1554. *Pedacii Dioscoridis de materia medica libri sex* (Venice); 1557. *I discorsi . . . ne i sei libri della materia medicinale di Pedacio Dioscoride Anazarbeo* (Venice).

Secondary: De Toni, Giovanni Battista, 1923. 'Pierandrea Mattioli' in Mieli, Aldo, ed., *Gli scienziati italiani dall'inizio del Medio Evo ai nostri giorni* I (Rome) pp. 382–387; *DSB.*

Giuseppe Ongaro

MAUDSLEY, HENRY   (b. Giggleswick, Yorkshire, England, 5 February 1835; d. Bushy Heath, Hertfordshire, England, 24 January 1918), *psychiatry.*

Born and raised in a gloomy Yorkshire farmhouse, suffering the deaths of his mother and three of his siblings when he was ten, Maudsley was educated privately thanks to his aunt, Elizabeth Bateson. Studying medicine at University College, London, qualifying MB (1856) and MD (1857), and obtaining by his report ten gold medals, on account of an extraordinary memory for anything he read, Maudsley initially planned a career in surgery or in the Indian Medical Service. Working as assistant medical officer at Wakefield, then Brentwood, County Asylums, attracted him to psychiatry, and he was appointed superintendent of the (private) Manchester Lunatic Asylum at Cheadle (1858).

Despite three successful years, with glowing testimonials, he became 'restless and desirous of change' and 'threw himself on London'. He became a physician to the West London Hospital (1864), a FRCP, and a professor of medical jurisprudence at University College Hospital (1869). More importantly, his writings (e.g., on Edgar Allen Poe and the genesis of mind) brought him to the attention of John C. Bucknill (1817–97), then editor of the *Journal of Mental Science*, and Maudsley became joint editor (1862) until resigning (1878). He was President of the Medico-Psychological Association (MPA) in 1870 and dominated British psychiatry during the 1860s and 1870s, as editor, writer, clinician, and critic, via a series of authoritative articles, books, and pamphlets.

In 1866 he married John Conolly's (1794–1866) youngest daughter, Anne, and a month before Conolly's death moved his work to Lawn House, a private asylum for six females. Thereafter, his private practice flourished, including likely aristocratic involvements (e.g., he was one of the three European experts appointed to the case of the Austrian Empress), such that in 1908 he could offer £30,000 for the foundation of a new hospital. This would provide early treatment and scientific research, as well as specialist training for psychiatrists, and became the Maudsley Hospital, eventually opening in 1914.

Intellectually, Maudsley was head and shoulders above his British contemporaries, being widely read in European philosophical, psychological, and scientific literature, though his favorites were Goethe and Shakespeare. He formulated a strongly materialist and nondualist view of the mind and mental illness, as outlined in his first and widely acclaimed publication *The Physiology and Pathology of Mind* (1867). This emphasized the neurological basis of mental activity and malfunction and the unity of mind and body. Further writings were much influenced by Auguste Comte, T. H. Huxley (1825–95), and Herbert Spencer (1820–1903) in terms of their positivist and social scientific views. He was a vociferous critic of the law's attitudes toward mental illness in terms of attributing responsibility, he regarded asylums as not much more than prisons, and he despaired the decline of nonrestraint. His views as to the essentially organic processes of the mind relied on inductive science rather than experimentation, and later works such as *Body and Will* (1883) and *Natural Causes and Supernatural Seemings* (1886) were received critically by metaphysicians and empirical scientists alike.

Maudsley's combination of polymath, 'non-Christian' doctrines, and Yorkshire melancholy gave him a reputation for not suffering fools gladly. By 1879 he had given up Lawn House (concerned about his integrity as a private asylum owner), the editorship, and his chair. He moved increasingly away from the MPA philosophically and practically, decrying the institutional world of large asylums, legalism, and the general torpor of British psychiatry in the fin-de-siècle. Increasingly cynical and contentious, though reputed as an entertaining companion by those who knew him, his childlessness, his few friendships, and the slow decline of his wife, Anne, led to isolated retirement. His last (posthumous) work on 'war psychology' was both portentous and pessimistic. He destroyed his papers and was never knighted, but remained the most quoted of English psychiatrists for several decades.

Bibliography

Primary: 1867. *The Physiology and Pathology of Mind* (London); 1874. *Responsibility in Mental Diseases* (London); 1918. *Religion and Realities* (London).

Secondary: Collie, M., 1988. *Henry Maudsley: Victorian Psychiatrist. A Bibliographical Study* (Winchester); Turner, T. H., 1988. 'Henry Maudsley—Psychiatrist, Philosopher and Entrepreneur.' *Psychological Medicine* 18: 551–574; *Munk's Roll*; Oxford DNB.

Trevor Turner

AL-MAWṢILĪ, ʿAMMĀR IBN ʿALĪ (fl. *c.* 1010), *medicine, ophthalmology.*

The biographical material about ʿAmmār al-Mawṣilī that has come down to us is not very extensive; his epithet, al-Mawṣilī, indicates that his origins lay in Mossul, now northern Iraq. According to Ibn Abī Usaybiʿa's lexicon on Arab physicians, he moved to Egypt under the reign of al-Ḥākim (r. 996–1020/21); ʿAmmār himself mentions several journeys that took him to Khorasan, Mesopotamia, Syria, and other parts of the Near East.

ʿAmmār al-Mawṣilī was a famous eye doctor whose field of expertise included pharmaceutical treatment and surgical procedures—for instance, cataract operations. Two texts, both dealing with ophthalmology, have been transmitted under the name of al-Mawṣilī, one of which is genuine.

The Selection on Ophthalmology

The treatise *Kitāb al-muntakhab fī ʿilāj al-ʿayn* [Selection on Ophthalmology] survives in the Arabic original and a Hebrew translation by Nathan ha-Meathi (thirteenth century). The transmission of this treatise seems to be rather complicated, also because the Hebrew text differs widely from the Arabic and contains several additional chapters.

The structure of the treatise follows classical Greek models; the book begins with a description of the anatomy of the eye (followed by some additional chapters in the Hebrew translation explaining its functions). This is followed by an extensive description of the pathology and therapy of the eye arranged in anatomical order; i.e., the diseases of the eyelids form the first part and are followed by the diseases of the conjunctiva and so on.

The most interesting part of the book is his management of cataract treatment toward the end of the treatise. Whereas some other chapters seem to be part of a canon of ophthalmological knowledge and probably repeat earlier Greek sources, the description of surgical procedures and diagnosis are likely to be original and written by al-Mawṣilī.

In contrast to other parts of the treatise, here the theoretical instructions for treatment of a disease—in the case of the cataract—are followed by narrative accounts of operations performed by the author himself. All four histories describe complications and unusual or unexpected events during or following an operation, and they emphasize the importance of experience for medical practice.

The Tractatus de oculis canamosali

Several details, in particular the title and the name of the author given by the manuscripts, suggest the short Latin text on the eye by a certain Canamosali is also a work of al-Mawṣilī. In fact, it does not bear any similarity to the selection on ophthalmology described above; the treatise is divided into seven books, which are mostly devoted to recipes of eye salves and pharmaceutical ingredients. The text focuses on frequent diseases and humoral theory and does not attempt to be comprehensive.

Bibliography

Primary: 1904. 'Magistri David Armenici compilatio in libros de oculorum curationibus Accanamosali et diversorum philosophorum de Baldach' in Pansier, P., ed. *Collectio ophtalmologica* [sic] *veterum auctorum,* fasc. IV (Paris) pp. 1–56; Hirschberg, J., J. Lippert, and E. Mittwoch, eds., 1905. 'Ammār ibn 'Alī al-Mawṣilī. Das Buch der Auswahl von den Augenkrankheiten. Halifa al-Halabi Das Buch vom Genügenden' in *Augenheilkunde Salah ad-Din Licht der Augen aus arabischen Handschriften übersetzt und erläutert* (Leipzig); Meyerhof, M., 1937. *Las operaciones de catarata de Ammār ibn 'Alī al-Mawṣilī oculista de el Cairo (Principios del siglo XI)* (Barcelona).

Secondary: Ullmann, M., 1970. 'Die Medizin im Islam' in *Handbuch der Orientalistik* I 4, 1 (Leiden and Cologne); Scalinci, N., 1934. *Il liber pro sanitate oculorum di M.o Davide Armenio occulista Salernitano del secolo XII (noto come tractatus de oculis Canamosali)* (Naples); Hirschberg, J., 1905. *Die arabischen Lehrbücher der Augenheilkunde, ein Capitel zur arabischen Litteraturgeschichte, unter Mitwirkung von J. Lippert und E. Mittwoch* (Berlin).

Barbara Zipser

MAYO, WILLIAM JAMES

MAYO, WILLIAM JAMES (b. LeSueur, Minnesota, USA, 29 June 1861; d. Rochester, Minnesota, USA, 28 July 1939), *surgery, gastrointestinal surgery.* **MAYO, CHARLES HORACE** (b. LeSueur, Minnesota, USA, 19 July 1865; d. Chicago, Illinois, USA, 26 May 1939), *surgery.*

William ('Will') Mayo was the eldest child of William Worrall Mayo, a general practitioner and gynecologic surgeon. At the age of nineteen (1880), he began his medical school education at the University of Michigan. Upon graduation from medical school in 1883, Will joined his father in practice in Rochester, Minnesota. His brother Charles ('Charlie') did likewise upon his graduation from Chicago Medical College in 1888. The brothers spent their entire professional career in Rochester.

When Will joined his father's practice, it was already a large one; W. W. Mayo was considered to be one of the finest operative gynecologists in Minnesota. Most of the surgery performed by the Mayos during the early 1890s was gynecological in nature, and during that early period, the brothers continued to devote most of their time to general practice.

Will and Charlie soon became frustrated with the uselessness of the medical remedies of the period. Meanwhile, Listerian methods of antisepsis were allowing surgeons to enter the internal cavities of the body for the first time. This fact made surgery a much more exciting and promising field of endeavor to the Mayo brothers. The large volume of procedures they came to perform, and the skillfulness with which they carried them out, soon brought them recognition within the profession. For example, at the age of twenty-seven, Will presented a masterful report on diseases of the appendix, based on his already broad experience, to the Surgical Section of the Minnesota State Medical Society. So impressed was the assemblage that, despite his young age, they immediately elected him chairman of that section.

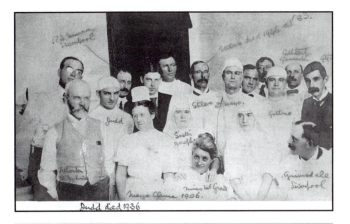

Group portrait at the Mayo Clinic, 1906. William Mayo stands sixth from the right. Halftone reproduction, Wellcome Library, London.

As their father began limiting his practice hours, and the number of patients referred to them for surgery continued to grow, Will and Charlie found it necessary to associate with physicians who could attend to the nonsurgical aspects of their work. This was the beginning of the Mayo cooperative practice, which was eventually to become the Mayo Clinic. The first physician to join them was A. W. Stinchfield in 1892. The second was Christopher Graham in 1894. Others followed, the most notable early addition being Henry Plummer in 1901.

The Mayo brothers took great pains to stay abreast of new developments in their field. Even early in their careers, when they could ill afford the time and money required to do so, they spent several weeks each year traveling to surgical centers throughout the United States. Their first trips were to New York, to see the work of Arpad Gerster, Robert Abbe, Charles McBurney, and others. From them the brothers learned several procedures, including the McBurney method for removing impacted gallstones and Abbe's 'string-saw' procedure for dilating esophageal strictures.

For years Will and Charlie made weekly trips to Chicago to attend Christian Fenger's Thursday clinics. Other Chicago surgeons providing the brothers instruction during these early years included Nicholas Senn, Albert Ochsner, and John Murphy. From the latter Will learned of the 'Murphy button' for intestinal anastomosis, which he used successfully for ten years. The brothers were also frequent visitors to Johns Hopkins University in Baltimore. From William Halsted they learned of a procedure for repairing inguinal hernias and another for the radical removal of breast cancer. It was also from Halsted that they learned the intricacies of Listerian technique and the use of rubber gloves during surgery.

During the first decade of their career, the Mayo brothers often operated as a team, but in the late 1890s, they took on assistants and began to operate separately. Will took an early interest in intra-abdominal procedures, and in the years to come, he became famous for his reports of large series of such cases in the medical literature. So sudden was his appearance on the surgical scene that when Will first submitted such a 'blockbuster' series of cases for publication in 1899 (105 surgeries for gallbladder disease), the journal's editor found it impossible to believe and immediately rejected the manuscript. Only after personal visits to Rochester by Carl Beck and others did their fellow surgeons come to realize that the Mayo brothers' reports were legitimate.

The most important of the large case series reported by the Mayo team include a report of 303 operations on the stomach and first portion of the duodenum (Mayo, 1903), 500 cases of gastroenterostomy (Mayo, 1905), 100 gastric resections for carcinoma of the stomach (Mayo, 1906a), and 1,500 cases of gallbladder surgery (Mayo, 1906b). The experience reflected in these reports was unmatched by any other surgeon of the period, and by 1905, Will Mayo was considered the foremost authority on stomach surgery in the United States.

The Mayo brothers not only devised new procedures, such as the overlapping of abdominal wall tissue in the treatment of umbilical hernia, but more importantly, they also expanded upon and perfected many of the procedures of others. For example, in the 'no-loop' gastroenterostomy, they included a lengthwise incision utilizing Moynihan clamps and shifted the angle at which the jejunum was joined to the stomach. Such modifications were facilitated by the fact that the Mayos performed surgery on such a large number of cases that their experience with a particular procedure often became greater than that of the surgeon who originally designed it. One of Will's main interests was stomach cancer, and he was the chief advocate of his generation for gastrectomy in cases of early disease, rightly seeing this as the only possible means of cure. Later in his career, he became known for his kidney and spleen surgery in addition to his gastrointestinal work.

When World War I interrupted the routine workings of the Clinic, both Will and Charlie assisted in the war effort. Will was appointed chairman of the Committee of American Physicians for Medical Preparedness in 1916 and later became Chief Consultant of the (American) Surgical Services. The Clinic, by now a sizable institution, also contributed manpower and materials in the form of a base hospital.

Many honors were bestowed upon Will Mayo in the course of his career. He was elected chairman of the Surgical Section of the American Medical Association at the age of thirty-seven (1898) and fellow of the Royal College of Surgeons of Edinburgh in 1905, and the next year, he was elected president of the American Medical Association. In 1907 Will was elected to the Board of Regents of the University of Minnesota, and in 1918 he was made president of the American College of Surgeons. He also received numerous honorary degrees from universities throughout the world.

Will Mayo continued to perform surgery until the age of sixty-seven. He performed his last procedure on 1 July 1928. Charlie performed his last surgery a year and a half later. Both brothers died in 1939. Ironically, Will died of a disease he had battled in so many of his patients: stomach cancer.

The Mayo Clinic and Affiliated Clinics and Hospitals

Throughout his professional life, Will Mayo served as chief administrator for the clinic that he and his brother had founded. The Mayo Clinic is, without a doubt, his greatest legacy.

Several factors converged to make the growth of the early Mayo practice unprecedented in the history of modern medicine. The newly described Listerian techniques allowed them to perform the intricate and invasive procedures for which they became famous. Also, the building of St Mary's Hospital in 1889 offered them a central 'base of operations' for their work, and the Sisters of St Frances provided their patients excellent nursing care. The reputation of their father as a great surgeon, coupled soon with their own reputations, brought them increasing numbers of patients from throughout Minnesota. The development of an efficient and extensive railway system also allowed patients from the 'new western frontier' states, especially North and South Dakota, relatively easy access to their skills. Will himself emphasized the importance of these factors in the growth of the Clinic when he advised his biographer to 'stress the unusual opportunity that existed in the time, the place, the general setup, not to be duplicated now' (Clapesattle, 1941, p. 270). But it must be stressed that the most important single factor in the early success and growth of the Mayo venture was the tremendous surgical skill of the brothers and their carefully chosen associates.

The number and variety of surgical procedures performed each year by the Mayos rose exponentially. They performed 655 surgical operations between the years 1889 and 1892. By 1904, the year prior to the opening of the third operating room at St Mary's, the brothers and their assistants were performing a total of 3,131 operations annually. The demand for surgical procedures became such that the medical practice during the early years virtually vanished, with the physicians in the group spending almost all of their time serving as diagnosticians, sorting the surgical from the nonsurgical patients. From 1889 to 1905, the brothers had only interns and assistants helping them in their operative work. They began associating with other surgeons in 1905, usually after having trained these men themselves. The first such associate surgeon to work with the Mayo brothers was E. Starr Judd. Numerous others soon followed. The internal medicine practice at the Clinic came into its own in the 1920s, research in medicine being greatly expanded by the first chairman of medicine of the Mayo Foundation, Leonard Rowntree, who brought with him a core group of medical researchers. Since the Rowntree years, progress in medicine has kept step with progress in surgery at the Clinic.

As the number of patients and staff expanded over the years, a series of ever-larger Clinic buildings were built to accommodate them. The first of these (now demolished) was erected in 1914, the second in 1928, and the third and fourth in 1950 and 2001, respectively. St Mary's (later renamed 'St Marys') Hospital, established by the Sisters of St Francis, opened its doors in 1889 with a capacity of forty-five beds and a single operating room. Since that time, it has seen numerous expansions and at present has a total of 1,157 inpatient beds and sixty operating rooms.

During the early years of the twentieth century, as the need for hospital beds in Rochester continued to grow, several smaller hospital facilities arose in the downtown area close to the Clinic buildings. These several establishments (the largest of which was the Colonial Hospital) came to be administered by the Methodist Board of Hospitals in the early 1950s. In 1966 the Rochester Methodist Hospital became operational, incorporating the functions of the various smaller hospitals. At present this hospital has a total of 794 beds and forty-one operating rooms.

Mayo now has affiliations with numerous medical centers in the Rochester area. The Mayo Health system, which had its beginnings in 1992, comprises a network of clinics and hospitals in sixty-four communities in Minnesota, Iowa, and Wisconsin. Also, to further accommodate Mayo patients living in other parts of the country, two additional Mayo sites were opened in Jacksonville, Florida, and Scottsdale, Arizona, in 1986 and 1987, respectively. In 2005 Mayo employed a total of 2,929 staff physicians and scientists and 1,924 residents, fellows, and temporary professionals. It employed a total of 46,836 people.

The Mayo founders are no longer present at the Clinic, but their legacy lives on. Although a great deal of research and education is conducted within the institution, its primary function remains the provision of excellent patient care. It is this excellence that has allowed its continued growth.

Bibliography

Primary: 1903. 'A Review of 303 Operations upon the Stomach and First Portion of the Duodenum, with Tabulated Report of 313 Operated Cases.' *Annals of Surgery* 38: 38–46; 1905. 'A Review of 500 Cases of Gastro-Enterostomy, Including Pyloroplasty, Gastroduodenostomy and Gastrojejunostomy.' *Annals of Surgery* 42: 641–655; 1906a. 'The Surgical Treatment of Cancer of the Stomach; with Report of 100 Gastric Resections.' *JAMA* 46: 999–1006; 1906b. 'A Review of 1500 Operations upon the Gallbladder and Bile Passages, with Special Reference to the Mortality.' *Annals of Surgery* 44: 209–216.

Secondary: Holmes, William, 1984. *Dedicated to Excellence: The Rochester Methodist Hospital Story* (Rochester); Clapesattle, Helen, 1941. *The Doctors Mayo* (Minneapolis); Anon., 1926. *Sketch of the History of the Mayo Clinic and the Mayo Foundation* (Philadelphia); *DAMB.*

John L. Graner

MAZZA, SALVADOR (b. Rauch, Buenos Aires Province, Argentina, 6 June 1886; d. Monterrey, Mexico, 9 November 1946), *rural medicine, epidemiology.*

Son of Sicilian immigrants, Mazza attended prestigious primary and secondary schools in Buenos Aires. Not having an affluent family, he had to work to pay for his college education. He became an aide in two laboratories and, over summer breaks, he worked as a vaccination assistant and a public health inspector in his hometown, Rauch. There, away from the capital city, he noticed how epidemic outbreaks resulted from the lack of preventive measures. Thus, he set up a vaccination office.

After graduating as a doctor from the School of Medical Sciences of the University of Buenos Aires (1910), he worked as a bacteriologist at the National Hygiene Department. There, at the leprosarium on Martín García island, he set up a laboratory where he examined immigrants, who were quarantined before entering Argentina, and screened them for the cholera bacillus. His efficiency, evidenced by his detection of the organism in two people that seemingly presented no symptoms, aroused the interest of German bacteriologist Rudolph Kraus, who called on him to work at Instituto Bacteriológico (1913–15). There, they both found out that the typhoid fever vaccine could be administered as a single dose, a reduction from the customary three injections prescribed until then (1919).

Mazza was in charge of the bacteriology department at Hospital Militar Central (1915–20). In 1916, during World War I, he was sent to Europe to study preventive measures against transmissible diseases in combatant armies.

Between 1920 and 1922, he combined his teaching activities as professor of the bacteriology chair at the University of Buenos Aires with his job as head of the laboratory at Hospital de Clínicas. In 1922 he undertook his second study trip to Europe, representing the University of Buenos Aires. He remained there for two years, which were instrumental in his professional development. He visited research centers in Europe and in colonial territories in northern Africa. He also met Charles Nicolle, the future Nobel Prize winner, who ran the Pasteur Institute in Tunisia. In this location, Mazza was impressed with the science as well as the good relations between scientists and authorities.

After returning to Buenos Aires (1924), Mazza managed to get the government to invite Nicolle to Argentina. Both bacteriologists traveled to Jujuy, a province in northeastern Argentina. As a result of their hard work, they managed to isolate the *Leishmania braziliensis* strain, which caused leishmaniasis, a disease affecting the skin and mucous membranes. Also, they observed the precarious living conditions of the local inhabitants and the need to create a research center for regional endemic diseases.

This led Mazza to propose that the University of Buenos Aires create the Misión de Estudios de Patología Regional Argentina (MEPRA), with headquarters in Jujuy (1926). MEPRA's multidisciplinary team studied the regional diseases and conducted numerous therapeutic activities. Also, MEPRA became a training and information release center for the scientific community.

Mazza combined his theoretical background with a painstaking gathering of data about the different types of ailments affecting people and their animals. His studies identified cases of infection with *Trypanosoma cruzi*, a pathogenic agent of Chagas' disease. His research showed that the parasite, whose vector is known as 'vinchuca' (*Triatoma infestans*), propagated easily in poor dwellings in northwestern Argentina. The local scientific community had thought the disease spread only in Brazil and did not exist in Argentina. Thus, this finding fostered further studies on the local characteristics of the disease, which had been discovered by Carlos Chagas in 1909. Furthermore, Mazza showed his peers the biological and environmental bases of other infectious processes, such as brucellosis and infantile kala-azar.

Bibliography

Primary: 1926. *Recuerdos médicos y otros recuerdos de Argelia y Túnez* (Buenos Aires); 1949. *Enfermedad de Chagas en la República Argentina* (Buenos Aires).

Secondary: Leonard, Jonathan, 1992. 'Research in the Argentine Outback: The Health Quest of Salvador Mazza.' *Bulletin of the Pan American Health Organization* 26(3): 256–270; Ivern, Andrés, 1987. *Vida y obra de Salvador Mazza: historia de una epopeya científica* (Rosario).

Karina Ramacciotti

MCBURNEY, CHARLES (b. Roxbury, Massachusetts, USA, 17 February 1845; d. Brookline, Massachusetts, USA, 3 November 1913), *surgery.*

McBurney's name is ineradicably associated with the diagnosis of appendicitis and the operation to cure that common disease.

McBurney was born in Roxbury, Massachusetts, and obtained his secondary school education at the renowned Boston Latin School. From there, he went on to Harvard College, from which he obtained BA and MA degrees. Following this, he enrolled at the College of Physicians and Surgeons in New York, at that time officially associated with Columbia University, but in fact an autonomous school owned by members of its faculty. After an internship at Bellevue Hospital, he followed the course taken by so many young American physicians, by extensive travel and study at European medical institutions, in his case London, Paris, and Vienna. At the age of twenty-eight, he returned to New York and opened his surgical practice.

McBurney's closest institutional affiliation was with Roosevelt Hospital in Manhattan, though he was at various times on the staff at Presbyterian, Bellevue, New York Hospital, St Luke's, and the Hospital for the Ruptured and Crippled (now the Hospital for Special Surgery). He served on the faculty of his alma mater for much of his career, as professor of surgery from 1889 to 1894 and then as clinical professor from 1894 until 1907. In 1888 he was appointed chief of surgery at the Roosevelt Hospital, remaining in that position for the next twelve years.

In 1886 Reginald Heber Fitts published the first major paper on the pathophysiology of appendicitis in the *Transactions of the Association of American Physicians*, not only giving the disease its name and calling attention to its characteristics, but also exciting considerable interest in its clinical manifestations. Within three years, McBurney had written a paper destined to become a classic in the history of medicine, 'Experience with Early Operative Interference in Cases of Disease of the Vermiform Appendix', in the *New York Medical Journal*, vol. 50, 1889. It was in this paper that he described what would come to be called McBurney's point: 'in every case the seat of greatest pain, determined by the pressure of one finger, has been very exactly between an inch and a half and two inches from the anterior spinous process of the ilium on a straight line drawn from that process to the umbilicus.'

Because of the size of McBurney's private practice and the many patients he saw in his capacity as a teacher, as well as his advocacy of early operation, he treated many people with appendicitis. In 1894 he was the first to describe the so-called gridiron incision earlier developed by L. L. Mc Arthur of Chicago, which would become the standard approach to opening the abdomen directly over the affected structure with minimal damage to the overlying muscular layer. By this technique, the fibers of the external and internal oblique muscles were separated by the process of splitting instead of by being cut, allowing them to fall back into normal position when the wound was closed, providing maximal strength during the healing phase. As with the famous point, the name of McBurney became the eponym for the incision.

Shortly after William Halsted described his first use of rubber gloves during aseptic surgery in 1889, McBurney took up the practice and became one of its strongest advocates, writing a paper in 1898 in the *Annals of Surgery* describing its good results in many operations, having presented those results at a meeting of the New York Surgical Society earlier that year. His papers in the surgical literature were written in a clear and direct manner that made them models of technical exposition, and his teaching was of a similar nature.

During much of his career, McBurney was the leading surgeon of Manhattan, and he developed a reputation for his early advocacy of asepsis, the wide variety of his surgical endeavors, and the vast extent of his operative experience. But to the generations that followed, he would always be the man who introduced his colleagues to McBurney's point and McBurney's incision.

Bibliography

Secondary: Thien, V., 2000. 'Charles McBurney: Reflecting upon His Life's Work.' *Journal of Investigative Surgery* 13: 3–5; Smith, D.,

1986. 'Appendicitis, Appendectomy and the Surgeon.' *New York State Journal of Medicine* 86: 571–583, 639–647; 1966. 'Charles McBurney (1845–1913)—Point, Sign, and Incision.' *JAMA* 197: 1098–1099; *DAMB*.

Sherwin Nuland

MCDOWELL, EPHRAIM   (b. Rockbridge County, Virginia, USA, 11 November 1771; d. Danville, Kentucky, USA, 25 June 1830), *surgery*.

Born to prominent and wealthy parents, Samuel and Mary (McClung) McDowell, Ephraim moved with his family to Kentucky in 1783. McDowell received the best liberal education Kentucky had to offer, and after studying medicine under Alexander Humphreys for several years, he enrolled as a medical student at the University of Edinburgh. McDowell left Edinburgh in 1795 sans diploma and began practice at his home in Danville, Kentucky. The practice of medicine without a degree was common at that time, and McDowell prospered under the empowerment of influential connections cast in the halo of his Edinburgh studies. In 1802 those connections were further strengthened when he married Sarah Hart Shelby, daughter of Kentucky's first governor, Isaac Shelby (1750–1826). They had six children: two sons and four daughters.

McDowell's fame rests upon a case in December 1809 that called him to examine Jane Todd Crawford (1764?–1842). Her distended abdomen was at first thought to be a pregnancy, but after more than the usual nine-month term elapsed, a physical disorder was suspected. Upon examination, McDowell confirmed that the problem was an ovarian mass. After some hesitation, he concluded that only an operation could save the woman. The procedure needed to be performed at McDowell's residence, some sixty miles from Crawford's home. Despite the discomfort and dangers of travel, Crawford made the trip. On Christmas Day, McDowell, with the assistance of his physician nephew, James McDowell, and Alban Smith, removed a cystic and partly solid tumor weighing a total of twenty-two and a half pounds. The operation took only twenty-five minutes. Five days later, McDowell surprisingly found his patient up and making her bed; about three weeks later, he sent her home in good health.

Because this was a time when every abdominal surgery to date had resulted in peritonitis and death, McDowell's success deserves comment. Undoubtedly, a good deal may be attributed to his scrupulously clean habits and his meticulousness. His 1817 report details how he removed blood from the peritoneal cavity, bathed the intestines in warm water, and carefully drained the remaining blood from the area once the intestines were returned to the cavity. Adhesive plaster was placed between stitches to aid in wound closure and healing.

This procedure would serve him well. By the time McDowell published a report of his path-breaking ovariotomy some seven years later, he had successfully performed the procedure on two black women as well. But fame was not immediate. Prominent University of Pennsylvania surgeon Philip Physick (1768–1837) dismissed and even disparaged McDowell's achievement, as did James Johnson, editor of the *London Medico-Chirurgical Review*. These detractors notwithstanding, the Medical Society of Philadelphia publicly recognized McDowell's contribution in 1817, and eight years later, he received an honorary degree from the University of Maryland, an accomplishment that had eluded the gifted surgeon since his Edinburgh days. McDowell would perform the lifesaving operation another ten times. He lived out the remainder of his life in his beloved Danville.

Today McDowell is internationally renowned. His image appears on the official seal of the Southern Surgical Association, and on 3 December 1959, the U.S. Postal Service honored McDowell with a four-cent stamp bearing his image. With no formal degree and working under crude pioneer conditions, he epitomized the characteristics and professional qualities of a surgeon *par excellence*.

Bibliography

Primary: 1817. 'Three Cases of Extirpation of Diseased Ovaria.' *Eclectic Repertory and Analytical Review* 7: 242–244; 1819. 'Observation on Diseased Ovaria.' *Eclectic Repertory and Analytical Review* 9: 546.

Secondary: Tan, S. Y, J. D. Wong, and C. Wong, 2005. 'Ephraim McDowell (1771–1830): Pioneer of Ovariotomy.' *Singapore Medical Journal* 46(1): 4–5; Othersen, H. Biemann, Jr., 2004. 'Ephraim McDowell: The Qualities of a Good Surgeon.' *Annals of Surgery* 239 (May): 648–650; Van Doren, Charles, ed., 1984. *Webster's American Biographies* (Springfield, MA); Schachner, August, 1921. *Ephraim McDowell: "Father of Ovariotomy" and Founder of Abdominal Surgery* (Philadelphia); *DAMB*.

Michael A. Flannery

MCGRIGOR, JAMES   (b. Cromdale, Inverness shire, Scotland, 9 April 1771; d. London, England, 2 April 1858), *military surgery, military medicine*.

James was the eldest of three sons of Colquhoun McGrigor (d. 1797), general merchant of Aberdeen and founder of the Aberdeen Gaelic Church. McGrigor was educated at Aberdeen Grammar School and then Marischal College, Aberdeen, where he graduated MA (1788). He was apprenticed to Dr French in Aberdeen, but because there was no formal instruction in medicine in Aberdeen, he walked to Edinburgh, where he attended medical classes from 1789 to 1791, but did not graduate. Shortly after he returned to Aberdeen (1792), the French Revolution broke out. It was then his wish to become an army surgeon. He journeyed to London and attended Mr Wilson's lectures on Anatomy. In September 1793 he purchased the post of surgeon in De Burgh's Regiment, later called the 88th or Connaught Rangers, and served with them in Flanders. In 1795 he was posted to the West Indies, but was shipwrecked on the way there. He later served in Grenada and St Vincent, and then in Bombay. In 1801 he proceeded to Ceylon. He was put in medical charge of 8,000 Indian and European troops sent to join the army in Egypt under Major-General David Baird.

On returning to England, McGrigor transferred to the Blues (Royal Horse Guards) and served with them in Canterbury and Windsor. He proceeded to finish his MD at Marischal College, Aberdeen (1804). In 1805 he was promoted to inspector general of hospitals based at York and then was transferred to Winchester. He took charge of the troops who had returned from Corunna in 1809. Later that year, he was sent to Walcheren, Netherlands, where many of the men either died of or suffered from malaria. Shortly afterward, he was promoted to inspector general of hospitals there and in 1811 was appointed physician in charge of the barracks in Portsmouth. On the recommendation of the Duke of York, he was sent early in 1812 to join the Duke of Wellington in the Peninsula. He introduced long-needed reforms into the administration of the army, and for this he was knighted (1814). In 1815 he was appointed director-general of the army medical department.

After Waterloo, all candidates for entry into the medical service sat for an entrance examination and were interviewed to determine their suitability. McGrigor was particularly involved in the education of army medical officers and insisted that advance would only be achieved following evidence of merit or enthusiasm. He advocated that medical officers should, where or when possible, gain a university degree and that physicians and surgeons should pass the Fellowship or equivalent examinations of their appropriate specialty. Many attended the three-month winter lecture courses on military surgery offered at the University of Edinburgh or attended Guthrie's lectures on surgery given in London.

McGrigor established the Museum of Natural History and Pathological Anatomy and Reference Library, at Fort Pitt, Chatham. He inaugurated the system of medical reports and returns from all military stations that twenty years later became the *Statistical Returns of the Health of the Army*. He organized the efficient removal of the wounded from the battlefield, basing his system on the work of Jean Dominique Larrey (1766–1842) during Napoleon's campaigns. He emphasized the need for the assistance of the widows and dependants of medical officers and believed that medical officers should be awarded military decorations like other meritorious serving officers. He was created a baronet in 1831, but it took until 1850 before a number of army surgeons were awarded the military division of the Order of the Bath.

He was director-general of the army medical department for thirty-five years and was only eventually allowed to retire from this post in 1851.

Bibliography

Primary: 1816. *Sketch of the Medical History of fhe* [sic] *British Armies in the Peninsula of Spain and Portugal, During the Late Campaigns* (London); 1861. *The Autobiography and Services of Sir J. McGrigor Bt., Late Director-General of the Army Medical Department*.

Secondary: McGrigor, Mary, ed., 2000. *Sir James McGrigor: The Scalpel and the Sword: The Autobiography of the Father of Army Medicine* (Dalkeith, Scotland); Blanco, R. L., 1974. *Wellington's Surgeon General—Sir James McGrigor* (Durham, NC); *Oxford DNB*.

Matthew Howard Kaufman

MCKEOWN, THOMAS

MCKEOWN, THOMAS (b. Portadown, Ulster, Northern Ireland, 2 November 1912; d. Birmingham, England, 13 June 1988), *epidemiology, social medicine, demography.*

Born in Portadown into the divided society of Ulster, McKeown was the second of three sons born after a daughter to William McKeown and Matilda Duff. Both parents were officers in the Salvation Army, and William, a builder, was also a Presbyterian preacher. When McKeown was nine years old, the family emigrated to Vancouver, Canada, where McKeown went to Burnaby South High School, entering the University of British Columbia so young that he had graduated with a first in chemistry by the age of nineteen. His precocious trajectory was sustained with a national research scholarship to McGill University, where he completed a doctorate in endocrinology under Hans Selye (1907–82) by age twenty-two, thence moving to Trinity College, Oxford, on a Rhodes scholarship. Here he completed his second doctorate in physiology (1938), coauthoring publications (on ferret reproductive physiology) with Wilfred Le Gros Clark (1895–1971, organizer of The Committee against Malnutrition at that time) and Solly Zuckerman (1904–93).

He commenced medical studies at Guy's Hospital, London (1939), while employed there as a demonstrator in physiology and also continuing research in endocrinology. He graduated MB BS in 1942, by which time he had also been working as part of a team, under his Oxford mentor Zuckerman, on an influential official investigation into the effects of enemy bombing on the population and morale of Londoners. In 1937 he had met Esmé Joan Bryan, daughter of Thomas William Widdowson, a consultant in dentistry at King's College, London, and in 1940 they married. They had a son, Michael (b. 1947), and a daughter, Suzie (b. 1951).

In 1944, at age just thirty-two, he applied for the chair of anatomy at Birmingham University. He so impressed the interviewing panel (who appointed Zuckerman himself to this Chair) that the following year he was invited by the Dean, Leonard Parsons (1879–1950), to apply for a new chair in social medicine at Birmingham University, funded initially for three years by the Nuffield Foundation, following the precedent set by Nuffield at Oxford, where John Ryle (1889–1950) had been appointed to the first such chair in the country. McKeown was to remain in this post until his retirement in 1977, though he traveled and lectured internationally; he was also a consultant and committee chairman at the WHO for many years after his retirement until his death from cancer.

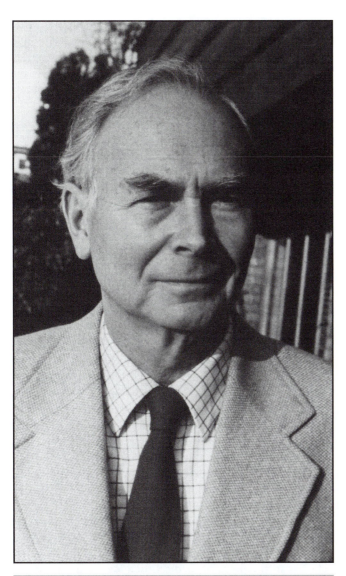

Thomas McKeown, 1988. Photograph, Wellcome Library, London. Reproduced with permission of Mrs Esmé McKeown.

The new discipline of social medicine was a highly ambitious project in all senses. Intellectually born of the egalitarian left of the Socialist Medical Association in the 1930s, politically—like the NHS itself—it was a child of postwar reconstructive, liberal humanitarian ideals. Social medicine sought to replace and massively expand the scope of 'public health' medicine. Public health was unnecessarily limited in scope to the administration by one isolated section of the profession— the local medical officers of health (MoHs)—of the statutory controls legislated by Parliament to prevent infectious and sanitary diseases. Instead, social medicine would offer all doctors a comprehensive view of the full diversity of medical needs of all in society, notably including the chronic sick, the disabled, the elderly, and those with mental health problems. Relevant research would be pursued to guide health policy and services through the investigation of population health patterns, using epidemiological techniques to analyze the health implications of the changing social and economic environment and of people's changing behavior.

As the new professor of social medicine, McKeown was sent by the Nuffield Foundation on a comprehensive, eight-month tour of medical departments and institutions in the United States and Canada to survey new developments and ideas relevant to the emerging field (resulting in an exceptionally thorough and politically acute evaluation of the state of 'American Medical Services', which McKeown published in the second volume of the *British Journal of Social Medicine*, 1948). Once back at Birmingham, McKeown rapidly built a research-active department from scratch, commencing a number of highly productive epidemiological research collaborations with colleagues, often utilizing local Birmingham data. With (C. R.) Ron Lowe (1912–93) he analyzed the medical and social needs of the hospitalized elderly chronic sick, showing that 60 percent would be better placed, if suitably supported, in their own homes. With R. G. Record and B. MacMahon, he began a series of studies of congenital malformations, focusing particularly on infantile pyloric stenosis. The pioneering research explored environmental influences such as season of birth, maternal age, and birth rank and showed how the latter were related to socioeconomic status, as was differential incidence in the causes of stillbirth. With Record he also initiated the first population-based continuous register of malformations, providing the basis for valuable cohort-studies, which subsequently stimulated an international network of similar registers. With J. R. Gibson he analyzed medical records of all 23,970 births occurring in Birmingham in 1947 to investigate relations between duration of gestation, birth weight, prematurity, survival, and socioeconomic status. McKeown and Record were also subsequently able to follow up on the 1947 births, to produce studies of measured intelligence scores in this cohort at age eleven, including studies on sets of twins, finding an absence of relationship between intelligence scores and various prenatal factors, such as birth weight, but finding that the effects of postnatal influences of environment and socioeconomic status could be positively demonstrated. These projects and others produced an impressive flow of as many as ten high-quality research articles in some years throughout the 1950s and 1960s, published in premier research journals on both sides of the Atlantic

McKeown always played a leading institutional role in the new discipline of social medicine. He was a member of the editorial board of the *British Journal of Social Medicine* and joined F. A. E. Crew (1886–1973) and Lancelot Hogben (1895–1975, who rapidly became a great friend of the McKeowns) as co-editor (1951). Founded in 1947, the journal virtually defined the new field for a decade. It became the *British Journal of Social and Preventive Medicine* (1953) and subsequently the *Journal of Epidemiology and*

Community Health (1978), reflecting successive shifts in the dominant professional definitions of public medicine. McKeown was also one of the five members of the original steering committee of the Society for Social Medicine, founded in 1956, and he organized and chaired its first annual scientific meeting at his department in Birmingham University (1957). During the 1950s and 1960s, he took on an increasingly public role as a leading advocate of social medicine, as the new discipline struggled to make the impact it aimed for on the nation's health services. A number of high-profile lectures and articles culminated in his first book: *Medicine in Modern Society. Medical Planning Based on Medical Achievement* (1965).

McKeown argued for radical reform of the medical profession and its associated hospital and medical-education systems in order to achieve a set of structures best serving the requirements of a national health service, rather than the historic, commercial self-interests of hospital consultants. He was an early advocate for the application of economic-management principles within the NHS. In the past of private practice, hospital consultants had ensured the dominance of their curative specialties, offered to a wealthy paying minority. Now that citizens' taxes paid for the nation's health services in a liberal democracy, McKeown foresaw that the key economic criterion of 'opportunity cost' would be increasingly invoked to justify resources devoted to different medical activities, with the perceived needs of suffering patients playing an increasingly influential role. In particular he believed the voting public's priorities would require greater diversion of medical resources into traditionally low-status activities, such as care for the elderly and those with chronic illnesses, pain, and disabilities; services for the mentally ill; and comfort for the dying. He advocated a clear plan of reorganization, arguing that both the design of hospitals and the structure of medical education had to be simultaneously changed to effect the necessary transformation in the medical profession to fit the needs of a national health service. The subsequent 1974 changes to the nation's health services, boosting the role of social services and converting MoHs into consultant-grade members of the new faculty of community medicine, did not conform at all exactly to McKeown's blueprint, but certainly reflected the influence of his powerful advocacy for change.

McKeown's trademark approach was to argue both a general and a principled case for a superior system to the current one on the basis of clearly enunciated principles of need, justice, and efficiency, which were hard to dispute, while also demonstrating, through a historical account, that the medical profession had little justification to defend the status quo on the grounds of its past record of achievement. Overall, it was a devastating strategy, pulled off with great panache. McKeown was a formidable opponent for the conservative interests in the medical establishment to face, considering that he was not only an elegant and persuasive writer (reflecting and benefiting from his intellectual first love, which was in fact literature), but also a witty public speaker and ruthless debater. His obituary in *Lancet* pointedly noted that the medical elite had failed to nominate the profession's leading internal critic for a single civil honor during his lifetime.

It was the historically grounded research that he produced in a series of articles with R. G. Brown, R. G. Record, and R. D. Turner that eventually became his most well-known and long-lasting intellectual contribution to the disciplines of both medicine and history. The 'McKeown thesis' has remained a staple of textbooks for three decades since it was given its final, summary form in the academic best seller *The Modern Rise of Population* (1976). In fact there were two distinct McKeown theses, a negative and a positive one. The negative thesis constituted McKeown's most iconoclastic and enduring blow against the incumbent elite of the medical profession. This was the finding that scientific, clinical, curative, and therapeutic medicine could not claim to have played a significant role in most of the improvement in population health that had occurred from the time of the industrial revolution until the 1930s. This was for the very simple and compelling reason that, with the exception of smallpox, most medical advances in therapy, surgery, drugs, antibiotics, vaccinations, etc. had arrived far too recently to account for the long-term secular fall in mortality rates from most infectious diseases. This has remained an irrefutable finding and a permanent diminution in our evaluation of the historic achievements of medical science and the medical profession. The finding was also important in helping to open up the discipline of medicine itself to a more receptive attitude toward the reflective and critical approaches to its history, practices, and theories pioneered in the 1960s and 1970s by other scholars in the fields of medical sociology and the history of science and medicine.

McKeown's positive historical thesis has proved to be far more scientifically contentious and subject to revisionist challenge, but in so doing, it has also been highly productive, generating decades of consequent debate and research. McKeown argued that although medical science and the medical profession could take little credit for the modern fall in mortality rates, which, he believed, had primarily driven the modern rise of population, a review of the human historical record indicated that three identifiable factors were positively responsible both for the relatively high mortality suffered in pre-modern times and for the progressive alleviation of those problems during the post-industrial, modern era. These three factors were food supply, 'hygiene', and degree of 'crowding' of the population (invoking the Malthusian notion of tendencies to over-population). Before the industrial revolution, there had been problems in all three respects, whereas since industrialization, all three had been progressively optimized. McKeown argued that British historical evidence showed that the most significant single source of these historic mortality improvements had been the increasing per capita nutrition made available since the eighteenth century by the rapidly growing British economy. This was followed from the 1870s onward by the secondary factors of improved 'hygiene' (municipal sanitation, etc.) and new habits of contraception (a solution to the Malthusian problem). The demographic historians of the Cambridge Group have since shown, however, that, contrary to McKeown's assumptions, rapid population growth during Britain's industrialization was due mainly to fertility rising, not mortality falling, and that the modern British mortality decline in fact began in the 1870s, a whole century later than McKeown had supposed. Building on this, the Szreter critique has argued that McKeown significantly underestimated the importance of social intervention, in the form of the late Victorian public health movement's sanitary and environmental measures, in initiating Britain's modern mortality decline. On the other hand, the importance of nutrition has continued to receive strong support from two high-profile research projects during the last three decades, one conducted by the eminent economic historian Robert Fogel and the other by the leading medical researcher David Barker.

A major reason for the massive influence and continuing interest in McKeown's intellectual agenda is the wide scope of his synthesis and vision, which brought into dialogue core interests and debates in the distinct major disciplines of medicine, evolutionary biology, and economic history, while also showing that our historical and evolutionary interpretations link closely to major contemporary policy concerns in the health services. The kernel of his own radical and subversive perspective, as expounded in his Rock Carling lectures of 1976, *The Role of Medicine. Dream, Mirage or Nemesis,* was that 'it is assumed that we are ill and are made well, whereas it is nearer the truth to say that we are well and are made ill.'

McKeown challenged fundamentally the orthodox metaphors of modern medical science, which envisaged the body as a complex machine subject to breakdown and to attack, repairable and defensible through applied medical knowledge, the product of the separate, reasoning, scientific mind. Instead, McKeown argued, the human body should be seen as an essentially fit and healthy entity—thanks to evolution. However, the body was also a composite with the human mind and was enmeshed in the changing forms of social and economic activity created by human culture. History showed this generated potential threats to health because it created environmental conditions and associated behaviors different from those of humans' adaptive evolutionary past. It was the role of a humanist social medicine to monitor keenly these often human-created 'environmental' hazards to life, to understand the origins of the diseases they produced, to devise solutions through medical science where possible, and to provide care and comfort to the sick and dying when cure was not possible.

McKeown was an articulate and learned man of ideas, distinguished by his fearless willingness to utter in public the uncomfortable truth as he saw it—and to pursue it at length. He was not always right, but he was always highly stimulating, and he had a huge, constructive impact both on the practice of medicine and on the study of the history of human health. His approach exemplified exactly the tenets of the great Henry Sigerist (1891–1957), doyen of the history of medicine, who wrote, 'The historical analysis is a method that can be applied profitably in medicine as in other fields to clarify concepts, to make trends and developments conscious, so that we may face them openly and may act more intelligently.'

Bibliography

Primary: 1955. (with Brown, R. G.) 'Medical Evidence Related to English Population Changes in the Eighteenth Century.' *Population Studies* 9: 119–141; 1962. (with Record, R. G.) 'Reasons for the Decline of Mortality in England and Wales during the Nineteenth Century.' *Population Studies* 16: 94–122; 1965. *Medicine in Modern Society. Planning Based on Medical Achievement* (London); 1966. (with Lowe, C. R.) *An Introduction to Social Medicine* (London, 2nd edn. 1974); 1971. (ed. with McLachlan, G.) *Medical History and Medical Care* (Oxford); 1975. (with Record, R. G., and R. D. Turner) 'An Interpretation of the Decline of Mortality in England and Wales during the Twentieth Century.' *Population Studies* 29: 391–422; 1976. *The Modern Rise of Population* (London); 1976. *The Role of Medicine. Dream, Mirage or Nemesis* (London; republished in extended form, 1979, Oxford); 1988. *The Origins of Human Disease* (Oxford).

Secondary: Pemberton, J., 2000. 'Origins and Early History of the Society for Social Medicine in the UK and Ireland.' *Journal of Epidemiology and Community Health* 56: 342–346; 1988. Obituary. *British Medical Journal,* 9 July, p. 129; 1988. Obituary. *Lancet,* 2 July, p. 58; 1988. Obituary. *The Times,* 20 June; 1988. Obituary. *The Independent,* 21 June; Szreter, S., 1988. 'The Importance of Social Intervention in Britain's Mortality Decline c. 1850–1914: A Reinterpretation of the Role of Public Health.' *Social History of Medicine* 1(1): 1–37, note 102, p. 34; Porter, D., ed., 1997. *Social Medicine and Medical Sociology in the Twentieth Century* (Amsterdam); Leck, I., 1996. 'McKeown, Record and the Epidemiology of Malformations.' *Paediatr. Perinat. Epidemiology* 10(1): 2–16; *Oxford DNB.*

Simon Szreter

MCMICHAEL, JOHN (b. Gatehouse of Fleet, Kirkcudbrightshire, Scotland, 25 July 1904; d. Merton, near Oxford, England, 3 March 1993), *cardiology, clinical science.*

The youngest of five children of James McMichael and his wife, Margaret, from Gatehouse of Fleet on the coast of the Irish Sea, John remembered his father, a farmer and local butcher, as a God-fearing and kind-natured man who struggled to make ends meet. Up to the age of ten, McMichael was educated at a local school under the patronage of the Lady of the Manor. When this school was closed, he transferred to Girthon Public School, where his first teacher was William Learmonth, father of the Edinburgh surgeon Sir James Learmonth. At age fourteen his parents followed Learmonth's suggestion and sent their son to Kirkudbright Academy, where he blossomed. With a local scholarship and a Carnegie Scholarship, he went to Edinburgh, where he studied medicine and graduated (1927) with honors, a scholarship, and a gold medal.

After junior posts at Bradford Royal Infirmary and Paddington Green Children's Hospital in London, McMichael returned to Edinburgh as Sir David Wilkie's (1882–1938) house surgeon. He started research on splenic anemia, which was to become the subject of his MD thesis. In Wilkie's laboratory, he met Stanley Davidson (1894–1981), whom he accompanied to Aberdeen, supported by a Beit Memorial Fellowship, when Davidson was appointed Regius professor. Conditions in Aberdeen were poor for the experimental work to which McMichael was committed by this stage, and he was thrilled to move to London (1932) to work in Thomas Renton Elliot's (1877–1961) Medical Unit at University College Hospital (UCH), which was funded by the Medical Research Council as part of a program to establish in Britain an infrastructure for full-time clinical research. His time at UCH brought McMichael into contact with the pioneer of clinical science, Thomas Lewis (1881–1945), as well as members of his own generation who were to shape the field in Britain in subsequent decades, such as George Pickering (1904–80) and Harold Himsworth (1905–93). McMichael completed work on his MD dissertation on liver and spleen fibrosis, for which he was awarded a gold medal by Edinburgh University. His Beit Fellowship ended in 1934, and he returned to Edinburgh as a Lecturer in Human Physiology. Although faced with a large teaching load, he managed to undertake research on the physiology of the heart. In 1937 a research fellowship that assured his appointment to the Royal Infirmary Edinburgh as an assistant physician allowed him to return to clinical research.

In 1938 Francis Fraser (1885–1964), the first director of the department of medicine at the recently established Postgraduate Medical School at Hammersmith Hospital, persuaded McMichael to apply for a vacant readership. In the following year, McMichael found himself effectively in charge of the department of medicine when Fraser left to set up the Emergency Medical Service. The move to Hammersmith proved crucial for McMichael's further career and the development of clinical science in Britain. In the decades that followed, he turned the department at Hammersmith into a major center for clinical research on cardiovascular diseases and other medical problems. During the war, much research work in the department was dedicated to 'crush syndrome' and liver disease, which McMichael and Sheila Sherlock (1918–2001) addressed by applying the new method of liver biopsy. In 1942 McMichael and E. P. Sharpey-Schafer (1908–1963) established another new invasive technique at the Hammersmith—cardiac catheterization, for which they were much criticized by a clinical establishment that opposed such procedures as unethical. From 1946 to 1966, McMichael was professor of medicine and director of the School. He turned to work on the pathology and the pharmacology of heart failure, focusing particularly on the effects of digitalis and related drugs. In the 1950s (when his second wife, Sybil, developed severe hypertension), he became interested in the treatment of high blood pressure with the new drugs that were becoming available in these years. McMichael's students have praised him for the stimulating research environment he established at Hammersmith. He emphasized teamwork across disciplines and did not allow staff to work in private practice while affiliated with the department.

McMichael's many honors included FRS (1957) and a knighthood (1965). He was a member of the MRC from 1949 to 1953. After leaving Hammersmith in 1966, he continued to influence clinical science and medical education in Britain as director of the British Postgraduate Medical Federation until 1971 and as a Wellcome trustee until 1977.

Bibliography

Primary: 1950. *Pharmacology of the Failing Human Heart* (Springfield, IL).

Secondary: Dollery, Colin, 1995. 'Sir John McMichael.' *Biographical Memoirs of Fellows of the Royal Society* 41: 283–296; *Oxford DNB*.

Carsten Timmermann

MEAD, RICHARD (b. Stepney, Middlesex, England, 11 August 1673; d. London, England, 11 February 1754), *medicine, antiquarianism.*

Mead was the eleventh of the thirteen children of Mathew Meade (1628/9–99), a nonconforming minister, and his wife, Elizabeth Walton (d. 1707). Mead was educated at home and, while his father was in the Netherlands because of involvement in the Rye House plot of 1683, temporarily at a private school run by a dissenter in Clerkenwell Close. In 1689 Mead, who was already a noted student of the classics, entered the University of Utrecht, where he studied with Johann Georg Graevius, a recognized scholar of classical culture. On 18 April 1693, Mead registered to study medicine at the University of Leiden. There he lived in the house of Archibald Pitcairne (1652–1713), professor of medicine, along with Herman Boerhaave (1668–1713), with whom he remained friends.

Mead left Leiden in 1695 without taking a degree and toured Italy with a small group of friends and his brother Samuel. By this time Mead already had strongly developed antiquarian interests. He received his MD at Florence on 26 August 1695. He returned to England in 1696 and practiced medicine in London (probably largely among nonconformists) from his father's house in Stepney, in spite of having no license from the RCP. In July 1699 he married a merchant's daughter, Ruth Marsh (1683–1720), and his father gave him the Stepney House. Mead and his wife had eight children, of whom three daughters and a son reached adulthood. Soon after his father died (1699), Mead joined the Church of England.

In Leiden, Mead, along with Boerhaave, cultivated the iatromechanical philosophy, also an interest fostered by Pitcairne. His first work, *A Mechanical Account of Poisons* (1702), embodied this view. By invoking an attractive force in chemistry, he identified himself as a Newtonian. Mead had dissected vipers in Leiden, and much of the study centered on venomous snakes. He swallowed the venom of the viper without effect and confirmed Galen's view that a puncture wound was necessary for the poison to work. The *Mechanical Account* had its desired effect. He was recognized as one of a young group of Newton's disciples and was elected to the Royal Society in 1703. In the same year, he became a physician to St Thomas's Hospital, and around the same time, he was appointed as one of the readers in anatomy at the Barber-Surgeons' Company, in which position he remained until 1715. In 1704 Mead published, in Latin (English translation, 1708), a work on the influence of the sun and moon on the body, usually described as a fusion of Newtonianism, Hippocratism, and astrology. Mead later discarded attracting particles for the new, fashionable Newtonian doctrine of ethers.

Recognition and wealth flowed: he was made a DM of Oxford (1707), Newton appointed him a vice president of the Royal Society (1713), and he was elected FRCP (1716). He moved west, from Stepney to Crutched Friars, and, in 1711, to Austin Friars. He mixed with the most distinguished physicians of the era, notably John Freind (1675–1728), Hans Sloane (1660–1753), and John Radcliffe (1650–1714), whose gold-headed cane, Bloomsbury house, and practice Mead inherited. His patients included the Princess of Wales. In 1719 he entered into a public feud (at one point physical) and pamphlet war with John Woodward (1665–1728) over smallpox therapy. After his wife died in 1720, he moved to a house on Great Ormond Street, later occupied by the Hospital for Sick Children. A work on contagion was published in 1720, and seven editions appeared in a year. In 1721, with Sloane, he conducted successful trials of small pox inoculation (a practice he championed) on condemned prisoners at Newgate. He became a governor of three hospitals—St Bartholomew's, Bridewell, and Bethlem—and in 1727 was appointed physician to George II. He also attended Newton in his final illness. He championed the ventilation of ships and wrote a *Discourse on the Scurvy* (1749). By the 1720s, his income was around £5,000 per annum. Mead was one of those Augustan physicians who began to employ public display as much as *gravitas* as a way of drawing attention to their talents. Much of his practice was carried out in coffee houses.

Wealth allowed Mead to pursue his collecting and antiquarian interests. He was an excellent classical scholar and, like John Freind, devoted much time to the history of medicine. His Harveian oration of 1723 was an address on the status of physicians in ancient Greece and Rome. A pamphlet war ensued. He subscribed to a huge number of books, both medical and otherwise, and his library numbered 10,000 volumes and included many rare first editions. He also collected manuscripts, antique coins, medals, fossils, scientific instruments, and antiquities from Egypt and elsewhere. His paintings included works by Rembrandt and Breueghel. He owned thousands of engravings. Mead sponsored the printer Samuel Palmer to write his *History of Printing* (1732). In 1724 he married Anne, daughter of Sir Rowland Alston of Odell. Anne had no children. He had a coach and six horses to drive to his country house at Windsor. By his second marriage, he had possession of Harrold Hall in Bedfordshire. Physicians, natural philosophers, and men of letters gathered at his Great Ormond Street house. In spite of all this, he was rumored to be in financial difficulty late in life. His collections were auctioned and scattered after his death.

Bibliography

Primary: 1708. *A Discourse Concerning the Action of the Sun and Moon on Animal bodies; and the Influence which this may have in many Diseases* (London); 1720. *A Short Discourse concerning Pestilential Contagion, and the Methods to be Used to Prevent it* (London); *1748. A Discourse on the Small Pox and Measles / By Richard Mead . . . To which is Annexed, a Treatise on the same Diseases, by the Celebrated Arabian Physician Abu-Beker Rhazes. The whole Translated into English, under the Author's Inspection, by Thomas Stack* (London).

Secondary: Meade, R. H., 1974. *In the Sunshine of Life: A Biography of Dr. Richard Mead, 1673–1754 (Philadelphia); Oxford DNB.*

Christopher Lawrence

MECHNIKOV, ELIE (b. Ivanovka, Kharkov Province, Russia, 3 (15) May 1845; d. Paris, France, 16 July 1916), *comparative embryology, epidemiology, bacteriology, immunology.*

Mechnikov was born to Ilia Ivanovich Mechnikov, a Guards officer and landowner, and Emilia Nevahovich, daughter of the Jewish writer Leo Nevahovich. He began formal schooling rather late, at the age of eleven, at the Khar'kov gymnasium in 1856, but his intellect developed rapidly, and he wrote his first academic article in 1862, his last year of school. He graduated from Khar'kov University in 1864, just two years later.

Mechnikov made his first real scientific discovery in 1864 in Rudolf Leuckart's laboratory at Giessen when he discovered alternating generations (sexual and asexual) in nematodes. Mechnikov devoted many years to studying the comparative development of the embryonic stages of lower animals. His outstanding works on the embryogenesis, morphology, and taxonomy of lower animals confirmed the theory of the common origin of all animals, as a result of which many ambiguous and disputed questions of animal taxonomy were resolved.

When he was twenty-two Mechnikov defended his master's thesis ('History of the Embryonic Development of *Sepiola*', 1867), and at twenty-three his doctorate ('History of the Development of *Nebalia*', 1868), at St Petersburg University. From 1870 until 1882 he worked as a professor in the chair of zoology and comparative anatomy at Novorossiisk University (Odessa).

In December 1882, in Messina (Italy), Mechnikov made his greatest scientific discovery, the role of phagocytes in the defense of the animal body. He observed that the mobile cells in a starfish larva surrounded intruding foreign bodies, a phenomenon similar to the inflammatory response in animals with a vascular system, and reasoned correctly that these cells might serve in the defense of the animal against intruders.

That observation had wide implications. In 1883 the first of many papers appeared in which Mechnikov explored the newly developing field of immunology. He first used the term *phagocyte* in Carl Claus's *Arbeiten*. Mechnikov was the first in the history of science who came to the conclusion that the immune response is a function of specialized cells, united into a special physiological system that included free and fixed phagocytes of blood, lymph, and connective tissue, and the organs containing phagocytes.

In 1887 Mechnikov proposed his classification of leukocytes: 'microphages', 'macrophages', and 'lymphocytes'. While microphages always caused destruction, macrophages were also constructive. No one had previously connected these cells with the defense of an organism against alien elements. He changed the basic paradigm of pathology of his time, according to which inflammation was a disease of vessels, whereas according to Mechnikov it was a battle between phagocytes and alien cells.

This dispute was the main reason for the antagonistic attitude toward Mechnikov and his works. Mechnikov and his wife traveled to various centers in Europe in search of a congenial place to settle. Pasteur in Paris made them most welcome, and gave him a laboratory in his institute in which to work. Mechnikov worked there, starting from 1888, for twenty-eight years until the end of his life, and was elected deputy director in 1905.

In 1891 he published *Leçons sur la pathologie comparée de l'inflammation*, a magnificent review of the entire field of both comparative and human immunology. Mechnikov's investigations also started a new field, immunopathology, the study of diseases based on disorders of immune mechanisms. In 1908 Mechnikov and Ehrlich were awarded the Nobel Prize for their research illuminating the understanding of immunity.

During World War I Mechnikov was diagnosed with myocarditis, which progressed rapidly and with very strong pain and dyspnea, but despite all this he continued to work, writing scientific papers in his hospital bed up until his death on 16 July 1916.

Bibliography

Primary: 1891. *Leçons sur la pathologie comparée de inflammation* (Paris); 1901. *L'immunité dans les maladies infectieuses* (Paris); 1903. *Essays on Human Nature* (Moscow); 1950–64. *Academic Collection of Publications by Mechnikov, I. I.* (Moscow); 1968. (Starling, F. A., and E. H. Starling, trans.) *Lectures on the Comparative Pathology of Inflammation (1893)* (Paris).

Secondary: Ul'iankina, T. I., 2005. *Mechnikov Ilia Iliich (1845–1916). Bibliographia* [Bibliography] (Moscow); Tauber, Alfred I., and Leon Chernyak, 1991. *Metchnikoff and the Origins of Immunology: From Metaphor to Theory* (New York); Mechnikov, I. I., 1980. *Pisma k O.N. Mechnikov* [Letters to O. N. Mechnikov] *(1900–1914)* (Moscow); Gaisinovich, A. E., B. V. Levshin, and I. I. Mechnikov, 1978. *Pisma k O.N. Mechnikov* [Letters to O. N. Mechnikov] *(1876–1899)* (Moscow); Lepine, Pierre, 1966. *Elie Mechnikov et l'immunologie* (Vichy); Zeiss, Heinz, 1932. *Elias Metchnikow, Leben und Werk* (Jena); Mechnikov, Olga, 1921. (Lankester, E. Ray, trans.) *Life of Elie Mechnikov 1845–1916* (Boston); Bezredka, Alexandr, 1921. *Histoire d'une idée, l'oeuvre de E. Mechnikov* (Paris); *DSB*.

Tatiana Ul'iankina

MEIGS, CHARLES DELUCENA (b. St George, Bermuda, 19 February 1792; d. Hamanassett, Delaware County, Pennsylvania, USA, 22 June 1869), *medical education, obstetrics.*

Renowned in his day as an obstetrician, Meigs is remembered today as an opponent of important innovations in obstetrical care. Both characterizations ignore his broad range of interests, skills, and accomplishments.

Meigs's father was professor of mathematics at Yale and then the first president of the University of Georgia; the son had a classical education, graduating from Georgia in 1809. He served a two-year apprenticeship with Thomas H. M. Fendall of Augusta, Georgia. During the next six years, he took two courses in medicine at the University of Pennsylvania, twice set up practice in Augusta, and married Mary Montgomery of Philadelphia (1815). He was awarded his MB in 1817 and remained in Philadelphia for the rest of his career.

A prolific author, Meigs wrote on numerous topics: the state of blood vessels in fevers (1823), croup (1838), spasmodic cholera (1849), diphtheria and its treatment (1864), etc. His article on cardiac thrombosis as a cause of the sudden deaths in childbed ('The Heart-Clot', 1849), which had generally been attributed to syncope, made a seminal contribution. Meigs was also a voracious reader of contemporary German works, and he translated two major French texts into English. He made his own clay and wax models to illustrate his lectures. He drew and painted; the lithographs in Meigs's *Treatise on Acute and Chronic Diseases of the Neck of the Uterus* (1854) were made from his drawings.

In 1826 Meigs became an editor of the *North American Medical and Surgical Journal*; in 1827 he was elected a fellow of the College of Physicians of Philadelphia (he would serve as a College officer from 1841 to 1855). He began lecturing on midwifery at the School of Medicine in 1830. After being passed over for the professorship at the University of Pennsylvania in 1836 (Hugh L. Hodge was appointed instead), Meigs was made professor of obstetrics and the diseases of women and children at Philadelphia's Jefferson Medical College (1841). Some twenty years later, against his colleagues' wishes, he resigned.

Meigs's outspoken opposition to the hypothesis that puerperal fever was contagious led him to publish intemperate remarks about the paper in which the young Boston physician Oliver Wendell Holmes concluded that doctors themselves were carrying puerperal fever to their patients. Holmes was so infuriated by Meigs's *On the Nature, Signs and Treatment of Childbed Fever*, not least because of the mocking way Meigs characterized the contagion theory as 'the jejune and fizenless dreamings of sophomore writers' (Meigs, 1854, p. 113), that he responded to the attack by republishing his paper with a long introduction in which—among other things—he decried the widespread influence that Meigs and his Philadelphia colleague Hodge had over students of obstetrics.

Meigs also stubbornly opposed the operation of ovariotomy, largely on the grounds that it was neither necessary nor safe. He was not altogether wrong in this, or in his view that anesthesia in childbirth was dangerous, though he seems to have been unconcerned about the relative benefits of ether and chloroform. Highly regarded as he was by many physicians of the day, Meigs added to his future infamy by insisting that painful childbirth belonged to the 'natural and physiological forces that the Divinity has ordained' (Meigs, 1856, p. 368). Despite his conservative attitudes, however, this popular and skillful obstetrician did much to advance the field of obstetrics.

Bibliography

Primary: 1838. *The Philadelphia Practice of Midwifery* (Philadelphia); 1847. *Woman, Her Diseases and Remedies* (Philadelphia); 1849. *Obstetrics: The Science and the Art* (Philadelphia); 1854. *On the Nature, Signs and Treatment of Childbed Fever* (Philadelphia).

Secondary: Thoms, Herbert, 1936. 'Charles Delucena Meigs: A Leader in American Obstetrics.' *American Journal of Obstetrics and Gynecology* 31: 1049–1055; Meigs, J. Forsyth, 1872. 'Memoir of Charles D. Meigs, M.D.' *Transactions of the College of Physicians of Philadelphia*, n.s., 4(6), 1863–74: 417–448; *DAMB*.

Constance Putnam

MENNINGER, KARL (b. Topeka, Kansas, USA, 22 July 1893; d. Topeka, 18 July 1990), *psychiatry, psychoanalysis.*

Menninger was the oldest of three brothers. His mother, Flo, was devoutly religious and taught Bible classes. His father, Charles (1862–1953), was a homeopathic physician and had qualified at the Hahnemann Medical College in Chicago in 1889. Charles Menninger had a practice with Henry Robb, and in that practice, he combined homeopathic with allopathic medicine, taking postgraduate courses at the Kansas Medical College. His main interests were in internal medicine. Karl Menninger, after studying at the University of Wisconsin, went to Harvard Medical School, and after completing his medical studies, he took an internship at the Kansas City General Hospital. However, he became interested there in neurological cases and took up a residency at the Boston Psychopathic Hospital, where the chief superintendent was Elmer Southard. Through studying with Southard, he became committed to neuropsychiatry and acquired interest in the mental hygiene movement. At Southard's suggestion, he returned to Topeka to set up a medical practice with his father in 1919, specializing in neuropsychiatry. His younger brother, William (1899–1966), later joined them in the practice. The practice grew and became the Menninger Diagnostic Clinic.

William Menninger studied at Washburn University and graduated from Cornell University College of Medicine in 1924. He was an intern at Bellevue Hospital for two years and studied psychiatry at St Elizabeth's Hospital in Washington, D.C., in 1927.

In 1916 Karl Menninger married Grace Kaines, with whom he had three children. Around 1921, he met Smith Ely Jelliffe, who increased his interest in psychoanalysis. Karl Menninger had a few sessions of analysis with Jelliffe, and the latter encouraged him to experiment with analysis in his practice. Jelliffe maintained a broad conception of psychoanalysis, corresponding with Carl Jung up to the 1930s. In their practice, the Menningers found an increasing need to have facilities for inpatients. After initially boarding patients in various local hospitals, they purchased a farmhouse in 1925, which became the Menninger Sanitarium, a private asylum. The following year, they established the Southard School for disturbed children.

In 1930 William Menninger became director of the sanitarium. Following the reformulation of psychiatry by Southard, Adolf Meyer, and William Alonson White, the Menningers developed a progressive, melioristic view of its prospects, combined with an optimistic reformulation of psychoanalysis. As Karl Menninger later recalled, in the United States, psychoanalysis 'combined with the psychology of William James, the philosophy of Josiah Royce, the psychiatry of Ernest Southard and the psychiatry of Adolf Meyer'. In his view, psychoanalysis changed American psychiatry from a diagnostic to a therapeutic science. In stark contrast to Freud's pessimism concerning the prospects of Western civilization, in *Man against Himself*, Karl Menninger argued that the 'death instinct' could be tamed.

At their sanitarium, the Menningers developed a form of milieu therapy, believing that all aspects of the interaction with patients could aid their recovery. William Menninger drew from the nineteenth-century tradition of moral treatment, together with Adolf Meyer's psychobiology and the example of Ernst Simmel's psychoanalytic sanitarium at Schloss Tegel. A treatment program was drawn up for each patient, involving the physicians, attendants, and nurses. Karl Menninger maintained that a psychoanalytically inspired hospital would be run more like a college dormitory than a medical hospital.

In 1930 Karl Menninger published his first book, *The Human Mind*, which was based on his graduate course in mental hygiene at Washburn College. Because of its fluent and accessible style and sharply drawn and recognizable personality profiles, the work became a best seller and did much to popularize the new psychiatry and psychoanalysis. Between 1929 and 1942, he wrote a column in *Household Magazine* giving advice to parents troubled by their children's behavior. Between 1930 and 1932, he wrote a monthly column in the *Ladies Home Journal* on mental hygiene in the home and answered letters that were sent to the magazine. Karl Menninger stressed the continuity between mental health and disease, which he conceived as lying on a spectrum, and maintained that 'we all have mental diseases of different degrees at different times'.

In 1931 Karl Menninger commenced an analysis with Franz Alexander in Chicago, commuting from Topeka. He became the first graduate of the Chicago Psychoanalytic Institute. Both he and his brother William Menninger became presidents of the American Psychoanalytic Association.

In 1941 the Menninger Foundation was established, which facilitated the doctors' capacity to raise funds. William Menninger was responsible for the fundraising. All the Menninger properties and programs were consolidated under the umbrella of the Foundation.

In 1942 Karl Menninger established a psychoanalytic study group, which became the Topeka Institute for Psychoanalysis, affiliated with the Menninger Clinic. The combination of personal and training analyses and staff roles in a hospital setting led at times to the abuse of power through the utilization of intimate information. During the war, the Menningers actively recruited émigré European analysts, who flocked to Topeka to take up positions at the Menninger Clinic. However, the European approach to psychoanalysis, emphasizing the unconscious, symbolism, and symptomatic acts and chiefly concerned with cases of neuroses, frequently came into conflict with its American formulation, stressing ego psychology, defenses, relationships, reactions, and adaptation, and using an inpatient environment with chronic cases.

Karl Menninger became less enthusiastic about the therapeutic potentiality of psychoanalysis, compared with its educational value as an invaluable form of self-knowledge for those who taught psychiatry and the social sciences.

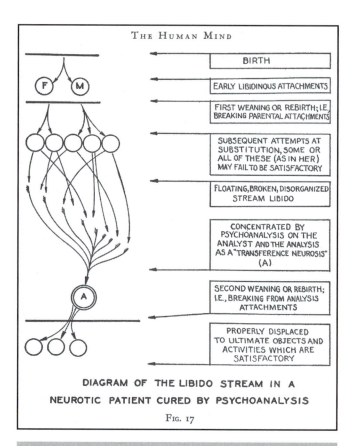

Diagram of the libido stream in a neurotic patient cured by psychoanalysis. Illustration from *The Human Mind*, New York/London, 1930. Wellcome Library, London.

The manner in which psychoanalysis was taken up at the Menninger clinic within psychiatry and combined with indigenous developments in psychiatry and mental hygiene led to its dominance within American psychiatry in the 1940s and 1950s. It was not that the majority of psychiatrists in America practiced psychoanalysis, but the domination of the teaching positions and positions of power ensured and indeed enforced a broadly psychoanalytic orientation within psychiatry.

In the 1930s, Karl Menninger had some affairs with staff members at the Clinic. Between 1938 and 1940, he moved to New York to be analyzed by Ruth Mack Brunswick. In 1941 he divorced his wife Grace and married Jeanette Lyle, a staff member.

During World War II, William Menninger served in the Surgeon General's Office and was put in charge of the Neuropsychiatry Division. In 1945 he laid the basis for a system of psychiatric classification for the army, which formed the basis of what in 1952 became the diagnostic and statistical manual (DSM-1) of the American Psychiatric Association. With its stress on syndromes and reactions, DSM-1 came to reflect the dynamic orientation of Menninger-style psychoanalysis. After the war, William Menninger persuaded the Veterans Administration to approve a psychiatric training establishment at the Winter General Army Hospital in Topeka, which became the Menninger School of Psychiatry, the largest psychiatric training center in the United States. In 1948 William Menninger, then president of the American Psychiatric Association, was the first psychiatrist to be featured on the cover of *Time* magazine and was described as 'psychiatry's US sales manager'. He went on to advise J. F. Kennedy on mental health policy.

In 1953 Charles Menninger died. The fact that the Menninger Foundation had two heads in Karl and William Menninger with overlapping authority at times led to frictions, and in 1965, Karl Menninger was deposed as chief of staff through internal machinations. In the following year, William Menninger died of cancer. In 1981 Karl Menninger, who had often been referred to as the 'dean of American psychiatry', was awarded the medal of freedom by President Jimmy Carter, the only psychiatrist to be so honored.

Bibliography

Primary: 1930. *The Human Mind* (New York); 1938. *Man against Himself* (New York); 1959. *A Psychiatrist's World: Selected Papers* (New York).

Secondary: Faulkner, Howard, and Virginia Pruitt, eds., 1997. *Dear Dr. Menninger: Women's Voices from the Thirties* (Columbia, MO); Friedman, Lawrence, 1990. *Menninger: The Family and the Clinic* (New York); Faulkner, Howard, and Virginia Pruitt, eds., 1988. *The Selected Correspondence of Karl A. Menninger, 1919–1945* (New Haven, CT); *DAMB* (also William and Charles Menninger).

Sonu Shamdasani

MERCADO, LUIS DE   (b. Valladolid, Spain, 1532; d. Valladolid, December 1611), *medicine, infant education, gynecology, obstetrics, orthopedic surgery.*

As can be deduced from his statements as a witness in litigation, Mercado was born in 1532. His father was Pedro de Ordás, a little-known surgeon from the mountains of León, habitually pursued by creditors, and his mother was María González de Mercado, from Valladolid. They left little in inheritance to their six children: to Luis de Mercado, a few books only.

It is thought that he studied arts and medicine at the University of Valladolid, after which he became a doctor (1560), financed by the money he received as the dowry of his wife Juana de Toro, daughter of a rich meat and wine merchant. In his will, the merchant confessed he had cheated Mercado, overvaluing a vineyard. But Mercado also confessed, at the time of making his own will, that he had also cheated his father-in-law by declaring himself well-off, when, at the time of the marriage, he possessed only a mule, some books, and the clothes he stood up in.

Thanks to the dowry money, he qualified as a doctor and entered the Senate of the University of Valladolid, where he became professor of medicine in 1572, occupying the chair until his retirement in 1592.

He was physician to Kings Philip II and Philip III from 1592 onward. Although he had perhaps had connections to the Royal Family since 1578, it would seem that Francisco de Valles brought him into the palace because of his profound talent, great learning, ample knowledge, acute shrewdness, good judgment, and excellent methodology and clarity of explanation, according to a panegyrist.

During the reign of Philip III, he became the most important physician in Spain, being named *Protomédico* (Chief Royal Physician) of all the Kingdoms, that is, director of the Spanish health service, which he reorganized in the years that saw the passage from the sixteenth to the seventeenth century, establishing new regulations for medical and surgical examinations.

He served as the King's physician and *Protomédico* until 1611, requesting retirement on the death of Queen Margarita. This incident tarnished the days that remained to him, as public opinion accused him of having poisoned the Queen on the orders of don Rodrigo Calderón, a minister put on trial for crimes against the state. It was said that she had been given the drug *Digitalis purpurea*, then unknown.

It is said that he left Madrid amid stones thrown by the crowds who recognized his carriage and returned to Valladolid to complete the chapel of San Jacinto in the monastery of San Pablo, which he had chosen as his resting place, decorating it with a rich collection of relics. His wife was interred there in October 1611, and he followed in December of the same year. According to Petrus Castellanus, he died of an inability to urinate. He left six children. Bernarda and Petronila were nuns, Bautista was a Jesuit, and Antonio de la Madre de Dios was a Carmelite friar. Isabel was wife of Juan Villagutierre, of the Council of the Indies. Finally, Luis, who later became a member of the Council of the Treasury, was heir to the title of lord of Santa Cecilia del Alcor—a title bought by his father in order to gain access to the nobility for his son.

From a young age, Mercado's ambition was to reorganize medicine, revising what ancient and modern scholars had written and rectifying their errors. What is more, he was convinced that physicians needed medicine to be organized differently and needed books that would be real tools, each specialized in a particular problem. A physician should have each subject in front of him, in a complete and manageable form, without having to spend hours searching through the mass of inherited literature. This was his great achievement, although he was criticized for preferring the ancient to the modern and for his penchant for using philosophical language and forms. Because of this, Kurt Sprenger cruelly called him 'Saint Thomas of Medicine'.

He is often described as one of the main European proponents of Galenism, hostile to the nascent scientific ideologies; or as one of the great figures of medical scholasticism, well-informed about the new discoveries of Renaissance medicine, but opposed to anything that might represent even the slightest attack on the old concepts.

His merits, however, are unquestionable and, as already pointed out, he carried out a restructuring of traditional medical knowledge. His first two works were *De communi et peculiari praesidiorum artis medicae indicationes* (1574), reedited in Cologne in 1589 and 1592; and *De essentia, causis, signis & curatione febris malignae. In qua maculae rubentes similes morsibus pulicum per cutem eruptum* (1574), reedited in Basel (1594) and Padua (1595). Incorporated by Vido Vidio into his *De Febribus libri septem* (1595), the latter includes one of the first known descriptions—along with those of Luis de Toro, Alfonso López de Corella, and Francisco Bravo—of the spotted or exanthematic fever that was called 'tabardillo' by the Spanish, because of the red spots in the area that would be covered by a 'tabard' or surcoat. Mercado is also the author of the first modern description of 'garrotillo', or croup, in a personal clinical history that has been called masterly. Here, the term 'garrotillo' referred to the means of execution, the *garrote*, because of the short time in which the illness took children's lives, as if it were an execution. Both nosological descriptions are the product of personal experience, which pervaded the *Consultationes morborum complicatorum & gravissiomorum* of his *Opera omnia*, which explains the respect they received in the following centuries.

Mercado deliberately chose a new illness with which to make his name as, in the sixteenth and seventeenth centuries, it was an aspiration of the Faculty of Medicine of Valladolid to replace the traditional philosophical-scholastic method with the new philosophical-Hippocratic method, in which doctrine was mixed with the daily exercise of the profession. That is why the books of the physicians of Valladolid, such as Mercado, usually contain many personal clinical case histories.

He put great interest in grouping medical knowledge by subject, splitting medicine into what today we call 'specialties'. Thus from his pen there arose texts edited separately or as part of his *Opera omnia*, the best edition of which is that published in Frankfurt (1608–14) with a preface by Johann Hartmann Beyer.

Belonging to this group are a monograph on the illnesses of women, *De mulierum affectionibus* (1579), which was so successful that it became the most widely sold treatise on obstetrics in Europe, with nine editions in less than fifty years; another work on pediatrics, *De puerorum educatione* (1611); and a third on hereditary illnesses, *De morbis hereditariis* (1605), which was among the first titles of its kind. His published observations on the most common affections of the skin also have a thematic organization.

In addition, he wished to write a series of works to facilitate the practice of medicine for young physicians. These would be books with the fundamental things a physician with little experience ought to learn: *De pulsus arte & harmonia libri duo* (1584), *De morborum internorum curatione*

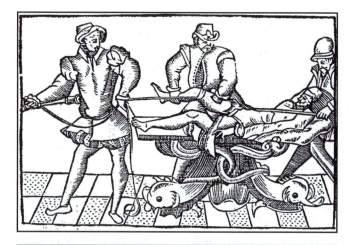

Technique for reducing a fracture. Woodcut from *Instituciones que Su Magestad mando hazer el doctor Mercado . . .* Madrid, 1599. Rare Books, Wellcome Library, London.

(1594), and two manuals for self-examination to obtain the title of physician and surgeon before the Protomedicato Tribunal, entitled *Institutiones medicae iussu regio factae pro medicis in praxi examinandis* (1594) and *Institutiones chirurgicae iussu regio factae pro chirurgis in praxi examinandis* (1594). To these he added in 1599, by the King's request, a short treatise for bonesetters on fractures, luxations, and dislocations: *Instituciones que su magestad mandó hazer al Doctor Mercado su Médico de Cámara, y Protomédico general, para el aprovechamiento y examen de los algebristas* (1599), which was later translated into Latin and edited in Frankfurt by Charles Lepois as *Institutiones ad usum et examen eorum, qui luxatoriam exercent artem* (1625).

Also by request of the crown, he wrote a book on the plague (1599), with advice on the necessary measures to be taken to prevent and combat the last of the great epidemics of the Iberian peninsula, the so-called 'Atlantic plague', which in Valladolid alone was considered to have killed five thousand people out of a total population of thirty thousand.

Mercado's reputation is currently dominated by the fame as a scholastic imposed on him by Sprenger, yet even a little research into seventeenth-century European medicine shows he had a positive influence on some of the new areas that were developing. He was especially valued for his theory on febrile heat, presented in *De natura caloris febrilis* and *De febrium essentia, differentis, causa, curatione*; for his *Gynaeciorum s. De mulierum, virginum, viduarum, praegnantium &c, morbis libri IV* in the field of pregnant women's illnesses; for his *De morbis hereditariis* in the field of hereditary illnesses; for his *Liber de puerperarum & nutricum passionibus & morbis* in illnesses of wet-nurses; and in infant education, for his *De puerorum educatione & custodia libri II*.

His reflections can be found in Francesco Torti, *Therapeutice specialis ad febres quasdam perniciosas*, who declared that Mercado was the first to observe pernicious fevers. P. G. Werlhof, D. Sennert, and A. de Häen also read his works, and the latter accused G. van Swieten of having appropriated many of Mercado's opinions without quoting him. Johann Hartmann made a tribute to him in the Frankfurt edition of the *Opera omnia*, and H. Boerhaave declared that two of his works, *De Mulierum affectionibus* and *De Morbis puerorum*, were still worthy of study in the eighteenth century.

To sum up, it is to Luis de Mercado that we owe the most influential systematization of medicine in Europe. It took the form of a body of organized medical knowledge that spanned the totality of accumulated knowledge up to that time: a review of the ancient and the modern, as long as the latter did not enter into serious conflict with traditional medicine.

In 1752 King Fernando VI reformed the study of medicine in Spain. Among the models proposed were those of foreigners such as Sydenham, van Swieten, Morton, Duret, Mercurial, Baillou, and Piso; and, among the Spanish models, those of Francisco Valles, Luis de Mercado, and Pedro Miguel de Heredia. Why were they chosen? They had all explained medicine by imitating Hippocrates.

Bibliography

Primary: 1608–14. *Opera omnia in quatuor tomos divisa* 5 vols. (Frankfurt); 1574. *De essentia causis signis & curatione febris malignae in qua maculae rubentes similes morsibus pulicum per cutem erumptunt* (Valladolid); 1579. *De mulierum affectionibus. Libri quatuor. Quorum primus de communibus mulierum passionibus disserit. Secundis, virgunum & viduaru, morbos tractat. Tertius, sterilium & praegnantium. Quartus, puerperarum, & nitricum accedentia* (Valladolid); 1599. *Instituciones que su magestad mandó hazer al Doctor Mercado su Médico de Cámara, y Protomédico general, para el aprovechamiento y examen de los algebristas* (Madrid).

Secondary: López Piñero, José M., 1983. 'Mercado, Luis' in López Piñero, José M., et al., eds., *Diccionario histórico de la ciencia moderna en España* vol. II (Barcelona); Granjel, Luis S., 1980. *La medicina Española Renacentista* (Salamanca); Riera, Juan, 1968. *Vida y obra de Luis Mercado* (Salamanca); Alcocer Martínez, Mariano, 1931. *Historia de la Universidad de Valladolid. Bio-Bibliografías de médicos notables* (Valladolid).

Anastasio Rojo

MERCURIALE, GIROLAMO (b. Forlì, Italy, 30 September 1530; d. Forlì, 8 November 1606), *medicine, pediatrics.*

The son of Giovanni Mercuriale and Camilla Pungetta, Mercuriale started his medical studies at Bologna, then went to Padua, and finally on 17 April 1555 was awarded a degree in medicine by the College of Physicians of Venice. He moved to Rome in 1562 and remained there until 1569 under the patronage of Cardinal Alessandro Farnese (1520–89), with whom he traveled also to Sicily. He maintained a close friendship with the Farnese family for the rest of his life. During his stay in Rome he had the opportunity to study codices and ancient documents, thus collecting

material for his work *De arte gymnastica*. By a decree dated 6 October 1569 he was called to the first chair of ordinary practical medicine at the University of Padua, where he stayed for eighteen years, and in 1581 was paid the considerable annual salary of 1,150 florins. On the occasion of the plague of 1575, he fell into a serious professional error when the Senate summoned him to Venice, together with another Paduan physician, the well-known Girolamo Capodivacca, who occupied the second chair of ordinary practical medicine, as they had expressed their opinion on the epidemic, which had reached the city from Trento. The two professors, contrary to the opinions of the Venetian physicians, claimed that they were dealing with a serious but not a contagious disease; unfortunately the events that followed showed their mistake.

In 1587 Mercuriale was persuaded to leave Padua for the University of Bologna, where he was given the 'supraordinaria' chair of theoretical medicine, with a more flattering contract than any previously offered to a professor of medicine at Bologna, including a twelve-year tenure, an annual salary of 1,200 gold *scudi*, and three hundred *scudi* for the journey and the transfer of his effects from Padua, plus honorary Bolognese citizenship, all in addition to the customary exemption from all taxes. However, despite the obligation to respect the precise terms of the contract, after Mercuriale had completed just six of the twelve years he began to show signs of intolerance and talked about leaving Bologna and going elsewhere. In 1591 some disputes, the details of which remain obscure, made him unhappy with his situation at Bologna and induced him to look for a more congenial and better-paid position. For several years he had been in close contact with Ferdinando I de' Medici, Grand Duke of Tuscany (1549–1609), who now offered him an annual salary of 2,000 gold *scudi* if he would teach at the University of Pisa. Mercuriale accepted the Grand Duke's offer without hesitation and in November 1592 moved to Pisa, claiming the inclement climate affected his health and alleging some nonexistent irregularities regarding payment of his salary. The Grand Duke of Tuscany nominated Mercuriale as his personal and family physician, and he stayed there until he retired to his hometown in 1606. But obviously even Pisa could not satisfy him, for when he was almost seventy years old, he asked the 'Riformatori dello Studio di Padova' if they would once again give him the position of lecturer for the chair of practical medicine, vacant since Alessandro Massaria's death in November 1598. His request was turned down, probably for a variety of reasons: his advanced years, the distant but not forgotten abandonment of the Padua university twelve years earlier, and perhaps even his gross blunder concerning the plague of 1575–76, and not least of all, his exorbitant requests for money.

During his lifetime Mercuriale gained great fame as a capable practitioner of medicine; in 1573 he was summoned to Vienna to attend the Emperor Maximilian II

(1527–76), who, once cured, heaped favors on him, gave him the title of Count Palatine, and made him a knight.

A humanist and philologist physician, with a profound knowledge of Greek, Latin, and the ancient medical literature, he studied the authenticity of the Hippocratic writings (*Censura et dispositio operum Hippocratis*, 1583) and published the Greek text and Latin translation of the works of Hippocrates collated on codices (1588). In the four books of *Variae lectiones* (1571) he made a critical exegesis of many difficult passages in the Greek and Latin authors, which he corrected where corrupt or illustrated when obscure. In 1570 Mercuriale published for the first time the Greek text and Latin translation of the *Letter on Intestinal Worms* by Alexander of Tralles, which he had found in the Biblioteca Vaticana (Cod. Vat. Gr. 299); the same edition was added to the *Variae lectiones* (1571) and republished as an appendix to the second edition (1584) of the treatise *De puerorum morbis*.

The six books entitled *De arte gymnastica* (1569), the result of almost seven years of study and research in the museums and libraries of Rome, and Mercuriale's most original and well-known work, are in effect the first complete treatise on medical gymnastics, in which the gymnastics of the ancients were closely linked with their modern counterparts, of which Mercuriale was the true forerunner. The gymnastics were examined from a historical, medical, and finally a hygienic point of view. He recalled the exercises in agility, strength, and dexterity practiced by the ancient Greeks and Romans; he also explained various athletic exercises and the best way to perform them, discussing the beneficial effects on individuals, both healthy and diseased. Mercuriale valued gymnastics as a therapeutic instrument, in particular for rehabilitating paralyzed patients; he also dealt with balneotherapy (immersion in baths, often mineral) and medical hydrology, a theme he later returned to in his *De balneis pisanis*, published together with *Praelectiones Pisanae* (1597). The treatise *De arte gymnastica* had no illustrations in the first edition (1569), whereas the second (1573) was illustrated by twenty-six excellent woodcuts inspired by ancient medals and statues.

His work in practical medicine was vast and varied. He has been credited with the creation of medical specialties for having, for the first time, treated separately sectors of medicine that afterward assumed distinct identities. In fact, several of his works were originally courses of lessons appearing as monographs, rather than as systematic treatises, and the material was often collected by his students and then revised or rewritten by him. Notwithstanding the obvious limitations of his time, these attempts to arrange medical knowledge according to the various affected parts or systems in organic order, for didactic purposes as well as for practical ones, must be highly commended. He was among the first to take a special interest in puericulture and pediatrics; when he was still only a student he published a

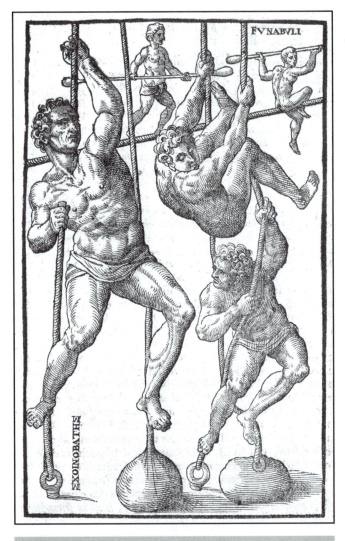

Gymnasts climbing ropes. Engraving from *De arte gymnastica . . .* Amsterdam, 1672. Rare Books, Wellcome Library, London.

small book *Nomothelasmus seu ratio lactandi infantes* (1552), where he set out the rules to be followed for breast-feeding infants, as well as other hygienic and dietetic suggestions for weaning and rearing children. In his *Nomothelasmus* (the oldest treatise on nursing), Mercuriale stressed the necessity of maternal breast-feeding and stated that a wet nurse should be employed only because of maternal agalactia. He also advised against giving the mother supposedly galactagogue medicines, for fear that they would affect the baby through the mother's milk.

The treatise *De morbis puerorum* (1583) was dedicated to the diseases of children and divided into three books, the third being devoted entirely to intestinal worms. The work was full of precise and perspicacious observations, amongst these being the distinction between measles and smallpox, the study of congenital syphilis, the description of feeding troubles in children, and the recognition—according to Rhazes—that hydrocephalus was sometimes caused by an intraventricular accumulation of fluid. This observation tended to upset the old classification in which the *caput succedaneum* was listed as external hydrocephalus. Of great interest too are his notes on stammering. Moreover, he recognized the contagious nature of pertussis, or whooping cough, and recommended the complete surgical excision of the ranula, or sublingual ptyalocele, in order to avoid a relapse. These two works should therefore be considered the starting-point for modern pediatrics.

Mercuriale also published the first systematic treatise on skin diseases (1572), which he classified according to a morphological criterion. However, the symptomatic nature of the majority of dermatological affections prevented physicians from constructing any new comprehensive view of the field. His lessons on diseases of the eye and ear (1584) represented the first clinical manual of otiatrics. Moreover, he clearly mentioned the ocular refractive defects and the possibility of correcting them: it was he who advised the use of concave lenses to counteract myopia. He was also interested in obstetrics and gynecology. The handling of the subject in his treatise *De morbis muliebribus* (1582) was traditional, even though the arrangement of the matter was rational.

Mercuriale was also concerned with epidemiology and hygiene. He described the symptomatology, course, complications, and aftermath of the pandemic influenza of 1580 with precision, admitting the disease's contagiousness. He also wrote on hydrophobia (1580), contributing his own observations and locating the anatomical seat of the illness in the front part of the brain, where he also located the imagination, of which rabies was a morbid form. His comments on the individual and social prophylaxis of the disease and on the symptomatology of canine rabies are noteworthy. He is also considered one of the most important toxicologists of the sixteenth century for his treatise *De venenis et morbis venenosis* (1584), where he contended that the only difference between poison and medicine was one of dosage. He was also interested in pharmacology and the composition of medicines; and lastly, in *Praelectiones Patavinae* (1601), he paid particular attention to mental illnesses, which he attempted to classify according to their etiology.

Of his many other works, *De decoratione* (1585) deserves special mention. In the first edition (Venice, 1585), Mercuriale reported on Gaspare Tagliacozzi's (1545–99) method of plastic repair of the nose. In response Tagliacozzi, sent a description of his method in a letter from Bologna dated 22 February 1586, which was later incorporated in the second edition of Mercuriale's book (Frankfurt, 1587), ten years before Tagliacozzi's own work, *De curtorum chirurgia per insitionem*, was published in Venice.

Bibliography

Primary: 1552. *Nomothelasmus seu ratio lactandi infantes* (Padua); 1569. *Artis gymnasticae apud antiquos celeberrimae, nostris temporibus ignoratae libri sex* (Venice) [1573, 2nd edn. entitled *De arte gymnastica libri sex* (Venice) illustrated; 1960, Italian trans. by Galante, Ippolito (Rome)]; 1572. *De morbis cutaneis et omnibus corporis humani excrementis* (Venice); 1582. *De morbis muliebribus praelectiones* (Basel); 1583. *De morbis puerorum* (Venice); 1584. *De compositione medicamentorum tractatus . . . de oculorum et aurium affectionibus praelectiones* (Frankfurt).

Secondary: Seneca, Federico, 1988. 'Un fallito tentativo di Girolamo Mercuriale di tornare nell'Ateneo patavino' in Rossetti, Lucia, ed., *Rapporti tra le Università di Padova e Bologna. Ricerche di filosofia, medicina e scienza* (Trieste) pp. 161–172; Ascanelli, Pietro, 1965. *L'opera pediatrica di G. Mercuriale* (Bologna); Simili, Alessandro, 1965. 'Gerolamo Mercuriale lettore e medico a Bologna. Nota II. Il soggiorno e gli insegnamenti.' *L'Archiginnasio* 60: 352–437; Paoletti, Italo, 1963. *Gerolamo Mercuriale e il suo tempo* (Lanciano); Greco, Enzo, 1961. 'Il posto di Gerolamo Mercuriale nella storia della ostetricia e ginecologia.' *Rivista italiana di Ginecologia* 45: 148–168.

Giuseppe Ongaro

MESMER, FRANZ ANTON   (b. Iznang near Radolfzell, Lake of Constance, Germany, 23 May 1734; d. Meersburg near Constance, Germany, 15 March 1815), *medicine*, 'animal magnetism', mesmerism.

Mesmer, son of a game warden in the service of the archbishop of Constance, visited the Jesuit school in Constance and from 1744–50 studied philosophy and theology at the Jesuit University of Dillingen and at the University of Ingolstadt. In 1759 he started to study jurisprudence and then medicine in Vienna, where he graduated 1766 with a dissertation on the influence of the planets on the human body (*Dissertatio physico-medica de planetarum influxu*) postulating a so-called animal gravity ('gravitas animalis'). In 1768 he married a rich widow, Anna Maria von Bosch (or Posch, 1725–90), and opened his doctor's practice in a suburb of Vienna.

As a general practitioner, Mesmer also tried to cure by electricity and steel magnets, which were considered efficient therapeutic agents in the early 1770s. In 1774, when Mesmer treated 'Jungfer Oesterlin', a twenty-nine–year-old lady, by magnets, he had the impression, that there was another and much more subtle power active than the magnetic one. He so 'detected' the 'animal magnetism'—a natural healing power, which he imagined as a special physical entity ('fluidum') flooding through the macrocosm and affecting the human body through the nervous system.

In 1777, after Mesmer treated the eighteen-year-old blind pianist Maria Theresia Paradis, he claimed that he had cured her by animal magnetism. Some of his colleagues from the medical faculty in Vienna accused him of fraud. This case caused a scandal, and Mesmer had to flee from Vienna. After three months of deep personal crisis, he arrived in Paris, where he became a famous charismatic healer in the years before the French Revolution.

In magnetizing, the magnetic power (fluidum) could supposedly be transferred from the magnetizer to the patient by different techniques: by laying on of hands, by

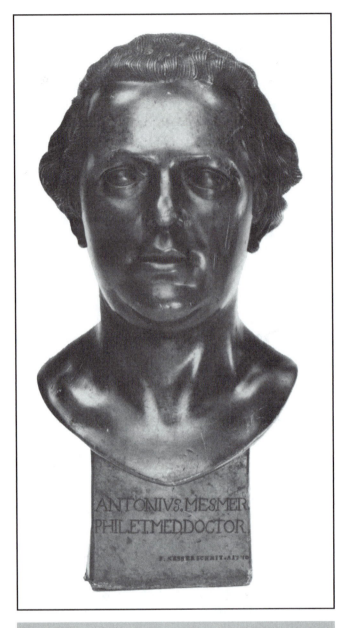

Bust of Franz Anton Mesmer by Franz Xaver Messerschmidt, 1770. Height 47cm, private collection. Photograph Heinz Schott.

manipulations over the surface of the body without touching it (French: 'passes'), by use of a wand, or by giving a glance (by means of beams out of the eyes). Mesmer also believed it was possible to magnetize at a distance, through walls, by means of magnetized trees or water, etc. In his house in Paris, Mesmer created a typical setting for his magnetic cures. The so-called magnetic tub (French: 'baquet') was supposed to work as an accumulator of the 'fluidum'. The patients surrounded it to get the animal magnetism transferred to them by iron sticks and ropes, while forming a human chain and singing and praying. Moreover, Mesmer recommended, as a means of reinforcing the 'fluidum', the use of mirrors on the walls and of improvised music, especially played on the glass harp, which he played masterfully (impressing even the young Wolfgang Amadeus Mozart in earlier times).

In 1784 Mesmer's theory was rejected after an official investigation by a special commission of the Royal Academy, which denied the existence of the animal magnetism and explained its effects by pure 'imagination' of the patients. But Mesmer never retracted his quasiphysical assumptions. He denied not only the psychological explanation of the effects of animal magnetism, initiated in 1784 by Marquis de Puységur's concept of 'artificial somnambulism', but also the incorporation of his doctrine by Romantic doctors and authors. Mesmer was much more committed to the ideas of the Enlightenment than to the speculations of romanticism. After the French Revolution, he retired from active business and went back to his home region. By the time of his death, the Romantics had made him into a leading figure of their movement.

Bibliography

Primary: 1779. *Mémoire sur la découverte du magnétisme animal* (Geneva) [German translation 1781, *Abhandlung über die Entdeckung des thierischen Magnetismus* (Karlsruhe)]; 1812. *Allgemeine Erläuterungen über den Magnetismus und den Somnambulismus. Als vorläufige Einleitung in das Natursystem . . .* (Halle and Berlin); 1814. (Wolfart, Karl Christian, ed.) *Mesmerismus. Oder System der Wechselwirkungen, Theorie und Anwendung des thierischen Magnetismus als die allgemeine Heilkunde zur Erhaltung des Menschen* (Berlin); 1980. (Bloch, George, trans.) *Mesmerism: A Translation of the Original Scientific and Medical Writings* (Los Altos, CA).

Secondary: Florey, Ernst, 1995. *Ars Magnetica. Franz Anton Mesmer 1734–1815, Magier vom Bodensee* (Konstanz); Gauld, Alan, 1992. *A History of Hypnotism* (Cambridge); Schott, Heinz, ed., 1985. *Franz Anton Mesmer und die Geschichte des Mesmerismus* (Stuttgart); Darnton, Robert, 1968. *Mesmerism and the End of the Enlightenment* (Cambridge, MA); Kerner, Justinus, 1856. *Franz Anton Mesmer aus Schwaben, Entdecker des thierischen Magnetismus. Erinnereungen an denselben, nebst Nachrichten von den letzten Jahren seines Lebens zu Meersburg am Bodensee* (Frankfurt am Main).

Heinz Schott

MEYER, ADOLF   (b. Niederweningen, Switzerland, 13 September 1866; d. Baltimore, Maryland, USA, 17 March 1950), *psychiatry*.

Meyer was the son of Rudolf Meyer, a Zwinglian minister, and Anna Walder. He studied with August Forel (1848–1941) at the University of Zurich, receiving his MD (1892) for a thesis on the reptilian forebrain. During the course of his studies, he spent a year abroad in England, Scotland, and Paris, where he worked with John Hughlings Jackson (1835–1911) and Jean-Martin Charcot (1825–93), among others. His early hopes for a research career in Switzerland were seemingly blocked, and concluding that his professional opportunities would be greater in the United States, he at once emigrated, settling initially in Chicago.

Unable to obtain a salaried university post, Meyer was forced to seek alternative employment, securing a position as a pathologist at the vast Illinois Eastern Hospital for the Insane at Kankakee, fifty miles south of Chicago. Trained in neurology, Meyer first attempted to correlate brain lesions with psychiatric diagnoses, performing large numbers of autopsies. He felt handicapped at the outset by the absence of systematically recorded observation of the patients' illnesses while they were alive, and this led him to a greater interest in studying the clinical course of disease in living patients. He began to train the hospital staff in systematic history-taking and record-keeping and devoted much less time to observations in the morgue. Assembling the hospital staff and employing a stenographer to take notes as he examined patients, Meyer created a standardized case record and began to emphasize the need for a comprehensive record of all aspects of the patients' mental, physical, and developmental history, features that would become standard elements in Meyerian psychiatry.

In 1895, wearying of the politics and the isolation of Kankakee, Meyer secured a new position at Worcester State Hospital in Massachusetts. Acquainted by now with the work of John Dewey and William James, Meyer had become heavily influenced by their version of pragmatism and was beginning to develop an approach to mental disease he labeled psychobiology. At Worcester, he succeeded in implementing a competition to attract small numbers of highly qualified new physicians to work on a common research program. Several of these early assistants went on to secure leading positions in American psychiatry, a number subsequently serving as presidents of the professional association. While at Worcester, Meyer lectured on psychology to students at Clark University, and he returned in September 1909 to speak at the famous conference where Sigmund Freud (1856–1939) gave introductory lectures on psychoanalysis, on the occasion of the latter's first and only visit to the United States.

In 1901 Meyer left Worcester to serve as the second head of the Pathological Institute of the New York State Hospitals, becoming professor of clinical medicine at Cornell University Medical College in 1904. He remade the Institute into a center for research and training for the hospital system, established an outpatient clinic, and standardized record-keeping and statistics state wide. In 1908 he was recruited to head the Phipps Clinic in Baltimore and to occupy the first chair of psychiatry at Johns Hopkins University, where he remained until his retirement in 1941. Hopkins's preeminence in American medicine in these years helped to ensure Meyer's status as America's most prominent psychiatrist of the first half of the twentieth century. His intimidating Teutonic manner, the prestige of the institutions at which he had trained, his neurological background, and his extensive knowledge of the European and especially the German literature helped to cement his status, as did the number of his former students who went on

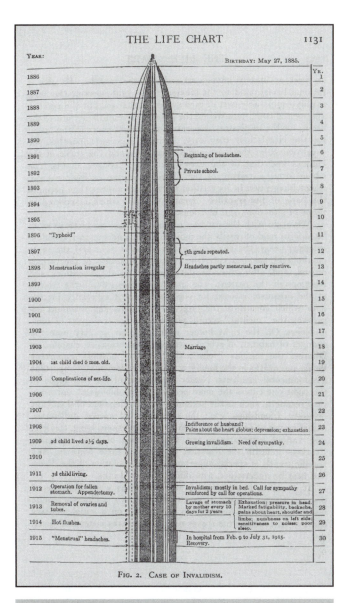

FIG. 2. CASE OF INVALIDISM.

Meyer's life chart of a chronic invalid culminating in removal of her ovaries at the age of thirty. From *Contributions to Medical and Biological Research*, New York, 1919. Wellcome Library, London.

to head departments of psychiatry across the United States. Other psychiatrists in training came from abroad, and two of them, in particular, D. K. Henderson (1884–1965) and Aubrey Lewis (1900–75), helped to extend Meyer's influence to the United Kingdom.

Meyer's prose is notoriously dense, almost impenetrable, and riddled with idiosyncratic jargon, so that providing any precise definition of his psychobiological approach is all but impossible. By temperament he was an eclectic. He embraced neither of the major competing psychiatric doctrines of his time: Freudian psychoanalysis and Emil Kraepelin's (1856–1926) emphasis on classification. For Meyer, mental illness represented a failure of functional adaptation to the demands of everyday life—dementia praecox or schizophrenia, for example, was a progressive disorganization of an individual's habits—and virtually anything might potentially explain that adaptive failure. For his critics, that was precisely the problem: Meyer emphasized the rigorous recording of everything that might have affected the patient's mental state—biology, medical history, social and familial context, psychological factors, environment (physical and social)—so the list was almost infinite, and without any criteria of relevance or any way to assign weights or significance to anything, the assembling of a life chart became almost an end in itself. At the same time, reinterpreting mental disorder as maladjustment and insisting that normal functioning, neuroses, and psychoses were simply variations along a continuum potentially opened up a far wider range of problems to psychiatric intervention: juvenile delinquency, crime, alcoholism, marital disharmony, and so forth could all be subsumed as medical problems.

Therapeutically, Meyer embraced psychotherapeutics, but also somatic treatments. Indeed, he provided crucial support in the 1920s when one of his protégés, Henry Cotton (1876–1933), adopted the notion that mental illness was the product of focal sepsis and required surgical intervention to remove infected teeth, tonsils, colons, and other organs; and he provided such support again in the 1930s, when Walter Freeman's announcement of the first American lobotomies was greeted with great hostility, a barrage of criticism that almost stopped the brain surgery in its tracks. Privately, Freeman claimed that Meyer's intervention had been decisive, and the Hopkins professor remained a major ally. Despite Meyer's reputation in some quarters as someone who emphasized the psychosocial, these and other episodes reveal a continuing fascination with the supposed biological roots of mental disorder. Moreover, the focal sepsis episode, in which Meyer deliberately suppressed unambiguous findings that proved Cotton's experiments were devoid of therapeutic value and instead were mutilating and even deadly, retrospectively casts a pall over Meyer's contemporary reputation for scientific probity. Alongside his academic duties, Meyer was regularly consulted by the rich and famous. His patients included, for example, Stanley McCormick, heir to the International Harvester fortune, and Zelda Fitzgerald.

Meyer is associated with a number of other major developments in psychiatry. He championed the use of social workers as adjunct members of the therapeutic team, with his wife, Mary Potter Brooks, serving as one of the pioneers. He was also closely associated with the mental hygiene movement. Becoming associated with the former mental patient Clifford Beers (1876–1943), he helped to steer Beers away from his initial desire to focus his energies on reforming mental hospitals, and when he was unable to sidetrack Beers's desire to operate on a national stage, he ultimately helped shape the National Committee for Mental Hygiene in directions that were largely congenial to his fellow psychiatrists. In the process, he did much to expand the arena in which the profession could ply its trade beyond the asylum and out into the community.

Meyer played a major role in the professionalization of American psychiatry. He was elected president of the American Psychiatric Association in 1927. Besides his role as a teacher and mentor, he was active in systematizing psychiatric training, and together with his student Franklin G. Ebaugh, he established in 1931 a Division of Psychiatric Education within the National Committee on Mental Hygiene to survey the state of psychiatric training in American medical schools. Meyer also played a major part in the establishment of the American Board of Psychiatry and Neurology in 1934, chairing its organizational meeting. Not the least of his motives in creating this specialty board was to reinforce psychiatry's links to general medicine and to expel nonmedical personnel from the psychiatric arena. Over the years, he likewise helped to encourage a major change in the locus of much psychiatric practice, away from the state hospitals and toward outpatient clinics and office-based practice. As the elite of the profession moved in this direction, the neglect of the hundreds of thousands of involuntarily confined patients in the state institutions worsened.

Meyer clung to his position on the faculty at Hopkins long past the normal retirement age. When he formally retired, he insisted on maintaining an office at the university, from which his influence continued to loom large. But shortly after his death, his reputation declined sharply. In part, Meyer's eclipse reflected the growing dominance of Freudian psychoanalysis in American psychiatry after World War II. It was also, however, a reflection of the intellectual deficiencies of his work and of his failure to make any significant scientific contributions during the course of more than three decades at Hopkins.

Bibliography

Primary: 1950–1952. *The Collected Papers of Adolf Meyer* (Baltimore); 1948. *The Commonsense Psychiatry of Adolf Meyer* (New York); 1910. 'The Dynamic Interpretation of Dementia Praecox.' *American Journal of Psychology* 21: 2–3, 119–157.

Secondary: Scull, Andrew, 2005. *Madhouse: A Tragic Tale of Megalomania and Modern Medicine* (London and New Haven); Leys, Ruth, R. Evans, and B. Evans, 1990. *Defining American Psychology: The Correspondence between Adolf Meyer and Edward Bradford Tichener* (Baltimore); Grob, Gerald, 1983. *Mental Illness and American Psychiatry, 1875–1940* (Princeton); *DAMB*.

Andrew Scull

MEYERHOF, MAX (b. Hildesheim, Germany, 21 March 1874; d. Cairo, Egypt, 20 April 1945), *ophthalmology, history of medicine.*

Meyerhof's family was of German-Jewish origin. It includes the famous gynecologist Otto Spiegelberg, the Egyptologist William Spiegelberg, and the Nobel Prize–winning (1932) chemist Otto Meyerhof. Max Meyerhof studied medicine in Heidelberg, Berlin, and Strassburg. He received his MD degree from the University of Strassburg in 1898. He specialized in ophthalmology and served as assistant to Guttmann in Berlin, Augstein in Bromberg, and Uhthoff in Breslau.

In 1900 he accompanied his cousin Otto Meyerhof to Egypt, became fascinated by Cairo, and settled there in 1903 as an ophthalmologist. Between 1903 and 1914, he served as chief of the Khedival Ophthalmic Clinic. As early as 1907, he began to study Arabic ophthalmology. He studied Arabic with Littmann and learned many other Semitic languages. Later he gained access to manuscript depositories in Egypt and therefore was able to publish a number of previously unknown documents, among which are medical works by Maimonides and ophthalmological treatises by Ḥunayn b. Isḥāq. He also published the *Edwin Smith Papyrus*, known as the world's oldest book on surgery. Between 1910 and 1912, he gave postgraduate courses.

In 1914 Meyerhof returned to Germany to serve as a voluntary medical officer in the German Army and in 1918 settled in Hanover working as an ophthalmologist. In 1923 he returned to Cairo, where he devoted himself to private practice and scientific research.

Meyerhof was a prolific medical writer and an authority on the history of Arabic medicine. Both his work as a medical professional and a historian was distinguished by many honors. He wrote about a hundred medical articles and books on a variety of subjects, which include bacteriology, ocular histopathology, tumors of the eye, diseases of the conjunctiva, leprosy, vernal catarrh, and ocular surgery. He also authored about 110 works on the history of Arabic ophthalmology and medicine, and sixty-six medical reviews. Among his best-known works are *Über die ansteckenden Augenleiden Ägyptens* (1909) and *Ten Treatises of the Eye, ascribed to Hunain-ibn-Ishaq* (1928).

Bibliography

Primary: 1909. *Über die anst kenden Augenleidens Ägyptens, ihre geschichte, Verbreitung und Bekämpfung* (Cairo); 1928. *Hunain ibn Ishâq's "Book of the Ten Treatises of the Eye"* (Cairo); 1929. 'L'oeuvre médicale de Maimonide.' *Archeion* 11: 136–155.

Secondary: Picard, H., 1995. 'Dr. Max Meyerhof, F.I.C.S.: A Tribute.' *Koroth* 11: 8–11; Sugar, H. S., 1980–82. 'Max Meyerhof, The Man and His Works: Contributions of the Arabic and Jewish Physicians to Medieval Medicine and Opthalmology.' *Historia opthalmologica Internationalis* 2: 381–394; Horin, U. B., 1944. 'The works of Max Meyerhof: A Bibliography.' Hebrew University School of Oriental Studies (Jerusalem).

Nikolaj Serikoff

MIKULICZ-RADECKI, JOHANNES VON (b. Czernowitz, Austria, [now Poland], 16 May 1850; d. Breslau, Germany [now Poland], 14 June 1905), *surgery.*

Mikulicz was the fourth of five surviving children from his father's second marriage. His family was impoverished Lithuanian gentry. His father, a local architect, opposed his studying medicine in Vienna (1869), and so he earned his way with piano lessons until obtaining a study grant. After graduation (1875) he worked in Theodor Billroth's surgical clinic. In 1879 Billroth partially financed Mikulicz's five-month tour through Germany, Switzerland, France, and the British Isles to study the highly disputed antiseptic wound management technique first described twelve years earlier. Its originator, Joseph Lister, impressed him as a person and as a surgeon. Mikulicz henceforth had a predilection for Britain. He found no trace of antisepsis in Paris.

After qualifying as Privatdozent (1880), Mikulicz became professor of surgery at the University of Cracow (then in Austria) (1882) and the Universities of Königsberg (1887) and Breslau (from 1890) (both then in Prussia).

Mikulicz was a second-generation nineteenth-century surgeon, meaning inhalation anesthesia (1847) was already routine. He grew up, however, amid discussions about chemical antisepsis. His organizational qualities had an impact wherever he worked. By the time of his early death, his new clinic counted twenty-six assistants and was probably the biggest and best equipped in Europe in terms of operating rooms and research laboratories.

His surgery was 'scientific' in new ways. As from the mid-1880s, it increasingly relied on the laboratory. First, as was the case with Ernst von Bergmann in Berlin and Theodor Kocher in Bern, his own bacteriological research prompted Mikulicz to 'scientify' empirical antisepsis and to develop asepsis. He created the notion of 'droplet infection' and consequently introduced nose and mouth masks and silence during operations. Such work was also the basis for his highly contested introduction of sterile cotton gloves (1896), notwithstanding the current use of thick rubber ones reserved for infectious cases—to protect the surgeon.

Second, like Kocher, Mikulicz fostered experimental surgery. He studied the influences of body temperature on brain circulation and invented heated operating tables in Breslau and Bern. To the surprise of American visitors, such as Nicholas Senn, William Halsted, and Harvey Cushing, both used intravenous saline in cases of operative 'shock' from the mid-1880s onward. Both Kocher and Mikulicz transplanted thyroid tissue to correct the 'metabolic' consequences of thyroid extirpation. Mikulicz also sent assistants to Bern to work with Kocher. He induced the former physics student, Ferdinand Sauerbruch, to tackle ways of overcoming negative endothoracic pressure. The result was Sauerbruch's famous hypobaric chamber, which introduced thoracic surgery into Germany. Mikulicz first tested it in man (unsuccessfully) in 1904.

Mikulicz invented the first functional, electrically operated esophago-gastroscope (1881), which he later used for biopsies. He continued work on the alimentary canal pioneered by the Billroth school: in Cracow he was the first to succeed in plastic reconstruction of the esophagus after resection of its cervical portion (1886). Present-day surgeons are familiar with his two-stage operation for colon cancer and with his gauze tamponade to pack off the abdominal viscera ('Mick pad'). Other eponyms recall his technical originality, extensive work and influence: Mikulicz's drains absorb secretions in large and deep wound cavities, and Mikulicz's disease is the syndrome of symmetrical inflammation of the lacrimal and salivary glands.

Mikulicz convinced Bernhard Naunyn, a leading German internist, to co-found the interdisciplinary periodical *Mitteilungen aus den Grenzgebieten von Medizin und Chirurgie* [Contributions from the Borderlands of Medicine and Surgery] (1896), which reflected his 'physiological' approach to surgery, and which brought him more recognition in Anglo-American countries than in Germany. As the Cavendish lecturer in London (1904), he spoke on experimental immunization against wound infection. His wide travels included visits to the United States (1903), leading to an exchange of collaborators with Halsted's clinic.

Bibliography

Primary: 1881. 'Über Gastroskopie und Oespohagoskopie.' *Zentralblatt für Chirurgie* 8: 673; 1903. 'Chirurgische Erfahrungen über das Darmkarzinom.' *Archiv klinische Chirurgie* 69: 28–47.

Secondary: Olch, Peter, 1960. 'Johann von Mikulicz-Radecki.' *Annals of Surgery* 152: 923–926; Kausch, Walther, 1907. 'Johann von Mikulicz-Radecki.' *Mitteilungen aus den Grenzgebieten der Medizin und Chirurgie* 3rd supplementary vol. pp. 1–64.

Ulrich Tröhler

MINKOWSKI, OSKAR (b. Aleksotas, Russia [now Kaunas, Lithuania], 13 January 1858; d. Mecklenburg-Strelitz, Germany, 18 July 1931), *medicine, endocrinology.*

Minkowski was born in Alexotas, a Jewish suburb of Kaunas in the Russian empire. His younger brother was the mathematician Hermann Minkowski, and his son, Rudolf, was a physicist and astronomer. His parents emigrated to Königsberg in 1872, and after qualifying (1881), he worked there with the famous diabetes specialist Bernhard Naunyn from 1882 to 1892. In 1884 he identified the acid in diabetic coma as beta-hydroxybutyric, a discovery made simultaneously by Eduard Külz. He was a skilled experimental surgeon and was the first to remove the liver (in geese), thus showing that it produced bile pigment.

Minkowski moved with Naunyn to Strassburg (1888), and it was there that he made his famous discovery that pancreatectomy in a dog caused severe diabetes. This happened in April 1889, when he met Josef von Mering and discussed the latter's research in patients with pancreatic

(exocrine) insufficiency. Minkowski asked whether he had done any experiments to prove that free fatty acids in the diet were beneficial; von Mering answered, 'No, because even ligating the pancreatic duct does not completely exclude digestive enzymes.' 'Well, then', said Minkowski, 'remove the whole pancreas'. They carried out the operation the same afternoon. What drew Minkowski's attention to diabetes was that a few days after the operation, the lab man told him that the dog, which had been house-trained, was now urinating all over the place. He tested the urine, which contained 12 percent sugar. He pancreatectomized three more dogs; the first two died, but the third survived and, from the second day after the operation, had persistent diabetes. Von Mering's part was peripheral, and he did not see the paper until it was at the proof stage; Minkowski put von Mering's name first for alphabetical reasons and out of courtesy to the older man. He admitted that the discovery of pancreatic diabetes was a lucky accident, but other circumstances were propitious. He was working in a department where diabetes was the main subject of study and experimental work was encouraged. His surgical ability made the discovery possible, and he understood the implications from the beginning. He followed it up over many years with further experiments, including injections of his own pancreatic extract, which were ineffective. In 1909 he tested the pancreatic extract produced by Georg Zuelzer, but although it reduced glycosuria, he concluded that the side effects were too severe for clinical use. Later, he regretted that if he had investigated side effects (hypoglycemia) more carefully, he would have shared the glory for discovering insulin.

His peers recognized that Minkowski was preeminent in combining clinical chemistry and bedside medicine. He was interested in many things other than diabetes and wrote monographs on diabetes insipidus, liver disease, gout, and poison gases. He was one of the first (1887) to emphasize that most patients with acromegaly had pituitary tumors—he reported a thirty-year-old violinist who had to change to the flute when his fingers got too big. The musician then abandoned the flute as well because of thickening of the lips, and finally his sight became so bad that he could not read the music. In 1900 Minkowski described hereditary hemolytic jaundice (Minkowski-Chauffard disease or spherocytosis).

Naunyn claimed that Minkowski lacked ambition and was continually passed over for important positions. He did not have his own department until the age of fifty, and he was then director at Greifswald (1905–09) and Breslau (1909–26). He was nominated unsuccessfully for the Nobel Prize in 1902, 1906, 1912, 1914, 1924, and 1925.

Bibliography

Primary: 1887. 'Ueber einen Fall von Akromegalie.' *Berliner klinische Wochenschrift* 24: 371; 1890. (with Mering, J. von) 'Diabetes mellitus nach Pankreasexstirpation.' *Archiv für experimentalle Pathologie und Pharmakologie* 26: 371–387.

Secondary: Medvei, V. C., 1982. *A History of Endocrinology* (Lancaster); [Anon.], 1958. 'Oskar Minkowski.' *New England Journal of Medicine* 259: 1276–1277.

Robert Tattersall

MINOT, GEORGE RICHARDS

MINOT, GEORGE RICHARDS (b. Boston, Massachusetts, USA, 2 December 1885; d. Brookline, Massachusetts, USA, 25 February 1950), *medicine, hematology.*

Minot contributed to a series of fundamental discoveries in blood disease, including the creation of a successful treatment for pernicious anemia that earned him the Nobel Prize in 1934. Minot directed the Thorndike Memorial Laboratory at Boston City Hospital for more than two decades, providing training in clinical research to a generation of American physicians.

Minot was born into a family of prominent physicians in Boston. His grandmother was the daughter of James Jackson, who was one of the founders of the Massachusetts General Hospital. Minot's father, James Jackson Minot, was also a physician at the hospital. Minot was educated in Boston's elite institutions, moving from private schooling in his Back Bay neighborhood to earn an AB from Harvard College in 1908 and an MD from Harvard Medical School in 1912.

Minot's interest in medicine dovetailed with his enthusiasm for investigation and inquiry. He published his first scientific paper at the age of seventeen, a note on a type of butterfly chrysalis for *Entomological News*. From the start of his medical training, Minot gravitated toward research, especially in the nascent field of hematology. After a year as a resident 'house pupil' at Massachusetts General Hospital in 1913, Minot joined the Johns Hopkins Hospital in Baltimore for two years as a resident physician, where he worked on laboratory projects associated with the identification by William Howell of the anticoagulant heparin.

Returning to Boston in 1915, Minot quickly affiliated himself with new medical institutions, becoming established there to foster a combination of clinical and laboratory researches. He met his longtime mentor, Francis Peabody, at the Huntington Hospital, founded in 1912 to promote research on patients with cancer. Minot later succeeded Peabody as the chief of the medical service at the Huntington in 1923, when Peabody left to become the first director of the new Thorndike Laboratory at Boston City Hospital. After Peabody's untimely death in 1928, Minot took over as the second director of the Thorndike Laboratory. During Minot's tenure as director from 1923 to 1948, hundreds of young physicians passed through the institution, gaining experience in medical research on the path to leading academic posts.

Minot's most notable contribution to medicine was the identification of an extract from beef liver to treat patients with pernicious anemia. In 1934 he shared with William P. Murphy and George H. Whipple the Nobel Prize for this discovery. Much of the necessary work took place on the

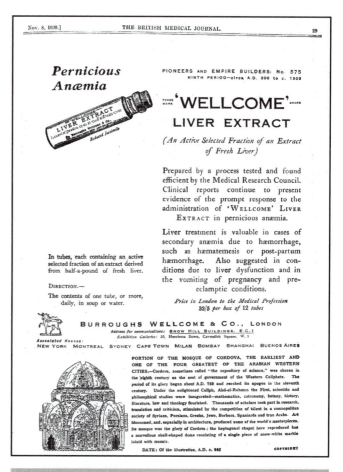

Advertisement for 'Wellcome' liver extract, a treatment for pernicious anemia. Halftone reproduction from the *British Medical Journal* (advert sets), 8 November 1930: 29. Wellcome Library, London.

wards of the Thorndike Laboratory, where physicians were able to follow patients carefully through laboratory assays and trials of treatment. Ironically, however, the initial observations concerning these successful dietary measures were made among Minot's own patients, whom he saw in a private office in his Back Bay neighborhood.

Minot stayed closely associated with the commercial development of more refined extracts of liver used to treat pernicious anemia, which eventually led to the isolation of vitamin B12. Minot served on the federal pharmaceutical formulary committee that approved Eli Lilly's production of the intermediate form of Extract G, which eliminated the need for patients to eat large quantities of processed beef liver. Minot's efforts at the Thorndike Laboratory resulted in the characterization of a number of critical bodily substances linked to the treatment of disease. His work on blood coagulation, for example, helped to isolate the protein whose absence caused a significant form of hemophilia. Subsequent treatments for the disease derived from Minot's fundamental advances.

Bibliography

Primary: 1926. 'Treatment of Pernicious Anemia by a Specialized Diet.' *Journal of the American Medical Association* 87: 470–476; 1935. 'The Development of Liver Therapy in Pernicious Anaemia: A Nobel Lecture.' *Lancet* i: 361–364.p

Secondary: Rackemann, Francis M., 1956. *The Inquisitive Physician: The Life and Times of George Richards Minot, M.D.* (Cambridge, MA); Castle, William B., 1952. 'Contributions of George Richards Minot to Experimental Medicine.' *New England Journal of Medicine* 247: 585–592; *DAMB*.

Christopher Crenner

MITCHELL, SILAS WEIR (b. Philadelphia, Pennsylvania, USA, 15 February 1829; d. Philadelphia, 4 January 1914), *neurology, psychiatry, literature.*

Mitchell's father was a distinguished professor of medicine in Philadelphia, interested in natural science and a pioneer in the use of ether in midwifery and suspension treatment for scoliosis. (After his father's death, Mitchell was to edit some of his contributions for a book.) John Mitchell sent his son to the University of Pennsylvania at the age of fifteen, and Weir then graduated from Jefferson Medical College in 1850. In this year he sailed with his sister to Europe—to England, where he met William Jenner and James Paget, and to France, where he was to study surgery in Paris at his father's wish. Here, however, he contracted smallpox, and on his return to the United States, he gradually moved into medicine, possibly because he had developed a (nonprogressive) tremor of the hands.

Publishing his first paper at the age of twenty-three, Mitchell threw himself into a variety of research projects, in both animals and man, many of which he presented at meetings of the Academy of Natural Sciences. Nevertheless, he was disappointed in his attempts to become a professor of physiology or medicine. He became intrigued by rattlesnake envenomation, starting research in 1858 and publishing a 145-page monograph two years later. In this work he collaborated with William Hammond, subsequently the Surgeon General of the Union Army in the American Civil War. During that war, many members of the Philadelphia College of Physicians served in the Union Army: one estimate in 1864 was that no fewer than 130 of the total of 174 had been involved. Mitchell himself served as a contract surgeon, remaining in his Philadelphia practice because he needed its income to support his widowed mother, who lost two of her other sons in the conflict. His first appointment was to the Filhurst Street Hospital, where he began to become interested in nervous diseases, malingering, and the results of wounds to nerves. He also encountered conditions such as hospital gangrene and erysipelas, while making what was to be a lifelong friendship with the bibliophile John Shaw Billings. Other duties including carrying out tours of inspection of military hospitals (though

these had high standards for cleanliness and organization) as well as visiting the Gettysburg battlefield and serving on a committee of inquiry into the medical aspects of scurvy.

Hammond then formed a new hospital in Philadelphia of 400 beds, all of them (save for one ward overseen by Jacob Mendes Da Costa for his studies on 'exhausted' hearts) devoted to patients with nervous diseases. This experience enabled Mitchell to write a monograph on nerve injuries; in 1872 this was subsumed into *Injuries to Nerves and their Consequences*, which, going into many editions, became the definitive reference work on the subject and was in use in the French Army until the outbreak of World War I. In 1895, moreover, he was to publish a book detailing follow-up histories of the surviving patients

During the Civil War, his elder son developed diphtheria and fatally infected Mitchell's wife (Mary Middleton Elwyn, whom he had married in 1858). Two years later, Mitchell had a breakdown and was granted two months' leave of absence in France and England, where he was additionally depressed by the seemingly universal support for the Confederate cause. In 1870 he was appointed to the staff of the Orthopedic Hospital in Philadelphia (where William Osler was a resident) and was instrumental there in setting up an infirmary for nervous diseases. In particular, he gradually began to develop the concept of the rest cure as a treatment for hysteria.

Aimed as much at the layperson as the physician, Mitchell's *Wear and Tear* was published in 1871, subsequently going through at least five editions. His theme was the effect of increasing urban pressures and the rise of 'nervous diseases'. Particular predisposing factors of 'American nervousness' included the lack of warning of mental exhaustion, the harsh climate of the United States, and the poor health of women. Apart from recognizing the potential for harm, the prevention included adequate daily exercise and vacations and diminishing the academic stresses on women. Another book, *Fat and Blood*, dealing with semi-invalid women who, though having no organic disease, suffered from nervous exhaustion, went through eight editions in the Untied States and was translated into French, German, Spanish, Italian, and Russian.

In 1875 Mitchell helped form the American Neurological Association, married again (this time into the aristocracy, joining them in holidaying in the exclusive seaside resort of Newport), and developed his theories on nervous diseases. These were seen particularly in women who 'lacked blood' and consulted many doctors, being treated for gastric, spinal, or uterine troubles, but remaining invalids. Mitchell's 'rest cure' worked best for those with agitated melancholia with periodic attacks of excitement with delusions. It centered on seclusion, bed rest (to the extent even that initially patients did not even move or turn themselves), a rich diet, massage or manipulation, and electrical stimulation. A physician with a forceful character was likely to be particularly successful, as was a well-trained professional nurse possessing firm kindness.

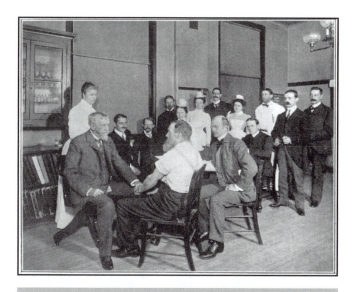

Silas Weir Mitchell examining a Civil War veteran at the Orthopedic Hospital, Philadelphia. Halftone reproduction from Anna Robeson Burr, *Weir Mitchell: His Life and Letters*, New York, 1929. Wellcome Library, London.

These principles were enshrined in *Lectures on the Disease of the Nervous System, Especially in Women*, dedicated to the London neurologist John Hughlings Jackson and published in 1881. Some of Mitchell's principles were to be adopted by Sigmund Freud, and notably his regimen was used by Sir George Savage for treating the novelist Virginia Woolf before World War I. Nevertheless, Mitchell was critical of psychiatry as practiced, pointing, in a lecture to the American Medico-Psychological Association, to its distance from general medicine and its lack of good original research. He was entitled to this opinion, for with the formation of the American Neurological Association, physicians began to vie with asylum superintendents as experts on mental illness, and for two or three decades many regarded Mitchell as the leading psychiatrist in the Untied States. And his popularity and the affluence of many of his neurotic patients were reflected in an annual income of $70,000 in his peak years.

Mitchell served as president of the Philadelphia College of Physicians on two occasions, while his output of publications (both professional and lay) was prodigious. Even at the height of his busy professional career, between 1870 and 1879, he published thirty-five papers and three books, and over the whole of his lifetime, the estimates are that he published 285 papers, nineteen novels, thirty or forty short stories, and 150 poems—many of the publications in these last three categories written during his vacations. His first paper was published at the age of twenty-three, and his last publication, the novel *Westways*, appeared some sixty years later. Many of his fictional pieces have medical backgrounds, with descriptions of doctors, patients, and epidemics, sometimes set against the American Civil War. Other subjects included the treatment of neurosis and have decay as a principal theme. The novels were well received by contemporary critics, who pointed out that, in contrast to Henry James, Mitchell's characters were recognizably normal—being mainly between twenty-five and forty-five, enjoying good food and drink, falling in love, marrying, and having children. His social life was also full, with distinguished friends from various walks of life, such as Oliver Wendell Holmes (author), William Osler (in whose appointment to the Philadelphia chair of medicine Mitchell had a central role), Andrew Carnegie (the millionaire philanthropist), William James (the philosopher), and George Meredith (English novelist and poet).

Above all, however, Mitchell's lasting contribution was to make mental illness respectable. Even if, say, Virginia Woolf's description of the rest cure in practice makes it seem rather harsh to today's opinion, there was little alternative until the practice was superseded by effective drug treatment—for, crucially, Mitchell was the first to take women's neurotic ailments seriously and to offer many patients amelioration of their problems. Although during the rest cure patients often poured out 'confessions', he did not use psychoanalytical techniques, but was concerned to shift some of the burden from patients onto the physician. To contemporary eyes his achievements, and especially his output of publications, may seem overprodigious, but several of his advances had a lasting effect on medical practice, and shrewd contemporaries considered him the most versatile American since Benjamin Franklin.

Bibliography

Primary: 1864. (with Morehouse, George R., and William W. Keen) *Gunshot Wounds and other Injuries of Nerves* (Philadelphia).

Secondary: Walker, R. D., 1970. *S. Weir Mitchell, M.D., Neurologist* (Springfield, IL); Earnest, Ernest, 1950. *Silas Weir Mitchell* (Philadelphia); Burr, A. R., ed., 1929. *Weir Mitchell: His Life and Letters* (New York); College of Physicians of Philadelphia, 1914. *S. Weir Mitchell: Memorial Addresses and Resolutions* (Philadelphia); *DAMB*; *DSB*.

Stephen Lock

MITSCHERLICH, ALEXANDER (b. Munich, Germany, 20 September 1908; d. Frankfurt am Main, Germany, 26 June 1982), *neurology, psychosomatic medicine, psychoanalysis*.

Mitscherlich was born into a family of academic chemists, the son of the chemist and entrepreneur Harbord Mitscherlich and Clara Heigenmooser. He started studying history in Munich in 1928, but did not complete his dissertation because his academic teacher P. Joachimsen died in 1932, and the successor was not willing to continue the supervision of research 'commenced under Jewish influence'. Instead, Mitscherlich opened a bookshop and pursued more political activities, supporting Ernst Niekisch and his 'National-Bolshevik' movement. After the Nazi takeover in 1933, he encountered the boycott of his shop by paramilitary SA activists several times.

In parallel to these events, Mitscherlich entered medical school, first in Munich, and from 1935 onward in Freiburg. In 1937 he was arrested at the Swiss-German border and taken to jail for eight months. After his release, he continued his medical training in Heidelberg, where he was attracted by the neurologist Victor von Weizsäcker. Weizsäcker was a proponent of the Heidelberg school of 'anthropological medicine', and attempted to develop a 'biographical method' intended to complement existing approaches to medicine, which he saw as much too oriented toward the natural sciences. In this context, Mitscherlich became acquainted with the work of Sigmund Freud, which at that time was banned from public libraries. After completing his dissertation on synesthetic perceptions in 1941, he worked as a member of Weizsäcker's team at the Heidelberg neurology department.

Immediately after the end of World War II, Mitscherlich was appointed a member of the regional civil government of Saar, Pfalz, and Rheinhessen by the American military authorities, but soon returned to his work and completed his Habilitation thesis on the origins of addiction (1946). On behalf of the West German chamber of physicians, Mitscherlich, together with the medical student Fred Mielke, acted as an official observer of the Nuremberg Medical Trial (1946–47) on the atrocities committed by Nazi physicians. In 1947 they published a first documentation of the Trial, which in 1949 was followed by a more comprehensive account (*Wissenschaft ohne Menschlichkeit*). These accounts also mentioned the active involvement in medical atrocities, or tacit acceptance of them, by leading German scientists, and as a consequence stirred heated debates in the medical community, including criticism of Mitscherlich as a whistle-blower.

From 1946 onward, Mitscherlich attempted to establish an academic unit for psychosomatic medicine and psychotherapy within the Medical School of Heidelberg University. This move met with much resistance in particular from representatives of academic psychiatry, but in 1950 was finally successful because of external political support and funding from the Rockefeller Foundation. The unit represented the first university department of its kind in Germany and became a model for later academic programs in the field. Mitscherlich was head of this department until 1967; in 1960 he was also appointed professor extraordinarius. He further initiated the independent Sigmund-Freud-Institute in Frankfurt and acted as its director from its opening in 1960 until 1976. This institute was devoted to research in and teaching of psychoanalysis, as well as to the development of its applications to psychotherapy, social psychology, and neighboring humanities. In 1966 Mitscherlich was appointed full professor of psychology at Frankfurt University.

With his writings on matters of social psychology and political affairs, Mitscherlich also became a prominent public figure who inspired the student movement of the late 1960s. The titles of some of his books (such as *Auf dem Weg zur vaterlosen Gesellschaft* [Toward a Society without Fathers, 1963] or *Die Unfähigkeit zu trauern* [The Inability to Mourn] 1967, together with Margarete Mitscherlich) have become standard formulas in public debates.

Bibliography

Primary: 1983. (Menne, Klaus, ed.) *Gesammelte Werke* 10 vols. (Frankfurt am Main); 1962. (with Mielke, F.) *The Death Doctors* (London).

Secondary: Dehli, Martin, 2004. 'Medizin zwischen Wissenschaft und Politik: Eine biographische Studie über den deutschen Arzt, Psychoanalytiker und Gesellschaftskritiker Alexander Mitscherlich (1908–1982).' PhD thesis, European University Institute, Florence; Roelcke, Volker, 2004. 'Psychotherapy between Medicine, Psychoanalysis, and Politics: Concepts, Practices, and Institutions in Germany, c. 1945–1992.' *Medical History* 48: 473–492.

Volker Roelcke

MIYAIRI, KEINOSUKE (b. Nishi-Terao, Nagano Prefecture, Japan, 15 May 1865; d. Fukuoka, Fukuoka Prefecture, Japan, 6 April 1946), *parasitology, hygiene.*

Miyairi is renowned for his discovery (1913) of the snail intermediate host of the parasite causing schistosomiasis japonica.

Miyairi was born as a son of a samurai in the Matsushiro province, now in Nagano Prefecture. After graduating from the School of Medicine at the University of Tokyo (1890), Mirairi took up teaching at the Dai-ichi High School (later, the foundation course of the Tokyo University). He joined the Home Ministry as a medical officer in 1897. Japan's first official classification of causes of death (1903) was elaborated by him together with Nikaidō Yasunori, his colleague at the Ministry. In 1902 Miyairi went to Germany to study under the bacteriologist Friedrich Löffler. After his return, he became the professor of hygiene at the University of Kyūshū in 1904.

Schistosomiasis japonica is a deadly chronic disease characterized by severe diarrhea, splenoma, ascites, and anemia. In Japan, it was endemic only in several zones, which were isolated from each other, notably Kōfu in Yamanashi Prefecture, Katayama in Hiroshima Prefecture, and Chikugo in Saga/Fukuoka Prefectures. The University of Kyūshū, where Miyairi got his post, was near the Chikugo area.

The disease had long been recognized in each area, but as a local enigma. From the mid-1880s scientific research was undertaken in earnest. In 1904 Katsurada Fujirō (1867–1946) of Okayama Medical School found a worm in the portal vein of cats showing signs of the disease in Yamanashi. Soon after Katsurada's discovery, Fujinami Akira (1870–1934) of Kyoto

University observed the same worm during his autopsy of a patient from the Katayama area. It was thus concluded that the worm, now called *Schistosoma japonicum*, was the causative agent of the disease. Yet the researchers were divided over the route of infection, oral or dermal. By the early 1910s, some researchers came to confirm the latter possibility: the larva of *S. japonicum* invaded through the skin and established itself in the portal system of the host. It was thought likely that many victims became infected during work, while parts of their bodies were in the water of rice paddies or rivers.

A question still remained: how to control the parasite. Miyairi's contributions were to solve this question. Suspecting that the parasite should need an intermediate host during its larval development, Miyairi, helped by his assistant, Suzuki Minoru, undertook thorough fieldwork in Chikugo. In September 1913, he finally found a suspect: it was a tiny snail of about seven millimeters in length, collected from an irrigation canal. After observing that the miracidia (first-stage larva) of *S. japonicum* swam into the snail, he concluded that it was indeed the intermediate host. His discovery opened the way to breaking the life cycle of the parasite by controlling the snails.

Outside Japan, many were afflicted with the same disease in Southern China and Southeast Asia, and with other types of schistosomiasis all over the world. Miyairi's work thus had an international significance. In particular, it prompted the discovery of the intermediate host of *S. hematobium* in the Nile delta, by Robert Leiper of the London School of Tropical Medicine (1914).

Since his discovery, the snail has commonly been called *miyairi-gai* (Miyairi's snail) in Japan. Projects for its extermination became vigorous after Miyairi's death (1946), by various means, such as dispersing chemicals, concreting riversides, and transforming rice paddies for nonwater uses. The snail has not been completely exterminated, but the Japanese authorities declared public safety from schistosomiasis japonica in the country by the mid-1990s.

Bibliography

Primary: 1913. 'Nihon-jūketsu-kyūchu no chūkan-shukushu' [The Intermediary Host of Japanese Schistosoma] *Tokyo iji shinshi*; 1914. (with Suzuki, Masatsugu) 'Der Zwischenwirt des Schistomum japonicum Katsurada' *Mitt. Med. Fak. Univ. Kyushu* 1: 187–197.

Secondary: Miyairi, Keinosuke Kinenshi Hensan Iinkai, 2005. *Jūketsu kyūchūshō to Miyairi Keinosuke* [Schistosomiasis and Miyairi Keinosuke] (Fukuoka); Sasa, M., 1972. 'A Historical Review of the Early Japanese Contributions to the Knowledge of Schistosomiasis Japonica' in Yokogawa, Muneo, ed., *Research in Filariasis and Schistosomiasis* vol. 2 (Tokyo) pp. 235–261.

Takeshi Nagashima

MOLEMA, SEETSELE [SILAS] MODIRI (b. Mafeking [now Mafikeng], South Africa, February 1891; d. Mafikeng, 13 August 1965), *medicine, politics.*

Molema matriculated in 1912 at Lovedale College in the Eastern Cape, the leading contemporary missionary educational institution for black students. Under Neil Macvicar, a Scottish medical missionary, he qualified as a medical orderly, the highest medical qualification blacks could then attain.

Of the Rolong-boo-RaTshidi royal clan at Mafikeng, Molema's father, Chief Silas Molema, was also a prominent local businessman and a co-owner (with Sol Plaatje) of the first Setswana-English newspaper (*Koranta ea Becoana*) and a Vice-President of the South African Natives National Congress (later the ANC). Keen to nurture similar ambitions in his son, Silas financed Molema's medical studies at Glasgow University, where he received the MB ChB (1919). Molema later became a Licentiate of Medicine at Dublin's Coombe Street Lying-in Hospital.

Molema returned to practice medicine in Mafikeng in 1921. Following Setswana custom, he married his cousin, Anna Moshwela (d. 1937). He later married Lucretia Hommel (d. 1991) and had two children. From the outset, his career was far from conventional. As a highly qualified black doctor in segregated Mafikeng, his presence in the Victoria Hospital's white wards aroused indignation. In 1927, despite his popularity amongst European residents, several white nurses went on strike against taking orders from a black doctor who examined white female patients. Molema sued the nurses successfully, but although he was one of the country's best-qualified doctors, he was still forced to leave the hospital under a cloud of scandal. Undeterred, he founded a private nursing home in white Mafikeng (closed in 1938 after racial difficulties) and a surgery in the African town, to improve medical care for African residents. White clients from throughout southern Africa continued to consult him.

Molema's historical interests began with the Siege of Mafikeng (1899–1900). He became the first black South African to publish a historical and ethnographic monograph on black South Africans: *The Bantu Past and Present* (1920), sadly overlooked by white historians and anthropologists until the 1990s. This strongly philosophical work tackled complex issues directly, including medicine and segregation. He also wrote two fine biographies of nineteenth-century chiefs, *Chief Moroka* (1951) and *Montshiwa, Barolong Chief and Patriot* (1966), and many essays, including one on Freud. His published one medical work, *Life and Health* (1924), providing basic advice on personal and community health care.

Like many contemporary black doctors, Molema believed people's medical needs were related to socioeconomic oppression, an approach honed in Scotland, where he and James Moroka formed the African Races of Glasgow with students from the African Diaspora. Molema joined the ANC in Kimberley (1914), becoming a lifelong member. From 1949–52, backed by the ANC Youth League's Nelson Mandela and Walter Sisulu, Molema became

Treasurer-General and Moroka President (Sisulu, 2002, p. 83). In 1950 Molema contributed £250 to the ANC's Defiance Campaign against the apartheid government's segregationist laws and its banning of the South Africa Communist Party.

His work as a doctor continued. He traveled to Cape Town to perform an appendectomy on his niece. Shortly after his return, he suffered a heart attack and died at the same Victoria Hospital that had once excluded him. Relevant archival collections include the Molema-Plaatje Papers (A979, 1978), University of the Witwatersrand Historical Papers (Johannesburg), and University of South Africa (UNISA), 'Molema Varia', Accounts, 1938–40.

Bibliography

Primary: 1920. *The Bantu Past and Present* (Edinburgh).

Secondary: Starfield, Jane, 2001. 'A Dance with the Empire: Modiri Molema's Glasgow Years, 1914–1921.' *Journal of Southern African Studies* 27: 479–503; Marks, Shula, 1994. *Divided Sisterhood: Race, Class and Gender in the South African Nursing Profession* (Johannesburg); Shapiro, Karin A., 1987. 'Doctors or Medical Aids—The Debate over the Training of Black Medical Personnel for the Rural Black Population in South Africa in the 1920s and 1930s.' *Journal of Southern African Studies* 13: 234–255.

Jane Starfield

MOLL, ALBERT (b. Lissa, Prussia, Germany, 4 May 1862; d. Berlin, Germany, 23 September 1939), *psychotherapy, sexology, medical ethics, occultism.*

Moll, son of a Jewish businessman, attended high school in Glogau (Silesia) and studied medicine from 1879 to 1884, at the universities of Breslau, Freiburg im Breisgau, Jena, and Berlin. He was awarded his MD in Berlin in 1885, based on a thesis on the effects of long-term immobilization of joints in experimental animals, supervised by the surgeon Julius Wolff. A two-year grand tour led Moll subsequently to the clinics of Vienna, Budapest, London, Paris, and Nancy. His stay at the Paris Salpêtrière clinic under Jean-Martin Charcot aroused his interest in treatment by hypnosis, which he studied further in Nancy according to the methods of Auguste Ambroise Liébault and Hippolyte Bernheim.

Returned to Berlin in 1887, he opened a neurological practice at the fashionable address of Kurfürstendamm 45. Moll lectured repeatedly about psychotherapy with hypnosis to the Berlin Medical Society, before publishing his textbook *Der Hypnotismus* in 1889. Based on numerous trials on patients and test subjects, it became the classic German introduction to the subject. As an early member of the Society for Experimental Psychology (founded in Berlin in 1888), Moll studied, alongside the psychologist Max Dessoir and several enthusiastic lay persons, the rapport between hypnotist and subject as well as several paranormal phenomena, such as telepathy, clairvoyance, and spiritism.

Keen to expose the tricks of 'mediums', Moll became an expert in the investigation of occultism and published widely in this then-fashionable field.

Starting with a monograph on homosexuality, *Die konträre Sexualempfindung*, published in 1891, Moll developed into one the founders of sexology, publishing further on the human sexual drive and on sexuality in children and editing the *Handbuch der Sexualwissenschaften* (1912; third edition, 1926). Like many of his medical contemporaries, Moll regarded homosexuality as a disease, which he treated with an 'association therapy' that aimed at learning heterosexual behavior. The then existing criminal status of homosexuality through §175 of the German Penal Code was in his view an anachronism. Moll was hostile toward Sigmund Freud's psychoanalysis, believing that it exaggerated the role of sexual conflicts as causes of neurotic conditions. In 1926 Moll chaired the first International Congress for Sexual Research in Berlin—Freud refused to take part.

Besides his leading role in the Psychological Society and the International Society for Sexual Research, Moll was active in the politics of the medical profession. Although he treated only private patients, he represented Berlin doctors in negotiations with the health insurance organizations. Appalled by reports of unethical experimentation on hospital patients, in particular the trials with syphilis serum performed without valid consent by the Breslau professor of dermatology Albert Neisser, Moll published in 1902 a comprehensive book on the doctor's duties, *Ärztliche Ethik*. In this work he derived the doctor's ethical conduct from a (tacit) contract with the patient. This implied the duty of the practitioner to consider first and foremost the interests of the individual patient (or in Moll's terminology, the 'client'). While Moll's work on ethics met a rather cool reception by members of the medical profession, it was appreciated by lawyers such as Melchior Stenglein, a former senior official at the Supreme Court of the German Reich.

Although Moll had converted to Protestantism in 1896 and had joined the nationalist Deutsche Vaterlandspartei in 1917, his license to practice medicine was withdrawn by the National Socialist regime in 1938, as it was for other doctors of Jewish origin. Unmarried and socially isolated, Moll died shortly after the outbreak of World War II in his Berlin flat.

Bibliography

Primary: 1889. *Der Hypnotismus* (Berlin) [5th edn., 1924, English trans. 1890 and 1913]; 1891. *Die konträre Sexualempfindung* (Berlin) [4th edn., 1914, English trans., 1931]; 1902. *Ärztliche Ethik. Die Pflichten des Arztes in allen Beziehungen seiner Thätigkeit* (Stuttgart); 1936. *Ein Leben als Arzt der Seele. Erinnerungen* (Dresden).

Secondary: Maehle, Andreas-Holger, 2001. 'Zwischen medizinischem Paternalismus und Patientenautonomie: Albert Molls "Ärztliche Ethik" (1902) im historischen Kontext' in Frewer, Andreas, and Josef N. Neumann, eds., *Medizingeschichte und Medizinethik* (Frankfurt am Main) pp. 44–56; Cario, Dorothea,

1999. *Albert Moll (1862–1939). Leben, Werk und Bedeutung für die medizinische Psychologie.* MD thesis, University of Mainz.

Andreas-Holger Maehle

MOLLESON, IVAN IVANOVICH   (b. Irkutsk, Russia, 22 February [6 March] 1842; d. Voronezh, Russia, 18 December 1920), *hygiene.*

Molleson was born into the family of a mining official, and attended Kazan gymnasium, followed by Kazan University (1860–65), where he was influenced by a supporter of preventive medicine, Alexander Vasil'evich Petrov. He started his career as a *Zemstvo* (elective district council) physician in 1865, a post that lasted almost half a century and largely coincided with the history of Russian *Zemstvo* medicine. During this period he was an ideologist and an active organizer, in different parts of the Empire, of social medicine that was free of charge and preventive.

At first he worked as a *Zemstvo* physician in the Buguruslan district of Samara province (1865–66), where he struggled against epidemics and traveled constantly across the countryside. Considering his activity inefficient, he wanted to reorganize the system of medical help for the rural population. But his suggestion ran counter to the understanding of the local *Zemstvo* administration that discounted physicians' opinions, viewing them as only hired workers. Therefore Molleson left Samara province and began work as a cholera physician in the Spassky district of Kazan province (August–November 1866).

In 1866–69 he was a factory physician in the '*Spasskii zaton*' plant of the 'Caucasus and Mercury' steamship company. He began there to research the living conditions and morbidity rates of workers and helped to establish libraries and Sunday schools.

After that he practiced as a *Zemstvo* physician in Viatka province, but his wish to establish sanitary organization again conflicted with the administrative interests of *Zemstvo* officials. In 1871 Molleson's principal work *Zemskaia meditsina* [*Zemstvo* Medicine] was published, where he depicted the unhygienic everyday life of peasants and formulated a program for the transformation of *Zemstvo* medicine. He proposed to establish stationary physician *uchastki* (districts) in the country, to introduce the position of sanitary physician everywhere, and to carry out meetings of *Zemstvo* physicians. The main aim for him was to eliminate the causes of disease.

On 1 February 1872 Molleson was the first Russian to be appointed as the sanitary physician of the Perm province *Zemstvo*. Molleson immediately asked that his own wage be reduced from 3,000 to 2,000 rubles a year. Shortly after that he went for three months to Kazan and St Petersburg to survey the organization of hospitals and laboratories, in which chemical and hygienic research was performed. On his initiative, the first meeting of *Zemstvo* physicians occurred in August 1872, at which he advocated the involvement of all the *Zemstvo* physicians in preventive activity.

After the conflict with the Perm administration, he served as *uchastkovoi* (district) *Zemstvo* physician in Shadrinsk district (1873–82). He organized there the first Russian Physician-Sanitary Council (1873–75), through which the guidance of *Zemstvo* medicine passed, in practice, to the physicians. After the closing of the Council he continued to work as a physician in Olkhovka village (near Shadrinsk) and to deal with the prevention of syphilis, cholera, and smallpox. To attract the attention of the educated part of society to the problems of sanitary medicine, he began medical-topographic researches in his district and after that passed on to sanitary statistics. By virtue of figures and commentaries, he systematically drew a dramatic picture of the mortality and the sick rate in a typical Russian province.

After work in Irbitsk district (1882–84), Molleson came back to the Perm province *Zemstvo* (1884–88) and there edited the *Permskii epidemiologicheskii listok.* After that he worked as a head of the sanitary bureau of the Saratov province *Zemstvo* and edited the *Saratovskii sanitarnyi obzor.* From 1896 to 1906 he directed the sanitary bureau in Tambov, and from 1906 to 1911 he worked in Kaluga, where he edited the *Kaluzhskii sanitarnyi obzor.* He lived in Voronezh over the last years of his life.

Molleson wrote about 250 scholarly works; these include essays about the sanitary condition of the population, works about the organization of *Zemstvo* medicine, papers about epidemics, and other publications. As a physician he was very much engaged in social work, and organized nutrition dispensaries and rural asylums for children and updated hospital work. Molleson was an organizer of more than twenty meetings of *Zemstvo* physicians and a participant of Pirogov meetings, in which he was often elected as a chair of the *Zemstvo* medicine division.

Bibliography

Primary: 1871. *Zemskaia meditsina* [*Zemstvo* Medicine] (Kazan); 1890. *Pervyi iubilei zemskogo vracha, 1865–1890* [The First Jubilee of the *Zemstvo* Doctor, 1865–1890] (Saratov); 1906. *Ocherk organizatsii i raspredeleniia zemskoi vrachebnoi pomoshchi v Kaluzhskoi gubernii k 1 iiulia 1905 g.* [Study of the Organization and Distribution of *Zemstvo* Medical Care in Kaluga Province to 1 July 1905] (Kaluga).

Secondary: Petrov, Boris Dmitrievich, 1972. 'Pervyi russkii sanitarnyi vrach I.I. Molleson.' [The First Russian Sanitary Doctor I. I. Molleson] *Gigiena i sanitariia* 7: 9–15; Kanevsky, L. O., 1947. 'I. I. Molleson—pervyi russkii sanitarnyi vrach.' [I. I. Molleson—The First Russian Sanitary Doctor] *Gigiena i sanitariia,* 5: 37–42.

Dmitry Mikhel

MONARDES, NICOLÁS BAUTISTA   (b. Seville, Spain, *c.* 1492–1508; d. Seville, 1588), *medicine.*

Born in Seville, Monardes was son of a bookseller of Genoese origin. The date of his birth is still unknown, but suggested dates oscillate between 1492 and 1508. His mother, Ana de Alfaro, was daughter of the physician and surgeon Martín de Alfaro. Perhaps this family influence decided his future profession. Few other facts about his life are known before 1533, when he returned to Seville after finishing his university studies.

In the University of Alcalá he graduated in arts and philosophy (1530) and medicine (1533). Returning to Seville, he spent his practical training years with Garcia Pérez de Morales, whose daughter Catalina he married in 1537. They had seven children, four of whom moved to America.

Monardes practiced medicine in Seville over more than fifty years. The medical experience allowed him to acquire social prestige and economic prosperity and enabled him to pursue his three other outstanding activities: the business related to overseas commerce, the publication of medical works on therapeutics and materia medica, and the acquisition of knowledge through the gathering of natural products and the cultivation of a medicinal garden.

His early publications appeared between 1536 and 1545. They concerned various matters, such as the most appropriate place to carry out bloodletting in the disease known as *mal de costado* (1539), or roses and their therapeutic uses (1540). In 1545 he published a Spanish edition of a medical treatise written by Juan de Aviñón at the end of the fourteenth century. This first stage of his life culminated in 1547, when Monardes attained the degree of Doctor in Medicine at the College of Santa María, Seville.

There are reasons to believe that, starting from the 1550s, his intellectual and commercial interests became oriented toward American medicinal products, a matter he would devote himself to from then onward. His most important work, *Historia medicinal de las cosas que se traen de nuestras Indias occidentales que sirven al uso de la medicina* [Medicinal History of Things Taken from West India Which Serve in the Use of Medicine], published in Seville between 1565 and 1574, twenty years after his former works, cannot be understood without bearing in mind the three activities with which Monardes was concerned (collecting natural products, commercial business, and medical practice).

With respect to his natural-historical collecting, it should be noted that from at least 1554 the Sevillian doctor cultivated a medicinal garden behind his house in Sierpe Street, in the commercial district of the city, where he sowed seeds of plants, native ones as well as those from the New World. In his work there are direct references to the cultivation of *carlo santo*, sunflowers, guajava trees, *cachos*, *cuentas jaboneras*, and tobacco. Although Monardes's garden never reached the dimensions of that of his friend Simon de Tovar, or that of Rodrigo Zamorano, nonetheless it was one of the most well-known of the period. The same could be said of the museum housed at his home. Although the collection was not as rich as that of his friend Argote de Molina, it was notable for being one of the first and for

containing numerous natural and exotic objects, desiccated animals, precious stones, minerals, woods, resins, barks, gums, seeds, and bezoar stones, of which he was an authentic expert in Europe, and to which he dedicated a treatise in 1565.

Monardes's commercial activities were related to America from 1533 onward, when his first commercial company with Juan Núñez de Herrera was founded. Herrera was a commercial agent in Nombre de Dios, a town in the continental American isthmus. The company plan was to ship African slaves out and bring back cochineal, dye products (which were in great demand by the European textile manufacture), and some American medicinal products that were of good economic value: guaiacum, holly bark, liquid amber, balsam, cassia fistula, and Mechoacan root. The prosperity of the business seems to have declined starting from 1563, when his partner Herrera died. Four years later when his creditors were pursuing him, he took refuge in the Sevillian monastery Regina Coeli to evade prison. From there he offered the authorities a negotiated solution as regards to his bankruptcy, promising terms of payment of the almost twenty-five million maravedis that he owed. He thus gained time, and at the end of 1568 or the beginning of 1569 they released him.

Over the following twenty years until his death, Monardes managed to repay more than sixteen million, which would indicate that he had managed to recover a certain economic position. Possibly Monardes used the publication of the *Historia medicinal*, initiated precisely in those years, as a way to increase his misused fortune. He planned a safer form of participation in the income reported from the commercial traffic of these products.

Without doubt, it is Monardes's experience as a practicing doctor that played the definitive role in the elaboration of the *Historia medicinal*. Besides the patients of the aristocratic elite (including the Archbishop of Seville and future General Inquisitor, the Duchess of Bejar, and the Duke of Alcalá) and the city clergymen, Monardes performed his medical practice in diverse spheres of Sevillian society. Because the city was the obligatory gate both to and from America, merchants, businessmen, pilots, and crews of sailors, priests, friars, and soldiers were all visitors to the city, and very often were Monardes's patients. All this provided many and diverse occasions to put into practice his medical knowledge, which included experimenting with the action of various drugs, of both local and American origin. This gathering of therapeutic experiences had another important consequence: his patients became, to a large extent, his principal sources of data when, nearly forty years after starting to practice medicine, he undertook the compilation of his work.

The first part of *Historia medicinal*, published in 1565 and dedicated to the Archbishop of Seville, was divided into four sections devoted to resins (*caraña*, copal, tacamahac, and the American substitute for the classical Greek *anime*); purges (especially the Mechoacan root, a substitute for other purges familiar to the Galenic materia medica); 'three medicines acclaimed throughout the world' (guaiacum, the root of China, also found in America, and the American spices of sarsaparilla); and finally a section devoted to the balsam of Peru (a substitute for the balsam known to the classic authors).

The success of the publication stimulated unsolicited informants who gave Monardes pieces of roots or seeds from plants with marvelous effects, or simply related a cure due to a singular remedy. These spontaneous testimonies nurtured the second part of the treatise, published in 1571 and dedicated to King Philip II. It began with a deep study about tobacco (the frontispiece being illustrated with an engraving of the plant) and continued with three long chapters about sassafras, *carlo santo,* and Indian caustic barley. The remainder of the book offered complementary notes to the chapters of the first part dedicated to sarsaparilla, resins, and purges. An outstanding example of the author's informants in the second part is Pedro de Osma, a soldier living in Lima, who decided in 1568 to send to Monardes, only known to him by his work, samples of medicinal products and descriptions of their properties. There are cases of medicinal uses of plants from Florida, referred by soldiers who arrived in Seville between 1567 and 1568. Other matters, such as commentaries describing the tree that gave 'Dragon's blood' and the virtues of the armadillo tail, came to light due to the bishop of Cartagena who arrived in the fleet in 1569 from America. He personally looked for the Sevillian doctor, because, as Monardes himself says, 'the bishop was very fond of the book which I did on materia herbaria'. The bishop provided him with a great amount of information and also with samples for his museum.

The third part, dedicated to Pope Gregory XIII and printed in 1574, together with a reissue of the first and second parts, almost exclusively contains complementary additions and notes concerning products described in the previous parts. The form in which they are assembled and organized shows quite clearly the ideas and concepts handled by the author, his method of work, and his sources of information, as well as his opinion with regard to the Indian knowledge about medicinal plants. The most representative example is perhaps that of the Mechoacan root, the principal focus of attention in the first part, as pointed out by its frontispiece. Its purgative action cured the illness of a Franciscan friar in a convent in the Mechoacan region. Because of his contact and 'very close friendship with Cazoncín, *cacique* [headman] and master of all those lands', the Indian chief asked 'one of his Indians who was a doctor' to administer 'some powder of a root', which finally cured the friar. The Franciscan Order then spread knowledge about the remedy in New Spain, which quickly reached Monardes in Seville thanks to a sick Genoese who, on being told he had to take a purge, replied to Monardes that if he had to, he would take the one he had brought with him from Mechoacan.

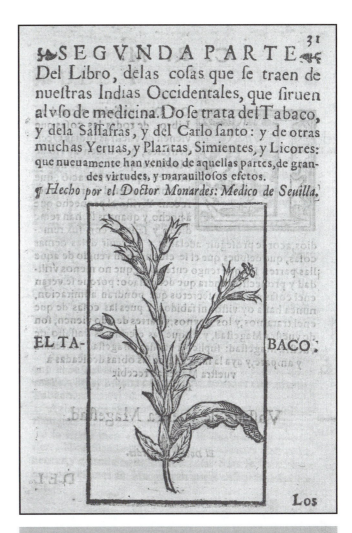

Use of the tobacco plant in medicine. Woodcut from part II of *la historia medicinal de las cosas que se traen de nuestras Indias Occidentales que sirven en medicina . . .* Seville, 1580. Rare Books, Wellcome Library, London.

This narrative schema was repeated again and again. The circulation of supposedly secret native knowledge, revealed to the settlers in a casual way, reached the metropolitan doctor. The 'hidden' explanation of the contents of the *Historia medicinal* is nothing else than the knowledge of the Indians. Nevertheless, they are almost always portrayed in the rhetorical context of accusations of maliciousness toward the conquerors and depictions of their secrecy concerning the properties of plants. This is the reason why Monardes took special care to disqualify the indigenous use of the remedies, accusing natives of empiricism and of being ignorant of rational methods befitting the European Galenic physicians, the only legitimate people allowed to experiment and to inform regarding the remedy, whatever it was.

The *Historia medicinal* was rapidly accepted and secured a position as a longstanding authority owing to three special reasons: the opportunity, the credibility conveyed to the new medicines by virtue of the practical experiences of the author himself, and the author's coherence and expressive ability, which he used to establish a practice according to the rationale of the Galenic medical system. Monardes succeeded in producing an authoritative reference source for Europe that integrated empirical information from the American cultures and therefore provided rational explanations for the therapeutic action of the new remedies.

Monardes died of an apoplexy at 9 or 10 P.M. on 10 October 1588 while staying with his daughter Jerónima in Seville. By then, the *Historia medicinal* had been reprinted in Seville (1580) and had been translated into four languages, and printed, in whole or in part, on seventeen other occasions: six in Italian, five in Latin, three in French, and three in English. Moreover, in the next hundred years there would be many other European editions: seven in Italian, ten in French, two in Latin, one in English, and one in German.

Bibliography

Primary: 1536. *Diálogo llamado pharmacodilosis* (Seville); 1539. *De secanda vena in pleuriti* (Seville); 1540. *De rosa et partibus eius* (Seville); 1545. [Juan de Aviñón] *Sevillana medicina* (Seville); 1565. *Dos libros. El uno trata de las cosas que se traen de nuestras Indias occidentales que sirven al uso de medicina . . . el otro . . . de dos medicinas maravillosas que son contra todo Veneno* (Seville); 1571. *Segunda parte del libro de las cosas que se traen de nuestras Indias Occidentales que sirven al uso de la medicina . . . va añadido un libro de la Nieve* (Seville); 1574. *Primera segunda y tercera partes de la Historia Medicinal de las cosas que se traen de nuestras Indias Occidentales que sirven en medicina . . . y el Diálogo del Hierro* (Seville).

Secondary: Pardo-Tomás, José, 2002. *Oviedo, Monardes, Hernández. El Tesoro natural de América. Colonialismo y ciencia en el siglo XVI* (Madrid); López-Piñero, José María, 1989. *La Historia Medicinal de las cosas que se traen de nuestras Indias Occidentales* (Madrid); Guerra, Francisco, 1961. *Nicolás Bautista Monardes. Su vida y su obra* (Mexico); Rodríguez-Marín, Francisco, 1925. *La verdadera biografía del Doctor Nicolás Monardes* (Madrid); *DSB*.

José Pardo-Tomás

MONDINO DE' LIUZZI (aka LIUCCI, LUZZI, MONDINUS DE LEUCIIS, DE LEUTIIS) (b. Bologna, Italy, *c.* 1270; d. Bologna, 1326), *medicine, anatomy.*

Mondino, son of Rainerio de' Liuzzi and Bella di Guidone Gonelli, was born into a prominent Florentine family of medical professionals who had settled in Bologna by 1259. His grandfather, Albizzo de' Liuzzi, and uncle, Liuzzio, were the owners of a pharmacy in Bologna, and Liuzzio was both a physician and lecturer at the Faculty of Medicine. It is likely that Mondino was introduced to medicine and trained by Liuzzio, although he was also a pupil of Taddeo Alderotti. It is not known when Mondino completed his studies; estimates range from *c.* 1290 to 1300. Although he was teaching by 1307, he is first referred to as a lecturer at the medical faculty in 1321. Mondino spent his

career teaching and practicing medicine in Bologna, and was buried at the Bolognese church of SS. Vitale e Agricola.

Mondino's principal contribution is his *Anatomy*, an anatomical treatise written *c.* 1316. The text was intended to illustrate anatomy to students of medicine during university-sponsored dissections, performed on the bodies of executed criminals. The *Anatomy* is therefore organized according to the stages of the anatomy lesson, which spanned four consecutive days. The abdomen was dissected on the first day, since its organs are prone to rapid decay, while the remaining days were dedicated to the chest, to the head, and lastly, to the back and limbs.

The *Anatomy* was the first treatise to consider human dissection for the purposes of medical training, and the work established a standardized method of anatomical instruction based on the cadaver. Before the advent of human dissection, anatomical knowledge was demonstrated through texts, illustrations, the dissection of animals, and possibly surgery and postmortem examinations. For this reason, Mondino has often been praised as the 'restorer of anatomy', and his work remained the textbook of anatomy until the early sixteenth century.

Modern scholarship has re-evaluated Mondino's achievement and significance to the development of anatomical study. Initially, neither the *Anatomy* nor the practice of dissection at Bologna furthered anatomic knowledge, and the text is replete with the errors of ancient and Arabic authorities. Furthermore, it is likely that Mondino did not institute dissection at Bologna, but merely responded to a procedure that was already taking place during his tenure. That he himself practiced or even supervised numerous dissections has also been questioned. On the other hand, Mondino worked in an age when the citation of ancient and Arabic sources was evidence of an author's erudition and modernity; his anatomies were intended to illustrate, not supplant, text-based medical education. Additionally, Siraisi notes Mondino's central role in the development of practical demonstration as a teaching tool, a major innovation of Bologna's medical faculty. He must therefore be credited for recording and propagating the practice of demonstrative dissection, which ultimately led to the innovations of the sixteenth century.

In spite of the practical nature of his *Anatomy*, Mondino was also interested in medical theory. He wrote commentaries on Hippocrates's *Prognostics* and *Regimen of Acute Diseases*, Avicenna's (Ibn Sīnā) *On the Generation of the Embryo*, Galen's *Tegni*, and Mesue's (Ibn Māsawahy) *General Canons*. In addition, he was the author of a series of *consilia*, or individualized recommendations, for patients, as well as of treatises concerning various topics, including medicinal doses, fevers, and weights and measures.

Bibliography

Primary: 1925. *Anathomia Mundini* in Joannes de Ketham, *Fasciculo di medicina* (ed., Singer, Charles) (Florence); 1992. (Giorgi, Piero P., and Gian Franco Pasini, eds.; trans. Cavazza, Albertina, and Gian

Franco Pasini) *Anothomia* (Bologna); 1993. (Martorelli Vico, Romana, ed.) *Expositio super capitulum de generatione embrionis canonis Avicennae cum quibusdam quaestionibus* (Rome).

Secondary: Siraisi, Nancy, 1981. *Taddeo Alderotti and His Pupils: Two Generations of Italian Medical Learning* (Princeton); Singer, Charles, 1925. *Evolution of Anatomy* (London); *DSB*.

Caroline Hillard

MONDOR, HENRI (b. St Cernin, France, 20 May 1885; d. Paris, France, 6 April 1962), *surgery, literature.*

Born in a small village in the central French mountain region of Auvergne, Mondor grew up in an area where the conditions of life were at that time very difficult, but which instilled in him the value of hard work. His father, the local school headmaster, raised him with a sense of probity and self-discipline. Following secondary education at the Aurillace lycée, he went to Paris in 1903 to enroll at the Faculté de medicine.

After completing basic medical studies, he joined Paul Lecene's department as an 'interne des hôpitaux' in 1909, progressively acquiring surgical techniques and judgment under the authority of this master that he admired so much. In 1913 his doctoral thesis on 'Cancer du rectum' was awarded a gold medal, the highest distinction. He returned to this subject in 1924, showing that the main lymph node invasion was located proximally, thus justifying the necessity of an abdominal approach.

His academic career was interrupted by World War I, during which he served as an auxiliary doctor for over five years; in 1917 he lost his only brother on the battlefield. During this difficult period, he was confronted by a wide range of surgical emergencies, an experience that he would later use in civilian practice, especially in his famous textbook *Diagnostics urgents de l'abdomen* (1930). The book was an immediate success and was translated into several languages; the most recent edition was reprinted in 1977. Two other noteworthy monographs were published in the next decade: *Les avortements mortels* (1936) and *Radiodiagnostics urgents* (1943), in which he demonstrated the increasing value of radiology in emergency situations.

During the same period he wrote more than 300 short papers covering many aspects of general surgery, including the eponymous 'Thrombophlebites et periphlebites de la paroi thoracique antérieure' (1939), revisited in 1951.

Mondor pursued his academic career within the Paris hospital system, as associate professor in 1923, and then successively as head of the surgical departments at the Broussais, Bichat, Hôtel Dieu, and Salpêtrière hospitals. He was named full professor of surgical pathology in 1941, teaching anatomy and pathology until his retirement in 1955. Recognition by his peers led to his election to the Academy of Medicine in 1945 and to the Academy of Sciences in 1961.

Mondor's ability to write clearly and simply was exceptional; he served as co-editor of the *Journal de chirurgie* and of the *Presse médicale*, and also as a member of the editorial boards of the *Revue de chirurgie* and of *Gynécologie et obstétrique.*

Mondor's literary achievements are as well known, if not more so in some circles, as his medical career. As a medical historian, he began in 1932 with a formal elegy to his master Paul Lecene, followed by biographies of Pasteur, Dupuytren, and his contemporary Leriche. His literary activities were quite extensive, including twenty-five works devoted to French poets such as S. Mallarmé and Paul Valery and to other writers such as Paul Claudel and M. Barrès. In his first literary title, *Lettres et images pour G. Duhamel* (1937), he showed great talent as a graphic artist, drawing dozens of plates and exhibiting a gift that he continued to develop in sixteen other books. He was elected to the Académie Française in 1947. He died in 1962 and was laid to rest in his native region at Aurillac.

In recognition of this unique career, Mondor's name was given to a new university hospital on the outskirts of Paris in 1968, and in 1970 to a square in the Latin Quarter, near his beloved medical university.

Bibliography

Primary: 1928. *Diagnostics urgents de l'abdomen* (Paris); 1960. *Doctors and Medicine in the Work of Daumier* (Paris).

Secondary: Kyle, R. A, and M. A. Shampo, 1986. 'Henri Mondor: Biographer and Surgeon.' *Mayo Clinic Proceedings* 61: 563; Ober, W. B., 1972. 'Henri Mondor, M.D. (1885–1962). Surgery and French Letters.' *New York State Journal of Medicine* 72: 222–227.

Jacques Philippon

MONGE MEDRANO, CARLOS (b. Lima, Peru, 13 December 1884; d. Lima, 15 February 1970), *high-altitude physiology.*

First Studies

Monge Medrano's initial studies and career were a remarkable case of upward social mobility and achievement. He came from a poor family; his father died when he was a child and his mother's determination, and piano lessons, enabled her four sons to graduate from the university. Upon completing his education in a public secondary school, he entered San Marcos University in 1902, and after two years he began his medical studies in what was then the only school of medicine in the country. The school was experiencing some changes with the inauguration of a new building, the creation of new chairs in areas such as bacteriology and tropical medicine, and the promotion of laboratory work in the first years of study. Like other Peruvian medical researchers of the turn of the twentieth century, Monge Medrano was attracted to study two diseases that—erroneously—were considered unique to the Andes: Carrion's disease (or Bartonellosis) and Leishmaniasis. In 1911 he wrote his medical thesis on the hematological dimension of Carrion's disease, and some years later he submitted a study on Leishmaniasis for his doctoral degree. While still in medical school he joined the Peruvian Army as a part-time physician.

which he became president some years later. In the same decade, he consolidated his university position at San Marcos's Medical School and a position as a physician of the newly inaugurated Hospital Loayza in Lima. His definitive appointment came in 1931 when he was appointed to the chair of clinical medicine, one of the main chairs of the school. For the rest of his career his clinical acumen and skill would mark his scientific studies on high-altitude physiology. Monge Medrano was self-taught in modern physiology.

High-Altitude Medicine

In 1927 Monge Medrano initiated the local high-altitude physiological studies that would give him a name in international medicine. In that year he organized the first scientific expedition to the Andes to study the adaptation of native dwellers to high altitudes. The enterprise was a response to a British scientific team led by the prestigious Cambridge physiologist Joseph Barcroft, which in 1921 visited Cerro de Pasco, a mining center located 14,200 feet above sea level. Two of the main conclusions of Barcroft—which appeared in a 1923 issue of the *Philosophical Transactions of the Royal Society*—were that humans found it difficult to adapt to an environment with little oxygen and that the native Andean Indians had 'impaired' physical and mental powers.

In contrast, Monge Medrano's expedition emphasized the exceptional physical performance of native Indians, who had been adapted for centuries to high altitudes. Monge was also responsible for the definition of a new clinical entity, the loss of acclimatization. Referred to as the 'disease of the Andes' or 'Chronic Mountain Sickness', it later became known as 'Monge's disease'. The symptoms were related to alterations in mental capacity and the nervous system; sufferers are cured when they descend to sea level. Monge Medrano believed that although most of the high-altitude natives were fully adapted to their environment, some individuals lost their acclimatization abilities.

After returning from the expedition, Monge Medrano actively promoted the findings of the emerging research in Peruvian high-altitude medicine and physiology. He delivered papers on this theme at national and international meetings. In 1929 he presented his results to the Paris School of Medicine and secured the publication in French of a book on high-altitude physiology. The event was significant because for many Latin American physicians French was the true language of medicine, and there had been only one prior medical book in French by a Peruvian physician. Upon his return to Lima in 1930, Monge Medrano and his associates organized new expeditions to the Andes and in 1931 created the Institute of Andean Biology, the first research center of San Marcos's Medical School. The Institute included an important high-altitude laboratory at Morococha, located in the central Andes. It attracted many visiting foreign scientists. Monge was director of the Institute, a position he held until 1956.

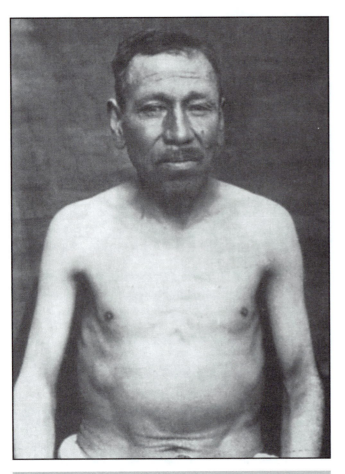

A **fifty-year-old inhabitant of the Peruvian Andes with polycythemia rubra vera with lowered oxygen tension of the blood associated with living at high altitude. Halftone reproduction from** *Les erythremies de l'altitude . . .* **Paris, 1929. Wellcome Library, London.**

European Experience

Shortly after obtaining his medical degree, Monge Medrano traveled to Europe thanks to a fellowship provided by the Peruvian government. He took courses at the School of Medicine of Paris, which was considered a mecca for many Latin American students, and at the London School of Tropical Medicine. He received a diploma from the British institution and authored two short papers on the infectious diseases of Peru (these appeared in 1912 issues of the journal of the London School). After two years in Europe he returned to his home country. Despite his experience abroad it was not easy for Monge Medrano to secure a permanent position at San Marcos's Medical School. Only in 1919, after a student strike that broke the resistance of traditional professors of medicine, did Monge Medrano and other young, talented physicians receive permanent appointments. In addition, some medical education reforms, including more laboratory work, were allowed.

In the 1920s Monge Medrano was admitted to the National Academy of Medicine, a prestigious association of

During most of his career Monge Medrano was assisted by Alberto Hurtado, a young Peruvian physician who graduated from Harvard University in 1921. Hurtado became the second leading figure in Peruvian high-altitude physiology. The Institute began with an ambitious program that dealt with the social and biological aspects of life in the highlands. The investigations went beyond the scope of physiology and examined the anatomical features of Peruvian Indians as well as their physical performance at sea level and in the Andes. In addition, a number of medical specialties, such as cardiology and hematology, derived benefits from the work of the Institute. The Institute also examined the physical and physiological compensatory mechanisms to high altitudes. Monge Medrano believed that his studies established a new scientific specialty: Andean biology. He thought that the mistake of earlier physiologists, such as Barcroft, had been to study life at high altitudes using life at sea level as a standard for normality. He complained about the tendency in medicine to ignore the reality that thousands of people, animals, and plants had acclimatized (by the late 1930s it was estimated that 12,000,000 people lived in the Andes at an altitude where the oxygen pressure is 85 millimeters, as contrasted with the sea-level pressure of 150 millimeters). It is interesting to note that his son, the physician and researcher Carlos Monge Casinelli and a graduate of Johns Hopkins, became a respected high-altitude scientist in his own right and challenged many of the original ideas of his father.

Monge Medrano's medical ideas on the capabilities of the Andean Indians also had the nationalistic overtones of the political and cultural milieu of Peru of the 1920s and early 1930s. During that period, Monge Medrano's medical advocacy on behalf of the native Indian can be considered as part of a revival and positive reconsideration of indigenous culture and people. Eventually, after the mid–twentieth-century nationalism waned in the country, the field originally named 'Andean biology' was redefined as 'high-altitude physiology', obliterating its original cultural dimension.

Monge Medrano's example remains as a model of how scientific research should be organized in a developing country. He believed that researchers in a poor country, such as Peru, should not seek sophisticated and expensive technology, but concentrate on areas of study related to national, natural characteristics, such as the high-altitude areas of Peru. The Andes was an excellent natural laboratory for physiological experimentation because very few countries had extensive populations located at more than 9,800 feet above sea level. In addition, a diversity of sick and healthy individuals, in their own environments, were readily available.

Monge Medrano's high-altitude studies were supported by various local and foreign interests, such as the government, which became interested in population issues; the mining companies, which had a significant number of workers in high-altitude locations; and even the U.S. Air

Force's School of Aviation Medicine. In addition, commercial aviation, which had to test the ability of its pilots to endure physical stress, and Andean landowners also followed and supported Monge Medrano's studies (for example, there were studies on animal fertility from the 1940s that discovered that the sterility manifested in some ram species transported to high altitudes was due to the lack of acclimatization).

Medical Practice

Monge Medrano never abandoned the practice of medicine, as Hurtado and a few Peruvian physicians who became full-time researchers in the laboratory did. Thanks to his reputation as an outstanding healer, his charismatic personality and his interlocking relationships with politicians, intellectuals, and journalists, he was able to obtain adequate support for medical research in Peru. He was also able to attract to research a number of young, talented medical students who pursued graduate studies in U.S. universities thanks to Rockefeller Foundation fellowships. His Institute also received valuable research grants from the Foundation under the assumption that basic medical science was essential for a reform of local medical education.

In 1941 Monge Medrano received his highest recognition: an honorary degree from the University of Chicago, made as part of the fiftieth anniversary of the university. Some years later the American Physiological Society elected him an honorary member. During the 1940s, Monge Medrano became less involved with the active direction of the Institute and played a prominent role in several university positions, such as dean of medicine and acting president of San Marcos University. Monge Medrano was also instrumental in UNESCO's decision to hold a meeting of high-altitude research centers in 1948 in Interlaken, Switzerland. A year later Monge Medrano and Hurtado organized a remarkable international symposium on high-altitude biology in Lima that was attended by scientists from all over the world.

Medicine and Anthropology

In the late 1940s, Monge Medrano's attention turned to anthropology and to a historical examination of acclimatization to the Andes (which resulted in a book published by Johns Hopkins University Press). His historical studies argued that the Incas had a wise organization for the Andean inhabitants that took into consideration the different ecologies marked by altitude. His enthusiasm with anthropology led to sociomedical projects in applied anthropology. He was also the head of a Peruvian commission on the social and cultural dimension of coca chewing by Andean Indians, assembled in response to a United Nations report. In 1950 he became director of a new organization, the Instituto Indigenista Peruano, an official institution that, with the aid of Cornell University, the Carnegie Foundation, and later the U.S. Peace Corps, carried out a pilot project for the modernization of Vicos, a peasant community located in rural northern Peru. This was a significant attempt to move an Indian community of about 2,500 inhabitants from low standards of living and subsistence agriculture to self-government, ownership of the land they worked, and participation in the market economy. The experiment preceded agrarian reform attempts implemented by Peruvian governments during the 1960s. In 1961 Monge Medrano was part of a new medical university in Lima, of which Hurtado and later his son Carlos Monge Casinelli would be presidents, and which after a few years was named Cayetano Heredia.

Monge Medrano was an example of a medical scientist from a developing country who became an authority in his field of research. He was also a champion in creating original medical research that was both locally and internationally significant.

Bibliography

Primary: 1928. *La Enfermedad de los Andes (síndromes eritrémicos) Estudios Fisiológicos sobre el hombre de los Andes* (Lima); 1930. *Les érythrémies de l'altitude* (Paris); 1942. 'Life in the Andes and Chronic Mountain Sickness.' *Science* 95: 79–84; 1948. *Acclimatization in the Andes. Historical Confirmations of Climatic Aggressions in the Development of Andean Man* (Baltimore).

Secondary: West, John B., 1998. *High Life: A History of High-Altitude Physiology and Medicine* (New York); Cueto, Marcos, 1989. 'Andean Biology in Peru: Scientific Styles in the Periphery.' *Isis* 80: 640–658; Dill, Bruce, 1973. 'Carlos Monge, Pioneer in Environmental Physiology.' *Physiologist* 16(1): 103–109.

Marcos Cueto

MONRO, ALEXANDER *SECUNDUS* (b. Edinburgh, Scotland, 20 May 1733; d. Edinburgh, 2 October 1817), *anatomy, medicine, medical education.*

Monro was the son of Alexander Monro, *primus* (1697–1767), professor of medicine and anatomy at Edinburgh University, and Isabella MacDonald. He attended James Mundell's school in Edinburgh and began taking his father's anatomy course in 1744. He took courses in Latin, Greek, philosophy, mathematics, and history at Edinburgh University from 1845 to 1849 and attended medical lectures from 1750 to 1753. He graduated MD in 1755.

Monro was destined to inherit his father's professorship from a young age. He began his teaching career by taking over the elder Monro's summer anatomy class (1753), and in 1754 he was named joint professor of medicine and anatomy at Edinburgh University. Immediately after finishing his MD, he went on an anatomical grand tour, studying in London under William Hunter (1718–83) and in Berlin with Johann Friedrich Meckel (1724–74). He also studied in Leyden, but returned home in 1757 to assume the professorship on his father's retirement. In 1762 he married Katherine Inglis, and the couple had five children.

In the fifty years he taught at Edinburgh University, Monro *secundus* became the most influential anatomy professor in the English-speaking world, lecturing daily from 1:00 to 3:00 P.M. during the six-month winter session. Virtually every anatomist of note attended his classes at least once, and he was the anatomy professor for founders of medical schools from Philadelphia to St Petersburg. Although his course did much to secure the position of anatomy as a scientific discipline, he resisted the growing movement to teach surgery as a separate subject in its own right, successfully fending off a professorial chair in surgery sponsored by the RCS of Edinburgh. Nor did he teach practical courses in dissection, which led many Edinburgh students to attend private lecturers or travel abroad for practical instruction.

Monro began his detailed anatomical studies in his MD thesis, when most theses were based only on printed sources. His next publication was *De venis lymphaticus valvulosis* (Berlin, 1757), in which he argued that the lymphatic system was absorbent and separate from the circulatory system. This led him into controversy with his former teacher, William Hunter, who accused Monro of plagiarizing the idea from him; Monro responded with a counter-accusation of plagiarism. Careful examination of the controversy has shown that though Monro published first, Hunter had in fact been teaching the idea for some years; both, however, had been preceded by Friedrich Hoffman (1660–1742) and Francis Glisson (1597–1677), among others. In this and other controversies, Monro defended his position vigorously, in person and in print.

The many extant copies of Monro's lecture notes remain the best source for a 'state of the art' assessment of anatomical and physiological knowledge in the second half of the eighteenth century. In addition, Monro frequently contributed anatomical papers to the Philosophical Society of Edinburgh. In 1764 he described to the Society the anatomical research that secured his posthumous reputation: the description of the communication between the lateral ventricles of the brain now known as the foramen of Monro. He later published an account of it, *Observations on the Structure and Functions of the Nervous System* (1783).

The 'famous Dr Monro', as his students knew him, was an integral part of the Edinburgh medical faculty during its golden age in the eighteenth century. His careful research and systematic lectures contributed to ever-increasing precision in the study of human anatomy.

Bibliography

Primary: 1781. (Monro, Alexander, ed.) *The Works of Alexander Monro, MD* (Edinburgh); 1783. *Observations on the Structure and Functions of the Nervous System* (Edinburgh).

Secondary: Eales, N., 1974. 'The History of the Lymphatic System, with Special Reference to the Hunter-Monro Controversy.' *Journal of the History of Medicine and Allied Sciences* 29: 280–294; Wright-St. Clair, R. E., 1964. *Doctors Monro: A Medical Saga* (London); *DSB*; *Oxford DNB*.

Lisa Rosner

MONTAÑA CARRANCO, LUIS JOSÉ

MONTAÑA CARRANCO, LUIS JOSÉ   (b. Puebla, Mexico, 20 October 1755; d. Mexico City, Mexico, 26 June 1820), *medicine, medical education.*

As was customary during his time, Montaña was unable to attend good schools because he was an orphan. However, as a small child he showed great intelligence and interest in studying, qualities that eventually won him admission to the finest schools. He studied humanities and philosophy at the Seminario Palafoxiano in Puebla, and theology at the Seminario San Ignacio. He earned a Bachelor of Arts degree and his bachelor's and doctoral degrees in medicine at the Real y Pontificia Universidad de México. In 1777 the Real Tribunal del Protomedicato awarded him his license to practice medicine.

Montaña left his imprint on Mexican medical education and the history of medicine by openly arguing that the medicine of his time was anachronistic, obsolete, and scholastic, a situation he attempted to change. To become a physician in New Spain, one had to take classes on traditional medical topics in the morning and in the afternoon, including ones in a few nonmedical subjects such as astronomy, but Montaña held that new sciences should be included, together with the ideas of Vesalius, Harvey, and Boerhaave. Thus, he sent his students to study chemistry and physics at the Royal Mining Seminary (1797) and established courses in botany (1802) and biology (1813) at the University, even organizing classes at his home.

Montaña believed that medicine had to be scientific and should incorporate the research methods of other sciences. A skilled clinical physician, he recognized that the principles of the art of curing required 'functional' physiology and perceived the need to interpret ancient clinical observations in a modern way. He reorganized the Aphorisms of Hippocrates by topic so that students would no longer just recite them by memory, but would apply them logically in their approach to patients. However, as a man of his time, he was unable to extricate himself totally from contemporary ideas, and presented a chemical interpretation of the theory of humors.

Montaña played an important role as a physician in Mexico City. He was commissioned by the Viceroy and the municipal government to perform inoculations during the smallpox epidemics of 1779 and 1797 and to combat the *matlazahuatl* epidemic (1813). He attempted unsuccessfully to organize the first medical clinic based on observation at the Real Hospital de Naturales, and later taught clinical medicine at the Hospital de San Andrés. Much later, he was named to teach Vísperas, although he soon lost that appointment for political reasons, as he believed in the liberal ideas current in the United States and modern philosophy. He was well versed in Latin, English, Italian, Greek, and Náhuatl, and translated John Brown's *Elementa medicinae* (1780), a text that served as the basis for the later extension of the *Elements* by José Ma. Mociño.

Concerned about the health conditions in the country, Montaña wrote reports on public baths, drainage from lakes, and black vomit in Veracruz, as well as various treatises on the care of patients with fever.

Montaña confronted serious political problems because he believed that people lived in misery and Indians in slavery, and that both were victims of European monopolies and injustices. Due to his background, and because people remembered that he was an orphan, upon his death he was buried in secret, without the honors normally afforded to deceased physicians. However, such was his prestige that published eulogies soon appeared in Mexico, Spain, and the United States.

Bibliography

Primary: 1817. *Praelectiones et concertaciones medicae pro Hippocratis Magni Aphorismis* (Mexico).

Secondary: Izquierdo, José Joaquín, 1956. *El brownismo en México. Un estudio crítico, seguido de la primera edición castellana que hizo en México hacia 1800 el doctor Luis José Montaña de los elementos de medicina del doctor Juan Brown* (Mexico); Izquierdo, José Joaquín, 1955. *El Hipocratismo en México* (Mexico); Izquierdo, José Joaquín, 1955. *Montaña y los orígenes del movimiento social y científico de México* (Mexico).

Ana Cecilia Rodríguez de Romo

MONTOYA LAFRAGUA, MATILDE PETRA

MONTOYA LAFRAGUA, MATILDE PETRA   (b. Mexico City, Mexico, 14 March 1859; d. Mexico City, 26 January 1938), *midwifery, general practice.*

Upon finishing school, Montoya, daughter of José María Montoya, a military man, and Soledad Lafragua, studied to become a schoolteacher but was not allowed to take the license examinations because she was still a minor. She then studied professional midwifery at Mexico's National School of Medicine (1870–73) and, after receiving her diploma, continued her training at the San Andrés General Hospital and the Maternity and Infancy Hospital with two important obstetricians: Manuel Gutiérrez and Luis Muñoz. In 1875 she moved to the city of Puebla and attracted a large clientele. However, she was resented by physicians, who felt threatened by her success, and so decided to move to Veracruz. On the insistence of her patients, she returned to Puebla, her mother's hometown, in 1880 and subsequently decided to study medicine (eventually becoming the first female Mexican doctor). Originally, she envisioned studying in the United States because she felt it would be less difficult there than in Mexico, but obstacles, such as the cost of these studies, impeded her from doing so. Thus, she enrolled in the Puebla School of Medicine, an institution created in 1834, where she achieved brilliant results in her first examinations. Once again, the harsh criticism she faced caused her to abandon her studies. Almost immediately she registered in the National School of Medicine in Mexico City. During her years of study there (1881–87)—in which she had detractors and supporters—she obtained remarkable grades. Her thesis dealt with bacteriology, a relatively unknown field in Mexico at that time. Her professional examination (24–25 August 1887) was attended by reporters, students, and professors, not to mention Porfirio Díaz, the president of the Republic.

Montoya stands out in the practice of general medicine, obstetrics, gynecology, and pediatrics. Throughout her professional life she was denied membership in allopathic medical associations, though she was highly esteemed in the country's academic circles and by homeopathic medical societies. This recognition might explain her use of homeopathic medications. She was a member and a leader of the Association of Mexican Women Physicians, created in 1925, and of a number of women's organizations. In addition, she contributed to the magazine *Las Hijas del Anáhuac*, and served as one of the Mexican representatives to the Second Pan-American Conference of Women (Mexico City, 1923).

She always maintained two offices: one free and a second one for paying patients. Though she never married, she adopted several children, boys and girls. One of her adopted daughters, Esperanza Herrera Vega, was an outstanding musician who was taken prisoner during a tour in Europe and spent the years from 1939 to 1945 in a concentration camp. Montoya continued to attend her patients during the Mexican Revolution (1910–17) and remained active until she was seventy-three years old. The 'Matilde Montoya' medal was established in 1979 by the Federation of Associations of Mexican Women Physicians to honor female physicians. Some years later, in commemoration of the centennial of Montoya's professional examination, a statue was erected near the National Medical Center.

Montoya was the first Mexican woman to register in a professional school, and her examination is deemed as a watershed that established Mexican women's rights to study, to obtain university degrees, and to exercise professional careers. Her work as a physician and as a member of women's medical associations also set an example.

Bibliography

Primary: 1887. *Técnicas de laboratorio en algunas investigaciones clínicas* (Mexico).

Secondary: Carrillo, Ana María, 2002. *Matilde Montoya: primera médica mexicana* (Mexico); Fernández del Castillo, Francisco, 1982. 'Matilde Montoya.' *Revista de la Facultad de Medicina* 3: 41–45; Wright de Kleinhans, Laureana, 1910. *Mujeres notables mexicanas* (Mexico) pp. 534–542.

Ana María Carrillo

MOREAU DE TOURS, JACQUES-JOSEPH (b. Montrésor, France, 3 June 1804; d. Paris, France, 26 June 1884), *psychiatry.*

Moreau (de Tours) was the son of a highly decorated soldier of the revolutionary and Napoleonic wars. He was educated at first in Chinon and then in Tours, where he completed his first two years of medical studies. Moreau then moved to Paris and, in 1826, interned under Esquirol at Charenton. He defended his medical thesis on Esquirol's concept of monomania in 1830. Twice in the 1830s, Esquirol chose Moreau to accompany private patients on long therapeutic voyages. The second journey, a three-year tour of the Middle East, enabled Moreau to study the treatment of mental illness in Muslim countries. He often adopted the local costume in order to facilitate his research. In 1840 Moreau obtained a position as asylum physician at Bicêtre. When Esquirol died in December 1840, Moreau and his colleague Jules Baillarger also assumed the direction of Esquirol's private clinic at Ivry, a situation that ensured Moreau's financial security. In 1861 Moreau was appointed to the Salpêtrière, where he remained until his death.

Moreau published widely, but his reputation rests on his research on hashish and his contribution to the development of the psychiatric theory of degeneration. Moreau had been introduced to hashish during his travels in the Middle East. When he returned to Paris, he continued his experiments with the drug, both on himself and with his medical students, in an attempt to understand mental illness through an analysis of drug-induced hallucinations. His experiments brought him into contact with leading artists and writers, such as Théophile Gautier, and he was a member of the famous Hashish Club. In 1845 Moreau published his major work *Du hachich et de l'aliénation mentale,* in which he argued that all mental disorders were the result of manic excitement. He maintained that the hallucinations produced by hashish were a type of madness and, more controversially, that dreams and madness were identical psychic states. The book also contained a chapter on the therapeutic uses of hashish. Moreau continued to experiment with drugs that affected the brain, including belladonna and chloroform, in the hope that they could be used to treat mental illness. This research has established Moreau's reputation as a pioneer of psychopharmacology in France.

In the 1850s Moreau began to concentrate his research on heredity and mental illness. In 1851 he drew on his experience in treating a large group of epileptics at Bicêtre to emphasize the importance of heredity as a primary cause of the disorder. He argued that a predisposition to a variety of nervous problems could cause epilepsy and that, for example, alcoholic or tubercular parents could have epileptic children. In 1859 he published his book on heredity and degeneration, *La psychologie morbide dans ses rapports avec la philosphie de l'histoire,* a work that was praised by Bénédict-Augustin Morel. Moreau argued that mental illness was somatic in origin, caused by functional lesions that were primarily the result of a morbid heredity. He also maintained that madness and genius were closely associated and had common hereditary origins, an assertion that provoked great controversy.

Moreau published his last book, on hysteria, in 1869. He never retired from the Salpêtrière and would visit the hospital until shortly before his death, occasionally seeing patients but also recounting his memories of Esquirol to a younger generation of psychiatrists.

Bibliography

Primary: 1845. *Du hachich et de l'aliénation mentale* (Paris); 1859. *La psychologie morbide dans ses rapports avec la philosphie de l'histoire, ou de l'influence des névropathies sur le dynamisme intellectuel* (Paris); 1973. *Hashish and Mental Illness* (New York).

Secondary: Dowbiggin, Ian, 1991. *Inheriting Madness. Professionalization and Psychiatric Knowledge in Nineteenth-Century France* (Berkeley); Semelaigne, René, 1930. *Les pionniers de la psychiatrie française avant et après Pinel* vol. 1 (Paris) pp. 294–301; Ritti, Antoine, 1887. 'Eloge de Moreau (de Tours).' *Annales médico-psychologiques* 6: 112–145.

Patricia E. Prestwich

MOREHEAD, CHARLES (b. Edinburgh, Scotland, 5 February 1807; d. Wilton Castle, Yorkshire, England, 24 August 1882), *medical education.*

Morehead, second son of Reverend Robert Morehead, a minister, had his early education in Edinburgh. He studied moral philosophy at the University of Glasgow and medicine at the University of Edinburgh, where he won honors and attracted notice for his devotion to clinical medicine (1828). After joining the Indian Medical Service in 1829, he had two years in regimental duty and then joined the staff of Sir Robert Grant, Governor of Bombay. He served as surgeon in the European General Hospital. Morehead was secretary of the Bombay Medical and Physical Society (established in 1835) for twelve years and regularly contributed to the *Transactions*, and was Secretary to the Board of Education, Bombay (1840). With the support of Grant, Morehead planned and set up the Grant Medical College (1845). He served as principal of the college for the next fifteen years and as surgeon at the adjacent Jamsetji Jejeebhoy Hospital.

The aim of the college was not merely to train subordinate personnel for government service, but to create scientific Indian professionals of medicine. Importance was given to clinical instruction and examination at the bedside of the sick. He maintained that the college provided an education 'scarcely second' to any similar institution in Europe, and in the late 1850s it had reached a standard to which the British General Medical Council (GMC) was striving. Though he had a large private practice among Indians in Bombay, he gave it up when the first batch of graduates left (1851) because he wanted to leave the field to his students. He held that Indian doctors should perform many of the medical duties in connection with Indian troops and the promotion of smallpox vaccination. He wrote *Clinical Researches on Disease in India* (1856) primarily for

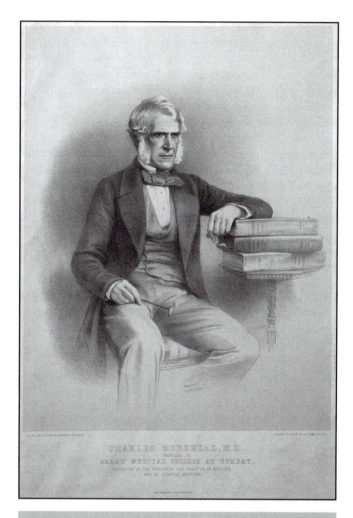

Charles Morehead. Lithograph by R. J. Lane after H. Watkins. Iconographic Collection, Wellcome Library, London.

Indian graduates, to show 'the present state of medical practice' and modify the application of its principles to the 'peculiarities' of Indian habits and constitutions. Like his contemporaries, he believed that the Indian climate was a predisposing cause of disease.

Morehead was also associated with the founding of the Obstetrics Institution (1852), which provided medical relief to poor women during childbirth, the first facility of its kind in western India. By the time he left India, thirty-three of his graduates practiced in Bombay, two practiced in the districts, and nineteen were in government employment or with princely states in different regions of western India. His influence on his students was long lasting, and even at the end of the nineteenth century they recalled his sense of dedication.

Along with his colleague John Peet, Morehead founded the Grant College Medical Society (1851) as a forum for interaction among the teachers and alumni of the college. The objectives were the improvement of its members' knowledge of medicine and its collateral branches, through reading and discussion at periodic meetings. The members presented papers on the topography, customs, amusements, superstitions, and diet of the people in the regions they served in, exchanged notes on the cases they had treated, and discussed the progress of smallpox vaccination.

Morehead was elected FRCP (London) (1860), appointed honorary surgeon to the Queen (1861), and was awarded Commander of the Indian Empire (1881). After his return to Edinburgh, he continued to write about his beloved college in Bombay. He believed in autonomous development and hence disapproved of the increasing bureaucratic control over medical education and the control of epidemics. He objected to the education department taking over the college inasmuch as he contended that it was not military officers but the medical authorities on the spot who knew what to do in the prevention and treatment of cholera. He participated as a disputant on many medical questions, discussing the pathology of enteric fever, pneumonia, and hepatitis, and suggested that for communicating with those with impaired hearing, finger sign language was most suitable.

Bibliography

Primary: 1856. *Clinical Researches on Disease in India* (London) (2nd edn., 1860).

Secondary: Ramanna, Mridula, 2002. *Western Medicine and Public Health in Colonial Bombay, 1845–1895* (New Delhi); Haines, Hermann, ed., 1884. *Memorial of the Life and Work of Charles Morehead* (London); *Munk's Roll*.

Mridula Ramanna

MOREL, BÉNÉDICT-AUGUSTIN

MOREL, BÉNÉDICT-AUGUSTIN (b. Vienna, Austria, 22 November 1809; d. Rouen, France, 30 March 1873), *psychiatry.*

Morel was born in Vienna, the son of a supplier to Napoleon's armies. From a young age, he was raised and educated by a French cleric. After a brief, unhappy period in a seminary, Morel went to Paris in 1830 to work as a journalist and tutor. He later enrolled in the Faculty of Medicine, where his fellow student and close friend was Claude Bernard. Morel defended his medical thesis in 1839, but was unable to earn his living as a physician. Thanks to Bernard, he found work translating German medical texts for the noted alienist Jean-Pierre Falret, and this experience convinced Morel to devote himself to psychiatry.

Morel's financial situation was precarious until 1848, when he was appointed as physician-in-chief to the public asylum of Maréville in Nancy. At Maréville, Morel abolished the cells, arguing that such confinement only produced violence. He established a course on psychiatry for medical students, and his lectures, entitled *Études cliniques*, were published in 1852–53. They included the first description of a condition Morel termed *démence précoce*. Morel also pursued his study of cretinism, a subject that had interested him since the 1830s. In 1856 he was appointed as the director of the Saint-Yon public asylum in Rouen, where he was able to observe a large working-class population and its many medical and social problems, including alcoholism.

Morel's *Traité des dégénérescences physiques, intellectuelles et morales de l'espèce humaine* (1857) was a work of primary importance in establishing degeneration as an influential doctrine within French psychiatry for the next sixty years. Morel argued that degeneration was a hereditary and progressively morbid deviation from a primal norm. He redefined heredity to mean not simply the transmission of a specific disease, but a predisposition to a variety of disorders. He discerned four progressively more serious stages of hereditary transmission, from nervous disorders in the first generation to idiocy, cretinism, and sterility in the fourth and final generation.

In his textbook *Traité des maladies mentales* (1860), Morel proposed a new classification of psychiatric disorders based not on symptoms, as was the practice, but on causes. He argued that most mental illnesses were the result of a primary functional lesion that could produce a variety of mental disturbances. His largest and most innovative classification was that of hereditary madness. Morel's theories were well received by many psychiatrists in part because they offered a plausible explanation for the seemingly intractable nature of many mental illnesses.

Although Morel's theory portrayed the grim decline of a compromised heredity, he was not a therapeutic nihilist. He maintained that hereditary madness could be cured through the early intervention of a qualified physician. He was also a strong advocate of preventive measures that might eliminate specific factors, such as alcoholism or environmental pollution, that could trigger an inherited predisposition to mental problems. He argued for an expanded social role for the alienist, both as an expert adviser on public health to governments and as a counselor to families.

Morel was a pioneer of forensic medicine in France, with an international reputation as an expert witness. Throughout his life, he was also an advocate of asylum reform, including the abolition of restraints and the establishment of aid societies for patients. Morel died from diabetes while still in practice at Saint-Yon.

Bibliography

Primary: 1852, 1853. *Etudes cliniques* 2 vols. (Nancy and Paris); 1857. *Traité des dégénérescences physiques, intellectuelles et morales de l'espèce humaine* (Paris); 1860. *Traité des maladies mentales* (Paris).

Secondary: Dowbiggin, Ian, 1991. *Inheriting Madness. Professionalization and Psychiatric Knowledge in Nineteenth-Century France* (Berkeley); Martin, Claude, 1985. 'La dégénérescence dans l'oeuvre de B.A. Morel et dans son postérité.' 2 vols. Doctoral thesis; Friedlander, Ruth, 1973. 'Bénédict-Augustin Morel and the Development of the Theory of Degenerescence.' PhD thesis, University of California (San Francisco).

Patricia E. Prestwich

MORGAGNI, GIOVANNI BATTISTA   (b. Forlì, Italy, 25 February 1682; d. Padua, Italy, 5 December 1771), *medicine, anatomy, pathological anatomy.*

Morgagni, the son of Fabrizio Morgagni and Maria Tornielli, began his studies in his hometown, but when he was sixteen he enrolled at the University of Bologna on 18 November 1698. He stayed there until the beginning of 1707, his principal teachers being Giacomo Sandri (d. 1718), Ippolito Francesco Albertini (1662–1738), and Antonio Maria Valsalva (1666–1723). All had been Marcello Malpighi's (1628–94) pupils and followers, and they duly taught him Malpighi's methods and the principles of rational medicine. Valsalva, who noticed his young pupil's interest and determination, especially influenced Morgagni. He was very soon chosen as Valsalva's personal assistant during his anatomical demonstrations. Of all of Malpighi's followers, Valsalva most distinguished himself by his experimental passion, and Morgagni remained closely bound to him throughout his studies and subsequent research. Some aspects of Morgagni's method of study explained the exceptional amount of painstaking and methodical work he carried out. From the very first public anatomy he attended, held by Sandri, Morgagni began to keep a daily medical-scientific journal. Here he noted down all the interesting facts he had read, heard, or observed: a method he continued and which enabled him to collect and classify, for the period 1699–1767, all the clinical and anatomical observations, postmortem examinations, records of conversations and discussions, and critical summaries of lectures, together with revisions, comparisons, and comments, sometimes made many years afterward.

After obtaining his degree in philosophy and medicine on 16 July 1701, Morgagni regularly attended the three leading Bolognese hospitals, where he was especially interested in postmortem examinations and through them gained a wide medical and anatomical experience. He and Valsalva collaborated closely not only in the latter's anatomical demonstrations, but also in the preparation of his treatise *De aure humana* (1704). Soon after his arrival in Bologna, Morgagni was admitted into the Accademia degli Inquieti, of which he became the 'prince' in 1704, resolutely occupying himself with the reform of the Accademia (later incorporated into the Istituto delle Scienze founded by Luigi Ferdinando Marsili in 1714). Morgagni dedicated his first work, *Adversaria anatomica prima* (Bologna, December 1706), to the Accademia, part of which he had already presented there in 1705 and 1706. It won him international fame as an anatomist at the age of only twenty-four.

When in 1704 the influential Giovanni Girolamo Sbaraglia (1641–1710)—Bologna's principal exponent of empirical medicine and the author of harsh polemics against Malpighi and the supporters of rational medicine—published a violent refutation of Malpighian thought (*Oculorum et mentis vigiliae ad distinguendum studium anatomicum*

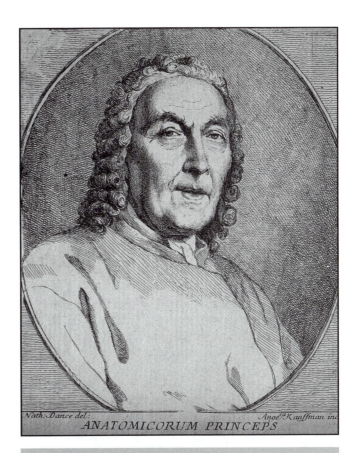

Giovanni Battista Morgagni. Etching by Angelica Kauffman after Sir Nathaniel Dance-Holland. Iconographic Collection, Wellcome Library, London.

et ad praxin medicam dirigendam), Morgagni joined the debate with two *Epistolae* published in 1705 under the assumed names of Luca Terranova and Orazio de Floriani. In effect this was a passionate defense of Malpighi's moral and intellectual figure and of minute or 'subtle' anatomy and the importance it offered for practical medicine.

Thereafter the Bolognese environment became very hostile for Morgagni, suspected of authoring the pseudonymous anti-Sbaraglia *Epistolae*, and the hostility intensified when in 1706 Morgagni officially substituted for Valsalva (who had been invited to Parma) at the public anatomy. His enemies imagined a preconceived plan that would assure Morgagni Valsalva's place when be left. Morgagni himself realized the impossibility of crowning his years of preparation and study with a chair at the University of Bologna; even Valsalva was aware of this when he returned from Parma, and thus he suggested a move to Venice. Most probably there was an understanding with Domenico Guglielmini (1655–1710)—Malpighi's former pupil, an influential supporter of the new science and especially of rational medicine, whom Morgagni had already met—about a transfer to Venice and the possibility of a chair at the University of Padua. In 1698 Guglielmini was asked by the University of Padua to occupy the chair of mathematics. In 1702 Guglielmini moved to the first chair of ordinary theoretical medicine, where he had begun his new teaching with an inaugural lecture expressively entitled *Pro theoria medica adversus empiricam sectam.*

The *Adversaria anatomica prima* was published before Christmas 1706. At the beginning of 1707 Morgagni abandoned Bologna, thus concluding an extraordinary period of study and research, which left its mark on his successive activity as a scientist and teacher. It was in Bologna, applying Malpighi and Valsalva's teaching, that he conceived the bold project of a work 'of diagnoses based on the anatomies of morbid cadavers', as he wrote to Eraclito Manfredi (*c.* 1682–1759) in a letter from Padua dated 5 May 1707. He had first announced it to the Accademia degli Inquieti on 11 December 1704, explaining that he had already begun a work 'circa Sepulchretum Anatomicum', i.e., referring to Théophile Bonet's (1620–89) first broad attempt in 1679 to compile a systematic collection of anatomo-medical histories from previous and current literature. This project was reconfirmed in the *Adversaria anatomica prima*, thus outlining a lifelong program, completed in 1761 with the publication of *De sedibus et causis morborum per anatomen indagatis.*

Morgagni moved to Venice, secretly hoping to obtain a chair at Padua, attracted by the freedom and protection the Republic of Venice offered to its university's teachers. He reached Venice around 12 January 1707 and stayed until May 1709, taking the opportunity to obtain a deeper knowledge of chemistry from chemist and pharmacist Giangirolamo Zannichelli (1662–1729). He established close and very profitable relationships for study and research, especially with the anatomist Giovanni Domenico Santorini (1681–1737), at that time dissector and lecturer in anatomy at the Venetian College of Physicians, with whom he performed a number of dissections on human cadavers. He conducted research in comparative anatomy and put together a collection of rare and choice books. During his stay in Venice, Morgagni visited Padua several times to attend public lectures and to learn about the Paduan academic environment, leaving us with some important comments on the anatomical and medical teaching of that time.

In June 1709 Morgagni returned to Forlì, where he practiced medicine with great success. However, during his Venetian and Paduan period (1707–09), he had made enough contacts and acquired such a reputation that a chair in the not-too-distant future was assured. By a decree dated 8 October 1711 he was called to the second chair of ordinary theoretical medicine at the University of Padua, vacant after Antonio Vallisneri's (1661–1730) transfer to the first chair in the same subject on Guglielmini's death. On 17 March 1712 Morgagni began teaching with an inaugural lecture *Nova institutionum medicarum idea*, once again presenting his anatomical-clinical project, claiming

that 'it is not possible to suggest the nature and the causes of a disease without the confirmation of cadaveric sections'. Morgagni's lessons on theoretical medicine held between 1712 and 1715 were published posthumously (from 1964 to 1981). He was appointed to the first chair of anatomy by a decree dated 8 October 1715 (following the death of Michelangelo Molinetti) and began teaching on 21 January 1716. Morgagni occupied this position up to his death, never losing his exceptional lucidity of mind.

Anatomy

The *Adversaria anatomica prima* was a series of researches on fine anatomy carried out according to the Malpighian tradition, even though Morgagni was more attentive both to anatomical artifices and the use of the microscope, aware of the illusory images compound microscopes sometimes created. Despite its modest title [Notes on Anatomy] the work was a continuous succession of discoveries of minute organic mechanisms, such as the glands of the trachea, the male urethra (Morgagni's glands), and the female genitalia. These were new contributions to the mechanical interpretation of an organism's structure, as were those contained in the following five *Adversaria anatomica* (1717–19), the *Epistolae anatomicae duae* (1728) published in Leiden by Herman Boerhaave (1668–1738), and the *Epistolae anatomicae duodeviginti* (1740) on Valsalva's writings. He made innumerable original observations on many anatomical structures, several of which bear his name, including the laryngeal ventricles (Morgagni's ventricles), cuneiform cartilages of the larynx (Morgagni's cartilages), pyramidal lobe of the thyroid (Morgagni's appendix), the sebaceous glands of the areola of the breast (Morgagni's tubercles), the nodules of pulmonary semilunar valves (Morgagni's nodules), frenula or retinacula of the ileocecal valve, rectal columns (Morgagni's columns) and sinuses (Morgagni's rectal crypts), hydatids of the testis and epididymis, the stalked hydatid in women, urethral lacunae, navicular fossa of the male urethra, the middle lobe of the prostate especially when enlarged (Morgagni's caruncle), superior turbinate bone (Morgagni's concha), *foramen singulare* of the petrous pyramid, and sublingual minor ducts.

During his Paduan period Morgagni also wrote on medical history, history, and erudition, gathering these together in *Opuscula miscellanea* (1763) along with others, including the *Epistolae Aemilianae* in which he discussed his native land from various points of view (e.g., geological, geophysical, archeological, and historical).

The Seats and Causes of Diseases Investigated by Anatomy

Morgagni's most important work was the *De sedibus et causis morborum per anatomen indagatis* (*The Seats and Causes of Diseases Investigated by Anatomy*) (1761), a title summarizing the anatomic-clinical method associated with his name. *Morbus*, or the disease, was the clinical phenomena presented by the patient; *causa*, indeed *causa per anatomen indagata*, referred to the organic alterations inside the patient's body revealed by a postmortem examination. In other words, the postmortem discovery of a breakdown at some point within the mechanical complex of the organism meant the recognition of the seat and cause of a disease or, rather, of its clinical manifestations presented while the patient was still alive, which could be conceived as a functional impairment and open to anatomical investigation.

For example, the first case in *De sedibus* concerned a boy of thirteen, whose brother and sister had died of consumption. He was affected by a rapidly ingravescent neuropsychic symptomatology: headache, delirium, convulsions, coma, and death. During the autopsy, when the cerebral meninx was torn, 'a little sanious serum burst forth': a finding that, thanks also to the presence of a caseous subclavicular infiltrate in the course of colliquation, allowed the identification of the lesion now called tubercular meningitis. Since 1882 Koch's bacillus has been considered the cause of the disease, and therefore responsible for the boy's death, but this was not what Morgagni intended, given that the *Mycobacterium tuberculosis* is certainly the cause of the tuberculosis, but not *per anatomen indagata*. For Morgagni, on the contrary, both the cause and seat of the disease lay in the meningeal lesion, responsible for the complex neuropsychic phenomena and death. Morgagni's objective was to identify with precision the lesions corresponding to the clinical symptomatology, which he believed were the immediate cause of disease. He therefore considered observations in the cases where death was determined by a common and frequent morbid process, rather than by a rare disease, to be much more useful.

The *De sedibus* was the result of sixty years of daily work. It comprised two large folio volumes of 750 closely printed pages arranged in two columns, and included seventy 'anatomic-medical letters' arranged topographically in five books: the first dealing with cerebral affections; the second with respiratory and cardiac dysfunctions; the third with diseases of digestion and the genito-urinary tract; the fourth with fevers, tumors, traumatic, and surgical conditions; and the fifth with miscellaneous entities and reconsiderations of previously discussed material. Each of the five books was dedicated to one of the five principal academies of Europe to which Morgagni belonged and prefaced by a letter to an illustrious physician in which the fundamental problems of anatomicopathological research were discussed. Every 'anatomic-medical letter' took a morbid entity or syndrome—'Of pain in the head'; 'Of the apoplexy in general', etc.—into consideration, and presented a certain number of cases, complete with postmortem findings and the epicritic discussion. Altogether, no fewer than 700 cases and postmortem examinations were reported, mostly conducted by Morgagni, although some were

Valsalva's and Santorini's, which he had attended during his sojourn in Bologna and then in Venice; also, some of the cases taken from the previous literature were the work of authors whom he considered credible. In each 'anatomic-medical letter' Morgagni carried out an almost complete revision of the previous literature, systematically comparing it with his own observations. His synthesis was therefore the result of a process of continuous comparative examination, first between anatomical findings and clinical symptoms and then establishing the correlations between the two orders of phenomena. The four indices, which occupied seventy-eight pages and included exhaustive cross-references, above all between diseases, symptoms, and lesions observed in cadavers, made Morgagni's work much more useful and easy to consult.

The parallelism between anatomical lesion and clinical symptom is the basis of the anatomic-medical histories of *De sedibus*, which is founded on a clinical and not an anatomical point of view. Like Bonet's *Sepulchretum*, the *De sedibus* was in effect arranged as a *practica medicinae*, the traditional treatise of special pathology with the typical organization of the matter *a capite ad calcem* [from head to foot]. The radical difference lies in the fact that Morgagni made wide use of the new knowledge about the structure and function of a mechanically devised organism, correlating the clinical record with postmortem findings and establishing the causal meaning of the lesion only when the coexistence between morbid phenomena and anatomical alteration were demonstrated to be constant and characteristic of that group of cases. Morgagni also acknowledged an iatrochemical as well as an iatromechanical conception, deducing the local lesion from an altered chemistry and tracing back mechanically from this to the functional alteration, namely to clinical phenomena.

The lesion of an organ was therefore the cause determining the clinical aspect of the disease. Unlike our modern conceptions, for Morgagni etiology included 'external' causes, namely the traditional environmental factors, including what we call 'lifestyle', and the type of work done by the patient, as suggested by Bernardino Ramazzini (1633–1714). This explains Morgagni's interest in meteorological observations and his meticulous notes, made from 1740 to 1768 and now housed in the archives of the Osservatorio Astronomico, Padua. His interest in meteorology was purely medical. When the doctrine of the contagium vivum was still in its early stages, a preeminent etiological role was attributed to environmental factors, which were seen to be associated with the outbreak of a disease. According to the iatromechanical interpretation, these external factors affected the 'fibers', which were considered—as later were the cells—the fundamental constitutive element of the body.

Morgagni's work is a true mine of original clinical and anatomo-pathological observations. He gave the first descriptions of several pathological conditions, including the syndrome characterized by epileptiform seizures with a slow pulse, described again in 1827 by Robert Adams (1791–1875) and in 1846 by William Stokes (1804–78) and today referred to as the Morgagni-Adams-Stokes syndrome; cirrhosis of the liver, which was more extensively described in 1819 by René Laennec (1781–1826); articular chondromatosis; and hyperostosis frontalis interna and its association with obesity and virilism in old women, called Morgagni's syndrome by Folke Henschen (1936). Other masterly descriptions concerned various kinds of aneurysms, gastric ulcer, lobar pneumonia with the description of hepatization, acute yellow atrophy of the liver, renal tuberculosis, the rule that in hemiplegia the lesion is in the contralateral cerebral hemisphere (Valsalva's rule), and the frequent otitic origin of intracranial suppurations, revealing the anatomical basis of several important diseases. However, the significance of Morgagni's work lies more in the epistemological break he achieved than in the individual contributions, so that, after him, no one would think and write as they had done previously. His magnificent synthesis led to the recognition of pathological anatomy as an integral part of medicine and showed the way for its further development.

Morgagni's work had an immediate influence on the world of medicine. Just a few years after its publication, *De sedibus* was translated into English (1769) and German (1771–76). The subsequent French (1820–24) and Italian (1823–29) translations almost sixty years later showed that the work retained its preeminence in Europe. The anatomicoclinical method was to be employed in all the principal medical centers in Europe, particularly Leiden and Vienna.

The next stage was represented by the identification of anatomicopathological entities similar to the morbid species identified by empirical nosology, for instance the typing of organ lesions found in Matthew Baillie's *Morbid Anatomy of Some of the Most Important Parts of the Human Body* (1793–95), representing anatomical pathology in the strictest sense. The *Morbid Anatomy* was the first treatise in which pathological anatomy was considered as an independent discipline, describing the alterations of every organ in systematic succession. Examples of anatomicopathological entities were cirrhosis of the liver and pulmonary emphysema, named by Laennec, whose treatise *De l'auscultation médiate* (1819) was a faithful continuation of Morgagni's work.

Today Morgagni is recognized as the founder of organ pathology, with which he profoundly influenced medicine. Rudolf Virchow (1821–1902) definitively recognized (1894) the significance and importance of Morgagni's work: for the founder of cellular pathology, *De sedibus* was a great methodological work, representing the successful introduction of the concept of localism in medicine.

Bibliography

Primary: 1764. *Opera omnia* 5 vols. (Venice); 1706. *Adversaria anatomica prima* (Bologna); 1712. *Nova institutionum medicarum idea* (Padua); 1717. *Adversaria anatomica altera et tertia* (Padua); 1719. *Adversaria anatomica quarta, quinta et sexta* (Padua); 1728. *Epistolae anatomicae duae novas observationes, et animadversiones complectentes* (Leiden); 1740. *Epistolae anatomicae duodeviginti ad scripta pertinentes celeberrimi viri Antonii Mariae Valsalvae* (Venice); 1761. *De sedibus et causis morborum per anatomen indagatis* 2 vols. (Venice) [English trans., 3 vols., 1769 (London), repr. 1980 (New York), German trans., 5 vols., 1771–76 (Altenburg), French trans., 10 vols., 1820–24 (Paris), Italian trans., 15 vols., 1823–29 (Milan)]; 1763. *Opuscula miscellanea* (Venice); 1935. (Benassi, Enrico, ed.) *Consulti medici pubblicati da minute inedite* (Bologna) [English trans. Jarcho, Saul, 1984 (Boston)]; 1964–92. *Opera postuma* 9 vols. (Rome).

Secondary: Ongaro, Giuseppe, 2002. 'Giambattista Morgagni' in Casellato, Sandra, and Luciana Sitran Rea, eds., *Professori e scienziati a Padova nel Settecento* (Treviso) pp. 20–30; Ongaro, Giuseppe, 1988. 'Morgagni a Bologna' in Rossetti, Lucia, ed., *Rapporti tra le Università di Padova e Bologna. Ricerche di filosofia, medicina e scienza* (Trieste) pp. 255–306; Cappelletti, Vincenzo, and Federico Di Trocchio, eds., 1986. *De sedibus, et causis. Morgagni nel Centenario* (Rome); Ongaro, Giuseppe, and Renato G. Mazzolini, 1985–86. 'Morgagni Revisited: The Papers at the Biblioteca Palatina of Parma Re-examined.' *Clio medica* 20: 160–162; Barile, Elisabetta, and Rosalba Suriano, eds., 1983. *Il 'Catalogo di libri' di Giambattista Morgagni* (Padua and Trieste); Belloni, Luigi, 1971. 'L'opera di Giambattista Morgagni dalla strutturazione meccanica dell'organismo vivente all'anatomia patologica.' *Morgagni* 4: 71–80; Ongaro, Giuseppe, 1970. 'La biblioteca di Giambattista Morgagni.' *Quaderni per la storia dell'Università di Padova* 3: 113–129; DSB.

Giuseppe Ongaro

MORGAN, JOHN (b. Philadelphia, Pennsylvania, USA, 10 June 1735; d. Philadelphia, 15 October 1789), *medical education, medicine, surgery, military medicine.*

Morgan—a 1757 graduate (the first class) of the College of Philadelphia (later the University of Pennsylvania)—in 1765 founded colonial America's first medical school in that city. His appointment to teach the theory and practice of medicine (subsequently also materia medica, pharmacy, and pharmaceutical chemistry) made him the first professor of medicine in a chartered college in the colonies. He was furthermore the first physician in the colonies who wrote prescriptions for qualified apothecaries to fill rather than concocting and dispensing his own medications.

The significance of Morgan's *Discourse upon the Institution of Medical Schools in America*, delivered at the College of Philadelphia's commencement in May 1765, can hardly be overestimated. His bold plan called for establishing a university-attached department of medicine, regularizing the practice of 'physic', and setting minimum standards for physicians. Conscious that he was laying a foundation for the future of medical education in the English-speaking New World, he detailed the contemporary condition of medical science in America and the obstacles faced by those wishing to study medicine, and he convincingly clarified why medical schools were needed. (His effort to separate the work of doctors from that of apothecaries was less successful, and he failed—he was twenty years too early—when he attempted to establish a Philadelphia 'College of Physicians'.)

Apart from Morgan's pioneering role in medical education, he is probably best known for his long-running feud with William Shippen, Jr., another Philadelphia physician. Shippen claimed priority in instituting formal medical instruction in Pennsylvania, on the strength of his private course. The Trustees' public affirmation (in 1770) of Morgan's claim to precedence angered him. Then George Washington appointed Morgan director general of the military hospitals during the Revolutionary War, and Shippen—also in the army—found himself subordinate to his nemesis. Morgan believed (probably correctly) that Shippen was primarily responsible for the charges subsequently raised against Morgan's handling of affairs, which forced Morgan's resignation; Shippen was appointed in his stead. Morgan, his pride wounded, responded by publishing a lengthy *Vindication*. That and more politicking led to his eventual reinstatement.

Focusing on these quarrels mars the picture of Morgan as perhaps the most erudite physician of his day in the colonies. Following college, he was apprenticed to John Redman of Philadelphia for six years and worked as apothecary to the Pennsylvania Hospital. Having served as a medical officer in the French and Indian War (his friend and early student Benjamin Rush later praised him for his skill as both physician and surgeon), Morgan traveled to London with letters of introduction from Benjamin Franklin. There he spent time under the tutelage of Fothergill, both Hunters, and Hewson prior to studying in Edinburgh (only the tenth American to enroll). Awarded his MD in 1763 after two years' work (primarily under Cullen) and a Latin thesis on the formation of pus, he studied anatomy briefly in Paris and met the eighty-two-year-old Morgagni in Padua. A more complete medical education was not possible.

A Licentiate of the Royal College of Physicians in both Edinburgh and London, Morgan was further honored with membership in the Royal Society of London, the Académie Royale de Chirurgie de Paris, and the Belles-Lettres Society of Rome. Rush later wrote that Morgan's name once filled half the world.

Bibliography

Primary: 1765. *A discourse upon the Institution of Medical Schools in America* (Philadelphia); 1776. *A Vindication of His Public Character in the Station of Director-General of the Military Hospitals and Physician in Chief to the American Army* (Boston).

Secondary: Bell, Whitfield J., 1965. *John Morgan, Continental Doctor* (Philadelphia); Corner, George Washington, 1965. *Two Centuries of Medicine: A History of the School of Medicine, University of Pennsylvania* (Philadelphia); Wilbert, Martin I., 1904. 'John Morgan: The Founder of the First Medical School and the Originator of Pharmacy in America.' *American Journal of Pharmacy* 76: 1–15; *DAMB*.

Constance Putnam

MORI, RINTARŌ (aka MORI, ŌGAI) (b. Tsuwano, Iwami domain [now Shimane Prefecture], Japan, 27 February 1862; d. Tokyo, Japan, 9 July 1922), *military medicine, literature.*

Mori Rintarō is much better known by the name of Mori Ōgai, under which he wrote novels and essays that are now major classics in modern Japanese literature. His career in military medicine was no less illustrious, including service as the surgeon general from 1907 to 1916. No modern Japanese intellectual has ever achieved such a feat of combining eminent medical and literary careers.

Mori was born in 1862 in Tsuwano-machi in the Iwami domain (now Shimane Prefecture) as the first son of Mori Seitai (later Shizuo) and his wife Mine. Generations of the Mori family had served as court physicians to the local daimyō. In 1872 Mori's family moved to Tokyo, where the father started a private practice and Rintarō started to learn German, preparing for a career in medicine. In 1874 he matriculated in the preparatory course of the Medical School of the University of Tokyo (then called Tokyo School of Medicine) at the age of twelve, two years below the lower age limit. In 1881 Mori graduated from the Medical School and entered the army medical service. In 1884 he was ordered to study military medicine and hygiene in Germany, fulfilling his ambition to join the medical and intellectual elites in Japan. In Germany he studied hygiene under three professors—Franz Hoffmann (1843–1920) at Leipzig, Max von Pettenkofer (1818–1901) at Munich, and Robert Koch (1843–1910) at Berlin—as well as studying military medicine at Dresden. The choice of hygiene and military medicine showed that Mori's ambition was to serve the state and the public, and that he was attracted by the scientific rigor and the intellectual prestige of experimental laboratory medical science.

His return to Japan in 1888 was soon followed by the prodigious combination of literary and medical outputs. As well as publishing widely-read and influential novels, essays, and translations, he assumed the position of editor-in-chief of *Tokyo iji shinshi* [Tokyo Medical News], a major medical weekly at that time. In this and other journals, he conducted active controversies over various medical matters, such as the nature of medical statistics and the role of medical associations. For the army, he conducted physiological experiments on the food of soldiers, which was a key question at that time when Takaki Kanehiro (1849–1920) in the navy and other eminent doctors were preaching the harm of polished rice. In 1897, with his colleague in the army medical service Koike Masanao (1854–1913), Mori published *Eisei shinpen* [New Hygiene], a two-volume textbook on military and civil hygiene, which went through five editions until 1914. After serving in the Sino-Japanese War (1894–95) and Russo-Japanese War (1904–05), he succeeded Koike as the surgeon general of the army medical service in 1907. As surgeon general, he promoted vaccination against typhoid in the army, which was implemented in 1910 and had a dramatic result. He was also responsible for major historical projects of the army, such as the history of the medical service in the Russo-Japanese War and the history of military hygiene in Japan. These historical projects perhaps directed Mori's creative literary energy toward history and historical novels, which resulted in several masterpieces in those genres. He died from tuberculosis in 1922.

Mori managed to combine prominent literary activities with the successful performance of military medical service. Mori is thus largely seen as an embodiment of the ideals of Japanese intellectuals, combining science and literature, at home with both modern Western science and traditional Japanese humanistic learning, casting a critical eye on the present and keeping a keen interest in history.

Bibliography

Primary: 1971–. *Ōgaizenshū* [Collected Works of Mori Ōgai] 38+ vols. (Tokyo).

Secondary: Asai, Takuo, 1986. *Gun'i Mori Ōgai no shōgai* [The Life of Mori Ōgai as a Military Surgeon] (Tokyo); Date, Kazuo, 1981. *Ishi to shiteno Mori Ōgai* [Life of Mori Ōgai as a Doctor] (Tokyo); Date, Kazuo, 1989. *Zoku ishi to shiteno Mori Ōgai* [Life of Mori Ōgai as a Doctor, Part II] (Tokyo).

Akihito Suzuki

MOROKA, JAMES SEBEBUJIWASEGOKGOBONTHARILE
(b. Thaba 'Nchu [Black Mountain], Free State, South Africa, 16 March 1891; d. Thaba 'Nchu, 10 November 1985), *medicine, political activism.*

Moroka's great-grandfather was the illustrious Chief Moroka II of the Setswana-speaking Rolong-boo-Seleka royal line. After schooling at Lovedale College, Eastern Cape, Moroka studied medicine on a church scholarship at Edinburgh University because South African universities excluded black students. He graduated MB ChB (1918) and was still one of just six black medical doctors in South Africa in 1946. Moroka and his lifelong colleague and friend, Modiri Molema, then studying medicine at Glasgow University, felt culturally captive as 'the only two Batswana here in Scotland' during World War I (MPP, A979 Ad1, 27 Aug 1915, Modiri Molema, Glasgow to ST Molema, Mafikeng).

Returning to Thaba 'Nchu in 1919, Moroka established a 'lucrative multiracial [medical] practice' (ACC142, Molema, 1952, '. . . Moroka'), where he practiced medicine until his retirement in 1976. Patients would travel vast distances to his Thaba 'Nchu and Johannesburg surgeries. Early in this productive period, he married his cousin,

Maggy Fenyang, who died young; he later married Susan Motshumi and had ten children.

Moroka dedicated himself to community health care, as state-funded treatment for rural blacks was lacking. In 1937 he and his father-in-law, Chief Fenyang, established Thaba 'Nchu's Moroka Methodist Institution (MMI): a Secondary Training School and the Moroka Missionary Hospital (MMH). The MMH's maternity, tuberculosis, venereal disease wards, and x-ray facilities improved the black and white communities' health care in Thaba 'Nchu and Lesotho. Although by 1948 it enrolled 450 patients annually, Moroka did not practice there, given the 'difficulties involved if a European nurse serves under a non-European doctor' (UNISA, Karis and Carter, 'Dr SJ Moroka', p. 1). His surgery often received buses 'packed with 50 or more patients' and he would work 'until the late hours of the night, never sparing himself' (Olivier and Kriel, 1978, p. 2).

Moroka could be politically 'militant', defying stringent land laws by owning farms in 'white areas'. In 1936 he became treasurer of the All Africa Convention, which united Africans, 'Coloreds', and Indians against segregationist laws.

The pinnacle of his career was his unorthodox election as African National Congress (ANC) President at the December 1949 Conference, unseating another doctor-politician, Alfred Bitini Xuma. The ANC Youth League (ANCYL), under Nelson Mandela and Walter Sisulu, adopted a Programme of Action, and sought a leader to steer their mass-based passive resistance against discriminatory legislation. Others declined, so the ANCYL approached Moroka. After his election, he launched the 1950 Defiance Campaign in Johannesburg, saying: 'Those who are keeping us down do so not because we are Communists . . . they want to exploit us, they want to eat the fat of the land alone' (Simons and Simons, 1983, pp. 604–605).

His medical practice echoed his nonracial politics. He declared in 1952: '. . . co-operation with Europeans [whites] is essential. It is impossible to have a lot of small and separate civilisations . . . in the same county' (*Drum*, February 1952, pp. 15ff). Moroka believed that large-scale medical improvements would only come through black political liberation. A vocal politician until the mid-1950s, Moroka demanded the abolition of all discrimination. Moroka's medical contributions are less well-acknowledged. Wealthy through farming interests, he supported numerous medical students, including '2 White Afrikaans-speaking South Africans' to qualify as medical doctors (Olivier and Kriel, 1978, p. 2). Archival collections relating to Moroka are housed at the University of South Africa (UNISA), Karis and Carter Papers [microfilm], 2: XM130: 961, 'Dr SJ Moroka, President of the ANC' (1952); UNISA, Pretoria, ACC142, Molema Varia [MV], SM Molema, 'Dr James Moroka, President-General: African National Congress' (1977); and the Molema-Plaatje Papers (1978) [MPP] University of the Witwatersrand (Johannesburg).

Bibliography

Secondary: Cobley, Alan, 1990. *Class and Consciousness: The Black Petty Bourgeoisie in South Africa, 1924 to 1950* (New York); Shapiro, Karin A., 1987. 'Doctors or Medical Aids—The Debate over the Training of Black Medical Personnel for the Rural Black Population in South Africa in the 1920s and 1930s.' *Journal of Southern African Studies* 13: 234–255; Simons, Jack, and Ray Simons, 1983. *Class and Colour in South Africa 1850–1950* (London); Olivier, L. R., and J. R. Kriel, 1978. 'A Job Well Done—A Short History of Dr James Moroka.' *South African Medical Journal* 54: 331–332.

Jane Starfield

MORQUIO, LUIS   (b. Montevideo, Uruguay, 24 September 1867; d. Montevideo, 9 July 1935), *pediatrics.*

Morquio was the oldest of ten children of Italian immigrant shoemaker José Morquio and second-generation immigrant Ana Bélinzon. He studied medicine at the University of the Republic of Uruguay (1887–92), interning with Pedro Visca, the country's founding medical clinician, and writing a dissertation on the treatment of typhoid fever.

After receiving his doctorate, Morquio went to Paris to study childhood diseases. He attended the Sick Children's Clinic under Jacques-Joseph Grancher and Antoine Marfan; frequented the clinics of Jules Comby, Pierre Potain, and others; and took classes at the Pasteur Institute, founded in 1887 to advance the study of infectious diseases.

Morquio's return to Montevideo in 1894 coincided with the establishment of the country's first chair in children's medicine at the Faculty of Medicine; he launched the Faculty's Children's Clinic and became medical director of external services at the national Orphanage and Foundling Home. There he oversaw an extraordinarily low—for its time—mortality rate of 7 percent of orphaned children, which he attributed to careful infant feeding and weekly visits to his clinic by wet nurses with their charges. In 1896 he married María Josefa Márquez; they had two children.

In 1900 Morquio assumed the pediatrics chair (a position he held until his death), marking Uruguay's inauguration of pediatrics as both a teaching discipline and a clinical specialty. Morquio went on to hold a series of administrative positions—including medical director of Uruguay's largest children's asylum, founder of the Uruguayan Society of Pediatrics, and organizer of the Institute of Pediatrics and Puericulture—all the while maintaining his clinical practice, public health activities, and international involvement. Morquio was a prolific contributor to work on infant mortality and childhood diseases, publishing several well-cited textbooks, authoring 335 articles in five languages (almost half of which were in foreign journals), co-founding the *Archivos Latino Americanos de Pediatría*, and frequently presenting analyses of Uruguay's children's health situation to (Latin) American and European congresses. Among many honors, he was named officer of the Légion d'Honneur and corresponding member of the Paris Academy of Medicine.

Morquio's work bridged the worlds of medicine, scientific research, and public policy. He became widely known for his 1917 book on gastrointestinal problems of infants, which was translated into several languages. In 1928 the Pan American Sanitary Bureau cited his work on infant mortality as bearing 'universal relevance'. He described in 1901 'complete atrioventricular block', known today as Morquio's disease. In 1929 he observed a severe form of 'familial skeletal dystrophy' in a rural Uruguayan family (now known both as Morquio's syndrome and as mucopolysaccharidosis IV). He was also a leading advocate of puericulture—positive eugenics aimed at enhancing prenatal and child-raising conditions.

In the late 1910s Morquio became involved with the Pan American Child Congresses, a Latin American network of reformers, feminists, physicians, and social workers devoted to improving the health and welfare of poor and working-class women and their children. As host of the highly successful second congress held in Montevideo in 1919, he proposed the founding of an International Institute for the Protection of Childhood (IIPI), a goal realized in 1927 with League of Nations backing. Under Morquio's directorship, the IIPI—the world's first such organization—published an influential journal, became a much-consulted clearinghouse for international legislation and policy on child well-being, and provided a worldwide platform for Uruguayan developments, such as its 1934 'Children's Code of Rights'. In 1930 Morquio was elected president of Save the Children in Geneva.

Bibliography

Primary: 1917. *Los desarreglos gastrointestinales del lactante* (Montevideo); 1929. 'Sur une forme de dystrophie osseuse familiale.' *Archives de Médecine des Enfants* 32; 1931. 'Conférence d'experts hygiénistes en matière de protection de la première enfance.' *Boletín del Instituto Internacional Americano de Protección a la Infancia* 4(3): 535–580.

Secondary: Gorlero Bacigalupi, Rubén, 1967. *Biografía de Luis Morquio* (Montevideo); Consejo del Niño, 1935. *Morquio 1867–1935 Homenaje* (Montevideo); Sergent, Emile, 1935. *Luis Morquio (1867–1935)* (Paris).

Anne-Emanuelle Birn

MORSELLI, ENRICO   (b. Modena, Italy, 7 July 1852; d. Genoa, Italy, 18 February 1929), *psychiatry.*

Morselli was three when his father died; he attended a private Catholic school, becoming as a result anticlerical and a Darwinist. He attended the Faculty of Medicine at the University of Modena and had as teachers the zoologist Giovanni Canestrini, considered the most Darwinian of the Italian scientists, the psychiatrist Carlo Livi, and the anatomist Paolo Gaddi. Morselli graduated in 1874 with a thesis on blood transfusion. Under the guidance of Livi, Morselli started his training as an alienist at the prestigious psychiatric hospital in Reggio Emilia with Augusto Tamburini. The three of them founded the *Rivista sperimentale di freniatria e medicina legale* in 1875, which became the organ of the Italian Society of Psychiatry. Also in 1875, Morselli got a research grant at the institute of anthropology in Florence, directed by Paolo Mantegazza, where he became involved in an international academic environment and worked at the Santa Maria Nuova Hospital among the followers of Maurizio Bufalini, the leader of experimental medicine.

At the age of twenty-five, Morselli was appointed director of a private psychiatric asylum in Macerata; in the meantime he worked on anthropological research in applying statistical methods and wrote his book on suicide, which was translated into English and German and won a prestigious award. In 1880 he became the director of the provincial psychiatric hospital in Turin. Such an appointment brought with it the chair of nervous and mental diseases at the university, which Cesare Lombroso also wanted. It was offered to Morselli, who had very capable assistants, such as Gabriele Buccola, an experimental psychologist, and the psychiatrist Eugenio Tanzi.

Morselli's handbook on the semeiotics of mental diseases enjoyed great success and was adopted by generations of psychiatrists. The first volume, in 1885, focused on the anamnestic, anthropological, and physiological examination of the mentally ill; giving priority to the suffering individual rather than to disease, it stated that the investigation of psychic processes represents the 'true intimate specificity of psychiatry'. Despite Morselli's tireless productivity, it took him nearly ten years to complete the second volume of his handbook, which dealt with the psychological approach to therapeutics. He criticized the Lombrosian psychiatry of measuring and stigmatizing, though Morselli himself had also been a supporter of criminal anthropological theories, when he was nominated as an expert in an internationally famous trial of child murder in 1877. This was just the first of several forensic cases in which he argued for diminished responsibility by reason of insanity.

The asylum administrators in Turin did not agree with Morselli's proposals for reform, and some of his colleagues, including Lombroso, blamed his somewhat unorthodox attitudes, such as his subjecting himself to a Belgian hypnotist's performances in 1886. Morselli decided to leave Turin, where he had also founded and directed the *Rivista di filosofia scientifica* (1881–89), a journal that was the most active voice of Italian positivism. He moved to Genoa in 1889, where his courses at the university included a wide variety of topics in psychiatry, sexology, psychology, and anthropology. He was also director of the psychiatric clinic, following Dario Maragliano. In Genoa he directed the neurological ward of the polyclinic; he also founded an outpatient mental health service with free consultations for the poor and a private clinic for upper-class patients. He described neurasthenia in adolescents and worked with mentally retarded children at the Paedagogium of Nervi,

near Genoa. During World War I, he specialized in psychiatric trauma among soldiers and the civilian population.

He encouraged the investigation of the unconscious, and engaged in experimental research on animal magnetism, hypnotism, and such pathological states as hysteria, as well as on exceptional states, such as the trances of the medium Eusapia Paladino, who attracted the attention of the Society for Psychical Research in England and the United States. He was well disposed toward the few psychiatrists, such as Edoardo Weiss, who tried to introduce Freudian theories to Italy, but Morselli never believed in psychoanalysis.

Bibliography

Primary: 1881. *Suicide. An essay on comparative moral statistics* (London) (first published Milan, 1879); 1882–83. *Il metodo clinico nella diagnosi generale della pazzia* (Milan); 1885–94. *Manuale di semejotica delle malattie mentali* (Milan).

Secondary: Guarnieri, Patrizia, 1993. *A Case of Child Murder. Law and Science in Nineteenth-Century Tuscany* (Cambridge); Guarnieri, Patrizia, 1988. 'Between Soma and Psyche: Morselli and Psychiatry in Late-Nineteenth-Century Italy' in Bynum, W. F., Roy Porter, and Michael Shepherd, eds., *The Anatomy of Madness* vol. 3 (London) pp. 102–124; Guarnieri, Patrizia, 1986. *Individualità difformi. La psichiatria antropologica di Enrico Morselli* (Milan).

Patrizia Guarnieri

MORTON, SAMUEL GEORGE (b. Philadelphia, Pennsylvania, USA, 26 January 1799; d. Philadelphia, 15 May 1851), *medicine, physical anthropology, craniometry.*

Morton, son of George Morton, a Quaker merchant, and Jane Cummings, was educated by the Society of Friends in Westchester County, New York, following the death of his father when Samuel was a child. With his mother's remarriage (1812) to Thomas Rogers, an amateur mineralogist, he returned to Philadelphia and was apprenticed to a city merchant (1815), although his stepfather encouraged his interest in natural history. After his mother died (1817), Morton left the business world to study medicine with the physician Joseph Parrish and attended lectures at Pennsylvania University, graduating MD (1820). Further medical studies at Edinburgh University (MD, 1823) were sponsored by a wealthy uncle in Ireland. Returning to Philadelphia (1824), Morton set up in medical practice and joined a number of medical and scientific institutions, including the Academy of Natural Sciences of Philadelphia (secretary 1825, president 1850), the American Philosophical Society (1828), and the Philadelphia Association for Medical Instruction. He was physician and clinical tutor to the Philadelphia Almshouse and professor of anatomy at Pennsylvania College (1839–43). His marriage to Rebecca Grellet Pearsall (1827) produced eight children, one of whom, Thomas George Morton, became a surgeon.

Although Morton published several medical books, specifically biased toward anatomy (1834, 1849), his chief interests lay in natural history. His *Synopsis of the Organic*

Remains of the Cretaceous Group of the United States (1834) was an important study of the fossils collected along the Missouri River by Meriwether Lewis and William Clark in a project commissioned by President Thomas Jefferson (1803). In 1830, while preparing to give an anatomy lecture on Blumenbach's five races of man (Caucasian, Mongolian, American, Ethiopian, and Malayan), Morton found himself two skulls short and decided to start his own collection. Through various scientific, phrenological, mercantile, missionary, and military contacts and personal expeditions (one to the West Indies, *c.* 1833), he eventually amassed the largest skull collection in North America (about 1,500 specimens). International contacts included James Cowles Prichard and Anders Retzius. Morton's intention, as with most craniometrists of this period, was to corroborate Blumenbach's racial classification, but he was also influenced by phrenology, which related skull contours to mental faculties. *Crania Americana* (1839), in which Morton claimed to have identified significant differences in cranial capacity (equated with intellect) among races, contained a chapter written by the Edinburgh phrenologist George Combe. In Morton's racial hierarchy, Caucasians and Mongolians possessed superior intellect to Ethiopians and Americans (i.e., Native Americans and Indians of Central and South America). In *Crania Aegyptiaca* (1844), Morton compared skulls from Ancient Egypt, concluding that the civilization's Pharaohs and dynastic rulers were of Caucasian stock, whereas the servants and slaves were Negroes, distinctions that had not changed over the millennia. He argued for immutability of racial characteristics and distinct biological types (polygenism).

Morton's work exerted a profound influence on American physical anthropology and 'race science' at a time of debate about the ethics of slavery and its reconciliation with the principle of equality fundamental to the Declaration of Independence. His supporters included Josiah Clark Nott and George Robins Gliddon, whose *Types of Mankind* (1854), dedicated to Morton, elaborated on the inferiority of the negro type. Nevertheless, the idea of polygenism conflicted with that of man's unitary origins as presented in Genesis, although some of Morton's detractors, including John Bachman, a Lutheran minister from South Carolina, defended slavery on other grounds. Bachman's argument that unity could be proven by the interfertility of Caucasians and Africans (1850) contradicted 'evidence' from physicians such as Nott that the mulatto was an infertile hybrid and that intermarriage between blacks and whites, if allowed, would exterminate both races. Morton himself produced a manuscript on the subject, 'Some remarks on the infrequency of mixed offspring between the European and Australian races' (1850), but died before its publication, having been ailing since an attack of pleurisy (1848).

Although best known for his craniometrical studies, Morton had wide interests in natural history, including botany, ornithology, mineralogy, and paleontology.

Bibliography

Primary: 1834. *Illustrations of Pulmonary Consumption, Its Anatomical Characters, Causes, Symptoms and Treatment* (Philadelphia); 1839. *Crania Americana, or, a Comparative View of the Skulls of Aboriginal Nations of North and South America* (Philadelphia); 1844. *Crania Aegyptiaca, or, Observations on Egyptian Ethnography Derived from Anatomy, History, and the Monuments* (Philadelphia); 1849. *An Illustrated System of Human Anatomy, Special, General and Microscopic* (Philadelphia).

Secondary: Luyendijk-Elshout, Antoine M., 1997. 'Opening Address: The Magic of the Skull: 'Commercium Cranorium' in the Nineteenth Century.' *International Journal of Osteoarchaeology* 7: 571–574; Haller, John S., 1975. *Outcasts from Evolution: Scientific Attitudes of Racial Inferiority, 1859–1900* (Urbana, IL); Stanton, William R., 1960. *The Leopard's Spots: Scientific Attitudes towards Race in America, 1815–59* (Chicago); Nott, J. C., and George R. Gliddon, 1854. *Types of Mankind, or Ethnological Researches . . .* (Philadelphia); Meigs, Charles D., 1851. *A Memoir of Samuel George Morton, M.D.* (Philadelphia); Bachman, John, 1850. *The Doctrine of the Unity of the Human Race Examined on the Principles of Science* (Charleston, SC); *DSB; DAMB.*

Carole Reeves

MORTON, WILLIAM THOMAS GREEN   (b. Charlton, Massachusetts, USA, 9 August 1819; d. New York, New York, USA, 15 July 1868), *anesthetics, dentistry.*

Morton, son of James Morton and Rebecca Needham, both farmers, entered the College of Dental Surgery, Baltimore, in 1840. After graduating in 1842, he went into practice with the dentist Horace Wells. He married Elizabeth Whitman in the spring of 1844, and in March of the same year, he entered Harvard Medical School. He attended the early lectures on anatomy, but after less than a year, he returned to dentistry.

In the first half of the nineteenth century, a number of surgeons and dentists began to experiment with ways of reducing the pain of surgery. By the 1840s, interest centered on two techniques: the inhalation of gases or volatile chemicals and the use of mesmerism or hypnotism. From 1842, Crawford Long, a surgeon in Georgia, used ether as an anesthetic in a series of surgical procedures, but did not report his work until the end of the decade. In December 1844, Wells had begun to use nitrous oxide for dental extraction, and in 1845 he demonstrated, with Morton's assistance, the use of nitrous oxide for minor surgery at Massachusetts General Hospital (MGH).

Wells's technique failed to provide pain relief, and the surgeons ridiculed his efforts, but the experience whetted Morton's interest in the idea of anesthesia. He had already used ether drops as a local anesthetic at the suggestion of his landlord and teacher Charles Jackson, professor of chemistry at Harvard. Now he began a series of experiments with ether vapor as a general anesthetic. In early September 1846, he met with Jackson to discuss the possibility of inhalational anesthesia, but (a crucial detail) did not mention his experiments.

Morton performed his first successful dental extraction under ether anesthesia on the morning of 30 September 1846. He was convinced of the importance and financial value of his work: by the end of the day, he had applied for a patent and had written to a surgeon at MGH to offer a demonstration of his technique. On 16 October, Morton's ether anesthesia was used successfully for the removal of a neck tumor. News of his success spread quickly across the United States and to Europe, and Morton began to manufacture a large number of the glass inhalers he had designed. He did not, however, reveal the details of his method, preferring to wait until his patent was secure.

Morton's success quickly unraveled. The surgeons at MGH, uneasy about Morton's secretiveness, insisted they be exempted from the terms of the patent. Jackson claimed a share of the patent, and by November 1846, he was describing ether anesthesia as his own invention. Wells also began to claim precedence over Morton. Morton's neglected dental practice began to fail, and in 1850 he took up farming. In April 1854 the U.S. Senate passed a bill to compensate the discoverer of anesthesia, but the large number of rival claimants—Morton, Bigelow, Jackson, Long—made this impossible. Morton attempted to sue the U.S. Army for breach of his patent, but his case was dismissed and the patent declared invalid.

It is not possible to identify one individual as the inventor of anesthesia. Morton certainly played an important part in its development and, more significantly, its dissemination. This has been obscured, however, by his desire to be seen as the 'father' of anesthesia and his unabashed pursuit of commercial success.

Bibliography

Primary: 1846. *Morton's Letheon: Cautioning Those who Attempt to Infringe upon his Legal Rights* (Boston); 1847. *Remarks on the Proper Mode of Administering Sulphuric Ether by Inhalation* (Boston).

Secondary: Wolfe, Richard J., 2001. *Tarnished Idol: William Thomas Green Morton and the Introduction of Surgical Anesthesia: A Chronicle of the Ether Controversy* (San Anselmo, CA); Duncum, Barbara M., 1994. *The Development of Inhalation Anaesthesia* (London); *DAMB*.

Richard Barnett

MOSHER, CLELIA DUEL   (b. Albany, New York, USA, 16 December 1863; d. Palo Alto, California, USA, 21 December 1940), *medicine, sex research.*

Mosher was born in Albany, New York, in 1863. She began her tertiary education in biology at Wellesley College but continued at Stanford University. For her master's thesis at Stanford, she studied variability in respiration between the sexes. Prior to her work, it was thought that women could only breathe high in the chest, whereas men breathed deeper with the diaphragm. Mosher showed that this difference was caused by women wearing constrictive clothing such as corsets and so challenged this idea of gender inequality. In 1900, when she was thirty-six years old, Mosher finished medical school at Johns Hopkins University, where she studied under William Osler.

After graduating in medicine, Mosher practiced medicine in Palo Alto, California, and she became the professor for hygiene and women's medical adviser at Stanford University. She continued her research into women's concerns, paying particular attention to women's posture, women's health, and proper exercise. One particular problem to which she gave attention was menstruation. Running against the grain that treated menstruating women as invalids, Mosher sought to aid women's health by developing a series of exercises to regulate menstruation and alleviate menstrual pain.

Mosher also served in France during World War I as a physician and associate medical director for the American National Red Cross, but she is most remembered for her contributions to the study of sexuality. Between 1892 and 1920, Mosher surveyed forty-seven women about their sex lives. Many of these women were the wives of faculty at Stanford or patients from her medical practice. These interviews were not published until they were uncovered in the library of Stanford University in the late 1970s. Her survey was detailed—nine pages in length—and asked explicit questions about sexual desire, marriage, contraception, masturbation, and suchlike. The findings were remarkable, and they stand as the most detailed investigation into the sex lives of Victorian women that we have. The reports stated that most (thirty-five of forty-seven) women actively desired sexual intercourse. Thirty-four women reported that they regularly had orgasms; some of those who did not reported feeling psychologically upset by this. These findings are in conflict with mythopoeic writings about female sexuality in the Victorian period. Also remarkable is the finding that two-thirds of the women used some form of contraception. Most of them used douching; others used withdrawal or had sex during the 'safe period'. Barrier methods used included condoms, and two of the women used either a diaphragm or cervical cap. One woman also used cocoa butter, presumably internally. These findings have been given much attention by contemporary historians.

When she died in 1940, Mosher was emeritus professor of hygiene at Stanford.

Bibliography

Primary: 1911. 'Functional Periodicity in Women and Some of the Modifying Factors.' *California State Journal of Medicine* 9 (1–2): 4–8, 55–58; 1921. 'Again in the Running. A Series of Sketches from Observations Made by the Author during Her Service in France.' *Medical Woman's Journal* 28: 128–130; 1921. 'All in the Day's Work.

A Series of Sketches from Observations Made by the Author during Her Service in France.' *Medical Woman's Journal* 28: 95–96; 1923. Woman's Physical Freedom (New York); 1927. *Personal Hygiene for Women* (Stanford); 1980. (Mahood, James, and Kristine Wenburg, eds.) *The Mosher Survey: Sexual Attitudes of 45 Victorian Women* (New York).

Secondary: Bullough, Vern, 1994. *Science in the Bedroom* (New York).

Ivan Crozier

MOSHER, ELIZA MARIA (b. Poplar Ridge, New York, USA, 2 October 1846; d. New York, New York, USA, 6 October 1928), *medicine, popular medicine.*

Mosher was born into a Quaker family in Poplar Ridge, a small town in Cayuga County, New York. After schooling at Union Springs Seminary, operated by the Society of Friends, she entered the New England Hospital for Women and Children as an apprentice intern in 1869, although she left this position after a year in order to nurse her sick mother. She maintained her medical contacts through assisting a female doctor in Boston, and in 1871 she resumed her studies by entering the first female intake of medical students at the University of Michigan in 1871, which included clinical experience during 1872–73 with Emily Blackwell (Elizabeth's sister) at the New York Infirmary. Mosher also undertook clinical studies at Bellevue and DeMilt Dispensary, as well as serving as assistant anatomy demonstrator to the women's section at Michigan. She took her MD from Michigan in 1875.

After graduation, Mosher opened and operated a joint practice with a fellow student from Michigan Medical School, Elizabeth Gerow, in Poughkeepsie, New York, for two years. She left private practice to serve as resident physician and later superintendent at the Massachusetts Reformatory Prison for Women in Sherborn, Massachusetts (1877–83), where she established a hospital ward. In 1879–80 Mosher and another fellow Michigan student, Amanda Sanford, traveled to London and Paris to further their medical studies. Mosher also began a private practice with Lucy Hall in Brooklyn, although they moved to take up a more lucrative position: alternating semesters as resident physician and associate professor of physiology and hygiene at Vassar College (1883–87).

This return to academic life encouraged Mosher's educative interests. In 1888 she organized a medical training course at the Union Missionary Training Institute in Brooklyn. In the following year, she commenced lecturing on anatomy and hygiene at the Chautauqua Institution in New York. She resigned these positions in 1896 when she was elected dean of women and professor of hygiene, sanitation, and home economics in the department of literature, science, and the arts at the University of Michigan—making her the first woman professor of this university. At Michigan, Mosher was the resident physician to female students and was director of physical education. She remained in this position until her retirement, which was brought on by an injury to her knee in 1902. After this time, Mosher remained in private practice in Brooklyn and lectured at various institutions.

In her educational work, Mosher maintained an interest in the relationship between physical education and fitness that would lead to a healthy lifestyle. She paid special attention to the medical aspects of posture, an interest that led to her founding the American Posture League. This organization encouraged further consideration of the design of children's furniture, rather than requiring the small bodies to fit themselves into adult-sized chairs. Mosher also wrote patents for an ergonomically beneficial streetcar bench, a comfortable bicycle seat, and a corset for women that did not impede breathing. From 1905 to 1928, Mosher was senior editor of the *Medical Woman's Journal*, in which she published a number of articles. Mosher was also Honorary President of the National Medical Women's Association (founded in 1915; renamed American Medical Women's Association). In 1912 she published her monograph *Health and Happiness*. Mosher died in New York in 1928.

Bibliography

Primary: 1912. *Health and Happiness: A Message to Girls* (New York and London).

Secondary: Tarolli, Janet, 2000. 'First Ladies in Medicine at Michigan.' *Medicine at Michigan* 2; Morantz-Sanchez, Regina Markell, 1985. *Sympathy and Science: Women Physicians in American Medicine* (New York and Oxford); *DAMB*.

Ivan Crozier

MOTT, VALENTINE (b. Glen Cove, New York, USA, 20 August 1785; d. New York, New York, USA, 26 April 1865), *surgery.*

When viewed in the light of the general state of surgical science in the first decades of the nineteenth century, the accomplishments of Valentine Mott are nothing less than astounding. Before the introduction of anesthesia or antisepsis, at a time when most surgical procedures were conducted with haste and a certain unconcern with niceties of technique, Mott performed operations of Herculean magnitude, involving meticulous dissection and sometimes taking hours to complete. His ability to succeed in such ventures was due to a combination of boldness, remarkable technical skill, exquisite patience, and meticulous knowledge of anatomy. The roster of procedures he introduced is long, particularly in regard to the ligation of aneurysms of major vessels, for which reason he has been called the 'Father of American Vascular Surgery'.

The son of a Quaker physician, Mott was born in Glen Cove, on Long Island, New York, and began his study of medicine as an apprentice to a relative, the surgeon Valentine Seaman. He took the two-year course of lectures offered by the medical department of Columbia College, receiving the MD degree in 1806, and continued for another year as Seaman's apprentice before traveling to England in 1807 to spend six months as dresser for London's leading surgeon, Astley Cooper. He was mightily influenced by watching Cooper successfully perform the first ligation ever done of the common carotid artery, for aneurysm. After two years of study with prominent surgeons in London and Edinburgh, Mott returned to New York in 1809 and began a flourishing practice that attracted large numbers of students and brought him the title of lecturer on surgery and demonstrator in anatomy at his alma mater. In 1811 he was elected professor of surgery at Columbia.

In 1818 a fifty-seven-year-old sailor presented himself to Mott with an aneurysm of the right subclavian artery, which the surgeon determined could only be cured by ligation of the innominate artery, an operation never before performed. Mott accomplished the procedure successfully, though the patient died twenty-eight days later of hemorrhage. In the following decades, he undertook a series of arterial ligations—of the common and external carotid; the subclavian; the common, internal, and external iliac; and the femoral and popliteal—of a magnitude that few surgeons of his time had the experience or skill to attempt, numbering 157 in all, at a time when major American hospitals were averaging fewer than one operation each week. In addition to his skill in the treatment of aneurysms, Mott became widely known for his lithotomy, the excision of stones from the bladder. In an era of high mortality, he performed 165 of these procedures with the remarkable record of only seven deaths.

Mott considered his most difficult operation to have been an excision of the left clavicle for osteosarcoma, which he did in 1828. Requiring that the subclavian and external jugular veins be dissected free of the mass, the tedious procedure took four hours and was successful, as were so many of the innovative and complex operations he did during his career, including a large number for the reconstruction of hare-lip.

Along with the rest of the faculty, Mott resigned from Columbia in 1826, to protest interference by the Board of Regents in Albany, the state capital. The group formed a new medical school associated with Rutgers University in New Jersey, but the experiment came to an end four years later, and Mott rejoined the Columbia faculty. Four years later, fatigued and in ill health, he set off on an extended European tour of seven years, during which time he visited many leading surgeons. Returning in 1841, he was named to the chair of surgery at the new University Medical College associated with New York University, where he remained for ten very productive years. Again in ill health, he traveled once more to Europe and then became emeritus at the school in 1853, though continuing to operate at a somewhat lessened pace. Having retired from teaching, he had more time for certain civic duties in

which he was interested, as well as his collection of pathological specimens. During the Civil War, he was active on committees of the U.S. Sanitary Commission and was consultant to the Surgeon General. The final six years of Mott's life were marred by angina pectoris, and he died of gangrene of the left leg. He had had an extraordinary career and a long and companionable marriage and was the father of nine children.

Bibliography

Primary: 1842. *Travels in Europe and the East . . .* (New York).

Secondary: Rutkow, I. M., 1979. 'The Father of American Vascular Surgery: A Historical Perspective.' *Surgery* 85: 441–450; Kelly, H. A., 1912. *Cyclopedia of American Medical Biography*, vol. 2, pp. 199–201 (Philadelphia); Gross, S. D., 1868. *Memoir of Valentine Mott* (New York); *DAMB*.

Sherwin Nuland

MOYNIHAN, BERKELEY GEORGE ANDREW (b. Malta, 2 October 1865; d. Meanwood, Leeds, England, 1 September 1936), *surgery.*

Moynihan was the son of Captain George Andrew Moynihan and Ellen Anne Parkin. He was educated in London at Christ's Hospital and the Royal Naval School and was planning for a career in the Navy. However, he changed track and enrolled at the Leeds School of Medicine, graduating MB BS (1887), before becoming MS London with gold medal (1890). In the same year, he became house surgeon to A. W. Mayo Robson (1853–1933) at the Leeds General Infirmary and then spent time in Berlin, before being appointed assistant surgeon at the Infirmary in 1896. Robson was an innovative surgeon who specialized in operations on abdominal organs, and Moynihan gained extensive experience. He also worked with Thomas Richard Jessop and developed a substantial private practice in the city. He was based in Leeds throughout his career, rising from assistant surgeon (1896) to surgeon (1906) and finally to consulting surgeon (1926) at the Leeds General Infirmary and holding the chair in surgery at the University of Leeds (1909). However, he also became a significant metropolitan and national figure. He built up a London consulting practice, which he ran with several assistants, and he was active in the RCS and elite medical circles more generally. His profile was evident by 1912, the year in which he was elected to the Council of the RSC and knighted.

From the early 1900s, Moynihan gained a reputation as a dexterous and scientific surgeon and one who published widely and wrote well. Following a visit to the American Surgical Association in 1903, he developed a friendship with William and Charles Mayo (1861–1939, 1865–1939) and George Crile (1864–1943), and their influence was evident in his first major book, *Abdominal Operations* (1905). Other books followed, which cemented Moynihan's reputation as a leading technical and scientific surgeon. He was innovative in pioneering new procedures and new techniques, not least the wearing of rubber gloves, and in creating a British surgical community beyond the RCS. He helped found the Provincial Surgeons' Club (1909) and the *British Journal of Surgery* (1913); he was also a founding member of the Association of Surgeons of Great Britain and Northern Ireland in 1920. The trajectory of his surgical work and his professional activities had the common theme of seeking to make surgery progressive and scientific, which after 1918 he pursued through the RCS. For example, he developed the idea and secured the funding for the RCS's research laboratory at Buckstone Browne Farm, opened in 1931. This followed his calls for surgeons to engage in 'vital' research (clinical research and experimental vivisection) rather than 'dead' research (pathology and morbid anatomy). Paradoxically, he came into conflict with Walter Morley Fletcher (1873–1933) and Medical Research Council policy, which tended to support laboratory scientists working in basic biomedical disciplines rather than research by clinicians.

Moynihan had wide interests within medicine and beyond. He was a keen student of medical history and a bibliophile. He had a distinguished record in World War I, in the organization of the medical services (1914–15), as chair of the Council of Consultants, and as a member of the medical advisory board. He was made CB (1917) and KCMG (1918), and he became Baron Moynihan of Leeds (1929). In the House of Lords, he spoke largely on medical matters, and just before his death, he introduced a bill on the treatment of road traffic casualties. In the early decades of the twentieth century, Moynihan emerged as one of the leaders of British surgery, and although he enjoyed great respect, he was not universally admired. Some surgeons felt that his undoubted skills in oratory, in print, and in self-promotion had played too great a part in his attaining this position. Nonetheless, he was a commanding figure in the profession—confident, tall, red-haired, and energetic—and eventually in national affairs. He had great organizational abilities and did as much as anyone in his generation to develop and promote British surgery. Upon his death, burial in Westminster Abbey—where he would have joined John Hunter and Joseph Lister—was offered to his family, but this was declined, and he was buried in his beloved Leeds.

Bibliography

Primary: 1901. (with Robson, A. W. Mayo) *Diseases of the stomach and their surgical treatment* (London); 1902. (with Robson, A. W. Mayo) *Diseases of the pancreas and their surgical treatment* (London); 1905. *Abdominal operations* (London); 1905. *Gall-stones and their surgical treatment* (London); 1910. *Duodenal ulcer* (London); 1932. *The Advance of Medicine* (Oxford).

Secondary: Moynihan, B., 1967. *Selected Writings of Lord Moynihan* (London); Bateman, D., 1940. *Berkeley Moynihan, Surgeon* (London); *Oxford DNB*; *Plarr's Lives*.

Michael Worboys

MÜLLER, JOHANNES PETER   (b. Koblenz, Germany, 14 July 1801; d. Berlin, Germany, 28 April 1858), *physiology, anatomy, zoology.*

Müller was born the eldest son of a shoemaker in Koblenz, a little town on the river Rhine. In 1801 Koblenz was occupied by Napoleon's soldiers and governed by France. His birth certificate was dated '25. messidor l'an 9' because during that time in Koblenz the calendar of the French revolution was in force. After primary school, his mother—a daughter of a coachman—supported her gifted child so that he could attend the gymnasium in Koblenz. His teacher Johannes von Schulze, later secretary to the Prussian Minister of Culture Baron Friedrich Stein zum Altenstein, further nurtured Müller's excellent ability in Latin and Greek with unpaid private lessons. Müller finished his schooling (1818) with a brilliant final examination. After one year of military service, he started his medical studies at the Friedrich–Wilhelm University at Bonn. This university had just been founded (1818), based on the idea of the university concept of Alexander (1769–1859) and Wilhelm von Humboldt (1767–1832) and Johann Gottlieb Fichte (1762–1814).

At the age of twenty-one (1822) Müller won a university award for his experimental study on the respiration of the fetus in the uterus. Müller's solution was an excellent example of his systematic work, whereby he carried out experimental studies. In the year 1823–24 he moved to Karl Asmund Rudolphi's (1771–1832) Institute of Anatomy and Physiology in Berlin. In Berlin Müller became acquainted with the latest scientific inventions of physiological chemistry, or animal chemistry as it was then known. The Swedish chemist Jöns Jacob Berzelius (1779–1848) greatly influenced Müller's views on physiology and animal chemistry. Müller finished his medical education in 1824 with the thesis 'De phoronimia animali' [On the Movement of Animals]. In the same year he became a university lecturer (Privatdozent) of anatomy and physiology at the University of Bonn. On 19 October 1824 Müller presented his inaugural lecture, *Über das Bedürfnis der Physiologie nach einer philosophischen Naturbetrachtung* [Physiology Requires a Philosophical Description of Nature]. This proved to be a turning point in the history of physiology. He there described his view of an 'accurate' way of physiological research. He argued that all physiological investigations have to be based on observation, experience—which requires also a good knowledge of the whole scientific literature—and experiment. However, only with a philosophical attitude can the scientist gain facts from nature, and from his philosophical background he is then able to interpret these facts. 'Der Physiolog erfährt die Natur, damit er sie denkt' [The physiologist experiences nature in order to think about it] (1826, p. 34).

Neurophysiology, Sensory Physiology

Within the next six years, Müller wrote four fundamental books and many papers. His two publications on sensory physiology in 1826 made him one of the most important sensory-physiologists in Europe, together with Jan Evangelista Purkinje (1787–1869), the Czech physiologist. In Müller's books *Über die phantastischen Gesichtserscheinungen* [On the Phantastical Apparition] and *Vergleichende Physiologie des Gesichtssinnes* [On Comparative Physiology of Visual Phenomena of Man and Animal], he addressed the problem of the physiology and anatomy of visual perception, and reported his comparative morphological investigations of the eye. Therein he formulated the law of specific sense energy, which is based on the simple but portentous following assumption: Every sensory stimulus affects the sensory nerves. But the sensation of 'light', for example, is quite different from the physical stimulus of light itself. The stimulus is the 'changing cause' [verändernde Ursache] of actions inside the sensory system. The sensory system itself 'creates' a specific sensory energy. Different stimulus qualities generate nothing else in the specific sensory organs than the specific sensory energy of the specific sensory organ, i.e., the stimulated eye replies always with a sensation of light and color indifferent to the stimulus quality. This basic law for sensory physiology opened the way for new research into the physiology and anatomy of the receptor organ, the sensory nerves, and the sensory cortex. One of the most important scientists in this field was his pupil Hermann von Helmholtz (1821–94), who explained color vision with his so called three-color theory (the Young-Helmholtz theory). He introduced the term 'Modalität' [modality] for Müller's law of specific sense energy and the term 'Qualität' [quality] for different nuances or graduations within the modality. The discussion of sensory perception forced Müller to the epistemological question of in what sense the outside world could be cognitively verified and experienced as reality. Müller did not advocate a simple theory of images but a theory of signs for reality. This means the perception through our senses gives us not an effective illustration of the external world, but signs of it, which we have to interpret with rationality and reason.

In 1830 Müller published a fundamental book on the glands. Based on comparative anatomy and physiological investigations he described the secretory function of the glands. In the same year his book on the ontogenesis of the genitals was published describing the 'Müllerschen Gang' (Müller's canal or the *ductus paramesonephricus*) of urogenital development. In the introduction of the *Bildungsschichte der Genitalien* Müller discussed several criteria for experimental observations in physiology and embryology.

Müller was nominated as university professor at the University of Bonn (1830). One year later he verified experimentally the Bell-Magendie law, which states that the anterior roots of the spinal cord have motor functions, whereas the posterior roots have sensory functions. That Alexander von Humboldt (1769–1859) met Müller in George Cuvier's (1769–1832) Institute in Paris, when Müller demonstrated (1831) his Bell-Magendie experiments, played an important role in Müller's nomination for the chair of anatomy and physiology in Berlin. Parallel to his experiments in neurophysiology and sensory physiology, Müller was engaged in biochemistry. He summarized his microscopic investigations and chemical experiments on the blood in sixty pages in *Poggendorff's Annalen* (1832).

Berlin

When his teacher Karl Asmund Rudolphi died on 29 November 1832, Müller offered himself for the chair of anatomy and physiology at the University of Berlin. Fortunately his former teacher in Koblenz, Johannes von Schulze, was at this time the secretary to the Prussian Minister of Culture, Friedrich Stein zum Altenstein, and Alexander von Humboldt voted positively for him. They expected him to bring forth new and significant directions for the institute in Berlin. Müller would not disappoint them. Three months later Müller was appointed as professor of anatomy and physiology at Berlin University. In April 1833 Müller moved from Bonn to Berlin with his beloved wife Nanny and their two children, Max and Maria.

In his first year in Berlin, the first part of the famous *Handbuch der Physiologie* [Elements of Physiology] appeared. The second part of the *Handbuch*, which included the great chapter on the 'Physiology of the Nerves', with the first description of the theory of reflexes, was finished in 1834. A year later a revised second edition was published, in which he discussed the important impacts of Marshall Hall's investigations of the theory of reflexes. Revised and enlarged third and fourth editions appeared in 1838 and 1844. The second part of the 'Elements' was published (1840) as a unique edition, in which Müller discussed the cell theory of his pupil Theodor Schwann. This book was a cornucopia of new physiological ideas. A whole generation of biomedical scientists was greatly inspired by Müller's 'Elements'. From 1833 until his death Müller edited the *Archiv für Anatomie, Physiologie und wissenschaftliche Medizin*, the continuation of the former journal of Johann Christian Reil and Friedrich Meckel, commonly called *Müller's Archiv*. After Müller's death the journal was divided in two parts: that on physiology was edited by Emil Du Bois-Reymond, whereas Karl Bogislav Reichert edited the anatomical part.

Müller was fascinated by marine biology from his first stay at the North Sea (1831). In the next decade he started to classify, with an unimaginable endurance, different species of fishes (*Myxinoiden, Ganoiden, Cycloxstomata*) and the whole species of *echinodermata*. Müller rediscovered (1840) 'Aristotle's smooth shark' by reading Aristotle's *De animarum* in Greek. He also verified that the *Amphioxus lanceolatum* is the early form of the vertebrates. Three years before his death he opened the door to a completely new field in marine biology: the life of the 'pelagischer Auftrieb' [pelagic upwelling]. The name plankton was introduced by the physiologist Victor Hensen (1854–1924) in 1889.

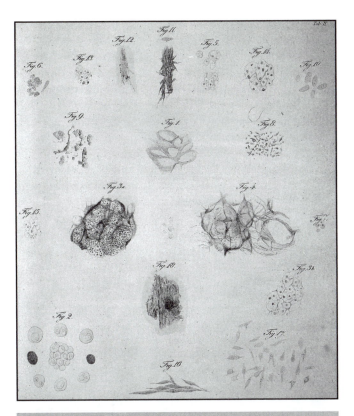

Microscopical appearance of various types of cancer cells. Lithograph from *Ueber den feinern Bau und die Formen der krankhaften Geschwülste . . .* Berlin, 1838. Rare Books, Wellcome Library, London.

Müller had many tasks besides his main scope of research, which would occupy him for weeks. He was in charge of the administration of the large institute and was dean of the faculty; twice he was chancellor of Berlin University. In the subsequent twenty-seven years, until his death, 233 further publications followed. His famous student Emil Du Bois-Reymond calculated that Müller produced 15,360 printed pages and in addition drew 350 tables with about twelve individual illustrations on each table. Furthermore, the Berlin collection was enriched with 12,000 anatomic objects during his professorship. This schedule might give a glimpse of Müller's incredible capacity for work and the extent of his knowledge in the fields of anatomy, physiology, and general biology.

Müller's exceptional position in the history of physiology, anatomy, and zoology is not only connected with his own research and investigations, but is also due to his epistemological reflections on scientific physiology and his experiments in biology and his role as an influential and important teacher. The list of his pupils reads like a roll-call of all the famous influential German scientists in medicine, biology, zoology, anatomy, and physiology in the second half of the nineteenth century. Müller's most famous pupils were Hermann von Helmholtz, Emil Du Bois-Reymond (1819–96), Theodor Schwann (1811–82), Jacob Henle (1808–83), Ernst Haeckel

(1834–1919), and Rudolf Virchow (1821–1902). Others include Ernst Wilhelm Brücke (1819–92), Friedrich Wilhelm Bidder (1810–94), Karl Vierordt (1818–94), Robert Remak (1815–65), Ludwig Wilhelm Bischoff (1807–82), Carl Bogislaw Reichert (1811–83), Nathanel Liebenkühn (1822–87), and Eduard Claparède (1832–70).

All Müller's students held him in the highest esteem and spoke of him with deepest admiration. Du Bois-Reymond accurately described the 'catalytic effect' Müller had on his colleagues and pupils. 'He allowed his students complete freedom . . . without exerting pressure, without declaring himself their master in word and deed, without even using the term "pupil". According to his own versatility, which cannot be transferred to his students, . . . Müller created objectively not only one, but . . . several branches in the biological sciences. But all his students queried nature according to his ways' (Du Bois-Reymond, 1858 [1887], pp. 289–90). All of them worked on crucial research problems that Müller identified and pointed out to them as open-ended questions, due to the inadequate methods of investigation. Müller's research method, epistemological view of biological sciences, and his open-minded personal style encouraged the development of new methods to be adapted to particular problems. The style and methodology of research that Müller's disciples shared arguably became their most important tool.

Bibliography

Primary: 1826. *Zur vergleichenden Physiologie des Gesichtssinnes des Menschen und der Thiere nebst einem Versuch über die Bewegung der Augen und über den menschlichen Blick* (Leipzig); 1830. *De glandularum secernetium structura penitorii earumque prima formatione in homine atque animalibus* (Leipzig); 1830. *Bildungsgeschichte der Genitalien aus anatomischen Untersuchungen an Embryonen des Menschen und der Thiere* (Düsseldorf); 1833–40. *Handbuch der Physiologie* (*Elements of physiology* trans. of 2nd edn. by William Baly, 1840–43) (Koblenz).

Secondary: Lohff, Brigitte, 2001. 'Facts and Philosophy in Neurophysiology. The 200th Anniversary of Johannes Müller (1801–1858).' *Journal of the History of the Neurosciences* 10: 277–292; Hagner, Michael, and Bettina Wahrig-Schmidt, eds., 1993. *Johannes Müller und die Philosophie* (Berlin); Haberling, Wilhelm, 1924. *Das Leben des rheinischen Naturforschers Johannes Müller* (Große Männer: Studien zur Biologie des Genies, vol. 9) (Leipzig); Du Bois-Reymond, Emil, 1887. 'Gedächtnisrede auf Johannes Müller' in Du Bois-Reymond, Estelle, ed., 1912. *Reden von Emil Du Bois-Reymond* vol. 2 (Leipzig) pp. 143–334; *DSB*.

Brigitte Lohff

MUKERJI, SUBHAS (aka MUKHOPADHYAY) (b. Hazaribagh, India, 16 January 1931, d. Calcutta [now Kolkata], India, 19 July 1981), *reproductive physiology.*

The son of a medical doctor, Mukerji spent his early childhood in Hazaribagh, in Bihar, and went to school in

Calcutta, graduating in 1945. He took his MBBS degree from the National Medical College (1955) and completed his DPhil under Sacchidananda Banerjee, of Presidency College, Calcutta, working on the biochemical changes in normal and abnormal pregnancies (1958). With a Colombo Plan scholarship (1960), Mukerji went on to work on reproductive physiology under John Lorraine at the MRC Unit of Clinical Endocrinology Research at Edinburgh. There he concentrated on developing new and sensitive bioassays for gonadotropins, using rats as his model system. He completed a PhD in reproductive endocrinology from Edinburgh (1963). Mukerji married Namita Banerji in 1960.

Mukerji returned to India in 1967, and joined the Sir Nil Ratan Sircar Medical College, Calcutta, and later became professor of physiology at Bankura Sammilani Medical College (1976). At Calcutta, he combined his considerable technical skills with his interest in innovative gynecological surgery. He worked on pharmacological methods of inducing ovulation and spermatogenesis, first on animals and later on human subjects. While in Calcutta, he worked on the luteotropic effects of DHEA (dehydroepiandrosterone) and testosterone in rats and humans. He developed bioassays and biochemical methods to demonstrate the presence of a substance similar to HCG (human chorionic gonadotropin) in the nonpregnant human endometrium and speculated on its possible role in fetal development. His investigations into the causes of the acyclicity of the menstrual cycle in amenorrhoeic women led to insights about polycystic ovaries. He was also among the first to link emotional stress with polycystic disease.

Mukerji, along with Sunit Mukerji, a cryobiologist, and the gynecologist Saroj Kanti Bhattacharya, worked on a method of *in vitro* fertilization that was used successfully on a patient with damaged fallopian tubes. On 3 October 1978 the team announced the birth of the world's second test-tube baby, in Calcutta. The announcement came sixty-seven days after R. G. Edwards and Patrick Steptoe had announced the birth of the first test-tube baby in England. Unlike his counterparts in England, Mukerji had used gonadotropins for ovarian stimulation, transvaginal colpotomy to harvest oocytes, and cryopreservation of the human embryo.

Mukerji presented his findings at the International Congress on Hormonal Steroids at New Delhi in 1978 and at the Indian Science Congress at Hyderabad in 1979. Despite his report to the Government of West Bengal entitled 'Transfer of *in vitro* Fertilized Frozen-Thawed Human Embryo' (19 October 1978), the achievement of the team was disbelieved. The Government set up a committee that investigated the claims and denounced them. Mukerji was also denied leave to write up a detailed report of his results and, later, to attend a meeting in Kyoto to discuss his work. In a final act of humiliation, he was transferred to the Regional Institute of Ophthalmology as professor of electrophysiology in June 1981. Frustrated, Mukerji committed suicide on 19 July 1981.

In 1997 Mukerji's papers and handwritten notes on his technique were assessed by T. C. Anand Kumar, formerly director of the Institute of Research in Reproduction, Mumbai. Kumar, who had played a key role in the birth of another test-tube baby born in Mumbai (1986), not only exonerated Mukerji of charges of fraud but also wrote extensively about his pioneering feat. Mukerji's method of combining in vitro fertilization and cryopreservation of human embryos is the currently preferred technique of medically assisted reproduction.

Bibliography

Primary: 1978. (with additional authors) 'The Feasibility of Long-Term Cryogenic Preservation of Viable Human Embryos: A Brief Pilot Study Report.' *Indian Journal of Cryogenics* 3: 80; Mukherjee, Sunit, et al., eds., 2001. *Architect of India's First Test-Tube Baby: Dr Subhas Mukerji* (Kolkata) (contains Mukerji's collected papers, notebooks, and correspondence).

Secondary: Anand Kumar, T. C., 1997. '"Architect of India's First Test Tube Baby: Dr Subhas Mukerji", Historical Notes.' *Current Science* 72(7): 526–531.

Indira Chowdhury

MUNTHE, AXEL FREDRIK MARTIN (b. Oscarshamn, Sweden, 31 October 1857; d. Stockholm, Sweden, 11 February 1949), *general practice, literature.*

Munthe was the son of the pharmacist Fredrik Munthe and his wife Aurora. Through his father Munthe became interested in medicine as a young boy. He finished high school (gymnasium) in Stockholm in 1874, after which he went through a preparatory medical education at the University of Uppsala. After receiving his 'medico-philosophical' degree in 1876, he wanted to continue to study medicine, but had to leave Sweden due to a lung disease. From 1877 to 1879 Munthe studied at the University of Montpellier, specializing in gynecology. In August 1880, he defended his doctoral thesis at the Sorbonne and was made doctor of medicine.

At the age of twenty-two, Axel Munthe was France's youngest ever doctor of medicine, and a foreigner to boot. Munthe stayed in Paris, which in the 1880s was teeming with Scandinavian artists. Munthe treated them all, he was appointed doctor to the Swedish-Norwegian legation, and at twenty-six he became a Chevalier of the Legion of Honor. His successful career was the result of a combination of his charismatic personality and his understanding that a doctor often does more good by listening and talking to a patient than by prescribing pills. Early on, he understood the psychosomatic character of many diseases. His interests moved gradually from gynecology toward the illnesses of the soul, and he studied Krafft-Ebing and other specialists in sexual pathology. He attended the lectures of Jean-Martin

Charcot, but there is no evidence that he worked with him, as he claims in *The Story of San Michele.*

Besides his empathic and psychological skills, Munthe's popularity as doctor was due to his conviction that the profession was a 'holy office'. He subscribed to a Robin Hood philosophy, according to which doctors should 'be welcome to take what they liked from their rich patients for their poor patients and for themselves, but they should not count their visits or write any bills.' An outbreak of cholera in Naples in 1884 gave Munthe the opportunity to practice his philosophy to the full. His reports from Naples made him a name as a writer as well.

After his divorce, Munthe spent two years on his beloved Capri. In 1889 he took up his practice again, this time in Rome, where he soon became a doctor of world renown. Patients from all over the world traveled there to seek his advice, among them the Swedish Crown Princess Victoria, with whom, in 1893, he entered a lifelong relationship. In 1901 Munthe moved to Capri, where his 'Villa San Michele' was by now as famous as its owner. He no longer maintained a medical practice, but had many patients among the European aristocracy and upper classes, who paid him well, and among the island's poor, whom he treated for free.

Munthe stayed in Capri until 1943, when he moved to Sweden. He was by then world-famous, not primarily as a doctor but as a writer. In 1929 he published *The Story of San Michele*, which was translated into dozens of languages and became one of the best-selling books of the 1930s. It is not an autobiography, and not a memoir, but a fanciful rendering of his rich and colorful life, intertwined with humorous stories with little connection to reality. Axel Munthe died in 1949 in the Royal Castle in Stockholm where he was staying as the king's guest. His royal patient, Queen Victoria, had then been dead for nineteen years.

Bibliography

Primary: 1880. *Prophylaxie et traitement des hémmorhagies post-partum* (Paris); 1887. *Letters from a Mourning City* (London); 1916. *Red Cross & Iron Cross* (London); 1929. *The Story of San Michele* (London).

Secondary: Jangfeldt, Bengt, 2003. *En osalig ande: Berättelsen om Axel Munthe* (Stockholm); Munthe, Gustafand Gudrun Uexküll, 1953. *The Story of Axel Munthe* (London); Nouaille, Henri, 1950. *Considérations médicales sur la vie et l'œuvre du docteur Axel Munthe* (Toulouse).

Bengt Jangfeldt

MURPHY, JOHN BENJAMIN (b. Appleton, Wisconsin, USA, 21 December 1857; d. Mackinac Island, Michigan, USA, 11 August 1916), *surgery.*

Like his contemporary in New York, Charles McBurney, Murphy is nowadays remembered primarily in association with the operation of appendectomy, although he made many other contributions to surgery.

Murphy was born on his parents' farm on 21 December 1857, the son of Irish immigrants from the potato famine. He attended a one-room grammar school and the Appleton High School, working part-time at the village drugstore. Above the store was the office of a general practitioner, H. W. Reilly, who kindled the boy's interest in medicine by taking him on house calls and having him assist in the office. After graduating, Murphy became Reilly's apprentice and shortly thereafter enrolled at nearby Rush Medical College, receiving his degree after a year of study, at the age of twenty-two. Following a year's internship at Cook County Hospital, he spent eighteen months studying in the great medical centers in Germany and Austria, coming under the influence of such surgical luminaries as Theodor Billroth of the University of Vienna, the greatest of the European innovators.

A year after returning to the United States, Murphy married Jeanette Plamondon, his patient and the daughter of a wealthy industrialist, with whom he would have five children. Upon opening his surgical office in 1889, he established an animal laboratory in a shed behind his house, beginning a pattern of experimental work that would go on throughout his career, often with his wife as assistant. In 1892, at the age of thirty-five, he was made professor of clinical surgery at Chicago's College of Physicians and Surgeons, later to become the College of Medicine of the University of Illinois. In time, he would serve as professor of surgery at Northwestern University (1901–05 and 1908–16) and Rush Medical College (1905–08). From 1895 until his death in 1916, he was chief of surgery at Mercy Hospital in Chicago. During his career, he received three honorary doctorates and numerous other awards and honorary foreign memberships for his many achievements.

Murphy was a controversial character, admired for his great surgical skill and clinical contributions, but reviled by accusations of being an opportunist, a self-promoter, and a fiercely competitive, money-hungry agitator. His early notoriety began in the immediate aftermath of the famous Haymarket Riot, in which a bomb was thrown into the midst of a crowd of strikers and policemen. Murphy, a twenty-nine-year-old staff surgeon at the Cook County Hospital, worked indefatigably through the night and until almost noon the next day to treat and operate on the many wounded. Though his feat was celebrated in the newspapers to the advantage of his growing practice, he became the focus of resentment by colleagues, who called him, probably not without justification, a publicity-seeker.

On 2 March 1889 Murphy performed what some consider the first operation for acute appendicitis before rupture, and he quickly became not only an advocate but even a missionary for the operation. By 1895, he had reported on 207 patients with a mortality rate of 10 percent, in contrast to the rate of at least 30 percent associated with delayed treatment. His results continued to improve, so that by 1904, he had performed 2,000 appendectomies with an astonishingly low mortality rate of under 2 percent.

Murphy made many contributions to the development of abdominal surgery, among which was a method of anastomosing bowel after resection, which had been an almost insuperable problem until he introduced a device that became known as the Murphy button. The button consisted of two circular metal rings fitting into each other so as to hold the inverted intestinal ends together until the ring sloughed through at the join, creating a lumen. This invention not only was an effective way to re-establish continuity of the gut, but also stimulated others to develop further techniques, resulting in an upsurge in safe intestinal surgery.

In addition to his work in abdominal surgery, Murphy introduced many new methods in vascular surgery, orthopedics, gynecology, neurosurgery, and thoracic surgery. Through societies, medical literature, and his own teaching, he had a major impact on the training of American surgeons and was one of the founders of the American College of Surgeons in 1913. After a long period of anginal attacks, he died of a heart attack, while on vacation at Mackinac Island, Michigan, the very place where another renowned American surgeon, William Beaumont, had begun his studies of gastric physiology almost a century earlier.

Bibliography

Secondary: Schmitz, R. L., and T. T. Oh, 1993. *The Remarkable Surgical Practice of John Benjamin Murphy* (Urbana, IL); Editors, 1968. 'John Murphy (1857–1916): Chicago Surgeon.' *JAMA* 204: 102–103; Meyer, K. A., and S. Hyman, 1960. 'John B. Murphy. An Inquiry into His Life and Scientific Achievements.' *Journal of the International College of Surgeons* 34: 118–126; Davis, L. 1938. *J. B. Murphy, Stormy Petrel of Surgery* (New York); Moynihan, B., 1920. 'John B. Murphy—Surgeon.' *Surgery, Gynecology, and Obstetrics* 31: 549–573; *DAMB*.

Sherwin Nuland

MUTIS Y BOSIO, JOSÉ CELESTINO BRUNO (b. Cadiz, Spain, 6 April 1732; d. Bogotá, Colombia, 2 September 1808), *botany, natural history.*

Mutis y Bosio was born in the spring of 1732 in the Atlantic port of Cadiz in Spain. He was the child of Julián Mutis and Gregoria Bosio. Mutis studied grammar and philosophy in his natal city and then moved to Seville to pursue studies in medicine, receiving his degree in 1757. In that same year, he traveled to Madrid to cultivate his knowledge of plants under the tutelage of Miguel Barnades, a prominent Spanish botanist. Mutis stayed in Madrid for three years, an experience that would shape his interests throughout his life; not only did he get acquainted with the new and prominent Linnaean system of classification, but his botanical interests would remain a central part of his work for years to come.

In 1760, when Mutis was twenty-eight years old, Pedro Messía de la Cerda, the recently appointed viceroy of New Granada—roughly present-day Colombia—invited him to become his personal physician in the New World. Mutis accepted the invitation and in October traveled to Cartagena, the viceroyalty's main port in the Caribbean. After a few days there, always escorting the viceroy, the convoy then journeyed along the Magdalena River to the city of Honda and then through land and mountains to their final destination, Santee de Bogotá. The trip gave Mutis the chance to see the different climates of the region and, as he revealed in his diary, he was overwhelmed by the variety of plant species and developed an interest in the medical practices of the natives.

The Americas

Mutis's plans in the Americas included much more than medicine and the good health of the viceroy; in 1761, just a few months after his arrival to Santee, he wrote a letter to the king of Spain, Carlos III, asking him to support a project to study the plants of New Granada. Mutis received no answer from the king, and his multiple duties as a physician kept him away from being able to pursue his studies in natural history. In 1763 and 1764, he once again requested help from the king, arguing that a botanical project would not only bring honors and wealth to Spain, but also immortal glory to its patron. However, support from Spain for a botanical expedition in New Granada did not come for another twenty years, and Mutis had to pursue his interests in natural history as a sideline of his medical practice.

In the 1760s, aided by his medical position, he tried to understand the medical benefits of some of the plants he found in Bogotá and began what would become an important collection of plants. He also initiated correspondence with Linnaeus, to whom he sent specimens and descriptions of plants he thought were unknown in Europe. At the same time, he became professor of mathematics at the Colegio Mayor de Nuestra Señora del Rosario, one of the most prestigious centers of higher education in Santee de Bogotá, and for many years initiated many of his students into Newton's approach to mathematics as well as Copernicus's controversial theories on the solar system.

However, Mutis remained strongly attached to the idea that the Spanish Crown should support a project on the natural history of the Americas, which he could use to spend all of his time studying the botanical richness of New Granada, rather than pursuing it only as a pastime. In the 1770s this idea slowly began to take shape. In 1772 Mutis was ordained priest. It is not clear why he took this decision, but it is possibly related to the fact that viceroy de la Cerda had to return to Spain, and Mutis, still with no official financial support for his project, wished to remain in America. The newly appointed viceroy for New Granada, Archbishop Caballero y Góngora, soon became a good friend of Mutis and interceded for him in his attempts to obtain royal support for his project.

In 1783 Carlos III approved the Royal Botanical Expedition to New Granada and appointed Mutis as the director.

This Expedition, together with Ruiz and Pavon's expedition in Peru, and Sesse and Mocino's expedition in New Spain, were the three largest natural history enterprises carried out by the Spanish Crown in America in the colonial period. These expeditions were, of course, only possible in the context of the late eighteenth century: the Spanish Bourbons were trying to restore the grandeur of the empire and expected not only a utilitarian outcome from the botanical exploration of the new world, but also wanted to show other empires that Spaniards were competent natural historians.

The Royal Botanical Expedition

Mutis did not choose Santee as the base for his expedition. Instead, he opted for Mariquita, a small town distant from the capital of the viceroyalty. Mariquita had a privileged position: it was 535 meters above sea level and had easy access to different habitats. It was also close to important silver mines and to Honda, an important port on the Magdalena River. Once established in Mariquita, the Expedition started its work analyzing medicinal plants, such as quinine, cinnamon, and tea, and domesticating bees, mining, and collecting birds and insects.

Mutis also began a massive and impressive attempt to draw and illustrate the plant specimens collected by the Expedition. In fact, the elaboration of one of the biggest iconographic collections in the history of botany became one of Mutis' main goals. Drawing and painting plants was an ideal form of appropriating the natural richness of the New World for the empire. Right from the beginning, Mutis employed some of the most famous artists in New Granada. He also requested artists from Madrid, but the only two artists that came from Spain in 1788 were a failure. However, Mutis himself trained the majority of painters that worked for the Expedition. He even started a school to teach young American artists how to draw plants properly in order to later recruit them for the Expedition. Overall, thirty-eight artists worked for the Expedition and two-thirds of the employees were painters.

In 1790, after seven years of intensive work in Mariquita, the Spanish Crown decided to move the Expedition to Santee. Mutis was not in good health at the time and the government in Madrid feared that Mutis was never going to finish the long-awaited *Flora de la Nueva Granada.* In 1791 Mutis moved the entire operation to the capital and continued directing the project for another seventeen years until 1808, when he died. By that time, the headquarters of the Expedition in Santee had become a center of astronomical, botanical, and zoological studies, and the Expedition had produced 5,393 plates representing 2,696 species of Colombian plants. After Mutis died, the Crown requested the plates, and archived them in Madrid's Botanical Garden.

Mutis's Legacy in New Granada

At the turn of the nineteenth century, members of the Creole elite of New Granada engaged in a revolutionary

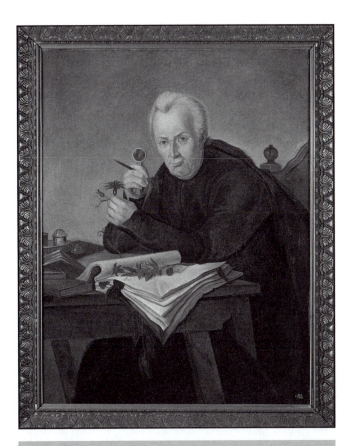

José Celestino Mutis observing plants through a magnifying lens. Oil painting by R. Cristobal, 1930. Iconographic Collection, Wellcome Library, London.

movement to obtain independence from the Spanish Crown. Important revolutionaries such as Francisco José de Caldas, Francisco Antonio Zea, or Jorge Tadeo Lozano, now seen as founding fathers and martyrs in Colombian history, were also important scientific figures who had been affiliated directly with the Royal Botanical Expedition. Mutis is often mistakenly studied as the teacher that initiated many of these characters into the revolutionary ideals that were rampaging Europe at the time, and that eventually led New Granada to declare its independence in 1810, two years after Mutis died. However, Mutis was a defender of the Spanish empire. The description, illustration, and naming of all the plants was done in the name of the Spanish Crown, and his detailed journal of all the matters related with the Expedition makes no reference to the insurgent character of many of his assistants in Santee. Mutis considered himself a European above all, and in one of his last statements before he died, he made clear that after he passed away, the position of director of the Royal Botanical Expedition should be extinguished and no one in America should replace him.

Rather than being a revolutionary instigator, Mutis's most important legacy in the Americas was the dissemination of important aspects of European culture. He trained a new generation of elite members in the ideas of the Enlightenment. As a teacher at the Colegio Mayor de Nuestra Señora del Rosario, Mutis insisted on the importance of mathematics, natural history, and natural philosophy to understand the natural world. He was the first in Colombia to teach the Copernican ideas of the cosmos, as well as Newton's and Linnaeus's systems, and he founded the first astronomical observatory of the Americas in 1803 in Santee.

Mutis also helped with the establishment of professional medical practice in New Granada. In the last years of the eighteenth century the low quality of medical practice, the unsanitary conditions among the population, and the high mortality rate from infectious diseases were perceived as the main obstacles in the development of a stable economy in the viceroyalty. Emissaries of the Spanish Crown informed the king of a lack of certified doctors. As a result, people often turned to indigenous and empiric doctors for help, a practice considered dangerous and pagan. Their solution was to bring certified doctors from Spain to offer the proper medical care to the population. Mutis however, offered a different solution. He insisted that there was no need for Spanish physicians in the colony. Instead, he offered to create a school to train American doctors in Santee. He had already trained one of his disciples, Miguel de Isla. Although Isla was not officially certified, Mutis guaranteed that he was as competent as any certified physician was. In 1802 Charles IV authorized Mutis to organize the first medical school in the capital of the viceroyalty, and he soon established a new curriculum in the Colegio Mayor de Nuestra Señora del Rosario. Botany, anatomy, and natural philosophy were included as crucial complements in the education of all the students.

Quinine

Throughout his life, Mutis remained proud of his role in Linnaeus's global project to classify and name plants in the eighteenth century. Mutis treasured the correspondence he had with the Swedish naturalist and believed this gave him more recognition as a natural historian. Mutis's studies of quinine, a famous plant in the history of medicine, are exemplary in this respect.

There is evidence that in the mid-seventeenth century Jesuits in Peru became interested in *Cinchona* (quinine), the bark of an Andean tree with properties to attenuate the attacks of malaria fevers. Up until the mid-eighteenth century, *Cinchona* was mostly a Peruvian product regulated by the Spanish Crown, and naturalists believed it did not grow north of the equator. Mutis tried to change this. He became acquainted with the fact that a type of quinine grew in the southwest of Colombia. In 1764 he sent a desiccated specimen of the plant to Linnaeus with a full description. Linnaeus had based his knowledge of the plant on the drawings of la Condamine. As a result, the 1767 edition of Linnaeus's *Systema naturae* included Mutis's additions as well.

Although Hipólito Ruiz, the director of the Royal Botanical Expedition in Peru, challenged the authenticity of Mutis's specimens of *Cinchona*, after 1780 Europe imported specimens from both Peru and New Granada. Both Mutis and Ruiz defended their specimens and their medicinal benefits. Mutis's studies on quinine were among the few complete scientific studies that he published before his death. Most of his work was published posthumously. In particular, the thousands of plates produced by the Expedition, which started to come out in 1954, are being released through the still ongoing joint effort of the Colombian and Spanish governments.

Bibliography

Primary: 1783. *Instruction sobre lass precautions, que debunk observers en la practical de la inoculation de lass virgules: formed de olden del Superior Oberon* (Santee de Bogotá); 1793. *Prospecto de los nombres y propiedades de lass quinas oficinales* (Santee de Bogotá); 1828. *El arcano de la quina: discurso que contiene la parte médica de lass cuatro especies de quinas oficinales, sus virtudes eminentes y su legítima preparación* (Madrid); 1947. (edición de Guillermo Hernández de Alba) *Archivo Epistolar del sabio naturalista don José Celestino Mutis* (Bogotá); 1954. *Flora de la Real Expedición Botánica del Nuevo Reino de Granada* (Madrid); 1983. *Escritos Científicos de Don José Celestino Mutis*, edición de Guillermo Hernández de Alba (Bogotá); 1983. (edición de Gabriel Fonnegra) *Mutis y la expedición botánica: documentos* (Bogotá); 1991. (edición de Marcelo Frías Nuñez) *Viaje a Santa fe* (Madrid).

Secondary: Pérez Mejia, Angela, 2002. *Le geografía de los tiempos difíciles: escritura de los viajes a Sur América durante los procesos de independencia, 1780–1849* (Medellín); Nieto Olarte, Mauricio, 2000. *Remedios para el imperio: historia natural y la apropiación del nuevo mundo* (Bogotá).

Camilo Quintero

MYA, GIUSEPPE   (b. Turin, Italy, 29 September 1857; d. Florence, Italy, 5 February 1911), *medicine, pediatrics.*

Mya graduated in medicine at the University of Turin in 1881, becoming Camillo Bozzolo's assistant in the medical clinic until 1890. He was named professor of medical pathology at the University of Siena, where he carried out his studies of pediatric pathology.

Mya moved to Florence, as full professor of special pathology at the Istituto di Studi Superiori, and taught an introductory course in clinical medicine. He was later appointed professor of clinical pediatrics. Following the didactic tradition started by Moisè Raffaele Levi in Florence, in 1882 Mya hospitalized ill children in the maternity ward of Santa Maria Nuova hospital. He was named full professor of pediatrics (1900) and became head of the pediatric clinic, which he moved in 1901 into the Anna Mayer pediatric hospital (opened in 1891).

At the third Italian Pediatric Congress, in 1898, he was elected vice-president of the new Italian Society of Pediatrics;

later, in 1905, he became the head of the society. Mya and his colleague Francesco Fede recommended that pediatrics should become a compulsory subject of study for medical students. This compulsory status in Italy began in 1906. In Florence, in 1903, in cooperation with Luigi Concetti, he founded the *Rivista di Clinica Pediatrica*. He joined the German pediatric society, becoming codirector together with Adalbert von Czerny of the *Monatsschrift für Kinderheilkunde*.

Together with Dante Cervesato, who had started the teaching of pediatrics in the University of Padua (1882), Mya was one of the pioneering figures who emancipated pediatrics from internal medicine and who struggled for the autonomy of the discipline. In those years, he was well aware of the passage from a 'sentimental' pediatrics connected to philanthropy, to a subject considered 'scientific' enough to gain the support of experimental researchers who could make observations in children's hospitals.

Mya's research touched on different sectors of pediatric pathology. He studied the diagnosis and therapeutic value of the lumbar puncture and the status of cerebrospinal fluid (CSF) in various pathologies and ages of life. He described the subtle threadlike fibrinous reticulum that takes shape in the CSF of patients affected by tubercular meningitis, which in some European countries was named 'Mya's reticulum'. He was among the first to report the congenital hydrocephalus and the congenital (aganglionic) megacolon, which is named Bettini-Mya's disease in Italy and is known outside Italy as Hirschsprung's disease. He also examined nutritive changes among nurslings and the cure of infective illness in the gastrointestinal tract. He studied the pathogenesis of infectious idiopathic amyotrophy early in life, congenital spastic diplegia (Little's disease), and diphtheria.

He was convinced of the necessity of transforming pediatrics on an outpatient basis. He became the head of the so-called *Aiuto materno*, the first in Italy, where mothers were encouraged to breastfeed their babies. It had been opened in 1900 by the obstetrician Ernesto Pestalozza, on the Boudin model, in the maternity ward of Florence, which was attached to the Foundling Hospital degl'Innocenti. There, weekly pediatrician checkups were carried out and poor mothers could receive support and education in infant care.

In Florence, Mya conducted a detailed inquiry into the living conditions of children in 1907. On the basis of these results, he requested the Italian state authorities to improve the level of health care services for poor children, illegitimate children, and orphans.

Bibliography

Primary: 1894. 'Sulla dilatazione ed ipertrofia congenita del colon.' *Lo sperimentale* 48; 1896. 'Idrocefalo congenito familiare con palese influenza dell'ereditarietà.' *Rivista di patologia nervosa e mentale* 1; 1909. *Inchiesta sulle condizioni dell'infanzia a Firenze* (Florence).

Secondary: Guarnieri, Patrizia, 2004. 'Dall'accoglienza alla cura. La riforma sanitaria nel brefotrofio degl'Innocenti di Firenze 1890–1918.' *Medicina & Storia* 7: 57–100; Società Italiana di Pediatria, 1937. *La Pediatria in Italia* (Milan).

Patrizia Guarnieri

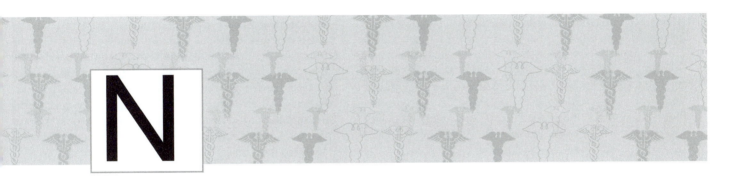

N

IBN AL-NAFĪS, ʿALĀʾ AL-DĪN ABU L-ʿALĀʾ ʿALĪ B. ABĪ L-HARAM AL-QURASHĪ AL-DIMASHQĪ

(b. Damascus, Syria, *c.* 1213, d. Cairo, Egypt, 1288), *medicine, grammar, logic, Islamic religious science.*

Ibn al-Nafīs was born in or near Damascus, perhaps in the village of al-Qurashiya, according to his patronimic. He studied medicine under Muhadhdhib al-Dīn ʿAbd al-Raḥīm b. ʿAlī al-Dakhwar, the founder of a medical school at Damascus. He was also trained in religious law, logic, and grammar; his lectures and writings on these disciplines were praised by his contemporaries. At an unknown date he moved to Cairo, where he developed a professional career as the chief physician of Egypt and as personal physician to Sultan Baybars I. Ibn al-Nafīs became rich and had a luxurious house built in Cairo. On his death, at the age of eighty lunar years, he bequeathed his house and books to the newly founded Mansuri Hospital there, which had been completed in 1284.

Among his works on logic and theology, Ibn al-Nafīs wrote *al-Risalat al-Kāmiliya fi s-sira al-nabawiya*, freely translated as The Theologus Autodidactus, that is, a counterpart to the philosophical novel by Ibn Ṭufayl (d. 1185), *Hayy ibn Yaqzān* [The Self-Taught Philosopher], which inspired Daniel Defoe's *The Life and Adventures of Robinson Crusoe* (1719). While Ibn Ṭufayl's purpose was to show the discovery of philosophical truths by an individual who had been created by spontaneous generation on a desert island, that of Ibn al-Nafīs was to show the discovery of independent reasoning of the main principles of Islamic religion and natural sciences under similar conditions.

With regard to medicine, Ibn al-Nafīs seems to have been a learned theorist rather than a practical physician. His extensive literary activity in this field focused mainly on commentaries, although he is said to have written most of his works out of his head without reference to books. Among them, he commented upon several works attributed to Hippocrates—such as *Aphorisms, Prognostics, Epidemics,* and *On the Nature of Man*—as well as the *Masāʾil fī ṭ-ṭibb* [Questions on Medicine] by Ḥunayn ibn Ishāq.

Ibn al-Nafīs wrote the *Kitāb al-Shāmil fī ṭ-ṭibb,* an encyclopedia of medicine said to consist in 300 volumes, of which only eighty were completed. He is also the author of a comprehensive compilation of medieval Islamic ophthalmological knowledge, entitled *Kitāb al-Muhadhdhab fī l-kuhl.* His most widely disseminated work in the Islamic medical tradition was the *Kitāb al-Mujiz* or *Mujiz al-Qānūn,* an epitome, or collection of extracts, in four sections from Avicenna's medical encyclopedia. This concise manual of medicine was commented upon by a number of later authors, and it was translated into Hebrew and several times into Turkish.

Ibn al-Nafīs's *Sharḥ al-Qānūn* is considered to be the reference book that threw light on the obscurities of Avicenna's (Ibn Sīnā's) *Canon of Medicine.* In this extensive commentary, he devoted a separate section to the passages relating to anatomy. Often copied as an independent book, the *Sharḥ Tashrīḥ al-Qānūn* by Ibn al-Nafīs contains the earliest known description of the lesser, or pulmonary, circulation of blood. Virtually ignored by later Islamic medical authors, his theory resulted from a logical deduction derived from knowledge about the impenetrability of the cardiac septum. Against Galen and Avicenna's accepted ideas, and anticipating part of William Harvey's discovery, Ibn al-Nafīs speculated that the blood must flow from the right ventricle of the heart through the pulmonary artery to the lung, and from there through the pulmonary vein to the left ventricle of the heart. A close parallel of this theory was formulated by Michael Servetus in his *Christianisimi restitutio* (Venice, 1553) and by Realdo Colombo in his *De re anatomica* (Venice, 1559). It is probable that these Western physicians had direct knowledge of Ibn al-Nafīs's theory through Andrea Alpago (d. 1522), who had lived more than thirty years in Syria collecting, translating, and editing medieval Islamic medical works—among them, the section devoted to compound drugs from Ibn al-Nafīs's *Sharḥ al Qānūn*—not all of which were printed posthumously.

Bibliography

Primary: Meyerhof, M., and J. Schacht, 1968. *The Theologus Autodidactus of Ibn al-Nafīs* (Oxford); Qatayah, S., and P. Galiyunji, eds., 1988. *Kitāb Sharḥ tashrīḥ al-Qānūn* (Cairo).

Secondary: Meyerhof, M., and J. Schacht, 2003. [*s.v.* Ibn al-Nafīs, 'Ala' al-Din Abu l-'Ala' 'Ali b. Abi l-Haram al-Qurashī al-Dimashqī], *The Encyclopaedia of Islam* (new edn., 11 vols., Leiden 1960–2002) vol. III, pp. 897–898; Savage-Smith, E., 1980. 'Ibn al-Nafīs's Perfected Book on Ophthalmology and His Treatment of Trachoma and Its Sequelae.' [edition, translation, and commentary] *Journal for the History of Arabic Science* 4: 147–206; Iskandar, A. Z., 1967. *A Catalogue of Arabic Manuscripts on Medicine and Science in the Wellcome Historical Medical Library* (London) pp. 38-42; Schacht, J., 1957. 'Ibn al-Nafīs, Servetus and Colombo.' *Al-Andalus* 22: 317–336; Meyerhof, Max, 1935. 'Ibn al-Nafīs (XIIIth cent.) and His Theory of the Lesser Circulation.' *Isis* 23: 100–120 (rpt. in Johnstone, P., ed., *Studies in Medieval Arabic Medicine* (London) 1984); *DSB*.

Cristina Álvarez Millán

NAGAYO, SENSAI (b. Ōmura, Hizen domain [now Nagasaki Prefecture], Japan, 28 August 1838; d. Tokyo, Japan, 8 September 1902), *public health, medical administration.*

Nagayo Sensai was an architect of Japan's modern medical and public health systems. He rendered distinguished services as the first chief medical officer to the Meiji government.

Nagayo was born to a family of medical practitioners in the Ōmura province, near the port of Nagasaki in Kyushu, the only port open to Westerners (the Dutch) until 1853. His grandfather and father were keen to introduce Western medical technologies, particularly smallpox vaccination, into their

practices. In 1854 he went to Osaka to study medicine at Teki-Juku, a school of Dutch studies founded by Ogata Kōan. Coming back to Nagasaki in 1860, he continued his study under Dutch physicians such as J. L. C. Pompe (1829–1908) and C. G. Mansvelt (1830–1912) and became the head of the Nagasaki Medical School in 1868.

The new Meiji government, which had replaced the Tokugawa shogunate in 1867, wanted talent for modernization of the country. In the sphere of medicine, Nagayo was selected and sent to the United States, England, Holland, and Prussia to investigate various systems for medicine and public health (1871–73). After his return, he was appointed the director of the Medical Affairs Bureau of the Education Ministry (1873–75) and then of the Sanitary Bureau of the Home Ministry (1875–91).

His first task as the country's chief public health administrator was the drafting of Isei (1874), a comprehensive law providing grand rules for public health administration, medical provision, education and qualifications, and pharmaceutical affairs. Among other things, it made the government's policy clear that the country should adopt Western medical sciences rather than traditional Kanpō (Chinese-Japanese) medicine.

When a cholera epidemic attacked Japan in 1877, Nagayo played a central role in the making of the Provisional Regulations for Prevention of Cholera. In 1880 this was transformed into a permanent and more comprehensive set of regulations: the Regulations for Prevention of Infectious Diseases, which prescribed preventive medical procedures such as notification, disinfection, and isolation, to be applied for six major acute infectious diseases: cholera, typhoid, dysentery, diphtheria, typhus, and smallpox. As for smallpox in particular, he was responsible also for the issue of the Vaccination Regulations of 1885.

While working in central administration, Nagayo was a keen promoter of local self-government. He was aware that a key to successful public health was the promotion of people's subjective cooperation as well as of preventive medical expertise at the local level. In 1879, under his initiative, elective sanitary committees were set up at each small unit of local administration, to let preventive medical works be subject to local democratic procedures. However, the committees were abolished, and their duties were transferred to the police forces in 1886, as part of the local-government reform initiated by the Cabinet, which wanted a local government system functioning smoothly according to directions from the central authorities. But Nagayo felt that public health movements were frustrated by these centralizing measures.

Outside government machinery, Nagayo, together with several other prominent medical men, formed the Japan Sanitary Society (Dai-Nihon Shiritsu Eisei-kai) in 1883. In his inaugural address, Nagayo, vice president of the Society, pointed to a penetration of public health ideas into the minds of people as its main objective. The Society was a voluntary organization, but with a quasi-official character, given that most of its founders were, like Nagayo, central government officials. Through speeches, discussions, and publications, it played an influential role in public health reform in late nineteenth-century and early twentieth-century Japan.

Entrusting his work as the top public health leader to Gotō Shinpei (1857–1929), Nagayo died at the age of sixty-four in 1902.

Bibliography

Primary: 1888. 'Eisei to jichi no kankei' [On the Relationship between Hygiene and Self-Government]. *Dai-Nhon Shiritsu Eisei-kai Zasshi* 6: 260–274; 1980. 'Shōkō-shishi.'[Autobiography] in Ogawa, Teizo, and S. Sakai, eds., *Matsumoto Jun Jiden, Nagayo Sensai jiden* (Tokyo) pp. 101–185.

Secondary: Ban, Tadayasu, 1987. *Teki-juku to Nagayo Sensai* (Osaka).

Takeshi Nagashima

NAIDOO, GONARATHNAM KESAVELOO (aka DR GOONAM) (b. Durban, South Africa, 24 February 1906; d. Durban, 21 September 1998), *general practice.*

The daughter of a well-off Indian merchant and his Mauritian-born Indian wife, Naidoo was encouraged by her progressive-minded mother to complete a full primary school education, the most an Indian girl could hope for in the South Africa of the 1910s. Overcoming her father's reservations about her studying further—this was regarded as superfluous in her socially conservative community, which firmly designated the home as the woman's sole terrain—she opted for a medical career so as to obtain the higher education that she craved.

Yet pursuing such a career then meant going abroad, for there was neither a high school for Indian girls in South Africa nor a local medical school willing to admit those who were not white-skinned. Accordingly, with the attention of the whole Indian community focused on such a radical step, in 1928 she traveled to Scotland alone, first to complete her schooling and then to enroll at Edinburgh University Medical School. The training she received there enabled her to gain the FRCP & S (Edin.), the LRFPS (Glasgow), and a licentiate in midwifery from Coombe Hospital in Dublin in 1936.

If her medical education was protracted, her political education while in Edinburgh certainly was not. Living for the first time in an environment where racial barriers were not the norm and mixing with politically aware students from India, she was exposed to the politics of anticolonialism, which triggered her own political awakening and social liberation.

Back in Durban starting in 1936, she initially remained on the fringe of local politics while trying to establish a private practice. The latter was easier said than done, for, particularly within her own Indian community, her gender,

Western clothing, lipstick, earrings, cigarettes, scorn for the community's traditional ideas about disease and medicine, and open criticism of conventions restricting Indian women weighed heavily against her acceptance as a doctor. Consequently, she found herself viewed ambivalently by many Indians, with pride for her achievements but with disapproval for her behavior and opinions, 'a novelty, but professionally . . . no draw', she recalled (1991, p. 58).

She therefore sought part-time institutional appointments to bolster her income, jobs that opened her eyes to the widespread poverty and squalor among the mass of Indians outside her elite circle. Nor did these appointments come without a political dimension, for not only did they heighten her social and political awareness, but through them she also experienced racial discrimination personally. From 1939 she thus began to become directly involved in Indian opposition to such discrimination in South Africa, her position as the sole Indian woman doctor in the country giving her actions a high profile, especially among Indian women. Strident and outspoken, she was at the forefront of the cadre of young Indian professionals who took over the conservative, male-only Natal Indian Congress and, between 1943 and 1948, steered it along a Gandhian path of passive resistance against the state's imposition of further residential restrictions on Indians. She was twice jailed for deliberately contravening segregationist laws.

Despite (or perhaps because of) this deepening political involvement, her private practice began to grow, both within the Indian community and beyond, and she was forced to take a partner, which allowed her to concentrate on her first love, gynecology and obstetrics. This juggling of her medical and political careers—to which she added lobbying Indian families to allow their daughters to train as nurses and doing voluntary medical work for welfare organizations—continued until 1955, when the juggernaut of apartheid made her leave South Africa, initially for Britain, but in 1956 for India, where her political connections secured her the post of assistant director of the national Family Planning Department.

However, the demands of her extended family took her back to South Africa in 1959, where her reopened private practice in Durban again had to coexist with her political activity. Once more, the latter eventually forced her to flee the country, this time (1978) to escape harassment and imprisonment by the apartheid authorities. Medical work in London was followed in 1983 by a return to her irresistible southern Africa, as a medical officer in a geriatric clinic in Zimbabwe. There she remained until the transition from apartheid to democracy drew her back to Durban in 1991, where, despite her age, she again did part-time sessions in clinics, concentrating, as ever, on the health of women and children.

Unorthodox and strong-willed in everything she did from her twenties onward, Naidoo—who re-named herself Goonam when she first returned to Durban because she felt her family name was too 'clannish, even casteish' (1991, p. 54)—had one daughter, though she never married, and also adopted a niece and a nephew. As one of her close associates said of her, 'It was clear that no man, or, for that matter, woman could dominate her' (Meer, 2002, p. 41).

Bibliography

Primary: 1991. *Coolie Doctor—An Autobiography of Dr Goonam* (Durban).

Secondary: Meer, I., 2002. *A Fortunate Man* (Cape Town); Romero, P. W., 1998. *Profiles in Diversity—Women in the New South Africa* (East Lansing, MI).

Howard Phillips

NEGOVSKII, VLADIMIR ALEKSANDROVICH (b. Kozeltce, Russian Empire [now Ukraine], 19 March [1 April] 1909; d. Moscow, Russia, 2 August 2003), *pathophysiology, neuropathology.*

The father of 'reanimatology' (the science of resuscitation medicine in the West) was born into a family of primary school teachers in a little town in the Ukraine. In childhood he fell ill with tuberculosis and spent a lot of time in hospitals; this later played an important role in his career choice. In 1928 Negovskii went to Moscow and entered the Second Moscow State Medical Institute, where he listened to the lectures of Fedor Andreev and Alexander Bogomolets, director of the Institute of Hematology and Blood Transfusion, both of whom had been working on the problems of near-death and revival for many years.

Under their influence, in 1933 Negovskii started the study of intra-arterial blood transfusion as a method of resuscitation medicine in the Laboratory of Experimental Physiology and Therapy, headed by Sergei Briukhonenko, also Andreev's student and inventor of the first heart–lung machine in 1925. But their cooperation was short-lived, and in 1936 Negovskii wrote to the Soviet government requesting permission to set up his own laboratory. Ever since the death of Bolshevik leader V. I. Lenin in 1924, the problems of immortality and resurrection were always a focus of Soviet rulers, and Negovskii's application was approved. In October 1936 the Laboratory of Experimental Physiology and Restoration of the Organism was established under his supervision in Moscow and became the first resuscitation research laboratory in the world. In 1985 it was renamed the Institute of Reanimatology in the USSR Academy of Medical Sciences, Negovskii remaining its director for more than half a century.

Negovskii regarded the concept of death as a gradual process consisting of two main stages, clinical death and biological death. He argued that the stopping of the heart and the end of respiration (i.e., clinical death) are only part of the transition to biological death. Only the death of the brain means irreversible death. The significance of the distinction between clinical and biological deaths was crucial for medi-

cal practice. Based on his concept, Negovskii and his collaborators started to use external cardiac massage, external defibrillation, and some other means of resuscitation many years before the clinical introduction of the method of emergency artificial circulation in the West.

World War II strongly reinforced and developed the clinical dimension of Negovskii's work. In 1943 he presented his doctoral thesis on the restoration of the vital functions of dying organisms, formed front-line resuscitation teams, and achieved effective resuscitation of a number of soldiers who were clinically dead. After the war Moscow hospitals were provided with a mobile team for emergency resuscitation, also for the first time in the world. On 2 March 1953, Negovskii and his team were invited to revive the most important patient in the USSR, Josef Stalin, but too late.

Negovskii devoted the second half of his life to the study of post-resuscitation disease and the training and mentoring of several generations of Soviet reanimatologists. He was the author or coauthor of more than 300 scientific publications and fourteen monographs; some of them have been translated into foreign languages. But many of his innovative ideas and procedures were unknown in the West because of language and Cold War barriers.

In 1975 Negovskii was elected a full member of the USSR Academy of Medical Sciences. In the 1990s he and the Western 'father' of critical care, Peter Safar, were jointly nominated three times for the Nobel Prize. The death of these two medical pioneers (2003) marked the end of the formative years of modern resuscitation.

Bibliography

Primary: 1943. *Vosstanovlenie zhiznennykh funktsii organizma, nakhodiashchegosia v sostoianii agonii ili klinicheskoi smerti* [The Restoration of the Vital Functions of the Organism in the Throes of Death and Clinical Death] (Moscow); 1983. (with Gurvich, A. M., and E. S. Zolotokrylina) *Postreanimatsionnaia bolezn,* trans. as *Postresuscitation Disease* (Amsterdam and New York).

Secondary: Negovskaia, A. V., and I. V. Molchanov, eds., 2004. *Padre della Rianimazione* (Moscow); Safar, Peter, 2001. 'Vladimir A. Negovskii, the Father of "Reanimatology".' *Resuscitation* 49: 223–229.

Marina Sorokina

NEŠIĆ, DJORDJE P. (b. Šabac, Serbia, 27 June 1873; d. Belgrade, Yugoslavia [now Serbia], 24 October 1959), *ophthalmology, military ophthalmology.*

The son of Petar (a civil servant) and Ljubica, Nešić (Nestich or Neschitch) was born in Šabac and educated in Moscow, where he developed his specialty under Kryukov. At his mentor's urging, Nešić attended lectures in physics and mathematics and later used this knowledge to devise and construct new instruments and devices. In 1899 he published the first ophthalmology textbook for military physicians and went on to become chief of ophthalmology at the

General State Hospital in 1904. In 1921 Nešić founded the Ophthalmology Clinic of the Medical Faculty and remained its chief until 1955.

Nešić was a participant in the Russo-Japanese war (1904–05), two Balkan wars, and World War I, when he served as commander of the Field Surgical Hospital on the Thessalonica Front from 1916 to 1918. There he studied hemeralopia (impaired vision during daylight), widely observed among exhausted Serbian soldiers retreating through Albania in 1915–16. His report, 'Étude sur l'Héméralopie', appeared in *Annales d'Oculistique* (1918) and brought him acclaim.

Nešić spent nearly six decades fighting against trachoma, once an endemic disease in Serbia; his most important work in that field was published in 1958. After 1906, Nešić focused largely on histopathologic research in ophthalmology and was deeply involved in efforts to combat tuberculosis, which had been the most lethal disease in Serbia during the first half of the twentieth century, accounting for nearly 30 percent of mortality. Nešić was particularly interested in the effects of tuberculosis keratoconjunctivitis in the form of stafyloma corneae.

Among the several ophthalmologic instruments Nešić devised, best known is a giant electromagnetic device for the removal of metal bodies from the eye (1940). Some of his electromagnetic devices were adopted in hospitals in Western Europe. His electromagnetic instruments, large and small, were used in military medicine as well. Their advantage derived not only from their power to extract and remove very small metal pieces, but also from the better visibility and great working space for the surgeon during an operation.

Throughout his career, Nešić published forty-three articles, twenty-two books, and eighteen popular medical texts, appearing in French, Italian, English, Russian, German, American, and Bulgarian medical periodicals. A lover of technology and machinery, Nešić was also a pioneer of automobile sport in Serbia and owner of the third car in Belgrade. As a student, he won several awards at bicycle races.

Bibliography

Primary: 1938. *Veliki elektromagnet konstrukcije Očne klinike.*

Secondary: Kecmanović, Zlatimir, 1998. 'Đorđe P. Nešić (1873–1959)' in *Život i delo srpskih naunčika* 3; 1972. *Spomenica Srpskog Lekarskog Društva* (Belgrade).

Jelena Jovanovic Simic and
Predrag J. Markovic

NETTER, ARNOLD-JUSTIN (b. Strasbourg, France, 20 September 1855; d. Paris, France, 1 March 1936), *pediatrics, bacteriology.*

Netter came from a Jewish family that had lived in Alsace for more than a century. With the German conquest, the family moved to Paris, where his father, a physician nearing the age of sixty, set about re-establishing a practice in the neighborhood. Although his father planned for him to enter the free military medical school at Val-de-Grâce, Arnold proved successful in the competitions in the Paris hospital and academic hierarchies. At age twenty-four, he distinguished himself in the concours for internship, received his MD degree in 1883, and earned the rank of hospital physician in 1888 and assistant professor of hygiene the following year. In 1897 he obtained the chair of experimental and comparative anatomy, and he was elected to the Academy of Medicine in 1903.

Netter combined bacteriological knowledge and epidemiological expertise with hygienic and therapeutic activism. He contributed to the reorganization of pathology on the basis of bacteriological findings. Named to the Trousseau hospital in 1895, he remained at that pediatric hospital for the rest of his career. His contributions to clinical bacteriology began with studies of the pathological action of the pneumococcus in childhood pneumonia and pleurisy. In 1908 he identified an epidemic of cerebro-spinal meningitis and investigated the frequency of the disease in Paris and other French cities. He drew attention to the importance of spinal tap for bacterial confirmation of the diagnosis. With his student Robert Debré, Netter showed the efficacy of anti-meningococcal serum from convalescent patients. He used sera for prevention of numerous other infectious diseases that were then frequent in children (and adults), such as polio and diphtheria, and he investigated epidemics of typhoid, typhus, and encephalitis. Nearly all of Netter's many publications appeared in medical journals, academic proceedings, and as chapters in textbooks.

Netter was known for his gentleness and kindliness to his pediatric patients and his staff. Debré likened his appearance to that of an Old Testament prophet, but a smiling one. Arriving early at the hospital daily, including Sundays and holidays, Netter was equally renowned for his erudition and immense culture extending to all the major European languages. He was active in the Jewish community and the Zionist movement. At the liberation of Alsace in 1918, he wept with joy, yet he was one of the first French scientists to re-establish contact with German colleagues. Netter died suddenly at the age of eighty while addressing a medical meeting.

Bibliography

Primary: 1883. *Diagnostic précoce d'une forme de tuberculisation pulmonaire à début pleurétique.* Thesis, Paris; 1911. (with Debré, Robert) *La méningite cérébro-spinale* (Paris).

Secondary: Debré, Robert, 1936. 'Éloge de Netter.' *Bull. de l'Académie de Médecine* 115: 419–422.

Anne Marie Moulin

NEWMAN, GEORGE (b. Leominster, Herefordshire, England, 23 October 1870; d. York, England, 26 May 1948), *public health.*

Newman was born into a Quaker family. He studied medicine at Edinburgh University, qualifying in 1892, before moving to the London Medical Mission as assistant physician. He pursued his interest in public health, lecturing and working part-time for the Medical Officer of Health of the Strand Board of Works. In 1894 he registered at King's College London to study for the Cambridge University Diploma in Public Health, which he passed in 1895. He was then appointed part-time demonstrator at King's College, teaching practical classes in bacteriology, which allowed him to undertake research for a book, *Bacteria* (1899).

In 1896 he was offered a position as a medical inspector at the Local Government Board, but turned it down as he wished for a position with the local authority as medical officer of health. He was appointed part-time Medical Officer of Health (MoH) to the Holborn Board of Guardians in 1897, while continuing to devote some of his time to Quaker societies (he edited *The Friend's Quarterly Examiner* anonymously from 1899 until his death). His first full-time position as MoH came in 1900, when he was appointed to the new metropolitan borough of Finsbury—a poor, overcrowded area with a high level of infant mortality. Newman spent the next six years instituting strict public health surveillance regimes, health education programs, and an infant milk depot. He published several key papers and books, and from 1905 lectured in public health at St Bartholomew's Hospital Medical School.

Through his association with Beatrice Webb (1858–1943), Newman presented evidence to the Royal Commission on the Poor Laws. He was appointed to the new post of Chief Medical Officer (CMO) to the Board of Education in 1907, the year in which a system of medical inspection and medical care of school children was established. His appointment was greeted with hostility from some in the medical profession, who took this as a sign of the state's restriction of private practice. Newman helped to create a comprehensive tuberculosis service out of the National Health Insurance legislation of 1911, and to found the Medical Research Committee (later Medical Research Council) in 1913.

From 1916 onward Newman participated in plans for a new Ministry of Health. On 1 April 1919 Newman was appointed as CMO to the Local Government Board, transferring two months later to the new Ministry alongside Robert Morant (1863–1920) as Permanent Secretary and Christopher Addison (1869–1951) as the first Minister of Health. They had hoped to create an administration in which the medical staff would have equal status and pay with the lay officials. His influence in the Ministry was reduced when Morant died suddenly from influenza in 1920 and when Addison was forced to resign as Minister in 1921.

Newman appeared to lack further creative energy, and his time in office did not produce significant policy developments. He did, however, work hard at developing a good relationship with the leading members of the medical profession, and by continuing as CMO to the Board of Education he ensured coordination between medical services. Newman also used his position at the Board of Education in the interwar years to pursue reforms in medical education, in particular urging that control of clinical training should be taken away from the elite private practitioners and placed with university-based academic teachers.

Bibliography

Primary: 1906. *Infant Mortality: A Social Problem* (London); 1907. *The Health of the State* (London); 1939. *The Building of a Nation's Health* (London).

Secondary: Sturdy, S., 1998. 'Hippocrates and State Medicine: George Newman Outlines the Founding Policy of the Ministry of Health' in Lawrence, C., and G. Weisz, eds., *Greater Than the Parts: Holism in Biomedicine: 1920–1950* (Oxford) pp. 112–134; Bynum, W. F., 1995. 'Sir George Newman and the American Way' in Nutton, V., and Roy Porter, eds., *The History of Medical Education in Britain* (Amsterdam) pp. 37–50; Hammer, M. A. E., 1995. 'The Building of a Nation's Health: The Life and Work of George Newman to 1921.' PhD thesis, Cambridge; *Oxford DNB.*

Sally Sheard

NEWSHOLME, ARTHUR (b. Haworth, Yorkshire, England, 10 February 1857; d. Worthing, Sussex, England, 17 May 1943), *public health.*

Newsholme was a prominent and internationally acclaimed champion of British public health. His time in office spanned the creation of a comprehensive state medical system, one only stopping short of universal access to free primary health care. Newsholme grew up in Haworth, Yorkshire, and was first apprenticed to a Bradford doctor. He then moved to London to train at St Thomas's Medical School, qualifying (1880) and receiving the MD (1881). His initial posts were hospital-based, before he moved to private practice in Clapham and took a part-time appointment as a district medical officer of health there in 1884.

After taking the new professional qualification in public health (the Diploma in Public Health), he moved to Brighton as a full-time medical officer of health (MoH) in 1888 (sustaining a loss of income in order to achieve his chosen medical career). Here Newsholme developed his practical public health techniques, gaining experience in controlling outbreaks of scarlet fever, diphtheria, and typhoid fever. His particular interests were in the welfare of infants and children and in the development of tuberculosis services. He also published a seminal text, *The Elements of Vital Statistics* (1889), which became a standard textbook for medical officers of health and went through several editions.

Newsholme was the first Chief Medical Officer (CMO) to be 'headhunted' for the post. When William Power's (1842–1916) retirement was imminent, he was approached by John Burns (1858–1943), president of the Local Government Board. Burns had considerable respect for Newsholme's pioneering work in Brighton and thought he would be a creative CMO, able to implement the Liberal welfare forms. He was the first 'outsider' to enter the medical civil service, and oversaw the transition in public health ideology from an essentially environmentalist approach to an emphasis on personal preventive medicine. Newsholme developed three new services—maternity and child welfare, tuberculosis medical services, and a service for venereal diseases. During his time as CMO much wider reforms to the welfare system were planned, following a Royal Commission on the Poor Law, and Newsholme's department also had to administer the consequences of the new National Insurance Act of 1911, although Newsholme had opposed some parts of Lloyd George's proposals because he feared they would compromise the valuable disease prevention work of local authorities.

World War I stifled some of Newsholme's plans at the Local Government Board, and his last year in office was marked by the influenza pandemic of 1918–19. He resigned on the eve of the creation of the Ministry of Health and immediately traveled to the United States, where he completed a large lecture tour to promote infant and child welfare. He spent some time lecturing on public health administration at Johns Hopkins University, Baltimore. During his time in America, while he was in his sixties, he also learned how to drive. He traveled widely in Europe on behalf of the Milbank Fund to make a major study of health care systems, which resulted in the publication of *International Studies on the Relation between Private and Official Practice of Medicine* (1931). On his return from Russia (1933) he coauthored a book entitled *Red Medicine* with John Kingsbury, secretary of the Milbank Fund. Newsholme was a prolific writer, with twenty-five books and over 160 articles and book chapters to his name, as well as many reports and pamphlets.

Bibliography

Primary: 1889. *The Elements of Vital Statistics* (London); 1935. *Fifty Years in Public Health: A Personal Narrative with Comments* (London); 1936. *The Last Thirty Years in Public Health: Recollections and Reflections on My Official and Post-Official Life* (London).

Secondary: Eyler, John M., 1997. *Sir Arthur Newsholme and State Medicine, 1885–1935* (Cambridge); Eyler, John M., 1992. 'The Sick Poor and the State: Arthur Newsholme on Poverty, Disease and Responsibility' in Rosenburg, Charles, and Janet Golden, eds., *Framing Disease: Studies in Cultural History* (New Brunswick, NJ); *Oxford DNB*.

Sally Sheard

NEWTON, ROBERT STAFFORD (b. near Gallipolis, Ohio, USA, 16 December 1818; d. New York, New York, USA, 9 October 1881), *medicine, sectarian medicine, eclecticism.*

Newton grew up in rural Ohio to farming parents of hardy pioneer stock. His father deemed a common school education sufficient for a life in agriculture, but Robert was an unhappy plowboy and resolved to study medicine. He subsequently left home to apprentice with a Gallipolis physician, Edward Naret. In 1839 Newton entered the Medical University of Louisville, graduating in 1841.

Although Newton earned his degree from a thoroughly orthodox medical school, he came to regard regular medicine as ineffective and inhumane. Convinced that regular physicians' practice of bleeding and purging was dangerous, he left orthodoxy in 1845 in favor of the eclectics, a group of herbal practitioners originally founded in 1827 by Wooster Beach in New York. By the 1840s, eclecticism had expanded throughout settled America, with Newton assuming a leadership role among eclectics almost from the beginning of his conversion. In 1848 he helped establish the National Eclectic Medical Association and served as its president at the 1851 and 1857 annual meetings. Newton was active in teaching as well, and from 1849 to 1850 was chair of surgery at the Memphis Institute. Following the death of Thomas Vaughan Morrow, founder of the Eclectic Medical Institute (EMI) of Cincinnati, in 1850, Newton was persuaded to accept the chair of surgery at this preeminent eclectic school. The following year he assumed that post along with duties as the school's chief administrator.

Newton adroitly managed the EMI through a serious faculty rift over contending ownership rights between his group and one led by self-styled 'psychometric' healer Joseph R. Buchanan. The disturbance escalated into a riotous attempt by Buchanan supporters, led by Charles Harley Cleaveland, to storm the building, culminating in Newton positioning a six-pound canon at the Institute's door to halt the assailants. Subsequent adjudication of the matter in 1856 decided the question of legitimate ownership on behalf of Newton and his colleagues. Victorious, Newton remained at the EMI until 1862. During that time he served as editor of the *Eclectic Medical Journal* and *Newton's Express*. Under Newton's leadership the EMI became one of the nation's more progressive medical schools. In an age when most schools—regular or otherwise—offered little clinical instruction, Newton's Clinical Institute gave EMI students much-needed practical experience.

He later shared controlling interest in the EMI with John Milton Scudder. After the dissolution of EMI, Newton went to New York City in 1863. There he organized the state Eclectic Medical Society and helped establish the Eclectic Medical College of New York City in 1865. Newton worked tirelessly to re-establish the National Eclectic Medical Association, which had disbanded after the eighth annual meeting in 1857. Finally, in 1870 he presided over the meeting in Chicago of the newly re-established association. In 1874 he assisted Alexander Wilder in editing the *Medical Eclectic*, the mouthpiece for the Eclectic Medical College.

Newton was man of forceful personality who assumed the mantle of leadership at a critical time for the eclectics. But for his able administration of the EMI, American eclecticism might well have perished with Thomas Vaughan

Morrow. Instead, the EMI carried on to enjoy some of its best years in the 1870s. The school would carry eclecticism on into the twentieth century until the forces of modernity demanded its final closure on 7 June 1939.

Bibliography

Primary: 1852. (with King, John) *The Eclectic Dispensatory of the United States of America* (Cincinnati); 1861. *An Eclectic Treatise on the Practice of Medicine, Embracing the Pathology of Inflammation and Fever, with Its Classification and Treatment* (Cincinnati); 1867. (with Powell, Byrd W.) *An Eclectic Treatise on Diseases of Children* (New York).

Secondary: Haller, John, 1994. *Medical Protestants: The Eclectics in American Medicine 1825–1939* (Carbondale, IL); Wilder, Alexander, 1904. *History of Medicine* (Augusta, ME); Felter, Harvey Wickes, 1902. *History of the Eclectic Medical Institute, Cincinnati, Ohio, 1845–1902* (Cincinnati); *DAMB*.

Michael A. Flannery

NICHOLAS OF POLAND   (aka NICHOLAS OF MONT-PELLIER) (b. Silesia, Poland, *c.* 1235; d. Cracow, Poland, *c.* 1316), *medicine, surgery, pharmacology.*

Although nothing is known of his early life, linguistic evidence suggests that Nicholas was a German of Silesian origin. A member of the Dominican Order, around 1250 he moved to Montpellier, where he taught in the Dominican *studium*. Around 1270, he returned to Silesia and entered the Dominican convent at Cracow, where, as part of the ministerial duties that attended his office as a friar, he provided medical as well as spiritual care to the people.

Nicholas was a popular and charismatic healer. Not long after his return to Silesia, he became the focus of an 'alternative' medical movement that flourished in Upper Silesia in the late thirteenth century. He was also a favorite in the court of Leszek the Black (Lestko Nigritius), the duke of Sieradz and one of Poland's more enlightened medieval princes. Nicholas's methods were certainly unorthodox. Urging a return to 'natural' methods of healing, he attributed extraordinary virtues to toads, scorpions, and lizards. His favorite remedy was serpents' flesh prepared according to detailed instructions contained in his treatise *Experimenta magistri Nicolai* [Master Nicholas's Experiments], a compilation of his medicaments. He urged all people, 'of whatever station, to eat serpents whenever it is possible to get them' (*Experimenta*, ed. Ganszyniec, 1920, p. 144). Evidently impressed by Nicholas's doctrine, Leszek ordered that serpents, lizards, and frogs be served at his court.

Nicholas elaborated on his doctrine in a fierce invective against scholastic medicine, a work whose title, *Antipocras* ('Against Hippocrates', *c.* 1270), reveals the principal target of his attack. In this versified polemic, Nicholas defended his empirical methods, which he claimed brought miraculous cures all over the Latin world, against the bankrupt methods of the physicians. Attacking the physicians' reliance on reason over experience, he rejected Galenic authority and extolled the 'wisdom of the people', to whom, he claimed, God had chosen to reveal the deepest secrets of nature. In fact, however, Nicholas's prescriptions were inspired not by folk medicine but by learned interest at Montpellier in the famous classical drug theriac, the principal ingredient of which was viper's flesh.

Educated at Montpellier during a period when Scholastic medicine was in full swing, Nicholas violently rejected the medical tradition being developed there. His strange and revolting arsenal of drugs was based on the principle that, although God had conferred marvelous virtues on all of nature, 'the more filthy, abominable, and common things are, the more they participate' in these marvelous virtues (*Antipocras*, ed. Ganszyniec, 1920, p. 60). Hence, remedies made of the most common and contemptible creatures contained far greater medicinal virtues than the 'precious and famous' drugs recommended by the physicians. Nicholas's radical critique of official medicine was grounded in an essentially religious doctrine calling for an acceptance of the marvelous; yet significantly, he invoked the authority of 'master Albert' to confirm his doctrine, a reference to the popular *De mirabilibus mundi* [On the Miracles of the World] attributed to Albertus Magnus.

A renowned surgeon, Nicholas also composed an influential treatise on surgery, the *Hübsch Chirurgia* [Fine Surgery]. The work is largely a compilation drawing from a complex of German and Latin texts that have their origins in the twelfth-century *Surgery* of the Lombard surgeon Roger Frugardi (fl. 1180). In 1316 King Władisław I Łokietek granted Nicholas a privilege, conferring on him feudal rights over three villages in Lesser Poland.

Bibliography

Primary: 1911. (Johnsson, John W. S., ed.) 'Les "Experimenta magistri Nicolai".' *Bulletin de la société français d'histoire de la médecine* 10: 269–290; 1916. (Sudhoff, Karl, ed.) 'Antipocras, Streitschrift für mystische Heilkunde' in *Versen des Magisters Nikolaus von Polen. Sudhoffs Archiv* 9: 31–52; 1920. (Ganszyniec, Ryszard, ed.) *Brata Mikotaja z Polski Pisma Lekarskie* (Posen).

Secondary: Jonecko, Antoni, 1993. 'Studien zum Dicterarzt Nikolaus von Polen. Eine Skizze des mittelalterlichen Arztes und Dichters unter besonderer Akzentuierung seiner "Antipocras"–Streitschrift, seiner "Experimenta", der "Chirurgie" sowie seiner Verbindungen nach Schlesien.' *Würzburger medizinhistorische Mitteilungen* 11: 205–225; Eamon, William, and Gundolf Keil, 1987. 'Plebs amat empirica: Nicholas of Poland and His Critique of the Medieval Medical Establishment.' *Sudhoffs Archiv* 71: 180–196; Keil, Gundolf, 1987. 'Nikolaus von Polen.' *Die deutsche Literatur des Mittelalters. Verfasserlexikon* 6: 1128–1133.

William Eamon

NICOLLE, CHARLES JULES HENRI (b. Rouen, France, 21 September 1866; d. Tunis, Tunisia, 28 February 1936), *bacteriology.*

Nicolle was born in Normandy, the middle son of Eugène (a doctor and teacher of natural history) and Aline Louvrier. Their eldest son Maurice became a noted immunologist at the Pasteur Institute, and Charles was expected to set aside his literary inclinations and follow in his father's provincial medical footsteps. After Eugène's death (1884), Charles complied. Partially to help care for younger brother Marcel, Nicolle completed his first two years of medical education in Rouen, continuing in Paris. In 1889 he passed the challenging Internat des Hôpitaux de Paris.

While working with patients, Nicolle discovered a physical limitation to his clinical future: hearing loss that grew increasingly profound throughout his life. Accepting his disability, he turned to Louis Pasteur's nascent Institute, where he studied under Emile Roux and Elie Mechnikov, producing a thesis on soft chancre (1893). The enthusiastic new 'pastorian' gladly accepted positions in Rouen as professeur suppléant in pathology and clinical medicine at the Ecole de Médecine and as médecin-adjoint to the city's hospitals. At the Ecole, Nicolle expanded a small bacteriology laboratory into a large serum-producing and microbial-testing facility. Appointed the laboratory's director (*c.* 1894), he conducted original research on the new Widal test (from 1896) and on variation in bacterial 'races'. In 1900 Nicolle was named chef de service in the venereal ward at the Hospice Général. His efforts to reform patient treatment there had, however, earned him few administrative friends and, moreover, had alienated the medical school's director, who blocked his bid for a permanent appointment. Frustrated, Nicolle accepted the directorship of the expanding Pasteur Institute in the French protectorate, Tunisia. He left Rouen in late 1902, accompanied by his wife, Alice Avice (married 1895), and children, Marcelle (b. 1896) and Pierre (b. 1898).

Under his guidance, the Institute flourished. During his time there, Nicolle started the Institute's *Archives* (1906), conducted important research on leishmaniasis and trachoma, discovered the parasite *Toxoplasma gondii*, and demonstrated that the organism responsible for the 1918–19 influenza pandemic was a filterable virus. Additionally, he conducted vaccine research, most notably developing a convalescent serum against measles.

Nicolle is best known for his work on louse-transmitted diseases: typhus and relapsing fever. When he began his research, typhus could not be cultivated outside the human body. In 1909 he successfully reproduced the disease in chimpanzees and then transmitted it to monkeys shortly thereafter, demonstrating its louse transmission. His typhus work led him to postulate the existence of a 'silent' (asymptomatic) but acute disease expression that he dubbed 'inapparent infection'. Nicolle was awarded the Nobel Prize in Medicine or Physiology (1928). He later returned to typhus after a rat/flea variety of the disease was identified. Ulti-

mately, his research in both relapsing fever and typhus informed his pioneering exploration of the 'birth, life, and death' of disease species, which he began articulating at length in 1932 as Chair of Experimental Medicine at Paris's Collège de France. In 1934 he contracted typhus in his Tunis lab. The illness exacerbated his tachycardia, resulting in his slow decline and eventual death. Still director of the Pasteur Institute of Tunis when he died, Nicolle was buried in his institute.

Nicolle never abandoned his literary aspirations, publishing seven novels and numerous essays and short stories. He also authored a number of philosophical books on medicine, biology, and civilization. In 1927 France awarded him its prestigious Osiris Prize, and in 1929 he was elected nonresident member of the Academy of Medicine. Both his children became doctors.

Bibliography

Primary: 1909. (with Comte, Charles, and Ernest Conseil) 'Transmission expérimentale du typhus exanthématique par le pou du corps.' *Comptes Rendus de l'Académie des Sciences* 149: 486–489; 1930. *Naissance, Vie et Mort des Maladies Infectieuses* [expanded (1933) as *Destin des Maladies Infectieuses* (Paris)].

Secondary: Pelis, Kim, 2006. *Charles Nicolle, Pasteur's Imperial Missionary: Typhus and Tunisia* (Rochester, NY); Huet, Maurice, 1995. *Le Pommier et l'Olivier: Charles Nicolle, une Biographie* (Paris); *DSB.*

Kim Pelis

NIGHTINGALE, FLORENCE (b. Florence, Italy, 12 May 1820; d. London, England, 13 August 1910), *nursing, sanitary science, hospital design.*

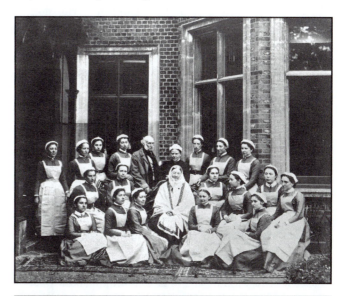

Florence Nightingale and Sir Harry Verney with nurses at Claydon House, *c.* 1890. Photograph, Archives and Manuscripts, Wellcome Library, London.

Family and Upbringing

Florence's parents, William Edward Nightingale and Frances Smith, were on the grand tour of Europe when she was born, and named her after the city of her birth. Her elder sister, born in Naples, was named Frances Parthenope. The Nightingales were of the prosperous upper middle classes, their income derived from commerce, and belonged to the Unitarian religious tradition. The family divided their time between their country houses, Embley Park in Hampshire and Lea Hurst in Derbyshire. There were trips to London and visits from the extended family. Mrs Nightingale was a celebrated hostess, and some of the most distinguished and intellectual figures of the day, including the future prime minister, Lord Palmerston, were among the visitors to her salon.

Nightingale was a conscientious local squire, providing schools for his tenants at his own expense among his other welfare activities. He personally supervised the education of his two daughters. Florence was an apt and responsive pupil and as a result enjoyed an education on a par with that of many upper-class men of the time. This intellectual development did not sit easily with her expected future role as wife and mother in a similar household. The enforced idleness of women of the leisured classes exacerbated her periods of depression and introspection.

At the age of sixteen (1837) she received what she described as a call to service from God. Her nebulous feelings, strengthened by a study of such mystics as St Teresa of Avila, crystallized into the desire to help the poor and sick. Her parents met with horror and refusal her request to train as a nurse at the nearby Salisbury Infirmary.

Early Travels

Her despair was tempered by parental permission to accompany Charles and Selina Bracebridge on their travels to Europe (1847–48). She formed a firm and long-lasting friendship with the Bracebridges. The trip was also significant because of her meeting in Rome with Sidney and Mary Elizabeth Herbert.

During a further trip with the Bracebridges (1850), she visited the community at Kaiserwerth-am-Rhein to observe the work of Pastor Theodor Fliedner. Women were trained at the Kaiserwerth Institute as deaconesses. Not only did they learn to nurse in an institutional setting, but the training also covered management, housekeeping, and home nursing. This gave Florence the idea to reform nursing by training suitably motivated women and creating a secular body of nurses, rather than a religious one.

Developing Knowledge of Public Health

She returned to England to face continuing family issues. She rejected a proposal of marriage from Richard Monckton Milnes, who had pursued her for nine years. Her sister Parthe was suffering from a nervous condition brought on by anxiety about Florence. Florence assuaged her ambitions by studying government reports, 'bluebooks', on public health and the Poor Law.

An opportunity to apply her burgeoning knowledge occurred when the Herberts suggested she accept the unpaid post of superintendent of the Institute for Sick Governesses in Distressed Circumstances, Harley Street, London. Her organizational flair was clearly demonstrated in her supervision of the Institute. During her time there, she revolutionized its management, installing piped water, lifts, and many labor-saving devices. Her skills were further illustrated by her assistance with the demands of a cholera epidemic at the nearby Middlesex Hospital.

In the Crimea 1854–1856

In the spring of 1854, the event occurred 'that made all that had gone before a mere prologue' (Baly, 1995, p.114): the start of the Crimean War, with Britain and France aiding Turkey against Russia. Dispatches from *The Times* correspondent William Russell criticized the poor medical provisions for the British wounded. They were in sharp contrast those of the French, which were managed by religious nursing orders. Many of the problems facing the British army were logistical rather than resource-based and were related to the fact that this was the first major European war for nearly forty years. Sidney Herbert, now Secretary of State at War, bore the brunt of the public indignation at the soldiers' situation. His response was to ask Florence to take a party of nurses to Scutari at the government's expense. With the help of Elizabeth Herbert and other women friends, applicants were interviewed and assessed, and thirty-eight nurses were assembled in the astonishing time of five days. The party consisted of a mix of nursing nuns, Anglican and Roman Catholic, and laywomen, and was supplemented by Florence's old friends, the Bracebridges. In November 1854 they reached the dilapidated barracks at Scutari on the Asian side of the Bosphorus, which had been taken over by the army medical service to serve as a hospital for the troops ferried across from the Crimea. Nightingale was to write later that Dante's words 'Abandon hope all ye that enter here' should have been inscribed over the entrance (Baly, 1995, p.115).

Initially the army doctors would not allow the nurses into the hospital; Nightingale, secure in her connections at home and in her possession of £30,000 and supplies, patiently bided her time. Later in the month the aftermath of the battle of Balaclava, with streams of wounded overwhelming the hospital, led the doctors to turn to the nurses for assistance. Applying the principles of sanitary science, Nightingale transformed the filthy barracks, where there had been at one stage four miles of patients on mattresses on the floor and 1,000 diarrhea cases, into something resembling a therapeutic institution. Her grasp of the importance of adequate nutrition is evident in her scheme to bring the society chef Alexis Soyer to the Crimea. Nightingale's personal dynamism was reflected in the hours she worked, and although her duties were predominantly administrative, she made a point of visiting the wards daily, often at the end of the day, hence the legend of the 'Lady with the Lamp'.

In May 1855 she crossed to the Crimea to visit the field hospitals. While there she contracted Crimean fever, which she referred to as typhus, but which was probably brucellosis (Young, 1995, pp. 1697–1700). Patients, staff, and the British public feared for her life, but she made a slow and painful recovery. The effects of the illness, characterized by relapses and remissions, were to dog her for many years to come and fuel a debate into its etiology. As a response to her work and recovery, in 1855, while Nightingale was still abroad, Herbert set up a committee to collect money from a grateful nation. A fund of £45,000 was established to enable Nightingale to train nurses. She was not enthusiastic about this, regarding the fund as a burden, which detracted from her real work.

Return to England

She returned to England in July 1856, emaciated and exhausted, but with a zeal to better the lot of the common soldier. The first step was participation in an investigation into the running of army medical services. The 1860 Royal Commission resulted in the establishment of an Army Medical School and improvements in barracks and army hospitals. She also prepared evidence for the 1861–63 sanitary commission on India. She became an expert on India, albeit from her sickbed. As part of her campaigns, she pursued lengthy correspondence with her network of immediate and extended family and friends, many of whom were influential figures in government and public life. Nightingale took advantage of her situation as an 'invalid', expecting them to visit her to discuss issues, including sanitary science, hospital design, and the reform of nursing.

Nursing Reform

Nightingale's reluctance to be involved with the reform of nurse training meant that initial plans were shelved until the late 1850s. Attracted by proposed plans to build a new St Thomas' Hospital on a suburban site, she entered into negotiations to establish a school of nursing at the new hospital. Ironically, the new hospital was built in Lambeth on the south bank of the Thames. The training school for nurses opened there in 1860. After an initial period when other matters occupied her, Nightingale began to devote more energy to the school, starting from the mid-1860s. The first ten years of the school were hardly spectacular. As Baly's analysis shows, comparatively few of the original probationers were nursing at the end of four years. The training and teaching of the probationers was done by the incumbent nursing and medical staff of the hospital. Although Nightingale was involved with inspections of the probationers' notebooks and had them visit her to discuss their progress, the probationers were ultimately used as a source of pliable, economical labor for the hospital as it increased its range of medical activities. The probationers lived on the hospital

premises in accommodations that Nightingale had hoped would be a home in a very rounded sense, but still facilitate their twenty-four-hour availability for duty. Contrary to its boasts, the school did not turn out generations of nurses who pioneered the Nightingale method. Some individuals did move on to other hospitals upon completing their training. As with most of Nightingale's ventures, publicity for the school was good, and by the 1870s most of the London teaching hospitals had a training school along the Nightingale lines. Perhaps its most successful achievements were its efforts with the reform of workhouse nursing—Miss Vincent had been sent to St Marylebone Workhouse Infirmary in 1882—and with district nursing. Nightingale could be said to have contributed more to the reform of workhouse nursing than to the school of nursing that bore her name. She was a key player in the investigations during the 1860s into provisions for the pauper sick.

In 1861 William Rathbone of Liverpool contacted Nightingale with the request to supply nurses for home nursing. Rathbone donated a new building to the Liverpool Royal Infirmary as a school of nursing. The resulting school began in 1862 to train nurses for care both at home and in hospital. Liverpool was divided into eighteen districts, each with a committee of lady volunteers and a trained nurse. In 1882 Queen Victoria, a great supporter of Nightingale, donated the greater part of the Women's Jubilee Fund to an extension of the district nurse scheme. Rathbone and Nightingale continued their work together until his death (1902).

Old Age and Death

Nightingale spent the last years of her life in her rooms at South Street near Park Lane, London. Her honors included being made a member of the Order of Merit (1907) (the first woman so honored) and the freedom of the City of London (1908). She became increasingly isolated as old colleagues died and her faculties gradually declined. She died in her sleep.

Nightingale Historiography

Despite her antipathy to the cause of state registration of nurses, early leaders of 'reformed' nursing held Nightingale as an exemplar of their aspirations to professional status, and overplayed the contrast between pre– and post–Nightingale School nursing. Nightingale was of interest to the generation after her; hence her inclusion in Strachey's *Eminent Victorians* and an early biography by Cook (1913). Her iconic status was perpetuated by Woodham Smith's 1950 biography and was popularized in the 1951 film *The Lady with a Lamp*, starring Anna Neagle. More recently, scholars, particularly F. B. Smith (1982), have challenged the almost hagiographic approach to Nightingale. A more balanced approach came with the extensive and thorough scholarship of Baly (1995, 1997, and *Oxford DNB*), who highlighted the complexity of Nightingale's character and achievements during a life of ninety years during a time of social, economic, and philosophical changes.

Achievements

Nightingale is most often popularly remembered for her work in the Crimea. This has tended to eclipse both the contributions of other women, particularly Mary Seacole (1805–81), to the care of the wounded in the Crimea and Nightingale's other achievements. The fruits of her endeavor were numerous. The range of her interests was extensive. Her research skills encompassed both the means of obtaining information and the method of displaying it. Many government departments adopted her model forms and her circular charts, or 'coxcombs' as she described them, bear a resemblance to the pie chart. In 1860 she was made a Fellow of the Statistical Society (the first woman). Her formidable intellect, nurtured by her classical education, is seen in her philosophical work *Suggestions for Thought to the Searchers after Truth among the Artisans of England* (1860).

Nightingale was an intensely religious person, and her beliefs and works are complexly intertwined. In this juxtaposition of religious conviction and social action she was a product of her time. In the posthumously published *Cassandra* (Strachey, 1928), which was originally volume two of *Suggestions,* she contributed to the debate on the place of women. Although doubtful of the value of women's suffrage, she argued that women's time was seen as an interruptible commodity set against the protected, waged time of male professionals. The demon that possessed her was embraced; she reckoned discontent a privilege (Strachey, 1928, p. 398). She stressed the vocational nature of nursing but expected nurses to earn a living wage. She was emphatic on the need for nurses to concentrate on nursing tasks and not be diverted by domestic chores (Nightingale, 1881). Her directions on how to nurse (Nightingale, 1859) have a universality that continues to resonate with succeeding generations of nurses.

Bibliography

Primary: 1859. *Notes on Nursing* (London); 1860. *Suggestions for Thought to the Searchers after Truth among the Artisans of England* (London); 1865. (with Liverpool Nurses' Training School Committee) *The Organisation of Nursing in a Large Town (Liverpool)* (London); 1881. *On Trained Nurses for the Sick Poor* (London); 1893. *Sick Nursing and Health Nursing* (London); Strachey, R., 1928. 'The cause': A Short History of the Women's Movement*—Appendix I: 'Cassandra by Florence Nightingale' (London).

Secondary: Baly, M., 1997. *Florence Nightingale and the Nursing Legacy* 2nd edn. (London); Baly, M., ed., 1997. *As Miss Nightingale Said . . . Florence Nightingale through Her Sayings* 2nd edn. (London); Baly, M., 1995. *Nursing and Social Change* 3rd edn. (London); Young, D. A. B., 1995. 'Florence Nightingale's Fever.' *British Medical Journal* 311: 1697–1700; Smith, F. B., 1982. *Florence Nightingale: Reputation and Power* (London and Canberra); Woodham

Smith, C., 1950. *Florence Nightingale 1820–1910* (London); Cook, E., 1913. *The Life of Florence Nightingale* 2 vols. (London); Strachey, L., 1918. *Eminent Victorians* (London); *Oxford DNB*.

Stephanie Kirby

NISSEN, RUDOLF (b. Neisse, Germany, 9 September 1896; d. Riehen, Basel, Switzerland, 22 January 1981), *surgery*.

Nissen's father had worked with leading German bacteriologists, such as Robert Koch and Emil von Behring, before turning to surgery with one of the top-ranking German surgeons, Ernst von Bergmann of Berlin. At Rudolf's birth, his father owned and practiced in a small hospital in his hometown. Preparing to succeed his father, Nissen read medicine at Breslau. During World War I he had to assume surgical responsibility before graduating (1920). Still in Breslau, he worked in internal medicine with Oskar Minkowski and later in pathological anatomy with Ludwig Aschoff in Freiburg. During his surgical internship with Ferdinand Sauerbruch in Munich and later Berlin (1921–33), Nissen became Privatdozent (1927) and, encouraged by his mentor, chose an academic career. Political inroads made this impossible in Germany. Forced to leave the country because his mother was Jewish, he became chairman of surgery at the University of Istanbul (1933), when the young Turkish Republic reformed its universities, hiring dozens of German Jewish professors. In 1939 Nissen further emigrated to the United States, where he worked at the Massachusetts General Hospital in Boston and later as chief surgeon of the (then) Jewish and Maimonides hospitals in New York. After World War II he accepted a call to the surgical chair of the University of Basle in neutral Switzerland (1952). He remained there until his retirement (1966), despite offers from Germany and the Vienna chair, prestigious since Theodor Billroth's time.

Through his wife's unremitting support, Nissen was able to cope with their burdens of life as emigrants; she thus stood behind his generous, broad-minded, and cosmopolitan personality.

His career was certainly facilitated by his early scientific and practical achievements. In Berlin he had already opened a new chapter in thoracic surgery when performing the world's first *successful* pneumonectomy (1931). The parents of his patient, a severely injured twelve-year-old girl, agreed to this daring operation. It was performed in two stages, by ligating the blood vessels of the pulmonary hilum and removing the necrotic lung two weeks later. Nissen was lucky, given the enormous technical obstacles to be overcome and the unknown pathophysiological consequences of the enormous empty space on the entire organism. American and Canadian colleagues followed his lead in the next two years.

In the United States, Nissen realized the superiority of intubation anesthesia and the use of sedatives over Sauerbruch's hypobaric chamber. In this respect, he far surpassed his mentor in the latter's own specialty of thoracic and pulmonary surgery, while such progress was systematically being thwarted in Germany because of Sauerbruch's authority. Among Nissen's later valuable accomplishments was fundoplication (1955), an operation for treating painful esophageal inflammation resulting from gastric reflux. It is still universally used.

Back in Europe, Nissen was instrumental in transferring not only technical, but also organizational, innovations to German-speaking lands. He was the driving force behind the transformation of academic surgery in Basle from a typically hierarchical Middle-European chair to a department, wherein he fostered subspecialties such as neurosurgery. Anesthesiology was to become an independent specialty. He also reformed clinical instruction, complementing the traditional *ex cathedra* lectures with bedside-teaching to small groups of students.

A master of the word, he authored an insightful autobiography (1969). As Billroth had done a hundred years before, Nissen wrote lucidly on general issues of contemporary medicine. Holding successively a German, Turkish, U.S., and Swiss passport, he was perhaps the most international surgeon of his generation.

Bibliography

Primary: 1931. 'Exstirpation eines ganzen Lungenflügels.' *Zentralblatt für Chirurgie* 58: 3003–3006; 1956. 'Eine einfache Operation zur Beeinflussung der Reflux-Oesophagitis.' *Schweizerische Medizinische Wochenschrift* 86: 590–592; 1969. *Helle Blätter-dunkle Blätter* [Autobiography] (Stuttgart).

Secondary: Schein, Moshe, Heidi Schein, and Leslie Wise, 1999. 'Rudolf Nissen: The Man behind the Fundoplication.' *Surgery* 125: 347–353; Harder, Felix, and Mario Rossetti, eds., 1997. *100 Jahre Rudolf Nissen* (Basel).

Ulrich Tröhler

NOGUCHI, HIDEYO   (b. Mistuwa, Fukushima Prefecture, Japan, 9 November 1876; d. Accra, Gold Coast [now Ghana], 21 May 1928), *microbiology.*

Noguchi was a son of a poor peasant in a small inland village in the northeastern region of Japan. The fingers on his left hand were maimed by a serious burn injury that he suffered at the age of one. Despite extreme poverty and this physical disability, his education was made possible by the self-sacrifice of his mother, Shika, and the benevolences shown by his teachers and friends, not to mention his own hard work. After his secondary education, he obtained an informal medical apprenticeship, first at a practitioner's office near his home and then at the Takayama Dental Clinic in Tokyo (1893–97). In 1897, after a brief attendance at the Saisei Medical School, he passed an examination and was qualified as a practitioner.

Noguchi then served as an assistant researcher at the Institute for Infectious Diseases (1897–1900), directed by Kitasato Shibasaburo (1852–1931), and held an additional post in the Yokohama Quarantine Office. When Simon Flexner (1863–1946) of the Johns Hopkins University came to the Institute in 1899, Noguchi conveyed to Flexner his desire to study in America.

In December 1900, helped financially by his friends, Noguchi visited the University of Pennsylvania in Philadelphia, where Flexner had just moved. There was, however, no formal place for him, and he started work as Flexner's personal assistant. His first work was on antitoxic sera for snake venom, which received wide recognition and brought Noguchi a formal research assistantship in the University (1902) and a one-year fellowship to study in Copenhagen with the Danish serologist Thorvald Madsen (1903).

In 1904 he was appointed a research assistant of the Rockefeller Institute for Medical Research, newly founded in New York with Flexner as its director. Noguchi rose to become its leading member through his researches on *Treponema pallidum,* the causative agent of syphilis. Noguchi claimed that he succeeded, for the first time in the world, in cultivating *T. pallidum* in a pure state (1911), although this was controversial given that no one could succeed in replicating this afterward. More credible was his detection of *T. pallidum* in the spinal cords of syphilis patients (1913), which greatly increased the knowledge of brain disorders associated with syphilis. This work made him a formal member of the Institute (1914).

He went on researching diseases whose causative agents had not yet been found. He successfully showed that verruga peruana was caused by *Bartonella bacilliformis,* the organism causing Oroya fever. On the other hand, he struggled in his research of diseases that are now known to have a viral cause, such as polio and yellow fever.

His biggest and final target was yellow fever. As a member of the Rockefeller Foundation's Yellow Fever Commission to Ecuador in 1918, Noguchi concluded that the disease was caused by a species of *Leptospira,* which he had detected in patients' blood. But those thinking that the causative agent should be a filterable organism, invisible with microscopic technology at that time, challenged this. In 1927 Noguchi went to Accra in West Africa to investigate and settle the controversies by himself. After six months of painstaking effort, however, he contracted yellow fever and died at the age of fifty-three, regrettably before a definite conclusion came out.

Noguchi made his only return to his home country in 1915. The moving reunion of a humble-boy-turned-internationally-famous-doctor with his old and barely literate mother has long been remembered in Japan as an example of an affectionate bond between mother and child.

Bibliography

Primary: Various dates. Collected Reprints of Hideyo Noguchi, M.D. (New York); 1909. *Snake Venoms* (Washington, DC); 1923. *Laboratory Diagnosis of Syphilis* (New York).

Secondary: Nakayama, Shigeru, 1978. *Noguchi Hideyo* (Tokyo); Eckstein, Gustav, 1931. *Noguchi* (New York); Flexner, Simon, 1929. 'Hideyo Noguchi. A Biographical Sketch.' *Science* 69: 653–660; *DSB*.

Takeshi Nagashima

NOTT, JOSIAH CLARK   (b. Columbia, South Carolina, USA, 31 March 1804; d. Mobile, Alabama, USA, 31 March 1873), *medicine, ethnology, medical entomology.*

Nott was the son of Abraham Nott, a judge and congressman from Columbia, South Carolina. The Nott family had the wherewithal to send several of their five sons to college, among them Josiah, who entered South Carolina College in 1824 before studying medicine at University of Pennsylvania. After graduating in 1827, Nott stayed in Philadelphia for two years. While in that city he studied under the prominent surgeon, Philip Syng Physick, and came under the influence of ethnologist Samuel George Morton (1799–1851).

In 1830 he returned to Columbia and started a medical practice there, marrying Sarah Deas in 1832. In 1835 Nott left for Paris, where he studied natural science, anthropology, and medicine before returning to Mobile in 1837. That year he gained first-hand experience with yellow fever when an epidemic struck the city. In 1848 Nott published a seminal paper proposing that yellow fever and malaria were transmitted by an insect vector. The work was disparaged and ridiculed by his colleagues, but today is considered a pioneer precursor to Albert F. A. King's fuller study of 1883.

Except for a brief year as chair of anatomy at the University of Louisiana in 1857, Nott maintained an active practice in Mobile. In 1859 he was instrumental in founding the Medical College of Alabama. Although classes were soon halted by the Civil War (1861–65), it resumed operations and eventually evolved into the University of Alabama School of Medicine, now located in Birmingham.

During the war Nott served as medical director for General Braxton Bragg. At war's end he moved north, where he took up gynecological surgery, first in Baltimore and then in New York City. Nott developed tuberculosis, and in 1872 he headed to the warmer climate of Aiken, South Carolina. In December he moved to the city he considered home, Mobile, and died there three months later.

Despite Nott's notable contributions to the etiology of disease and to medical education in the South, he is less favorably known for his views on ethnology. Opposed to the biblical view that all of humanity had a common ancestry, as described in the account of Adam and Eve in Genesis, Nott championed the notion that human races had developed independently in the localities of their origin. Moreover, Nott insisted that blacks were a separate species, distinct from and inferior to Caucasians. Nott's antibiblical views were extreme even for his day, but he nevertheless fit in well with other Southern physician-apologists such as Samuel Cartwright (1793–1863), who attempted to give a scientific justification for the institution of slavery. Nott's simplistic notions that cranial capacity correlated precisely with intelligence, that culture and socialization played little or no role in development, and that differences in appearance between races were both quantitative *and* qualitative presaged the misguided eugenics movement of the early twentieth century.

Nott is a paradoxical figure. He proved to be ahead of his time in suggesting the mode of transmission of yellow fever and malaria and was a progressive force for medical education, yet his dilettantish and self-serving work in ethnology validated a socioeconomic system based upon ideological presumptions of racial inferiority.

Bibliography

Primary: 1848. 'Yellow Fever Contrasted with Bilious Fever—Reasons for Believing It a Disease sui generic—Its Mode of Propagation—Remote Cause—Probable Insect or Animalcular Origin, &c.' *The New Orleans Medical and Surgical Journal* 4 (March): 563–601; 1857. (with Glidden, George B.) *Indigenous Races of the Earth* (Philadelphia).

Secondary: Horsman, Reginald, 1987. *Josiah Nott of Mobile: Southerner, Physician, and Racial Theorist* (Baton Rouge); Chernin, Eli, 1983. 'Josiah Clark, Insects, and Yellow Fever.' *Bulletin of the New York Academy of Medicine* 59: 790–802; Brace, C. Loring, 1974. 'The 'Ethnology' of Josiah Clark Nott.' *Bulletin of the New York Academy of Medicine* 50: 509–528; Holt, William Leland, 1928. 'Josiah Clark Nott of Mobile' *Medical Life* 35: 487–504; *DAMB*.

Michael A. Flannery

NÓVOA SANTOS, ROBERTO   (b. La Coruña, Spain, 6 July 1885; Santiago de Compostela, La Coruña, Spain, 9 December 1933), *medicine, pathology.*

Nóvoa Santos studied medicine at the University of Santiago de Compostela (1907). In 1911 he was awarded a grant by the Board for Advanced Studies and Scientific Research and visited Bordeaux, Paris, and Strasbourg, among other cities. In 1912 he won the chair of general pathology at the University of Santiago, where he remained until 1928. In 1929 he moved to the same position in Madrid, which he held until his death in 1933. He dedicated himself to politics for a brief period of his life and was a Deputy at the Constituent Assembly of the Second Spanish Republic in 1931.

Nóvoa was one of the most brilliant exponents in Spain of the new German pathophysiologic medicine. He was also very aware of other scientific currents of his time, such as psychoanalysis and Darwinism, which he used for some general explanations.

Like François Magendie, Nóvoa understood health status as a physico-chemical balance of the individual with the environment and saw disease as the disruption of this equilibrium—i.e., in the language of Charles Darwin, a poor adaptation to the environment. Besides the presence of an external cause, Nóvoa ascribed great importance to the predisposition of an individual to suffer morbid processes.

He also made notable contributions to the study of certain diseases, such as diabetes mellitus, liver disease, and nervous system disorders.

Nóvoa was a highly prolific author. In his twenty-five years of professional activity, he produced almost 200 works. One of his most important writings was his *Manual de Patología General*, a general pathology handbook, which ran to eight editions and was the textbook for several generations of Spanish physicians. Nóvoa offered a dynamic view of health and disease states, and this represented a revolution in the Spanish medicine of his time, which was wedded to a more static perspective on these processes. With his *Manual*, he established solid theoretical doctrinal foundations for Spanish pathology, which was still largely based on obsolete vitalist concepts or an excessively anatomopathologic approach.

Nóvoa was also interested in sexual function, which he understood as a process of adaptation of the individual to the environment. His defense of the lack of intellectual qualities of women, whom he considered only from a reproductive perspective, led him to reactionary positions that brought him into conflict with the feminist movements of his time.

Bibliography

Primary: 1916. *Manual de Patología general* (Santiago de Compostela); 1929. *La mujer, nuestro sexto sentido y otros esbozos* (Madrid); 1939. *Diabetes espuria y diabetes sacarina* (Madrid).

Secondary: Fernández Teijeiro, Juan José, 2003. *Roberto Nóvoa Santos. La imortalidad: Dolor y saudade* (A Coruña); Fernández Teijeiro, Juan José, 2001. *Más allá de la patología: la psicología de Nóvoa Santos* (Santiago de Compostela); Glick, Thomas. 'Nóvoa Santos, Roberto' in López Piñero, José María, et al., eds., 1983. *Diccionario histórico de la ciencia moderna en España* vol. 2 (Barcelona).

Guillermo Olagüe de Ros

NÚÑEZ BUTRÓN, MANUEL (b. Saman, Peru, 1 January 1900; d. Juliaca, Peru, 7 December 1952), *rural medicine.*

Núñez Butrón was born in a small town of the department of Puno, located in the southern Peruvian Andes. He was the illegitimate child of a Catholic priest and a middle-class mestizo woman. After completing his high school education at San Carlos, in the city of Puno, he pursued university studies, first at the Peruvian University of Arequipa and later at Lima's San Marcos University. In 1921 Núñez Butrón traveled to Spain to study medicine in Barcelona, enticed by the chance to study in Europe and prompted by the temporary closure of San Marcos. Núñez Butrón returned to Peru in 1925, and after working a few months in Lima, he returned to Puno, where he was appointed state physician in a number of provinces.

In the 1920s, the department of Puno was one of the poorest rural indigenous areas in Peru and was neglected by the State's health services. The miserable living conditions of

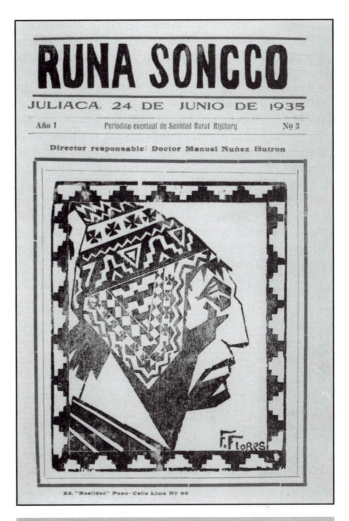

Cover of the first number of *Runa Soncco*, the journal founded by Núñez Butrón, 1935. Image supplied by Marcos Cueto.

the peasants in the rural estates had fostered endemic typhoid fever, dysentery, and, particularly, smallpox and epidemic typhus. Núñez Butrón went beyond the traditional role of provincial physicians. Because most of the sick could not go to his headquarters in Juliaca, he decided to travel to different locations first on a motorcycle and finally by car. He recruited local leaders, such as schoolteachers, who were ready to cooperate, and he organized them in 1933 into a brigade. The brigade was called *Rijchary* in Quechua—the main indigenous language—which translates as 'awaken'. Its members made themselves known at Sunday markets held in the main towns. They concentrated on smallpox vaccination and the promotion of hygiene to fight typhus. They also looked after childbirths, cut residents' hair, deloused people, gave purgatives, and built small stoves that killed the fleas afflicting humans without damaging the clothes. In 1937 the brigade comprised 122 members who looked after twenty-two different localities. A decisive step was the publication, in 1935, of the journal *Runa Soncco*, which meant 'Indian heart'. Although it was an irregular periodical, it persisted until the late 1940s. *Runa Soncco* described debates between the *rijcharys* and peasants on the magical origins of smallpox. Once, after the *rijcharys* convinced their rivals of the advantages of vaccination, all ended the meeting shouting, '*Viva*, Jenner, even though he is dead!'

This medical publication was linked to the *indigenista* movement, a cultural revival of Andean's indigenous history, people, and artistic expressions. Moreover, it was a sort of medical *indigenismo*. In the mid-1940s, Núñez Butrón launched his candidacy—with public health as the main theme of his proposal—to be a representative for a Puno province in the national congress. However, he lost the election. The latter was a general indication that his medical and political perspective found few supporters in Peru during the World War II period. As he grew older, Núñez Butrón began to suffer from chronic mountain sickness, an ailment characterized by the loss of tolerance for altitude in individ-uals who were previously acclimatized. He died when he was only fifty-two.

Núñez Butrón's brigade managed to make Western medicine and Indian culture cooperate and underscored the capacity of the rural poor in the Andes to participate actively in health programs.

Bibliography

Primary: 1935. 'Impresiones de un indio.' *Runa Soncco* 3 (24 June): 12–14; 1940. 'Qué es el Rijcharismo?' *Medicina Social* 2: 9–10.

Secondary: Cueto, Marcos, 1991. 'Indigenismo and Rural Medicine in Peru: The Indian Sanitary Brigade and Manuel Núñez Butrón.' *Bulletin of the History of Medicine* 65: 22–41; Frisancho Pineda, David, 1981. *Jatun Rijchari: Dr. Manuel Núñez Butrón, precursor de la sanidad rural en el Perú* (Puno, Peru).

Marcos Cueto

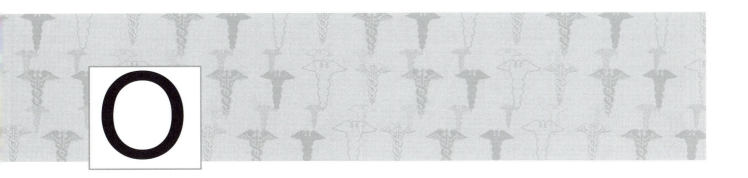

O

OBRADOR ALCALDE, SIXTO (b. Santander, Spain, 11 November 1911; d. Madrid, Spain, 27 April 1978), *neurosurgery.*

The surname Obrador comes from the island of Majorca, where his paternal grandfather and great-grandfather were born. He was the son of a railway employee and a cook from the mountains of Santander.

After doing his university preparation at the University of Salamanca, Obrador received his MD from the Central University of Madrid in 1933. He had several brilliant professors, such as Jorge Francisco Tello (Cajal's protégé), Juan Negrín, Severo Ochoa, and Carlos Jiménez Díaz, among others. His postgraduate education and training included the basic sciences—neurohistology and neurophysiology, and neurology and neurosurgery—and was obtained through his work at the Cajal Institute, Pío del Río-Hortega's laboratory, and Gonzalo Rodríguez Lafora's experimental physiology laboratory in Madrid. A research grant from the Board for Advanced Studies and Scientific Research allowed him to stay at the physiology laboratories of Charles Sherrington at Oxford University in 1934–35 and of John Fulton at Yale University in 1936. He prepared his first PhD thesis in Oxford, but the Spanish Civil War prevented its completion. He also visited several neurological and neurosurgical clinics: Otfrid Foerster's in Breslau (1934), Norman Dott's in Edinburgh (1937), and Hugh Cairns's in Oxford (August 1939–1940 and 1946).

From 1940 to 1945, Obrador lived in Mexico City, serving on the staff of the Spanish Hospital and the Mental Diseases Institute, thanks to the help of his Spanish colleagues López Albo and Rodríguez Lafora. His Mexican stay was very productive. He proceeded with his basic and neuropsychiatric training with Rodríguez Lafora and made several journeys to American neurological and neurosurgical departments, especially to the Johns Hopkins Hospital.

In 1946, thanks to his friend Jiménez Díaz, Obrador returned to Madrid where his expertise was used to develop several new public and private neurosurgical departments—to rival the best of the United Kingdom, the United States, Canada, and Germany. He served as physician-in-chief of neurosurgery services at the National Clinic of Labor (1946–63), Princess Hospital (1952–65), the National Institute of Cancer (1953–65), La Paz Hospital (1965–74), and Ramón y Cajal Hospital (1974–78)—all prominent centers within the National Healthcare System—and at the prestigious private Jiménez-Díaz Foundation (1955–74). In this capacity he directed the training of the neurosurgeons who later became heads of the newly founded neurosurgery departments throughout the whole of Spain.

Obrador introduced modern clinical sessions at the Princess Hospital. Although he continued his relationships with his international colleagues and his journeys to foreign hospitals, he turned solely to clinical practice, much to his later regret.

Obrador produced a large quantity of scientific work with more than 400 titles (including papers, books, and chapters of books) that covered his main topics of research: various types of brain tumors, different aspects of cerebral vascular and stereotaxic surgery, treatment of epilepsy by occipito-cervical hemispherectomy, head injuries, and intraventricular therapy. It is important to note that Obrador was the author of the first neurosurgical textbook published in Spanish (1951).

He was also secretary-founder of the Spanish-Portuguese Society of Neurosurgery, which was created in 1947, an honorary member of the main European and American societies of neurosurgery, and president of the Third European Congress of Neurosurgery (Madrid, 1967).

On 25 February 1936 Obrador married Margaret Blanchard Kennedy, whom he had met in Oxford.

Obrador played an important role in the introduction and development of neurosurgery in Spain thanks to his ambition and his major scientific-professional activities, including the development of modern departments of neurosurgery, the establishment of modern ways of training in the new specialty, and his contribution to the creation and support of neurosurgical societies and journals.

Bibliography

Primary: 1947. *Fisiopatología de las convulsiones epilépticas* (Madrid); 1947. *Las modernas intervenciones quirúrgicas en Psiquiatría* (Madrid); 1951. *Fundamentos de Neurocirugía* (Madrid).

Secondary: Gutiérrez Gómez, Diego, and José María Izquierdo Rojo, 1999. *El doctor Obrador en la Medicina de su tiempo* (Oviedo); Izquierdo Rojo, José María, 1985. *Sixto Obrador y la Neurocirugía de su tiempo* (Oviedo); Izquierdo Rojo, José María, 1979. *Historia de la neurología clínica española: 1882–1936* (Madrid).

María-Isabel Porras-Gallo

ODEKU, EMANUEL LATUDE (b. Awe, Nigeria, 29 June 1927; d. London, England, 20 August 1974), *medicine, neurosurgery.*

Odeku began his education in Lagos in 1932 and later graduated from the Methodist Boys' High School in 1945. Odeku's 'Baptist background might have stimulated his interest in America, as the American Baptist has contributed significantly to the development of education and medical care in Nigeria' (Adeloye, 1976, p. 13). Odeku left for the United States after 1945 and soon thereafter entered Howard University, Washington, D.C., from which he graduated first in his undergraduate class, with the BS degree, summa cum laude, in 1950. With a New York Phelps-Stokes Fund Scholarship for medical education, Odeku entered Howard University College of Medicine in 1950 and received his MD in 1954. During this period, he was an intern at the Freedmen's Hospital under a special program of the U.S. Public Health Service. From 1954 to 1955 he did his postgraduate medical internship in pathol-

ogy at the University Hospital, University of Michigan, Ann Arbor. During this time, Odeku was trained by neurosurgeon Edgar Kahn. Upon completion, Odeku went to the University of Western Ontario, from which he received the Licentiate of the Medical Council of Canada (1955) before returning to Nigeria. During 1955–56 Odeku was a medical officer at the Lagos General Hospital.

In 1956 Odeku returned to the University of Michigan as assistant resident in general surgery, and by 1960 had progressed from resident, to junior clinical instructor, and to senior clinical instructor. He occasionally acted as senior resident in neurosurgery at St Joseph's Mercy Hospital, at the Veterans Administration Hospital in Ann Arbor, and at the Wayne County General Hospital in Eloise, Michigan. In between these services, in 1959–60, Odeku was also a research training fellow in experimental neurosurgery at the University of Michigan. Kahn was Odeku's major mentor and in 1960 acclaimed Odeku as the 'most outstanding resident who passed through this service' (Adeloye, 1975, p. 19). Odeku went on to receive a Relm Foundation Special Grant of $3,400, and in July 1960 began work in neuropathology at the Armed Forces Institute of Pathology, Walter Reed Army Medical Center, Washington, D.C. He moved next to the Children's Hospital of Philadelphia in order to gain experience in neuropediatrics.

Odeku later returned to the College of Medicine, Howard University, where he taught neuroanatomy and neurosurgery during the academic year of 1961–62. In the same period, Odeku passed his examinations for the Diplomat of the American Board of Neurological Surgery at the Grace New Haven Hospital, Yale University.

Odeku returned to Nigeria in 1962, as the country's first neurosurgeon. His biographer noted 'the first difficulty he encountered was the prejudice of his British-trained colleagues who did not understand the details of the American residency training programme' (Adeloye, 1976, p. 25). In October 1962 Odeku suggested the establishment of a neurosurgical unit in the Department of Surgery, College of Medicine, Ibadan University. He appointed a consultant anesthetist through the Rockefeller Foundation, sought training for a corps of neurosurgical nurses, and acquired additional instruments for the eight-bed unit. Odeku operated each Thursday, supervised an outpatient clinic, and conducted his own neuroradiology and neuropathology.

In 1965 Kahn visited Odeku at Ibadan, and they performed surgeries together. As a result of this collaboration, Odeku published an article on brain tumors in *International Surgery* (1969). He also went on to publish several other pieces with Kahn at Michigan. Odeku became well-known as an important figure within the field of neurosurgery, and he published widely and belonged to numerous medical associations. Over time, Odeku's example helped to popularize American medical education among Nigerians.

Odeku died in 1974, of diabetes mellitus, at the Hammersmith Hospital, London. He married twice: first to Dr Mary

Gilda Marques, with whom he had a daughter Lenora and a son Peter, and next to Dr Katherine Jill Adcock Odeku, with whom he had two more children, a son, Alan, and daughter, Amanda.

Bibliography

Primary: 1965. 'Beginnings of Neurosurgery at the University of Ibadan.' *West African Medical Journal* 14: 85–98.

Secondary: Patton, Adell Jr., 1982. 'Howard University and Meharry Medical Schools in the Training of African Physicians, 1868–1978' in Harris, Joseph E., ed., *Global Dimensions of the African Diaspora* (Washington, DC) pp. 142–162; Adeloye, Adelola, 1976. *E. Latunde Odeku, An African Neurosurgeon* (Ibadan).

Adell Patton Jr.

ODIER, LOUIS (b. Republic of Geneva (now Switzerland), 17 March 1748; d. Geneva, 16 March 1817), *medicine.*

The Odiers came originally from Pont-en-Royans in the Dauphiné, but established themselves in Geneva when Antoine Odier (1698/99–1775), Louis's father, became a citizen on 11 December 1714. Antoine Odier was an established cloth-merchant, and he married Louise de Villas, also from a Huguenot family, in 1736. Louis was the eldest of four brothers. The Odier family lived frugally, and at first this was due to the poor state of the family business. With time, the family's income improved, although Odier complained in later life of the Protestant austerity of his youth and regretted both the Spartan upbringing, which left him and his siblings always hungry, and the coldness of his parents' attitude toward their children. At school his intellectual capacities were soon detected and he competed, sometimes successfully, for school prizes in prose and in piety. As a child and a teenager, Odier aspired to be a minister of religion. A defect in pronunciation deterred him from pursuing this ambition. In 1767 he completed a first cycle of studies in philosophy at the Academy in Geneva. His father, he later wrote, decided what he was to do next: he was to become a physician.

There was no medical school in Geneva, and medical students traditionally traveled to a French university (Montpellier or Valence) or to a German (Protestant) medical school. Louis Odier decided to study in Edinburgh. He set off in the summer of 1767. Among his tutors were John Gregory (1724–73), Joseph Black (1721–91), and William Cullen (1710–90). After the standard three years of study, Odier qualified as a doctor on 12 September 1770 with a thesis on musical sensations. He remained in Edinburgh an extra two years, and was elected president of two medical societies, the Medical Society and the Physico-Medical Society.

At this stage, after considering setting up practice in Britain, Odier decided to return to Geneva. He started a correspondence with a young lady he had not heard from for more than four years, Suzanne Baux. He continued

writing to her as he walked the wards of different hospitals, then a common practice after completing a theoretical curriculum; he was in St Thomas's Hospital in London for some months and in Leiden, La Haye, Amsterdam, and Utrecht, for shorter periods, before finally spending six months in Paris. As he completed his clinical experience, it became more and more apparent in his letters that his plans were to marry Baux and establish himself in Geneva. A year and two months after his first letter, Suzanne Baux, who had not seen him for almost six years, accepted his proposal of marriage.

On his return to Geneva in 1773 they married, and Odier established himself as a physician. After the death of Suzanne (1778), Odier married a second time, in 1780, a healthy young lady, Andrienne Lecointe. At this stage of his life, Louis Odier was a promising physician and a member of various medical societies. He was also ambitious: his main preoccupations were to make a name for himself and to open a medical school in Geneva.

In 1774 he was entrusted with teaching chemistry to the apprentices of the apothecary shops, and during the same period he published a series of articles on inoculation, offering in 1787 to inoculate the poor free of charge. He also formed a partnership with his friend and colleague Daniel De La Roche, with the aim of guaranteeing each of his patients a second opinion. This practice was not greeted with enthusiasm and was later abandoned. Starting from 1788, he was elected a member of Geneva's parliament, the *Conseil des Deux Cents*, and became secretary to the Consistory court and a member of numerous Genevese and foreign scientific academies, institutes, and societies. Over time, Odier became a respected practicing physician, and many patients recognized that he was a serious and caring healer. Besides his practice, he undertook the preparation of medical certificates for young ladies, in order to enable an investment company to choose those who could be included in the famous 'tontines', a system for investors to buy life annuities for groups (numbering thirty) of young girls living in Geneva. Along with many others, he invested much of the fortune he had inherited from his father in this system and in the French money market, which collapsed during the financial crisis caused by the French Revolution.

In the last years of the century, he could only count on the income generated by his failing practice—which was also affected by the Revolutionary years—to make a living, and decided to take in boarders. Odier was also a prominent member of the City elite. In 1789 he requested the endowment of a chair of medicine for himself, but his colleagues refused to approve, frightened to see a physician setting himself above the others. Nevertheless, in 1799, once both the Republic of Geneva and the medical guild had been overthrown by the Revolution and Geneva had been integrated into France, Odier was appointed by the consular government of France to an honorary chair of medicine. For six years he gave courses to surgeons and future medical students, and wrote a textbook, his successful *Manuel de médecine-pratique* (1803).

Odier was continually active as an author, publishing regular medical texts and writing a medical column in the *Journal de Genève* between 1787 and 1794. The author of more than forty medical publications, including a series of considerations on inoculation and vaccination, a *Pharmacopoea Genevensis* (coauthored with Daniel De La Roche), and a number of contributions on professional and ethical issues. One of his main achievements was his role as a founding member of the *Bibliothèque britannique* in 1796, a journal destined to spread the results of British science. The Napoleonic wars and the Continental blocs explain the success of the journal, which became an important means of communication between Britain and the French-speaking world. Odier was also central to the dissemination on the European continent of news of Jenner's discovery of vaccination against smallpox: Jenner's original paper was published in 1798, and Odier's translation and discussion of the discovery appeared in the columns of the *Bibliothèque britannique* in October of the same year. Letters and private papers of Odier are kept at the Bibliothèque Publique et Universitaire de Genève: Fonds Odier, and manuscripts are kept at the Musée d'Histoire des Sciences (Geneva): Fonds Odier (Z91: scientific manuscripts).

Bibliography

Secondary: Barblan, Marc-A., 1977. 'Journalisme médical et échanges intellectuels au tournant du XVIIIe siècle: le cas de la *Bibliothèque Britannique* (1795–1815).' *Archives des sciences* 30: 287–398 (especially pp. 291–323); Morsier de, Georges, 1975. 'La vie et l'oeuvre de Louis Odier docteur et professeur en médecine (1748–1817).' *Gesnerus* 32: 248–270; Gautier, Léon, 1906. *La médecine à Genève jusqu'à la fin du 18e siècle, Mémoires et documents publiés par la société d'histoire et d'archéologie* (Société d'Histoire et d'Archéologie de Genève) (Geneva) pp. 538–544 (contains a list of Odier's publications).

Philip Rieder

OGATA, KŌAN (b. Ashimori, Bicchū Domain [now Okayama Prefecture], Japan, 13 August 1810, d. Edo (now Tokyo), Japan, 25 July 1863), *Ranpō medicine, Rangaku education, medical education.*

Ogata was the fourth and last child of Saeki Koreyori and his wife Kyō. After using several names during his youth, he assumed the name Ogata Kōan in 1836. His father was a samurai serving the Ashiyori province in the domain of Bicchu. In 1826, while his father worked in Osaka at the Ashiyori province's financial office, Ogata started to study Dutch-style medicine and science at the private school of Naka Ten'yū (1783–1835). The Dutch-style medicine was called Ranpō medicine, and more comprehensive studies of the Dutch language and of scientific and technological

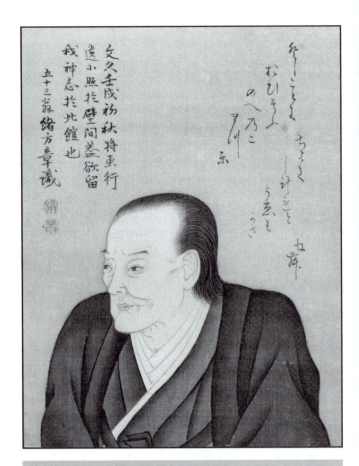

Ogata Kōan. Ink and watercolor, Ogata Kōan Memorial Museum, Osaka.

subjects were called Rangaku (Dutch studies). Soon he had read all available translations, and Ogata headed for Edo in 1831 to continue his study of Rangaku. He studied at the private school of Tsuboi Shindō (1795–1848), who was one of the most prosperous Rangaku scholars at that time. Ogata also learned under Udagawa Shinsai (1769–1834), another distinguished Rangaku scholar in Edo, and made acquaintance with Mitsukuri Genpo (1799–1863), who was to become the most distinguished Rangaku scholar and the first professor at Bansho Sirabejo [The Office for Examining Barbarian's Foreign Books], established by the shogunate in 1856. After staying in Edo for four years, Ogata made a short sojourn in Ashiyori and Osaka in 1835.

Ogata went to Nagasaki in 1836 to continue his training. He was already a mature scholar, and when he arrived in Nagasaki he made connections with other scholars in the city and together with two of them translated M. W. Plagge's work on therapeutics. In 1838 he left Nagasaki in order to start a practice and his own private Rangaku school in Osaka. In total, Ogata's training extended for thirteen years in three major cities: Osaka, Edo, and Nagasaki. At each place of abode, he forged close ties with major figures in Ranpō medicine and Rangaku studies. Although Ogata was a son of a provincial samurai with relatively small means and with virtually no medical and scholarly background, the extended networks of Rangaku scholars allowed Ogata to move around the country and climb the social latter of the late Tokugawa society.

In 1838, when he was twenty-nine years of age, Ogata settled himself at Kawara-machi in Osaka and started medical practice in the city. In the same year, he married Yae, who had been his fiancée for some time and was a daughter of Okugawa Hyakki, who, like Ogata, had studied medicine under Naka Ten'yū. In addition, Ogata had once helped Naka's son to run the Rangaku school when Naka died in 1835. Ogata's Osaka connections, as well as his own medical skill and fame as an eminent Rangaku scholar, must have helped his success in the highly competitive medical market of the city. In the year after he started to practice, his name appeared in a broadsheet-style list of popular and eminent doctors in Osaka. In ten years, he was at the top of the list.

His fame extended beyond the city and reached nationwide, as demonstrated by the great number of students who matriculated at his private medical school, known as Teki-juku. He started the private medical school in 1838 at the same time as he started his practice at Osaka. In 1845 he moved to a larger house, in order to accommodate a large number of students who had flocked to Osaka to study Rangaku under him. The surviving list of students (1844–62) records the names of about six hundred young men who came to study at Teki-juku from virtually all over the country. It is, however, not so much the number but the quality of the students that conferred on Teki-juku its lasting fame. The list of Teki-juku students includes giants in the modernization of Japan. The most famous are Ōmura Masujirō (1824–69), who became the founder of the modern army; Nagayo Sensai (1838–1902), who was the first director of the Sanitary Bureau and the founder figure in modern medical policy; and Fukuzawa Yukichi (1834–1901), who founded Keio Gijuku (now Keio University) and was the most influential spokesman of modernization. The fact that Ōmura and Fukuzawa each took up a career other than medicine is testimony both to the role of Ranpō medicine at that time and to the education offered at Teki-juku itself. Social expectations of Ranpō medicine were becoming higher and wider, especially in response to the mounting pressure to open up Japan to trade with Western powers and the ensuing intense political disputes. Learning Dutch medicine through Dutch books was becoming a gateway to Rangaku, a comprehensive program of Dutch-language education in European civilization, with special emphasis laid on its science and technology. In harmony with these expectations for Ranpō medicine and Rangaku, the curriculum at Teki-juku laid enormous emphasis on mastering the Dutch language, starting from Dutch grammar and syntax. Students were organized into eight classes according to their linguistic skill: their good performance in translation promoted them to a higher class. Reading materials included not only medicine, but also physics, chemistry, and military and civil engineering. Ogata himself wrote in 1854 (the year after Commodore Perry of the U.S. navy visited Japan to demand the opening of the country) that he was reducing his medical practice and focusing on teaching Rangaku. Teki-juku, the most famous and important of private Ranpō medical schools, accorded only secondary importance to medicine per se.

Among Rangaku subjects, military science and engineering were in particularly high demand, both from the Tokugawa Shogunate and from rich, progressive, and powerful provinces. Ranpō doctors were employed by the central and the local governments not just for their medical services; the doctors were also able to read and translate Dutch books on technology and to teach Dutch language at the Rangaku schools run by the provincial governments. Ogata responded to this new demand for scholars knowledgeable in Western sciences and technology, from governments keen on modernization, by encouraging his students to learn military and industrial technology. He at the same time found a new answer to the old question of the lowly status of medicine in Japanese society. Medicine had long been regarded as a 'small and mean art' vis-à-vis Confucian moral and political philosophy, and numerous doctors had struggled to improve medicine's standing in society. By expanding the study of Ranpō medicine to an all-inclusive Rangaku studies, Ogata and other Rangaku scholars in the 1850s and 1860s found a new role for the study of medicine via the Dutch language. Expanding Ranpo medicine into training in Rangaku to prepare for government service was a means to overcome traditional medicine's narrow focus on curing individual patients. Learning medicine at Teki-juku was a gateway to a broader project of societal reform and the building of a strong Japanese state. Behind Ogata's success at Teki-juku in overcoming the age-old limitations imposed on medicine as a personal service lay his vision of the wider role of medical learning in the new statecraft.

Although Teki-juku's medical teaching was nonsystematic, even perfunctory, this does not mean that Ogata is unimportant in the history of medicine itself. Ogata continued the work of translating and compiling Dutch medical texts. *Byōgaku tsūron* (1849) was a general pathology textbook that brought together Dutch texts on pathology. Ogata inherited this project from his teacher Udagawa while in Edo, and it took about fifteen years for him to finish. *Fushi keiken ikun* (1861) was Ogata's second major published work, in which he translated and annotated the Dutch translation of the second edition of C. W. Hufeland's *Enchiridion medicum*, originally published in 1836. A small work on cholera, which collated sections from several books on this disease, was published in 1858, when Japan and Osaka was hit by a cholera epidemic for the second time.

The most important of Ogata's contributions to medicine was the establishment of smallpox vaccination. Nakagawa Gorōji (1768–1858) learned smallpox vaccination in Russia and practiced it in the Northern provinces in 1825. This practice soon withered away, due to lack of support in the rural regions. The second successful vaccination attempt in Japan was performed in Nagasaki, in June 1849, by Otto Mohnike (1814–87), a German physician to the Dutch factory in Nagasaki. In September of the same year, a doctor in Kyoto successfully vaccinated a child and established a vaccination station in that city. In November, Ogata visited the station in Kyoto and arranged for reception of the lymph to start a vaccination station in Osaka. There was some resistance and noncompliance among the common people in the city, but this was overcome and the vaccination campaign in Osaka went on. The building of similar stations in other parts of Japan was facilitated by the strong and extensive networks of Ranpō doctors and Teki-juku graduates, many of whom were practicing medicine at their own hometown or village. Extension of stations into various locales helped to reduce smallpox epidemics and secured buffers on which each station could rely when the local supply of lymph ran out. The station at Osaka was maintained on a purely voluntary basis by Ogata and other practicing doctors until the business received an official sanction in 1858.

In 1862, when Ogata was fifty-three, his life took an unexpected turn. His fame as a Ranpō doctor and Rangaku scholar was at its zenith, after the publication of *Byōgaku tsūron* and *Fushi keiken ikun*, his two major and multivolume translations, and two decades of a flourishing Teki-juku school. Despite such eminence, he had remained a *machi-isha* [town doctor], a medical practitioner without any appointment to the office of the shogunate or *daimyōs*. In that year, however, he was appointed as the doctor to the Tokugawa Shogunate and the director of the Seiyō igaku-jo [Center of Western Medicine]. He now held, in a word, the most prestigious appointment in Japanese medicine, and was responsible for the state's policy on Ranpō medicine and Rangaku at the highest level. It would have been most interesting to watch Ogata in this new role. However, he occupied these appointments for only ten months. In June 1853 he suddenly vomited blood and died. The stress of moving from Osaka to Edo and adapting to rigid protocols at the court of the shogun were reputed to be the cause of this untimely and sudden death. His wife Yae and nine children survived him.

Bibliography

Primary: 1980-1996. (Ogata, Tomio, et al., eds.) *Ogata Kōan no tegami* [Letters of Ogata Kōan] 5 vols. (Tokyo).

Secondary: Umetani, Noboru, 1993. *Kōan Teki-juku no kenkyū* (Kyoto); Ogata, Tomio, 1977. *Ogata Kōan den* [Life of Ogata Kōan] (enlarged 2nd edn.) (Tokyo).

Akihito Suzuki

OGINO, GINKO (b. Tawarase, Musashi domain [now Saitama Prefecture], Japan, 3 March 1851; d. Tokyo, Japan, 23 June 1913), *women in medicine, obstetrics, gynecology.*

Gin (pronounced as in 'begin'; later she called herself Ginko) was a daughter of Ogino Ayasaburo and his wife, Kayo, in a wealthy farming family. She was brought up as respectable provincial women were; she was taught by a visiting tutor and at a *terakoya*, a temple academy for elementary education, and married a neighboring, prosperous, landed farmer in 1868. However, a year after the marriage she went back home with ill health caused by gonorrhea. While she was at home, she learned Chinese classics with local tutors. After divorcing in 1870, she went up to Tokyo for treatment. It is told almost as a legend that a clinical experience with male doctors during this hospitalization left her with the indelible impression of excruciating embarrassment, which developed into an empathy with the private suffering of other women.

Her own experience taught her the need for women doctors, which were virtually unheard of at that time, as the medical schools only accepted male students and only men could sit for the state exams. Extremely talented in academic pursuits, she made her way, step-by-step, as a pioneer, persuading others of the need and propriety of opening the profession to gifted women. In Tokyo, she first asked for tuition under Yorikuni Inoue, who was an established Japanese classical scholar and also a physician. After a period at the Tokyo Girls' Normal School (1875–79), personal recommendation enabled her to learn at the Kōjuin Medical School (1879–82). Her academic superiority won the sympathetic backing of progressive grandees, but now the obstacle she faced was formidable: the national system that conventionally refused women. Although there was no formal 'no-women' provision, her application was repeatedly turned down because of her sex. However, juridical history, as found in the medical regulation in a ninth-century official exposition to an eighth-century Yōrō statute, provided a justification for women doctors—though only in a limited capacity. Nagayo Sensai, director of the Sanitary Bureau, finally decided to allow women to apply. She grabbed the first opportunity, passing the primary examinations in September 1884 and the secondary in March 1885 to become the first woman doctor under the national license system. Thus Ginko opened the door of the system to women. She even maintained later that medical care is the vocation of women.

She began practice as an obstetrician and gynecologist in Hongo, Tokyo, in 1885 and soon moved to larger premises, where she could also provide accommodation for women medical students. Once authorized, a woman doctor could thrive in practice and also in society. Her profession and status led her to become involved in social reforms, including the suffrage movement and the campaign for abolition of licensed prostitution. Christians were prominent among her enlightened, well-educated contacts. She converted to

Christianity in 1886, joining the Christian Women's Society for Reformation of Manners. Meanwhile Shikata Yukiyoshi, a high-minded university student, sixteen years her junior, entered into her life. In spite of opposition on all sides, they got married in 1890. Shikata, driven by his missionary passion to build a Christian utopia, decided to take a chance in the reclamation scheme in Hokkaido, the northernmost part of Japan. Giving up her career and everything in the metropolis, Ginko followed and joined him. However, the land development work did not go as they hoped and expected. While in Hokkaido she resumed practice, organized women's social work, and started a Sunday school. In 1905 Shikata died. Ginko left Hokkaido in 1908 to join her sister in Tokyo. Her dramatic, idealistic and altruistic life has been fictionalized and staged.

Bibliography

Primary: 1893. 'Past, Present and Future of Women Doctors in Japan.' *Jogaku Zasshi* [Women's Learning Magazine].

Secondary; Japan Medical Women's Association, 1991. *Nihon joi shi* [History of Women Doctors in Japan] (Tokyo); Watanabe, Jun'ichi, 1970. *Hana uzumi* [Buried in Flowers: A Novel] (Tokyo); Ogino Ginko kenshōhi kensetsu kisei kai, ed., 1967. *Ogino Ginko* (Setana cho, Hokkaido).

Mika Suzuki

OKEN, LORENZ JOHANN ADAM (originally Okenfuß) (b. Offenburg, Germany, 1 August 1779; d. Zurich, Switzerland, 11 August 1851), *natural philosophy, zoology, natural history.*

As a son of a peasant, Oken grew up in an impoverished environment. His teachers at school realized his 'ingenium felix' and recommended him to the gymnasium (Stiftsschule) at Baden, the location of the famous spa where the European aristocracy met for holidays. His teacher Anton Maier inspired him to study mathematics and natural sciences. Oken then started his medical studies in Freiburg (1801). At the end of his fourth semester he wrote his preliminary thesis on *Abriss eines Systems der Naturphilosophie* [Short Scheme of Natural Philosophy], which was influenced by Schelling's natural philosophy. This paper was vehemently criticized by the dean of the medical faculty, Johann Matthias Alexander Ecker (1766–1829), as leading to mysticism and atheism. Oken's enthusiasm for scientific and philosophical research was not sufficiently supported at Freiburg. He longed to get into proximity to his idol, the famous idealistic philosopher Friedrich Wilhelm Joseph Schelling. After finishing his studies and publishing his thesis (1804) at his own expense, he traveled to Würzburg, where Schelling was teaching. On Schelling's request, Johann Friedrich Blumenbach obtained a lectureship for Oken at the University of Göttingen (1805). Two years later he received an appointment to the University of Jena, the center of romanticism.

Between the Napoleonic occupation and the liberation movement in Germany, the twelve years Oken spent as a professor of natural history in Jena (1807–19) were politically as well as socially tumultuous. Oken belonged to a group of politically active professors, and while lecturing he would often take the occasion to incite patriotism and liberalism from the lectern. As a result of the civil commotion accompanying the Wartburg Fest (1817) and the murder of the poet August von Koetzebue (1761–1819) by a student, Oken was expelled from his university position in 1819. Besides articles and books on natural philosophy and natural history, Oken also wrote political pamphlets and papers. His well-known journal *ISIS* (1817) and his foundation of the *Gesellschaft deutscher Naturforscher und Ärzte* (1822) were reflective of his concept of scientific and political education and enlightenment for all people and classes.

After supporting his family for eight years (1819–27) mainly through his activities as a journalist and as editor of his scientific journal *ISIS*, he then obtained the chair of physiology in Munich, and six years later (1833) he was appointed as rector and professor of the newly founded University of Zurich. During his final years Oken was undisturbed and scientifically productive. Academically well accepted by students and colleagues, he was seen as the much-honored key scholar of Zurich. During this time he wrote the thirteen volumes of his natural history, *Allgemeine Naturgeschichte für alle Stände*, which was based on his idea of a productive combination of empiricism and philosophical speculation in the sense of Schelling's natural philosophy. His explanation of the development of the earth was analogous to his idea of biological genesis. His explanations of natural history, as well as his theory of geological growth, were largely integrated into his theory of cranial evolution. Oken's natural-philosophical explanation of the development of species, with its attributes such as polarity, difference, and indifference, was extremely difficult for following generations of scientists to comprehend. In his *Origin of Species* Darwin classified Oken's theory of development as mystical. Despite this criticism, Oken's idea of microscopic 'vesicles' as the basic element of biological life can be regarded as a fruitful step toward the later description of the cell-theory by Matthias Schleiden (1804–81) and Theodor Schwann (1810–82).

Bibliography

Primary: 1805. *Abriss eines Systems der Biologie* (Göttingen); 1833–45. *Allgemeine Naturgeschichte für alle Stände* 13 vols. (Stuttgart).

Secondary: Engelhardt, Diedrich von, and Jürgen Nolte, eds., 2002. *Von Freiheit und Verantwortung in der Forschung—Zum 150sten Todestag von Lorenz Oken (1779–1851)* (Stuttgart); Breidbach, Olaf, Hans-Jürgen Fliedner, and Kurt Ries, eds., 2001. *Lorenz Oken (1779–1851). Ein politischer Philosoph* (Weimar).

Brigitte Lohff

ORENSTEIN, ALEXANDER JEREMIAH (b. USA, 26 September 1879; d. Johannesburg, South Africa, 7 July 1972), *occupational health.*

The son of Russian immigrants to the United States, Orenstein studied medicine at Jefferson Medical College, Philadelphia, where he was awarded an MD in 1905. After further study in tropical medicine in Hamburg and London, he joined the U.S. army as a medical officer. This specialized training in tropical medicine he soon put to good use, first as a member of Colonel Gorgas's team in the Panama Canal Zone (1906–13) and then as an adviser to the German East African government on malaria and plague (1913–14).

In 1914 Orenstein was chosen by Gorgas to head a program to reduce the soaring mortality from pneumonia among African mineworkers on the Witwatersrand. As chief medical officer of Rand Mines Ltd., Orenstein immediately tackled this problem, though it was not until the end of World War I that his drive and prodigious organizational talent were able to have full play. Brooking little opposition, he overhauled the overcrowded and unhygienic living conditions in the miners' compounds, improved their diet, and completely revamped mine hospitals, the provision of medical staff, and the underground rescue system. Virtually every aspect of the health of the company's miners became subject to his regimen, to good effect, for mortality from pneumonia and other communicable diseases fell markedly in his first decade there. Moreover, his model of health care was soon being followed by other mines, making the 'Orenstein method' the norm in subequatorial Africa.

His leadership and organizational capabilities were widely recognized by his peers, and in the 1920s he was successively elected president of the Association of Scientific and Technical Societies of South Africa, the Mine Medical Officers' Association, and the Federal Council of the Medical Association of South Africa. He also served on several official South African commissions of inquiry and standing committees on health, as a delegate to the International Labor Organization and as a member of its Industrial Hygiene Committee.

His skill in organizing large projects was harnessed by his adopted country's military authorities too, and for the latter part of World War I and the whole of World War II, Orenstein headed the South African Medical Corps. His enterprise in mobilizing Kimberley's population against the crisis of the 'Spanish' influenza pandemic in 1918 and in raising the medical corps almost from scratch in 1939–40 and turning it into a large, well-oiled force, and his zeal in implementing effective antimalarial strategies to safeguard South African troops, more than vindicated this confidence in him.

Orenstein's impressive track record in industrial health won him almost legendary status during his lifetime, and in the decade after World War II honors were showered on him in South Africa and abroad. Little deterred by advancing years, in 1956 he retired from Rand Mines, but then devoted the next three years to setting up the Pneumoconiosis Research Unit at the behest of the mining industry. This done, he went into an active semiretirement, continuing as a consultant to Rand Mines until his death.

Quick to grasp the nub of an issue, Orenstein was a man of strong views, not easily swayed or put off once he had reached a carefully considered conclusion. Contemporaries spoke of him as 'a respected tyrant' with 'an amazing knack for cutting red-tape and getting people to accept his views' (Coetzee, 1972, p. 1188). His determination and self-assurance ensured that he left a permanent mark within the field of mining health, a fact underlined by a mine hospital and an industrial medicine library still bearing his name today.

Orenstein had one daughter by Kate Bradbury, whom he married, divorced, remarried, and then divorced again.

Bibliography

Secondary: Coetzee, A. M., 1972. 'Alexander Jeremiah Orenstein.' *South African Medical Journal* 46(33): 1188-1189; Cartwright, A. P., 1971. *Doctors of the Mines* (Cape Town); Cartwright, A. P., 1960. *South Africa's Hall of Fame* (Johannesburg); *Munk's Roll.*

Howard Phillips

ORFILA I ROTGER, MATEO JOSÉ BUENAVENTURA (b. Mahón, Spain, 24 April 1787; d. Paris, France, 12 March 1853), *forensic medicine, toxicology.*

The son of an influential merchant, ship-owner, and banker of Minorca Island, Orfila began his studies of medicine at the University of Valencia in 1805, where he developed an early interest in chemistry through the classes taught by Pizcueta and through self-teaching by studying the works of the great French chemists, such as Lavoisier, Fourcroy, and Berthollet. A year later he moved to Barcelona, where he stayed for two years. His chemistry teacher was then Francisco Carbonell, a follower of Fourcroy and a major promoter of the then-new Industrial Chemistry. Thanks to the support of Carbonell, Orfila was granted a pension by *Junta de Comercio de Barcelona* to receive education as a chemist for four years, following which he should return to Barcelona to hold a chair of this discipline. He traveled to Paris in 1807, where he started his studies in physical and natural science, and also registered in medicine.

The outbreak of the War of Independence in 1808 resulted in the discontinuation of financial support by *Junta de Comercio* and the breaking of promises made regarding a chair at Barcelona; thus, upon completion of his studies, Orfila opened a private school, where he taught classes on chemistry. It was then that he discovered that most poisons, when mixed with animal or plant fluids, escaped identification by the means that had been used until then. This fact, which had not previously been recorded in the literature of legal medicine, revolutionized forensic techniques and gave birth to toxicology.

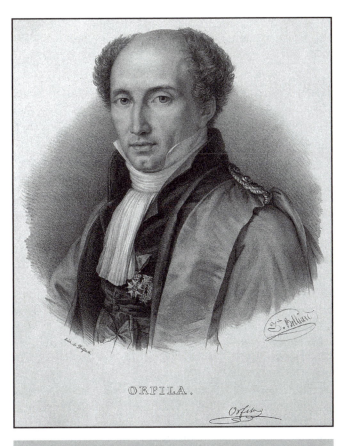

Mateo Orfila. Lithograph by Z. Belliard. Iconographic Collection, Wellcome Library, London.

His first publications, wherein he laid the foundations of the new toxicology, appeared in 1814, as did his student-oriented *Eléments de chimie médicale* (1817), which reached eight editions by 1851 and was translated into several languages.

In 1815 he married Gabrielle Lesueur, a youth from the Parisian bourgeoisie who introduced him to gatherings and *soirées,* in which Orfila stood out because of his charm and singing skills—the Italian entrepreneur Barilli even suggested that he make his début as a baritone, to no avail. Orfila lived an intense social life, which he managed to combine with his scientific activities and brought him appropriate social contacts to move up in the political and academic ranks.

Orfila's fame grew and spread across boundaries. In 1815 the Spanish government offered him a chair of chemistry in Madrid. The war had just come to an end and the absolute rule of Ferdinand VII had begun, a king not inclined to promote scientific advancement and progress. Orfila submitted to the government a report in which he set out the conditions by which he would accept office (resources for an eminently experimental teaching program, a training plan to provide all Spanish universities with chemistry professors within ten years, and so on). His proposal was rejected and Orfila stayed in France, where he was appointed physician to Louis XVIII.

In 1819 he was appointed to the chair of legal medicine at the Paris Faculty of Medicine, where he was also granted that of Chemistry in 1823. After his arrival at the university, his devotion to legal medicine became both well known and unswerving he first had to fill some gaps in his own knowledge, because his studies on poisons and their effects in the human body were only a part of the wide range of knowledge the forensic discipline demanded. As a result of his efforts he published *Leçons faisant partie du cours de médecine légale* in 1821, whose third edition (1835) became the definitive *Traité de médecine légale*. Similarly, he published a *Traité des exhumations juridiques* in collaboration with Octave Lesueur in 1831. In addition to these monographs, he contributed to a number of French medical journals, particularly *Annales d'hygiène publique et médecine légale*, a pioneering publication in its field whose first issue came out in 1829 thanks to the vigorous initiative of Orfila and Tardieu, among others.

Besides these contributions, which gained him fame and recognition in various intellectual circles, his involvement in law courts gave social prominence to his activities and, naturally, to himself. His views in cases of poisoning were considered infallible, and one trial even became famous only because a survey by the well-known toxicologist was required. One of the most significant proceedings in which Orfila participated was the 'Lafargue case'—Charles Lafargue, a resident in the town of Glandier, died of suspected arsenic poisoning on 14 January 1840. The necropsy yielded inconclusive results. A subsequent toxicological study revealed the presence of traces of arsenic in his stomach, on the basis of which his widow, Marie Capelle, was arrested and brought before court. The matter became further complicated when a new toxicological examination, requested by the defense and carried out by other experts, found no vestiges of poison. The first experts withdrew their report and recognized the poor reliability of their techniques, but a cloud of doubt still hovered over the case. In such a situation the only thing that remained to be done was to call for the arbitration of France's most prestigious toxicologist; Orfila demonstrated beyond doubt the presence of arsenic in Lafargue's body, which came neither from reagents used, nor from the earth around the coffin, nor from naturally-occurring traces within the human body. In short, by excluding a false positive result, it was demonstrated that Lafargue had been poisoned; the 'Lafargue case' entered the annals of crime, and placed Orfila at the summit of forensic science.

Besides his scientific accomplishments, Orfila should also be remembered for being the politician who managed France's health system during the 1830s. He was appointed dean of the Paris Faculty of Medicine on 1 May 1831, an office he held without interruption during the whole reign of Louis-Philippe of Orleans. The office of dean at an institution as prominent as this was mainly and above all political in nature, a government position signifying trust in the holder with regard to not only the administration of the conflicting dynamics in the university during those years, but also the direction and surveillance of medicine and health care in the country. In 1832 Orfila was appointed a member of the General Council for Hospitals, and in 1834 he became a member of Conseil Général de Seine and Conseil d'Instruction Publique; in the following years he gradually became involved in the Royal Academy of Medicine, Conseil de Salubrité, Conseil Municipal de Paris, and other organizations.

In the university setting Orfila favored a new teaching system, with the introduction of experimental practical classes, and he supported the definitive implementation of practical training within hospitals. His influence reached Spanish medicine through his disciple Pedro Mata, who held the first chair of legal medicine in Madrid and was also a reformer of university studies.

Reform of the organization of medical practice were intended to strengthen the power, fees, and social image of physicians, and would have led to dispensing with 'officiers de santé', the less well-qualified professionals who provided care particularly in rural settings and who were competitors to the regular medical profession.

During Orfila's term of office, which was not exempt from undeniable authoritarianism (in imitation of Louis XIV, he declared 'La Faculté c'est moi'), he surrounded himself with a select team of collaborators who undertook numerous organizational and administrative initiatives on matters of public health: compulsory establishment of archives in asylums and hospitals (1837), legislation for mentally ill people and asylums for the insane (1838), introduction of the metric system in medicine and pharmacy (1837), creation of a body of inspectors for foundling homes (1839), limitation of child labor in manufacturing (1841), requirement of a medical certification for paid wet nurses to be hired as such (1842), reinforcement of hygiene in cemeteries (1842), establishment of an inspectorate for poisonous substances (1845, 1846), express prohibition against the granting of invention patents by the Ministry of Commerce for unknown remedies or secret therapeutical means (1844), and other measures.

On 28 February 1848 Orfila was forced to resign from all of his posts, but continued to hold his chair of chemistry and remained a member of the Academy of Medicine, of which he became president in 1851. He died from pneumonia on 12 March 1853. His sumptuous funeral allowed Napoleon III and the Second Empire—which had established itself in France on 2 December 1852—to represent Orfila, in a masterful display of political skill, as one of the innocent victims of the Revolution of 1848.

Bibliography

Primary: 1814. *Traité des poisons tirés des règnes minéral, végétal et animal, ou toxicologie générale* (Paris); 1817. *Eléments de chimie médicale* (Paris); 1818. *Secours à donner aux personnes empoisonnées ou asphyxiées, suivis des moyens propres à reconnaître les poisons et les vins frelatés et à distinguer la mort réelle de la mort apparente* (Paris); 1835. *Traité de médecine légale* (Paris).

Secondary: Huertas, Rafael, 1988. *Orfila, saber y poder médico* (Madrid); Léonard, Jacques, 1982. *La médecine entre les pouvoirs et les savoirs. Histoire intellectuelle et politique de la médecine française au XIX siècle* (Paris); Fayol, Amedée. 1930. *La vie et l'oeuvre d'Orfila* (Paris); Beaudéant, Jean, and Armand Pasturel, 1913. *Etude juridique et psychologique d'un cause criminelle célèbre. Affaire Lafarge. Une réhabilitation qui s'impose* (Paris).

Rafael Huertas

ORIBASIUS OF PERGAMUM (b. Pergamum, Mysia, Asia Minor [now Bergama, Turkey], *c.* 320; d. ?, 390/400), *medicine.*

A pagan medical writer sometimes described as an 'iatrosophist', Oribasius belongs in the series of great epitomatists, scholastic-encyclopedic authors whose work consisted of summarizing and excerpting the authors of classical antiquity. This kind of work had no claims to originality and was of a theoretical character—features possibly associated with the scholasticism of medical education in late Hellenistic Alexandria, where Oribasius was trained under Zeno of Cyprus (Kudlien). This work is, however, of great importance to us, because it preserves material from earlier authors, especially the more obscure ones, that otherwise would have been lost. It is, for instance, the only extant source for large portions of the surgical treatises of Heliodorus and Antyllus, or of Herodotus's book on therapeutics. It also played a historical role from the early Middle Ages on, exerting a considerable influence on the shaping of medical traditions in the Latin West and in Islam.

The main source for Oribasius's life is Eunapius. Oribasius came from a distinguished family in Pergamum. There he became acquainted with Julian (351), who took him to Gaul (355). He was quaestor (magistrate) in Constantinople (360) and was involved in the proclamation of Julian as emperor (361). He enjoyed (though not without upheavals) a position of prestige and political power at the imperial court, and was entrusted with the leadership of the library and appointed as physician to the emperor, whom he accompanied until his death in Mesopotamia (363). Oribasius's subsequent banishment was followed by rehabilitation under Emperor Valens.

Oribasius wrote in Greek. His main work, *Collectiones medicae*, was a vast compilation in about seventy volumes of excerpts from the writings of the most famous Greek and Roman physicians; only twenty-five books survive. By and large, the excerpts tended to be close paraphrases rather than exact quotations. The model and inspiration for this encyclopedia was a collection (now lost) of summaries of Galen's writings. Both works were undertaken, at the emperor's suggestion, in an attempt to revive the classical past. Oribasius also composed two extremely popular summaries of the *Collectiones*—the *Synopsis ad Eusthatium* and *Ad Eunapium*, in nine and four books, respectively—which circulated in Latin, Syriac, and Arabic translations and can help with the reconstruction of some of the lost parts of the *Collectiones*. One of Oribasius' focal concerns was dietetics, a subject to which he devoted eight books of excerpts, arranged thematically under such topics as foods and their effects, spices and drinks, sleep and vigil, exercise, and baths.

Other writings include an *Anatomy of the Intestines*, a treatise *On Diseases*, a book entitled *To the Perplexed Physicians*, a work *On Royal Rule* (of which only the title now survives), and notes for a biography of Emperor Julian (also used by Eunapius for his own *Life of Julian*). However, the attributions of an *Introduction to Anatomy* and a *Commentary to the Aphorisms* to Oribasius are spurious.

Bibliography

Primary: Raeder, I., ed., 1964. *Oreibasii Opera* I–III (Amsterdam); Morland, H., 1940. *Oribasius Latinus* I (Oslo); Daremberg, C., and U. C. Bussemaker, eds., 1851–1876. *Oeuvres complètes d'Oribase* I–VII (Paris).

Secondary: Andorlini, I., 2004. *Medicina, medico e società nel mondo antico* (Florence) pp. 59–60, 86, 231; Grant, M., 1997. *Dieting for an Emperor* (Leiden); Baldwin, A., 1975. 'The Career of Oribasius.' *Acta Classica* 8: 85–98; Jones, A. H. M., J. R. Martindale, and J. Morris, 1971. *The Prosopography of the Later Roman Empire* I (Cambridge); Kudlien, Fr., 1968. 'Third Century—Black Spot' in Stevenson, L. G., and L. P. Multhauf, eds., *Essays for Temkin* (Baltimore) pp. 32ff; Schröder, H. O., 1940. 'Oreibasios' in Pauly, A., and G. Wissowa, eds., *Real-Encyclopädie der classischen Altertumswissenschaft* (Stuttgart) Suppl. VII, coll. 797–812; *DSB*.

Manuela Tecusan

ORR, JOHN BOYD

(b. Kilmaurs, Ayrshire, Scotland, 23 September 1880; d. Brechin, Angus, Scotland, 25 June 1971), *nutrition.*

Orr, son of Robert Clark Orr, a quarry owner, and Annie Boyd, attended Glasgow University, graduating MA (1902), BSc (1910), and MB, ChB (1912). After working as a ship's surgeon, he became a Carnegie Research Scholar under E. P. Cathcart (1877–1954) and a lecturer in chemical physiology, and received an MD in 1914. In 1915 he married Elizabeth Pearson.

In 1913 the Development Commission approved a proposal for an animal nutrition laboratory at Aberdeen and Orr was appointed director, taking up his post in April 1914. Construction began, but was suspended when Orr joined the RAMC. After serving as a sanitary officer in the southeast of England, he was sent to France, seeing action on the Somme and at Paschendaele, and receiving a MC and a DSO. After transferring to the navy (1918), he was seconded to study energy requirements of troops with Cathcart.

After returning to Aberdeen in December 1918, Orr raised funds for an alternative site for the animal nutrition laboratory, and new buildings were erected and named the Rowett Institute, after a major donor. Likewise, the Reid Library and Duthie Farm, as well as Strathcona House, a staff residence, were created later. The Imperial Bureau of Animal Nutrition was also located at the Institute, which published *Nutrition Abstracts and Reviews* starting in 1931.

During the 1920s, Orr developed a research program on minerals in farm animal nutrition, claiming that they were of greater practical importance than the recently discovered vitamins, and argued a similar line regarding human nutrition. One of the earliest mineral projects was conducted by the unionist MP and Glasgow medical graduate, Walter Elliot (1888–1958), who worked at the Institute in his spare time. Later in the 1920s, the Institute became a major beneficiary of the research grants committee of the Empire Marketing Board, chaired by Elliot. These funds supported an experimental farm in Kenya and studies on the mineral content of pastures, Kenyan natives' diets, milk supplements and the growth of schoolchildren, and minerals and disease resistance in Scottish highland sheep. The latter project produced few results before it was abandoned when the Empire Marketing Board was disbanded.

During the 1910s and 1920s, Cathcart and others argued that nutritional problems were the result of ignorance rather than poverty and were best tackled by educating housewives in efficient shopping and cooking. Orr initially accepted this position, but Isabella Leitch (1890–1980), his assistant, claimed that her arguments with him accounted for a change of heart. By the 1930s Orr was arguing that the solution to malnutrition lay in cheap food policies and in such schemes as school meals and milk. By this time he was also convinced of the practical importance of vitamins.

In 1930 Elliot introduced a private members' bill, which allowed Scottish local authorities to supply school milk regardless of children's circumstances. Later, as Minister of Agriculture, his Milk Act of 1934 introduced subsidized school milk nationally. Orr worked closely with Elliot's Market Supply Committee, which gathered data that could be used to support policies to increase food consumption. But in view of possible political consequences, Elliot balked at the release of a report based upon these data, which was instead published as *Food, Health and Income*, under Orr's name. This reanalysis of dietary survey data argued that about half the population was not consuming sufficient amounts of one or more nutrients. It was much quoted by campaigners arguing for changes in government policies and was the basis of a documentary film, *Enough to Eat*.

Food, Health and Income was not well received by the government, and the Ministry of Health's Advisory Committee on Nutrition (of which Orr was a member) felt that more data were needed. Orr set about a large-scale dietary survey and supplementation experiment, financed by the Carnegie Trust. However, the project was not completed before World War II, and the survey data were eventually published in 1955.

During the war, much of the Rowett's research was suspended, and Orr became professor of agriculture at Aberdeen University. He campaigned for scientific food policies and during 1940 was a leading member of the Scientific Food Committee, which reported to the Cabinet, and established the broad lines of wartime food policy. After this flurry of activity, however, Orr's wartime role was marginal, but it was upon his initiative that the Nutrition Society was founded in 1941. He retired from the Rowett in 1945 to his farm in Angus, but in the same year was elected MP for the Scottish universities and rector of Glasgow University (later becoming its chancellor, in 1946).

In the 1930s Orr became increasingly involved with nutritional issues on a world scale, through involvement in League of Nations initiatives. However, he was not a delegate to the 1943 Hot Springs conference, where it was agreed to establish the United Nations Food and Agriculture Organization, although he did attend a planning conference in Quebec (1945), as an unofficial adviser. He accepted the post of director-general, but resigned (1948) following the failure of his idealistic 'World Food Board' plan. He was elected FRS (1932), knighted (1935), and created Baron Boyd Orr and awarded a Nobel Peace Prize (1949). During the Cold War he traveled widely, campaigning for peace.

Bibliography

Primary: 1936. *Food, Health and Income* (London); 1966. *As I Recall* (London).

Secondary: Smith, David F., 2000. 'The Carnegie Survey: Background and Intended Impact' in Fenton, Alexander, ed., *Order and Disorder* (East Linton) pp. 64–80; Smith, David F., 2000. 'The Rise and Fall of the Scientific Food Committee during the Second World War' in Smith, David F., and Jim Phillips, eds., *Food, Science, Policy and Regulation in the Twentieth Century: International and Comparative Perspectives* (London) pp. 101–116; Smith, David F., 1999. 'The Use of "Team Work" in the Practical Management of Research in the Inter-War Period: John Boyd Orr at the Rowett Research Institute.' *Minerva* 37: 259–280. Kay, Herbert D., 1972. 'John Boyd Orr.' *Biographical Memoirs of Fellows of the Royal Society* 18: 43–81; *Oxford DNB*.

David F. Smith

ORTA, GARCIA DA (b. Castelo de Vide, Portugal, 1499?; d. Goa, India, 1568), *medicine, pharmacology.*

Da Orta was the son of Fernando da Orta and Leonor Gomes, both of them Jews expelled from Spain in 1492 and forced to convert to Christianity by the edict of the Portuguese king D. Manoel in 1497. Da Orta attended the universities of Salamanca and Alcalá de Henares, in Spain, where he received his MD in 1523. He returned to Portugal and in 1530 was appointed professor of logic at Coimbra University. Three years later, he became a member of the Coimbra University Senate.

In 1531 a papal bull established the Inquisition in Portugal, especially against the New Christians who maintained in secrecy the observance of the Jewish faith. In fact, the Inquisition began to act in Portugal only in 1536. During this period, da Orta, as a New Christian who kept his Jewish faith and practices, prepared his flight from Portugal. He went to Goa (then Portuguese India and a very important place of trade) in 1534 and worked there as a physician as well as a tradesman in the spice trade.

Da Orta became acquainted with the medical practices that took place in Goa, different from those in the Iberian Peninsula. He compared illnesses, realizing that some he saw in Goa also existed in Portugal, but others he had never heard about. He took part in the first autopsy carried out in Goa, during a cholera epidemic in 1543.

In connection with his spice trade, da Orta cultivated a garden with many medicinal herbs from Asia, herbs that he began to study, collecting information from various sources, including those outside the European medical tradition, as well as popular knowledge. He also made a new reading of the traditional European medical sources in the light of his Asian experiences.

The result of such enterprise was collected, classified, and published in a book (1563) written in dialogue form between two people: a newly arrived physician from Europe facing the materia medica and medical practices in India and another individual, who was acquainted with those practices.

The book did not particularly deal with clinical medicine. Its concern lay with describing new plants rather than detailing diseases and treatments. The fifty-seven dialogues, all of them in Portuguese, are each one dedicated to an item of materia medica—herbs, fruits, and minerals—in alphabetical order. This work, translated into French, Spanish, Latin, and Italian in the next two decades, showed, for the first time to European physicians, the therapeutic effects of plants effectively unknown before. Thus, it enhanced European knowledge about plants and medical practices from India and other parts of Asia.

Da Orta's work represents an awakening to the new. It required a skepticism able to doubt received wisdom and not reliant only on the ancient texts. It sought what can actually be found around us, fundamentally by observing and investigating nature itself.

The time and place in which da Orta lived was not so friendly to this kind of approach. The Inquisition reached Goa in 1560, and da Orta and his family suffered from persecution. After a long illness, da Orta died in 1568. Condemned posthumously by the Inquisition for the 'crime' of practicing Judaism, in December 1580, his bones were exhumed and burned.

Bibliography

Primary: 1563. *Colloquios dos simples e drogas e cousas medicinais da Índia* (Goa).

Secondary: Pearson, Michael N., 1996. 'First Contacts between Indian and European Medical Systems: Goa in the Sixteenth Century.' *Clio Medica* 35: 20–41; Fischel, W. J., 1974. 'Garcia da Orta—a Militant Marrano in Portuguese-India in the 16th Century'. *Salo Wittmayer Baron Jubilee Volume* (Jerusalem) pp. 407–432; Friedenwald, Harry, 1944. 'Medical Pioneers in the East Indies' in *The Jews and Medicine* (Baltimore); *DSB*.

Francisco Moreno de Carvalho

OSLER, WILLIAM

OSLER, WILLIAM (b. Bond Head, Ontario, Canada, 12 July 1849; d. Oxford, England, 29 December 1919), *medicine, medical education.*

The son of Reverend Featherstone and Ellen Picton Osler, Osler had his early schooling in the small schoolrooms of Bond Head, Dundas, and Weston, just outside Toronto. Although a good student and athlete, his enjoyment of pranks and practical jokes got him expelled from school on one occasion and a few days in jail on another.

Early Influences

At Trinity College School in Weston, Osler came under the influence of the founder, Rev William Johnson, who encouraged his love of nature and showed him the wonders to be seen through a microscope. He considered a career in the ministry and entered University of Trinity College, Toronto, in 1867, but continued with his interest in the natural sciences. At age nineteen he wrote his first paper on the microscopic life in a winter stream, called *Christmas and the Microscope* (1869). He was further influenced by James Bovell, a well-trained but disorganized physician who was enthusiastic about science and microscopy and had a large library. He invited Osler to attend some of his medical lectures and dissections. It was at this time that the young Osler found in Thomas Browne's *Religio medici* a means of resolving the ethical questions in science of the day, and this remained his favorite book throughout life.

Medical Education

Osler began medical studies at Toronto Medical School, but transferred to McGill University College of Medicine, where there was a well-established curriculum and better access to clinical experience at the Montreal General Hospital. Initially quiet and reserved, he did not stand out as a medical student, but was recognized as talented by many, including R. Palmer Howard, the third of his important mentors, who encouraged him and gave him opportunities to explore his interests. He graduated in 1872 with MD, CM, with a prize-winning thesis based on twenty postmortem studies.

With generous support from his brother, he traveled to Europe for further study. He considered a career in ophthalmology, but his teacher and mentor Howard said that others in Montreal were going into that field, so he should plan a

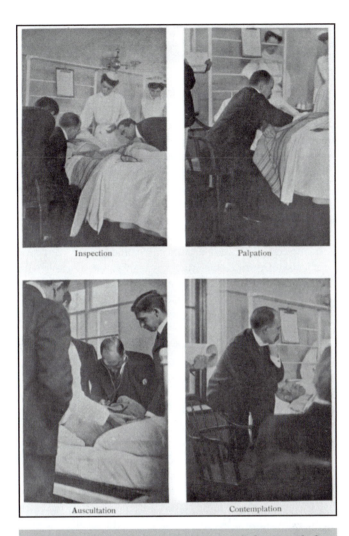

Inspection   Palpation

Auscultation   Contemplation

Sir William Osler at the bedside. Photographs by T.W. Clarke, from Harvey Cushing, *The Life of William Osler*, Oxford, 1925. Wellcome Library, London.

career in general medicine. He worked with John Burdon Sanderson and sampled the available teaching, clinical activity, and social life in London. He then traveled to Berlin and Vienna, seeking out those who were changing medicine, pathology, and laboratory sciences, learning firsthand the advances that put Continental medicine in the forefront of the profession.

Montreal

Osler returned to Canada without definite plans, but a sad event became a stroke of good fortune for him. A recently appointed professor of the institutes of medicine had to relinquish his new position due to heart disease, and the interim position went to Osler. He struggled with the heavy teaching load and hoped for some private practice to increase his meager income. He earned some additional salary by providing care at a smallpox hospital and used the experience to publish some original observations on the disease, and after treating eighty-one patients he himself developed a mild case.

He was not an impressive lecturer, but he worked at improving his presentations and was also beginning to see ways to develop innovative teaching methods. He organized a course on microscopy and histology, equipping the students with microscopes from Paris at his own expense, and developed a unique pathology demonstration course in the autopsy rooms of the Montreal General Hospital. He excelled as a teacher in the autopsy room and at the bedside. He offered to do all the autopsies for the staff, eventually documenting over 1,000 cases, which honed his skill in clinico-pathological correlation that would inform his later teaching and writing. He was also gaining confidence in his presentation skills and became a regular at the Montreal Medical-Chirurgical Society, showcasing autopsy cases with the clinical history and examination, and then showing pathological specimens. He later published many of these lectures, and the specimens were eventually added to the medical museum.

He gave formal lectures, taught the country's first course in clinical microscopy, and started a pathology laboratory. The next year he was formally appointed professor of the institutes of medicine and began bedside teaching at the Montreal General Hospital. In most medical schools, teaching was primarily through classroom lectures, but McGill had a tradition of bedside teaching, of which Osler would become a master.

For further income Osler taught at the Montreal Veterinary College, giving the first course in veterinary pathology in North America. He displayed an equal fascination with animal disease and became president of the local veterinary society and published cases in veterinary journals. He discovered a new parasitic disease in puppies caused by a nematode later known as *Filaroides osleri* and as *Oslerus osleri*.

He successfully campaigned for a position as an attending physician, and on the day he was appointed he sailed to Europe to again visit clinics and to meet and discuss with the prominent clinicians and academic medical men in England, something he would do often during his career. He visited England for the 1881 International Medical Congress, which was attended by 3,000 physicians, and in 1884 visited Germany. He admired the advances he saw in Germany, but, as a professional who was succeeding in academia as a teacher, he expressed concern about the imbalance in the rewards for research and teaching, with researchers achieving greater prestige, academic advancement, and recognition through their publications.

Philadelphia

While in Leipzig, Osler received a request that he let his name stand for the chair of clinical medicine in Philadelphia. Silas Weir Mitchell, the prominent Philadelphia clinician who was on the selection committee, was traveling in Europe, arranged a dinner with Osler and left impressed.

Others from Canada, England, and the United States also wrote references to assure the committee that they were looking at an outstanding young talent. The committee could not miss the fact that Osler had been selected that year as the prestigious Goulstonian Lecturer at the Royal College of Physicians in London and was the incoming president of the Canadian Medical Association. They offered the position and Osler accepted.

The Philadelphia students were underwhelmed by his first lecture but were enthralled by his teaching at the bedside and in the autopsy room. His academic income was still low, but his practice income was growing and his teaching opportunities were excellent, with access to a lot of autopsy material from 'Old Blockley', a huge chronic care facility. Osler had a fast-paced schedule, and although he socialized and became part of the social life of Philadelphia, he remained unmarried and committed to his work, also turning down offers from Harvard during this period. Through his teaching, his many publications, and the increasing number of his essays and philosophical addresses, his fame was spreading in North America and Europe. He delivered one of his most famous speeches at an evening celebration arranged for the retirement of one of Philadelphia's famous, the surgeon Hayes Agnew, during which the now-famous Eakins painting of Agnew performing surgery was unveiled. His talk, later published as *Aequanimitas*, became a classic essay in medicine.

Baltimore

Osler had warded off Harvard, but the plans for a hospital and medical school at Johns Hopkins University interested him as an opportunity to be in the forefront of a grand experiment in medical education and hospital care. Johns Hopkins, who died in 1873, had left his funds to develop a university and hospital of excellence, but the progress had been slow. Daniel Coit Gilman was recruited as the first president to develop the university and John Shaw Billings to form the hospital and medical school.

When Billings made Osler an offer, he quickly accepted the chair in the department of medicine at the new Johns Hopkins Hospital and Medical School in 1889, joining William Welch, a pathologist who had training in the classics and was enthusiastic about German science; William Halsted, an innovative and skilled surgeon; and Howard Kelly, a leading obstetrical surgeon. The 'Big Four' of Hopkins were all under forty, well-established in their specialties, and poised for great change.

When Osler arrived the hospital had still not been built, so he occupied himself with other activities: beginning his new consulting practice, publishing more clinical cases, and starting a textbook of medicine. Throughout his career he sent off spoof articles under the nom de plume Edgerton Yorrick Davis, MD, a reflection of his tendency to always have some fun when all around him was serious.

In 1890 he went on another of his busman's holidays to Europe, visiting clinicians and clinics in Germany, France,

Bavaria, Switzerland, and England. During 1890–91 he worked on his textbook, *The Principles and Practice of Medicine*, which was published in March 1892 by D. Appleton and Co. and was dedicated to his three teachers, Johnson, Bovell, and Howard. It was an immediate success, went into many printings, and over the following decades it ran to sixteen editions and was the most influential textbook of medicine for almost fifty years, providing him a comfortable financial cushion for the rest of his life.

During this time he was also courting Grace Revere Gross, widow of the famed surgeon Samuel Gross, but she encouraged him to finish the book before planning marriage. When the book was finished they married quietly and settled into Baltimore social life, entertaining at their large home at 1 West Franklin Street. He gave his house staff keys to the house so that they could use his library, and they became known as the latchkey students (the pin of the American Osler Society is in the form of a latchkey).

The couple went to England, Osler's eighth crossing, and his wife learned that she would have to adjust to his busy clinical and medically-related social life as he busied himself with his colleagues and their clinics and laboratories. His activities did change after marriage, however, and he became more the senior consultant and more philosophical in his writings and speeches, with a growing interest in the history and philosophy of medicine. Although he had a daily teaching schedule, he did few autopsies. His focus was enlarging as his views became more general and more oriented toward public health and global visions of medicine and health. Although still only in his forties, he was regarded as, and enjoyed the role of, a medical statesman.

When the medical school at Hopkins began, the first class of 1893–94 had eighteen students, which included three women, as the group of young, prominent Baltimore women who had helped the institution get over a funding block had insisted on equal entry opportunities for women. Some have criticized Osler for some comments that sounded chauvinistic, but in fact, even though he thought that a medical career was particularly difficult for a woman, he welcomed and mentored many women students.

The students were exposed to Osler's teaching when they entered their third year of study and could attend his clinical service and participate in his innovative bedside clinical teaching. He adopted the English concept of clinical clerkship that allowed senior students to learn as junior doctors under supervision. In this setting he was without equal, and his attention to his students and his positive and sparkling personality made him a popular and much-loved professor. As his reputation as a clinical teacher spread, he received constant requests from visitors to sit in on his sessions. He would invite two students to dinner each Saturday night, and after the meal they would be joined by a larger group of students to discuss books, medical history, and life in the profession, relaxing with beer and tobacco.

Honors were coming his way. He received honorary degrees from McGill, Michigan, Jefferson, Aberdeen, Edinburgh, Trinity College, and Toronto, and awards from medical organizations. His consulting practice put a strain on his schedule. His fees were often high, but not so outrageous as those of his surgical colleagues, and he treated many without charge. He also was generous in supporting the many charities and causes he worked for, and provided support for a number of family members.

In 1899, when Osler turned fifty, he became excited about a new passion. He had always maintained a good library and supported and fostered medical libraries and their associations, and he now began to collect the great books of medicine, buying hundreds of historical works wherever he could find them. Beginning with all the various editions of Thomas Browne's *Religio medici*, he began to acquire a library that would build to about 10,000 titles, not counting the many duplicates he purchased and regularly gave away to libraries and friends. His income was now sizable, $40,000 annually from all sources, and allowed him a comfortable life with ample travel as well as more books.

However, he and Grace knew that they needed a change. He seemed to recognize that medicine was rapidly advancing and that he was a man in the forefront of the previous age. His skill in clinical observation and reporting of cases was being overshadowed by scientific experimentation and laboratory sciences. He had often commented that a man was past his prime at forty, and he was now fifty-five, yet his pace of work did not lessen.

Oxford

After refusing many offers over the years, including the chair of medicine at Edinburgh, in 1905 Osler was offered the position of Regius professor of medicine at Oxford, which had great prestige but few responsibilities. Grace encouraged him to accept. His colleagues at Hopkins were devastated by the announcement of his departure, and he was feted at many dinners and celebrations. He gave three parting addresses, reflecting on his years and his profession. One, meant to be amusing, became a public controversy that dogged him the rest of his life, a parody on Trollop's *Fixed Period*, with the suggestion that a man was past his productive years at age forty, useless at sixty, and should be chloroformed at sixty-one, after a retirement year on double pension. A new term, Oslerizing, had entered the lexicon.

He spent the following years in the role of a senior statesman of medicine, busy as always, but with more opportunities for travel, vacations, book collecting, and reading the history of medicine. He became involved in organizations that fostered his interests, accepting the presidencies of the Classical Association, the British Hospital Association, the Fellowship of Medicine, the Ashmolean Natural History Society, and the new Section on the History of Medicine at the Royal Society of Medicine, a section he had initiated. He also turned down offers that just looked like new jobs, such as the presidencies of the University of Toronto and of the Royal Society of Medicine.

Osler traveled a lot each year, less to seek out the new advances in clinics and laboratories than to meet medical friends, to enjoy sights, and to haunt antiquarian bookstores. He revised his textbook regularly and could take pride in his role in the development of the Rockefeller Foundation and Institute and its support of medical research and medical education. Its inspiration came from Frederick T. Gates, assistant to John D. Rockefeller, who had read Osler's textbook while on vacation in 1897 and had been impressed by the positive view of medicine and the promise of medical advances that would benefit society.

At home in Oxford, which he loved, he entertained a constant flow of visitors to 13 Norham Gardens, known as the Open Arms. His main responsibility as the Regius professor was to examine the students who had completed their initial medical studies at Oxford and returned from their clinical years at major teaching hospitals in London and elsewhere. Another responsibility of the position, dating from 1618, was to serve as Master of Ewelme, an almshouse for thirteen elderly pensioners, and he visited them regularly. He did some consulting, organized teaching clinics at the Radcliffe Infirmary, and helped start the *Quarterly Journal of Medicine*. He started to write a history of medicine, but the organization of his library kept him busy. Honors continued to come, and a baronetcy was created for him in 1911.

Although Osler usually avoided politics on the local and national medical scene, he became embroiled in the controversy at Hopkins over whether clinical faculty should be on full salary or free to earn their incomes by private practice. His opinion was that the schools could never pay enough salary to attract and retain the best professors and that professors of medicine should always be involved in the daily practice of medicine.

He was sixty-five when World War I broke out and was swept into advisory roles for the war effort. His only son Revere signed up, first for an ambulance service, and then for a fighting unit. Always vocal about the joys and rewards that came to him through life, the tragedy of Osler's days came when Revere was killed by shrapnel, dying with Hopkins surgeon Harvey Cushing at his side and with George W. Crile administering transfusions while surgeons tried to close his wounds.

Osler continued to work at a constant pace to soften the sadness, editing and revising his textbook and other publications, consulting, visiting colleagues and the war injured, and entertaining visitors. In 1918 he suffered a bout of influenza, and on his seventieth birthday he developed a cough. He recovered and continued his daily schedule as before, making visits, writing, organizing his books, and working for a new medical grants committee. He battled the antivivisectionists. He criticized the Royal College of Physicians for their fellowship examination system with its very high failure rate, and he became more interested in postwar reforms to medical and postgraduate education.

After a tiring trip from Edinburgh during a rail strike, he developed another bout of bronchitis that was followed by a high temperature. After two months he still had not recovered and had his chest needled to drain off fluid, followed by a thoracotomy. It became evident that the pulmonary infection was overwhelming, and Osler died on 29 December 1919 of bronchopneumonia and empyema. Grace died in 1928, and the ashes of the couple rest behind a plaque in the Osler Library in Montreal.

Osler's Legacy

Bliss said that at the time of Osler's death there were questions about whether he was the greatest physician who ever lived or merely the greatest physician of his age. Either way, Osler's was a remarkable life in medicine, one that has had few if any rivals. Some had suggested during his career that he was being canonized, but the outpouring of praise after his death indicated that he had indeed been placed on a pedestal above all other physicians. Osler Clubs sprang up on every continent and in many medical schools, focused on the principles and subjects he espoused: professionalism, humanism, the humanities, and medical history. Three nations proudly claimed him as their own. Harvey Cushing produced a large biography of Osler in 1925, which won the Pulitzer Prize. Osler's words were kept alive for generations by the distribution of a collection of his essays to all medical students in North America, and in recent decades by the Hannah Institute of the History of Medicine. Osler Societies are active in Canada, the United States, England, and Japan. The Osler Library at McGill University, established when his personal collection of books arrived in eighty-six boxes in 1929, is an important and growing resource for the history of medicine and for Osleriana.

Osler's 1,628 publications encompassed clinical medicine, education, humanities, history of medicine, bibliography, and the philosophy of medicine. He was first a clinician, and although he did not make many original discoveries, he made many important clinical observations and his use of the laboratory was not for research but to answer clinical questions. His name lingers in the fading eponyms Osler-Weber-Rendu disease, Osler-Vaquez disease, Osler-Libman disease, Osler-Libman-Sacks Syndrome, Osler maneuver, Osler phenomenon, Osler nodes, Osler syndrome, and many others.

The memory of Osler waned with the passing of his students, but his status as an icon was revived in 1970 with the formation of the American Osler Society by a group of clinician-historians. Since then there has been a growing body of scholarship about Osler and his circle, which Roland called the 'Osler Industry' and which has encouraged many authors and collectors of Osleriana. A major collection of Osleriana, including the antiquarian books bequeathed by Osler, is maintained at the Osler Library, McGill University.

The Chesney Archives at the Johns Hopkins Medical Institutions also has a large collection of Osler papers and patient records.

Most great physicians are remembered for their discoveries. Osler is unique in that his star shines brighter than most because he was the complete physician and teacher, foremost in a profession he helped define and advance.

Bibliography

Primary: 1892. *The Principles and Practice of Medicine* (New York) (many subsequent editions); 1922. *Aequanimitas: With Other Addresses to Medical Students, Nurses, and Practitioners of Medicine* (Philadelphia); 1999. (Golden, Richard L., ed. and annotated) *The Works of Egerton Yorrick Davis, MD,* Osler Library Studies in the History of Medicine No. 3 (Montreal).

Secondary: Golden, R. L., 2004. *A History of William Osler's 'The Principles and Practice of Medicine'* Osler Library Studies in the History of Medicine No. 8 (Montreal); Barondess, J. A., J. P. McGovern, and C. G. Roland, 2002. *The Persisting Osler III: Selected Transactions of the American Osler Society 1991–2000* (Malabar, FL); Bliss, Michael, 1999. *William Osler: A Life in Medicine* (Toronto); Barondess, J. A., J. P. McGovern, and C. G. Roland, eds. 1994. *The Persisting Osler II: Selected Transactions of the American Osler Society 1981–1990* (Malabar, FL); Golden, R. L., and C. G. Roland, 1988. *Sir William Osler: An Annotated Bibliography with Illustrations* (San Francisco) (contains a complete list of Osler's 1,628 publications); Barondess, J. A., J. P. McGovern, and C. G. Roland, eds., 1985. *The Persisting Osler: Selected Transactions of the First Ten Years of the American Osler Society* (Baltimore); Nation, E. F., C. G. Roland, and J. P. McGovern, 1976. *An Annotated Checklist of Osleriana* (Kent, OH); Abbott, Maude, ed., 1926. *Sir William Osler: Appreciations and Reminiscence* (Bulletin No. 9, International Association of Medical Museums) (Montreal); Cushing, Harvey, 1925. *The Life of Sir William Osler* 2 vols. (Oxford); *Oxford DNB*; *DAMB*.

Jock Murray

OSTROUMOV, ALEKSEI ALEKSANDROVICH   (b. Moscow, Russia, 27 December 1844; d. Moscow, 11 July 1908), *therapeutics.*

Ostroumov, the son of a priest, attended theological seminary and Moscow University (1865–70). From 1870 onward he worked as a physician, first near Moscow, then in the clinic of Grigorii Antonovich Zakhar'in, thanks to whom he was brought back to academic life in 1871.

In 1873 Ostroumov defended his doctoral dissertation, *O proiskhozhdenii pervogo tona serdtsa* [On the Origin of the First Heart Sound], which was the result of his experiences with the exsanguinous heart and the electric stimulation of the cardiac muscle. In this work he discovered the role of oscillatory movements of valves in the genesis of the first sound.

From 1873 to 1879 he was in Germany, where he studied pathological anatomy and experimental pathology, working in the laboratory of Julius Cohnheim. Studying the tympanic sound of lungs, he argued for the role of bronchial tubes as resonators. He wrote in Russian and German periodicals about his discovery of the phenomenon of blood vessel enervation, observed in his experiences with dogs. Ostroumov explained the compression and expansion of blood vessels through the action of the nervous fibers. He also discovered that the activity of nerves of peripheral vessels does not depend on the central nervous system. He determined the phenomenon of sweat gland enervation and investigated the problem of nervous edemas.

From 1879 to 1900 Ostroumov headed the department of clinical therapy of Moscow University, at first as a sessional lecturer, then as a professor. He created, on his own initiative, a clinical laboratory (1884) and improved the process of therapy and the conditions for students. After moving the department to a new building in the small hospital settlement at Devich'e pole (1891), he created a well-equipped clinic that was exemplary for the time. He taught pathological anatomy and experimental pathology and gave lectures on clinical medicine, in which were discussed cases of cirrhosis of the liver, neurasthenia, sclerosis, chlorosis, typhoid fever, and other disorders. He analyzed the problem of early forms of tuberculosis especially successfully.

Ostroumov developed a doctrine of diagnosis, which, in his opinion, should be constructed with etiological, morphological, and functional data. In addition, by autopsying the deceased, the physician should reveal the role of environment in the illness of the organism. He recognized the significance of the microbe as a cause of mortality, but suggested that the condition of the organism should be the focus of attention.

Ostroumov was one of the first Russian physicians to raise the question of the value of biology for the development of medicine. He emphasized the constitutional features of the patient, considering that they played an important role in the development of pathology. He asserted that illness is a result of infringements of the adaptation of the human body to an environment, and that adaptations are hereditary. According to Ostroumov, the physician should be able to establish the congenital features of an organism. This was achieved by detailed inquiry of the patient. He thought it important to know how bodily organs function and about the health of relatives of the patient. Congenital features helped determine the purpose of treatment.

Ostroumov wanted to focus therapy on specific organs. He recommended baths, massage, application of electricity, and a change of climate. For the treatment of tuberculosis he advised milk, kefir (fermented cow's milk), and koumiss (fermented mare's milk), and in case of malaria, treatment by hydration. Ostroumov paid special attention to the condition of the nervous system and its role in the genesis of diseases, and therefore thought much of preventive actions and spoke about the importance of improving the material conditions of patients. While understanding the value of hospital therapy, he emphasized the importance of outpatient treatment and preventive maintenance.

Ostroumov was a chairman of the Moscow Medical Society (1879–89) and one of the organizers of the Pirogov Society. He was a deputy of the Moscow Municipal Duma (parliament), and participated in the political actions of university professors. Because he was ill, he lived in Batumi for a long time (1900–08), where he still worked as a physician. There he constructed general and maternity hospitals using his money and collected donations, and he was also engaged in the organization of a climate station for lung patients.

Ostroumov was an author of more than twenty works, published in *Moskovskii vrachebnyi vestnik, Protokoly Moskovskogo meditsinskogo obshchestva* and as lectures. At the Second Meeting of the Pirogov Society (1887) he reported on Pyelonephritis catarrhalis. Among his pupils there were many well-known physicians, including D. A. Burmin, V. A. Vorobiev, N. A. Kabanov, and A. P. Langovoi.

Bibliography

Primary: 1950. *Izbrannye trudy* [Collected Works] (Moscow); 1893. *O kholere i ee lechenii* [About Cholera and Its Treatment] (Moscow); 1903–04. *Arkhiv kliniki professora Ostroumova (1892–1900)* [Archive of the Clinic of Professor Ostroumov] 2 vols. (Moscow).

Secondary: Gukasian, Aram Grigorievich, 1950. *A. A. Ostroumov i ego kliniko-teoreticheskie vzgliady* [A .A. Ostroumov and His Clinical-Theoretical Perspectives] (Moscow); Zabludovsky, Pavel Efimovich, 1945. 'A. A. Ostroumov.' *Fel'dsher i akusherka* 1–2: 44–49; Kabanov N. A, 1927. 'Aleksei Aleksandrovich Ostroumov.' *Vrachebnoe delo* 1: 5–8.

Dmitry Mikhel

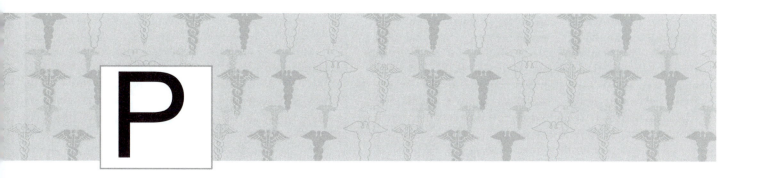

PACINI, FILIPPO (b. Pistoia, Italy, 25 May 1812; d. Florence, Italy, 9 July 1883), *medicine, anatomy, parasitology, microscopy, museology.*

Pacini was the son of Francesco Pacini, a cobbler, and Umiltà Dolfi. His parents wanted him to become a priest, and he was educated, with public assistance, at the Pistoia Episcopal seminary and later at the classical academy. As a boy he showed a great love for the natural sciences, and in 1830 he abandoned his ecclesiastical career and turned to medicine, enrolling in the Scuola Medica Pistoia, founded in 1666 in his native city and attached to the Ospedale del Ceppo. He graduated in surgery (1839) and in medicine (1840). In 1840, as a consequence of the reform of the medical studies in Toscana, Pacini went to Pisa, where he was appointed assistant to Professor Paolo Savi (1798–1871), in the Institute of Comparative Anatomy. He assumed a similar post at the Institute of Human Anatomy (1843) and became a substitute teacher there the following year.

In 1831, while he was dissecting as a student in the anatomy class in Pistoia hospital, Pacini saw the corpuscles that are now named after him, a large, sensory end organ consisting of concentric layers or lamellae of connective tissue surrounding a nerve ending. He discovered the corpuscles in a hand, around the digital branches of the median nerve, and suggested that they were the 'nervous ganglia of touch'. However, he soon found them also in the abdominal cavity.

In 1835 he presented his discovery to the Società Medico-Fisica Fiorentica. It was not accepted by the anatomical community, who considered these organs to be mere aggregations of fat. He continued his investigations, with an Amici microscope lent him by Niccolò Puccini and presented the results to the first national congress of Italian scientists held at Pisa (1839). The Congress established a commission to verify his assertions, but no final decision was taken. In the following year, Pacini published his results in *Nuovi organi scoperti nel corpo umano da Filippo Pacini*. In 1844 the German anatomists F. G. J. Henle and R. A. von Kölliker studied the corpuscles discovered by Pacini, defined their constitution and their anatomical specificity, and named them *Pacinische Körperchen*.

With a new microscope that he had perfected himself and built with Giovanni Battista Amici's (1786–1863) assistance, he investigated the human retina and published his results in 1844. The importance of his was work not recognized, and he met with animosity. In 1847 Pacini therefore began teaching descriptive anatomy at the Lyceum in Florence, where he also taught painting. Subsequently (1849), he became director of the anatomical museum and professor of general and topographical anatomy at the medical school (Istituto di Studi Superiori) and from 1859 also taught microscopic anatomy. In 1852 he published his works on the electric organ of the *Gymnotus electricus,* comparing it with the equivalent organ in other electric fishes.

As a teacher, convinced of the fundamental importance of the biological sciences to medical education, he initiated a number of new scientific programs, mainly based on the regular use of the microscope. In 1861, at the National Exhibition celebrating Italy's unification, he presented a collection of selected microscopic preparations. He was, however, occasionally frustrated and embittered by the antagonism of the clinician and pathologist Maurizio Bufalini (1785–1875), director of the department of internal medicine.

In 1854 epidemic cholera arrived in Florence. Pacini microscopically examined the blood and feces of living patients as well as changes in the intestinal mucosa of the dead. This work was done with the support of his assistant, and later professor of ophthalmology in Bologna, Francesco Magni (1828–88). These investigations proved the presence of millions of rod-shaped corpuscles, which Pacini considered to be microorganisms, naming them vibrions because of the S–shape and mobility. He provided drawings of the vibrions, observed in abundance in the cholera victims' intestines, and declared that these living corpuscles caused the intestinal injuries common to the disease.

In *Osservazioni microscopiche e deduzioni patalogiche sul cholera asiatico* (1854), Pacini stated that cholera was a contagious disease, characterized by destruction of the intestinal epithelium, followed by extreme loss of water and electrolytes. He recommended (1879) therapeutic intravenous injections of saline solution, later found to be effective. In 1865 he published another book, designating the vibrion as the 'specific cause' of cholera. Despite the significance of his research, Pacini was overlooked when the Italian government distributed medals for meritorious anticholera work after the 1866 epidemic.

In 1884 Koch rediscovered the cholera vibrion, naming it the 'Comma Bacillus'; by applying his rigorous postulates, he confirmed that the bacillus was the only cause of cholera. Koch presented his findings at the Cholera Commission of the Imperial Health Office in Berlin. However, the commission recognized Pacini's priority in discovering the microorganism, and in 1965 the international committee on nomenclature adopted *Vibrio cholerae* Pacini 1854 as the correct name of the cholera-causing organism.

Pacini also microscopically analyzed the structure of bone (1851). He studied the mechanism of respiration in humans (1847), from which he derived a method for artificial respiration (1870), based upon a rhythmic movement of the shoulders of the unconscious subject, to be used for 'reliving' victims of drowning and those poisoned with narcotic research.

In Florence, Pacini led the Physiological Museum of the Royal Anatomical Institute and devoted much attention to preparing and conserving anatomical specimens, creating special liquids for preserving the collection. Particularly important are his collections of histological preparations and microscopic slides (still preserved in Florence), including those of cholera vibrions made in 1854–55. His microscopic slides of the organism were clearly labeled, identifying the date and nature of his investigations.

Pacini never married, and his work was generally unrecognized. He died in a poorhouse, having spent all his money on scientific investigations and medical care for his sisters, and was buried in the cemetery of the Misericordia in Florence. In 1935 his remains were transferred with the remains of two other anatomists, Atto Tigri (1813–75) and Filippo Civinini (1805–44), to the church of Santa Maria delle Grazie in Pistoia.

Bibliography

Primary: 1835. 'Sopra un particulare genere di piccoli corpi globulari scoperti nel corpo umano da Filippo Pacini.' *Archivio delle scienze medico-fisiche toscana* 8; 1840. *Nuovi organi scoperti nel corpo umano* (Pistoia); 1845. 'Nuove richerche microscopiche sulla tessitura intima della retina.' *Nuovi annali delle scienze naturali* (July–August) (Reprinted separately 1845, Bologna); 1846. 'Sopra l'organo elettrico del Siluro del Nilo.' *Nuovi annali delle scienze naturali* (July); 1847. 'Sulla questione della meccanica dei muscoli intercostali.' *Gazzetta toscana delle scienze medico-fisiche* 5: 153–156; 1847. 'Cosa è ed a che è buona l'anatomia microscopica del corpo umano.' *Gazzetta toscana delle scienze medico-fisiche* 5: 193–199; 1851. 'Nuovo richerche microscopiche sulla tessitura intima delle ossa.' *Gazzetta medica italiana federative* (November); 1854. 'Osservazioni microscopiche e deduzioni patalogiche sul cholera asiatico.' *Gazzetta medica italiana federativa toscana,* 4 (December) (Reprinted 1924. *Lo Sperimentale* 78: 277–282); 1865. *Sulla causa specifica del colera asiatico, il suo processo patologico e la indicazione curativa che ne risulta* (Florence); 1866. 'Della natura del colera asiatico, sua teoria matematica e sua comparazione col colera europeo e con altri profluvi intestinali.' *Cronaca medica di Firenze* (August 10, November 10); 1870. 'Il mio metodo di respirazione artificiale per la cura dell'asfissia.' *L'Imparziale* 10: 481–486.

Secondary: Bentivoglio, M., and P. Pacini, 1995. 'Filippo Pacini: A Determined Observer.' *Brain Research Bulletin* 38: 161–165; Brancolini, L., and G. Niccolai, 1985. *Filippo Pacini con i lavori originali sui 'corpuscoli' e il colera, sul microscopio e sulla retina* (Pistoia); Crespi, M., 1975. 'Pacini, Filippo.' *Scienziati e tecnologi dalle origini al 1875* (Milan) p. 476; Coturri, E., 1957. 'Contributo alla storia della divulgazione della scoperta dei "corpuscoli del Pacini."' *Atti e memorie della Accademia di storia ed arte sanitaria* 23; *DSB*.

Bernardino Fantini

PAGET, JAMES (b. Great Yarmouth, Norfolk, England, 11 January 1814; d. London, England, 30 December 1899), *surgery, pathology.*

Paget was the son of Samuel Paget, brewer and ship owner, and one-time mayor of Great Yarmouth. His father's wealth had diminished by the time Paget reached school age, and unlike his three older brothers, he remained in Great Yarmouth for his early education. Paget initially contemplated joining the navy, but instead he was apprenticed (1830–34) to a local surgeon, Charles Costerton. After four and a half years of his apprenticeship, he was allowed to study in London and attended Costerton's former medical school, St Bartholomew's Hospital (1834–35). Self-taught in botany, chemistry, and zoology, Paget was ambitious for success, and in order to improve his knowledge of anatomy he taught himself German. Paget went on to win a series of prizes at the hospital and passed the MRCS (1836) after eighteen months in London. However, his lack of a classical and Oxbridge education continued to trouble him.

Early Career

During his time as a student, Paget built close links with the staff at St Bartholomew's, and after drifting to Paris on a medical tour (1836–37), he returned to the hospital to take up the post of curator of the anatomy museum (1837–39). The ambitious Paget had found English teaching hospitals better than Parisian hospitals and believed that it was important to remain connected with a 'good school' no matter how low he started. His intention 'to work my way if I could into better places' was well known, and many of the choices Paget made in his early career were shaped by this desire (Paget, 1901, pp. 92, 105). However, a series of disappointments in securing appointments followed, and he relied on medical journalism to bolster his standing and income. He was subeditor (1837–42) of the *Medical Gazette* and wrote for the *Medical Quarterly Review*. With several staff at St Bartholomew's feeling guilty about not finding him a better post, he was appointed demonstrator of pathology (1839–43). Paget used the demonstratorship to improve his position in the hospital, and he was appointed lecturer in general anatomy and physiology (1842–59) after conflict erupted between Edward Stanley (*c*. 1792–1862) and Thomas Wormald (1802–73). Paget now felt his 'fortune was made' (Paget, 1901, p. 139). Despite internal opposition, he was elected assistant surgeon (1847–61), surgeon (1861–71), and consulting surgeon (1871) to St Bartholomew's, as well as surgeon-extraordinary (1858–61), and Sergeant-surgeon-extraordinary (1867–77) to Queen Victoria. As his practice grew, he rose to international eminence as a surgeon and medical scientist, becoming a leading figure in the medical profession.

St Bartholomew's

Once established in a lecturing post at St Bartholomew's, Paget took a central role in shaping the teaching at the medical school, keeping in close contact with his brother, George, at Cambridge, a relationship that influenced Paget's work at the hospital. Concerned about the moral conduct of the students, he advised and then ran College Hall as warden (1843–51), the first halls of residence for medical students in London. Paget supported the entrance of Elizabeth Blackwell (1821–1910) to the hospital and was favorable to women becoming doctors. In the 1840s and 1850s his lectures on surgical pathology captivated students, who found his energetic style refreshing. His lectures were in sharp contrast to the monotonous lectures common in many teaching hospitals at the time, while many (such as those on masturbation or alcohol) tried to separate moral concerns from medical and physiological issues. As lecturer in physiology (1844–48) Paget encouraged a shift to physiology and pathology in the general anatomy and physiology courses. Although he felt the lectures did him little good professionally, he subsequently published them in the first edition of Kirkes's *Hand-book of Physiology* (1848)—a text many contemporaries felt had a considerable impact on the study of physiology.

By 1859 the austere Paget had become treasurer of the medical school and set about building up a system of prizes to promote scholarship, bringing the school's academic standards close to those of the University of London, and improving the disciplinary structure. He introduced surgical consultations (1868) so that surgeons could discuss their cases with their colleagues. Paget provided the leadership and administrative ability that had been lacking at St Bartholomew's since the 1820s. Under his influence the medical school reasserted its position as a leading London school through the emphasis he placed on academic performance and discipline.

However, Paget resigned his teaching posts at St Bartholomew's (1871) after contracting blood poisoning during the performance of a postmortem. Weakened by the protracted illness that followed, he felt unable to continue. By the mid-1870s he had ceased offering clinical lectures, pleading that it was impossible for him to find the time to prepare lectures that would be useful to students. He had become active in the RCS and felt constantly overworked. It was at the College rather than at St Bartholomew's that he had the greatest intellectual impact.

Medical Education

Paget was proud of his profession, serving on numerous professional bodies and becoming actively involved in reforming how medicine was taught and examined. He held numerous posts in the RCS, including member (1865–89), vice-president (1873–74), and president (1875) of the College council. He was president of the Royal Medical and Chirurgical Society (1875) and was the RCS's representative on the General Medical Council (1876–81), helping to negotiate the creation of the Conjoint Board. Paget also served on the senate (1860–95) and faculty of medicine (1876–95) of the University of London and as vice-chancellor (1883–95) of the University. Here he helped shape the examination requirements in medicine and supported moderate reform, carefully negotiating tensions between the University in its examining role and the teaching faculty.

Looking back, Paget noted that 'I had a full share in bringing about the improvements of the last twenty years in teaching and examining and in the general management of the affairs of the College and University' (Paget, 1901, p. 193). Critics argued that his moderate stance only put off major reforms.

Pathology

Paget is considered a founder of the science of pathology, a surgeon who 'advanced his art by showing how pathology might be applied successfully to elucidate clinical problems, when as yet there was no science of bacteriology' (*DNB, 1901, p. 241*). His studies of inflammation, diseases of the bone, and tumors were characterized by original observations. He made great use of the microscope to determine the nature of morbid growths, breaking from what he saw as a preoccupation with form, appearance, and structure in favor of an approach that sought to look at the teleological and morphological aspects of tissue (Paget, 1853).

Paget became renowned for his close observations. This was evident in his early discoveries while undertaking dissection work as a student in 1835. He noticed white specks in the muscles of his subject. On inspection, he found them to be cysts containing worms; the parasite later becoming known as *Trichina spiralis*. The anatomist Richard Owen (1804–92) confirmed his observations and took the first publication credit, causing tension between him and Paget.

Paget wrote extensively on surgical pathology and provided names for many of the conditions and structures he observed. Much of his work was shaped by his experiences as curator of the anatomy museum at St Bartholomew's. As curator he compiled a catalog of the museum (Paget, 1847, p. 1852), the style and content of which laid the foundation of his later work and reputation. He also prepared a catalog of the pathological specimens housed in the Hunterian Museum (Paget, 1846–49). Paget went on to publish over twenty articles on various aspects of pathology and surgery, combining his experience as a surgeon with his knowledge of clinical pathology, although it was his pathological work that was considered pioneering. His lectures as Arris and Gale Professor of anatomy and surgery (1847–52) at the RCS were subsequently published as *Lectures on Surgical Pathology* (1853). These provided a considerable stimulus to the study of pathology, which had been declining in England for some time.

Paget was a skilled diagnostician and emerged as an authority on diseases of the bones and joints. His name has become eponymously associated with several conditions. In 1876 Paget described five cases of 'osteitis deformans', a chronic inflammatory disease characterized by thickened bones and lesions in the neck and skull. He was the first to offer a clear description of the disease now referred to as Paget's disease of the bone. Although Paget believed it to be an inflammatory disease process, it is now known to result from an abnormality of bone remodeling, possibly due to viral infection. In 1870 Paget was also the first to

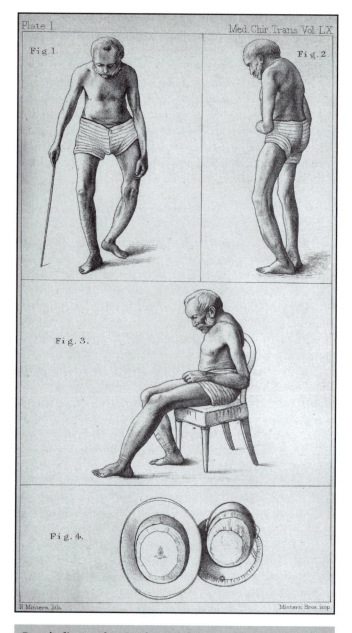

Paget's disease showing bone deformities and change in hat sizes in 1844 and 1876. Lithograph from 'On a form of chronic inflammation of bones (osteitis deformans).' *Medico-chirurgical Transactions* 1877, vol. 60.

describe osteochondritis dessicans, or multiple loose bodies in the knee joint. He also described several nonrheumatological conditions. In 1874 he reported a series of fifteen cases of chronic ulceration of the nipple (Paget's disease of the nipple), an eczema-like change in the skin of the nipple indicative of underlying breast cancer. He suggested that chronic ulceration induced the cancer. Paget's name has also been attached to other conditions, including Paget-von Schroetter (a form of thrombosis), Paget's recurrent fibroid, Paget's recurrent abscesses, Paget's test (to differentiate between solid and cystic tumors), and Paget's quiet necrosis (bone disease without signs of inflammation).

Science and Vivisection

Paget was a firm believer that doctors should always keep a mind for science in practice. He argued that the separation of science from clinical practice was nonsense. For Paget, the application of science to medicine was essential to improve learning, a stance he articulated in his presidential address to the International Medical Congress in London (1881). In this context, experimentation on animals acquired a central role, and Paget defended the importance of vivisection, becoming embroiled in the antivivisection debate. Paget believed that more knowledge was needed on how the human body worked. He defended vivisection, explaining that most animal experiments were undertaken with the animal anesthetized, removing much of the problem of pain. He believed that vivisection had a utility that went beyond any suffering that may have been caused to the animals, arguing that more pain was inflicted on animals for sport. For Paget, medicine had to be made more scientific through pathology, physiology, and animal experimentation in order for it to progress.

Contribution

The ambitious Paget was part of a small but highly visible group of Victorian clinicians who spent much of their time engaged in medical research and teaching. He was one of the most prominent surgeons of the late-Victorian period and a leading figure in the profession, traveling the length and breadth of Britain to speak to professional bodies and to operate. He acquired an international reputation as a surgeon, although it was his clinical pathology that had the greatest impact, with his published work providing a vital stimulus to the study of pathology.

Bibliography

Primary: 1846–49. *A Descriptive Catalogue of the Pathological Specimens contained in the Museum of the Royal College of Surgeons*, 5 vols. (London); 1847–52. *A Descriptive Catalogue of the Anatomical Museum of St Bartholomew's Hospital*, 2 vols. (London); 1848. (by Kirkes, William Senhouse, assisted by James Paget) *Hand-book of Physiology* (London); 1851. *Lectures on Tumours* (London); 1853. *Lectures on Surgical Pathology, delivered at the Royal College of Surgeons of England* (London).

Secondary: Waddington, Keir, 2003. *Medical Education at St Bartholomew's Hospital, 1123–1995* (Woodbridge, and Rochester, NY); Paget, Stephen, ed., 1901. *Memoirs and Letters of Sir James Paget* (London); *Oxford DNB*.

Keir Waddington

PAGET, (MARY) ROSALIND   (b. Greenbank, Liverpool, England, 4 January 1855; d. Bolney, Sussex, England, 19 August 1948), *midwifery, nursing.*

Rosalind Paget, daughter of John Paget, a London police magistrate, and Elizabeth Rathbone, entered Westminster Hospital to train as a nurse in 1875. She studied under the Nightingale disciple Miss Luckes at the London Hospital (1882–84), where she obtained her nursing certificate. She then gained her London Obstetrical Society certificate for midwifery at Endell Street Lying-in Hospital (1885).

Although Paget worked for some years at the London Hospital, her main interest lay in the reform of midwifery. Along with many women of her class and generation, she wanted to do something 'purposeful' with her life. Her family had a strong interest in social reform, and she acknowledged the influence of her uncle, William Rathbone MP, who initiated a district nursing scheme in Liverpool, on her choice of career. A turning point for Paget came in 1886, when she accompanied her matron, Miss Freeman, to a meeting of the Matron's Aid Society, soon to be renamed the Midwives' Institute and, later still, the Royal College of Midwives. The Institute aimed to raise the efficiency and status of midwives by seeking better training and education for them, protect the interests of midwives as a professional group, and work to improve the conditions under which working-class women gave birth. Paget was one of a small group of well-educated, middle-class women who provided the driving force behind the development of the Institute from the mid-1880s onward. She founded the Institute's journal, *Nursing Notes*, in 1887 and held the unpaid post of treasurer from 1890 to 1930. Her financial support enabled the Institute to have a permanent headquarters for meetings, a club, and a library, and she persuaded some of the most prestigious medical names of the day to give lectures on midwifery. She also had a long association with the Queen Victoria Jubilee Institute for Nursing (QVJIN), a group that promoted district nursing and midwifery services in country districts. Paget acted as first chief officer for a year (1890–91) and was a member of Council with special responsibility for midwifery. During the 1890s she played an active role in the campaign for midwife registration, giving evidence in 1892 to the select Committee on Midwifery. When registration was finally achieved with the Midwives' Act of 1902, Paget served as a member of the regulatory body, the Central Midwives' Board, between 1902 and 1924, representing the QVJIN.

Paget engaged in a broad range of activities designed to further the cause of midwifery reform, speaking to numerous women's groups, such as the Women's Liberal Federation and the Women's Co-operative Guild. She also linked her campaign to the broader aims of the contemporary women's movement, believing that women would never be able to influence policymaking without the vote. In 1908 she led twenty members of the Midwives' Institute in a suffrage procession under the banner of Florence Nightingale (1820–1910). Her political astuteness and communication skills, coupled with a lively sense of humor, ensured that she was an influential figure in the Institute until she retired in 1930.

Paget, described by Edith Pye, the president of the Institute in 1929, as the 'Florence Nightingale of midwifery', played a key role in ensuring the survival of the Midwives' Institute and in enhancing the professional status of the midwife in Britain. In recognition of her services she was appointed a Dame of the British Empire in 1935.

Bibliography

Secondary: Hannam, June, 1997. 'Rosalind Paget: The Midwife, The Women's Movement and Reform Before 1914' in Marland, Hilary, and Anne Marie Rafferty, eds., *Midwives, Society and Childbirth* (London) pp. 81–101; Cowell, B., and D. Wainwright, 1981. *Behind the Blue Door: The History of the Royal College of Midwives, 1881–1981* (London); Rivers, J., 1981. *Rosalind Paget: A Short Account of Her Life Work* (London); *Oxford DNB*.

June Hannam

PALFYN, JAN (b. Kortrijk [Courtrai], Belgium, 28 November 1650; d. Gent [Ghent], Belgium, 21 April 1730), *anatomy, surgery, obstetrics.*

Palfyn, the son of Margaretha De Roore and Egide Palfyn, learned the rudiments of the trade from his father, a barber-surgeon. In order to improve his knowledge of anatomy—to him the keystone of surgery—he went to Ghent in 1670 and became the apprentice of a surgeon connected with the medical school (*Collegium Medicum Gandavense*). This gave him the opportunity to attend lectures and witness dissections and operations at the School of Surgery.

Having passed the examination for master surgeon (1673), he left for Paris, where he worked for three years with Joseph Duverney, professor of anatomy and surgery at the Jardin du Roy. In 1676 he returned to Kortrijk, moved to Ieper (Ypres) in 1685, and finally, in 1697, settled down in Ghent. During these years he had made journeys to Holland and France, harvesting scientific information from leaders of the profession—like Ruysch, Van Leeuwenhoek, Duverney, and Tollet—and perfecting his knowledge and experience. Ghent, the capital city of Flanders, gave her lost son a hearty welcome, granting him burghership and admittance to the barber-surgeons' corporation.

In 1701 his first book was published: *Nieuwe Osteologie*, a thorough exposé of the nature, structure, function, and diseases of bones. Impressed by the author's erudition, the Collegium added a new course to the curriculum of the School of Surgery in 1708 and appointed the sworn surgeon Palfyn lector of osteology and surgery. Palfyn, taking his task to heart, published a surgical textbook for his students in 1710.

Following the resignation of Anthone van Breughel, *medicinae licentiatus* and professor of anatomy at the School of Surgery, the directors of the Collegium took an exceptional step in electing Palfyn, a surgeon, to succeed Van Breughel, an academic, as professor of anatomy at the School of Surgery.

Historians consider Palfyn's *Heelkonstige Ontleeding van's Menschen Lighaem*, which passed through numerous editions and was translated into French, German, and Italian and made the link between surgery and anatomy, to be his *opus princeps*. Velpeau wrote in 1834, 'To Monsieur Palfin belongs the honor to have introduced the title "surgical anatomy"'. A prolific writer, Palfyn made contributions to anatomy, surgery, teratology (his report of the dissection of Siamese twins (1703) was a first), and gynecology, as his monograph of the female organs of generation (1708) shows.

His name remains attached eponymously to the parallel forceps (the 'Iron Hands' or *Manus ferreae Palfini*), the precious instrument he presented at the Académie royale des Sciences de Paris around 1722 of which he offered many a colleague a copy. Unlike his predecessors—the Chamberlens in England and the Roonhuysens in the Dutch Republic—Palfyn did not keep his nondestructive tractor a secret. He never published his invention, a first picture of which was published in Lorenz Heister's *Chirurgie* (Nuremberg, 1724).

In recognition of his services to science and mankind, Kortrijk and Ghent erected a statue to his memory, and in 1931 Professor DeLee affixed a stone plaque with the name of his hero on a wall of the Chicago Lying-in Hospital.

Bibliography

Primary: 1701. *Nieuwe Osteologie ofte Waere, en zeer Nauwkeurige Beschrijving der Beenderen van 's Menschen Lichaem* (Ghent); 1710. *Nauwkeurige Verhandeling van de voornaemste Handwerken der Heelkonst, zoo in de harde, als sagte deelen van 's menschen lichaem* (Leiden); 1718. *Heelkonstige Ontleeding van 's Menschen Lighaam* (Leiden).

Secondary: Blondeau, R.-A., 1997. *Jan Palfijn. Een Vlaams Heelmeester in de 17de en 18de Eeuw* (Tielt); Stein, John Bethune, 1913. 'Jan Palfyn.' *Medical Record* 83: 47–55; Voisin, Auguste, 1827. *Notice sur la Vie et les Travaux de Jean Palfyn* (Ghent).

Michel Thiery

PALMER, BARTLETT JOSHUA (b. What Cheer, Iowa, USA, 10 September 1881; d. Sarasota, Florida, USA, 27 May 1961), *chiropractic.*

The son of Daniel David Palmer (1845–1913), the founder of chiropractic, and Lavinia McGhee, Palmer was educated at the Palmer School of Chiropractic in Davenport, Iowa, graduating in 1902. In 1904 he married Mabel Heath; they had one child.

Palmer exerted a commanding influence on the early evolution of chiropractic. In 1904 he took over operation of the Palmer School from his father, and served as the institution's president until his death. Under his entrepreneurial leadership, enrollment at the Palmer School grew from twenty-one students in 1904 to more than 2,000 by 1920; indeed, during the 1920s it was the largest educational establishment of any system of healing in the world.

Palmer authored numerous treatises on chiropractic and edited the journals *The Chiropractor* (1904–58) and *The Fountain Head News* (1914–61). He also founded the profession's first national organization, The Universal Chiropractors Association (1906), and was the pioneer in adopting the new x-ray technology for chiropractic diagnosis. In addition, Palmer was the chief defender of 'straight' chiropractic, which adhered strictly to the procedures of musculoskeletal manipulation that had been introduced by his father. Straight chiropractic attributed virtually all illness to the pressure of displaced vertebrae upon nerves exiting the spinal column, an impingement that disrupted the flow of a presumed nervous fluid called 'Innate Intelligence'. 'Adjustment' of the misaligned vertebra to return it to its normal position allowed Innate Intelligence to move freely and restored the body to health.

During the 1910s, however, reliance on vertebral adjustment exclusively came under challenge by revisionists, who advocated the use of supplemental drugless therapies such as heat, massage, and hydrotherapy. Palmer vigorously attacked these 'mixers', in lecture and in print, as traitors to true chiropractic. In furtherance of the cause, from 1914 onward he directed a weeklong event on the Davenport campus that became famous throughout the profession as the Lyceum. A gathering resembling a revivalist camp meeting, the Lyceum was aimed at confirming straight practitioners in their faith and drawing mixers back into the fold.

Palmer's success at attracting students and practitioners into the field earned him the title within the profession of 'The Developer': a designation that recognized not just his charismatic leadership, but also his business acumen. A master of advertising and salesmanship, he made the teaching of those skills a major component of the curriculum at the Palmer School of Chiropractic. The stereotype of the chiropractor as a mercenary self-promoter, a popular image that has dogged the profession through most of its history, was created largely by B. J. Palmer.

The most notable illustration of Palmer's commercial bent was his introduction at the 1923 Lyceum of a diagnostic device he named the neurocalometer. A standard part of the chiropractic examination theretofore had been palpation along the spinal column to locate areas of elevated temperature, evidence of inflammation caused by a displaced vertebra. The neurocalometer was purported to detect 'hot spots' electronically, thus removing subjectivity and guesswork from diagnosis. The instrument was of dubious value, but more disturbing was Palmer's demand that practitioners pay him exorbitant fees for its use. Many even among the straight practitioners denounced him for his greed, and The Developer's reputation never recovered. Although the Palmer School would continue as the chief educational institution in the profession, Palmer himself would be regarded as the black sheep in the chiropractic family for the rest of his life.

Bibliography

Primary: 1906. *The Science of Chiropractic* (Davenport, IA); 1920. *A Text Book on the Palmer Technique of Chiropractic* (Davenport, IA).

Secondary: Keating, Joseph, 1997. *B. J. of Davenport: The Early Years of Chiropractic* (Davenport, IA); Moore, J. Stuart, 1993. *Chiropractic in America. The History of a Medical Alternative* (Baltimore); Wardwell, Walter, 1992. *Chiropractic: History and Evolution of a New Profession* (St Louis); DAMB.

James Whorton

PALMER, DANIEL DAVID (b. Port Perry, Ontario, Canada, 7 March 1845; d. Los Angeles, California, USA, 20 October 1913), *chiropractic.*

Palmer was one of six children born to Thomas Palmer and Catherine McVay. Receiving only sporadic schooling in childhood, he immigrated to the United States in 1865, eventually settling in Iowa and pursuing a variety of jobs that included beekeeping and running a grocery.

During the early 1880s Palmer developed an interest in Mesmerism, or magnetic healing, and in 1886 began to practice the craft himself. Operating out of Davenport, he spent nine years providing magnetic therapy, until making the chance discovery in 1895 that he could cure more effectively by manually restoring displaced vertebrae to their correct position. To describe this technique, he adopted the name chiropractic, a term derived from Greek roots for 'done by hand'.

Palmer soon formulated a theory to account for the efficacy of his skeletal manipulations. A displaced vertebra, or vertebral 'subluxation', impinged upon nearby nerves exiting the spinal column, thereby interfering with the free flow of a presumed nervous fluid that regulated all vital functions. This fluid—what he called 'Innate Intelligence'—was believed to be the individual's allotment of the spiritual power that pervaded all creation, and its unimpeded movement through the body was essential for health. In virtually all cases, he maintained, illness was the result of a subluxated vertebra interfering with the flow of Innate Intelligence. Chiropractic therapy involved finding the misaligned vertebra and manually restoring the bone to its anatomical position through an 'adjustment'. With its freedom of action restored, Innate Intelligence would quickly return the body to full health.

The new healing method began to attract students in 1898, with the opening of the Palmer Institute and Chiropractic Infirmary in Davenport (to be renamed the Palmer School of Chiropractic in 1905). In 1903 Palmer moved from Davenport (leaving his school in the hands of his son, Bartlett Joshua) to Portland, Oregon, where he opened the Pacific College of Chiropractic; the institution survived only two years. Other educational ventures that he subsequently launched in Oregon, California, and Oklahoma were even less successful. During this period, Palmer also spent a short period in jail for practicing medicine without a license.

In 1910 Palmer published his *The Chiropractor's Adjuster*. A rambling hodgepodge of fatuous hypotheses, extravagant therapeutic claims, and petty polemics, the volume purported to be the final word on the principles and practice of a revolutionary method of healing. But the fact that chiropractic did ultimately evolve into a profession with demonstrated skill at relieving musculoskeletal ailments owes nothing to the baffling theoretical musings of its founder's textbook. Palmer's contribution was a practical one, the empirical development of basic procedures of skeletal manipulation. He pioneered the chiropractic 'thrust,' a maneuver distinguished by the abruptness and speed of 'racking' vertebrae back into position. For this he was revered within the profession as 'The Discoverer' and as 'Old Dad Chiro'.

Palmer's last years were plagued by the sight of many of his followers turning to 'mixed' chiropractic, i.e., the addition of various drugless modalities (massage, heat, hydrotherapy, vibration) to vertebral adjustment. He remained a staunch defender of the 'straight', adjustment-only version of chiropractic. Palmer died of typhoid fever in 1913, two months after Kansas became the first state to license chiropractors to practice. Palmer was married five times.

Bibliography

Primary: 1910. *The Chiropractor's Adjuster: Text Book of the Science, Art and Philosophy of Chiropractic for Students and Practitioners* (Portland, OR).

Secondary: Moore, J. Stuart, 1993. *Chiropractic in America. The History of a Medical Alternative* (Baltimore); Wardwell, Walter, 1992. *Chiropractic: History and Evolution of a New Profession* (St Louis); Gielow, Vern, 1991. *Old Dad Chiro. A Biography of D. D. Palmer, Founder of Chiropractic* (Davenport, IA); Rehm, William, 1980. 'Palmer, Daniel D.' in Lints-Dzaman, Fern, ed., *Who's Who in Chiropractic International* (Littleton, CO), pp. 271–272; *DAMB*.

James Whorton

PANDIT, CHINTAMANI GOVIND (b. ?, 1895; d. New Delhi, India, 10 July 1991), *preventive medicine, tropical medicine.*

Pandit, a brilliant student in school and college, joined Elphinstone College, Bombay, in 1910. Later he went to London and was the first Indian to be awarded a PhD in bacteriology from the University of London. On his return, he joined the Medical Research Department of the British Government in India and was posted to the King's Institute, Guindy, Madras, in 1924. During his years at the King's Institute, Pandit began investigations into a number of tropical diseases. His research into the manufacture of vaccine lymph derived from human variola was standardized for the first time at the institute. For a short time, he was also the first professor of bacteriology at the Madras Medical College. Pandit went on to become the first Indian director of the King's Institute.

As director of the Pasteur Institute at Shillong in northeast India, he pursued his research into rabies as well as the epidemiological dimensions of frequent cholera outbreaks in the Brahmaputra and Surma valleys. A Rockefeller Fellowship brought him in touch with numerous bacteriologists in the United States. Awarded a Ford Foundation Fellowship in virology, he studied techniques in tissue culture and micromanipulation. He also spent time at the Marine Biological Laboratories at Woods Hole, Massachusetts, USA, and at the Strangeways Laboratories at Cambridge, England.

Pandit's training in virology and his talent for seeking out new techniques resulted in pioneering work on the adhesion phenomenon in filariasis in 1928. The 'Pandit Reaction', or the intradermal test for filariasis, remained valid even after thirty-five years. Pandit also carried out epidemiological studies of older diseases like plague, tuberculosis, and leprosy but also 'new' diseases such as meningoencephalitis and, later, viral diseases such as poliomyelitis and sandfly fever, as well as trachoma. His article in 1940 was among the first that traced the causes of endemic fluorosis to the consumption of drinking water with high fluoride content.

The government of the Madras Presidency, as well as the British government in India, which had to deal with several outbreaks of epidemic disease, sought Pandit's evaluation. He represented India at the Far Eastern Congress of Tropical Medicine and Malariology, held in Nanking, China, in 1934. Five years later, he was awarded the Minto Gold Medal for his work in tropical medicine. In 1943 recognition for his scientific contributions from the British government came in the form of an OBE. During World War II, the British government in India deputed him to visit the United States to study yellow fever and its prevention.

After the war, Pandit and Dr Bennet Hance were assigned the task of studying various models of medical institutions in the UK, United States, and Canada in order to advise the government on the setting up of a similar institution for medical treatment and research in India. Pandit and Hance chose Johns Hopkins as the institutional model for the All India Institute of Medical Sciences, finally established in Delhi (1956) after Indian independence.

Apart from finding support for clinical research, Pandit remained an influential institution builder. The Indian Research Fund Association, to which Pandit was appointed secretary in 1948, was redesigned into the Indian Council of Medical Research in 1949 with Pandit as its first director. Before his retirement in 1964 he published a report on the workings of the ICMR.

Pandit inspired a generation of scientists and epidemiologists and actively shaped and recast medical research in independent India.

Bibliography

Primary: 1928. (with Pandit, S. R., and P. V. Seetharama Iyer) 'The Adhesion Phenomenon in Filariasis: A Preliminary Note.' (reprinted 1991) *Indian Journal of Medical Research* 93: 946–953; 1940. (with Raghavachari, T. N. S., D. S. Rao, and V. Krishnamurthi) 'Endemic Fluorosis in South India: A Study of the Factors Involved in the Production of Mottled Enamel in Children and Severe Bone Manifestations in Adults.' *Indian Journal of Medical Research* 28: 533–558; 1961. (with Rao, K. Somerwara) *Indian Research Fund Association and Indian Council of Medical Research, 1911–1961: Fifty Years of Progress* (New Delhi); 1982. *My World of Preventive Medicine* (Delhi).

Secondary: Sriramachari, S., 1991. 'A Homage to C. G. Pandit.' *Indian Journal of Medical Research* [A] 93 (November) pp. v–viii.

Indira Chowdhury

PANUM, PETER LUDVIG (b. Rønne, Denmark, 19 December 1820; d. Copenhagen, Denmark, 2 May 1885), *physiology, epidemiology.*

Son of a regimental surgeon, Panum attended the University of Copenhagen and gained his MD in 1845. For five years Panum worked at hospitals in Copenhagen and as a navy doctor during the war with Germany 1848-50. In 1846 the Danish State sent Panum to the Faroe Islands in the North Atlantic, where measles had appeared for the first time in sixty-five years. His report, 'Observations at the Faroes', was a very accurate study of the epidemic, which affected 6,000 out of 8,000 inhabitants, and it became a classic work in medical epidemiology. Relying on observations, case-tracing, and simple analysis of data, Panum demonstrated an unknown regularity of the epidemic disease. He showed that the skin rash appeared thirteen to fourteen days after exposure and that the disease was contagious as no cases indicated a miasmatic origin. This view was supported by Panum's effective quarantine arrangements, which protected fifteen villages and more than 1,000 people from contracting the disease.

Panum's accurate observations on the Faroe Islands were related to his early dedication to the natural sciences. He taught physics and chemistry at a grammar school while he was a medical student. His doctoral thesis on the coagulation of the blood (1851) argued in favor of a new medical science built on the laboratory and its practices. To gain knowledge about these he went abroad from 1851 to 1853 to study in Würzburg in Germany, where Joseph Scherer and Rudolf Virchow influenced him, and in Paris, where he served one year as a scientific assistant to Claude Bernard.

In 1853 Panum was appointed as a professor at the University of Kiel, at that time belonging to Denmark, and founded the first laboratory of physiology in Denmark. In 1864 he left Kiel, half a year before Kiel was lost to Germany, and became professor and director of a new labora-

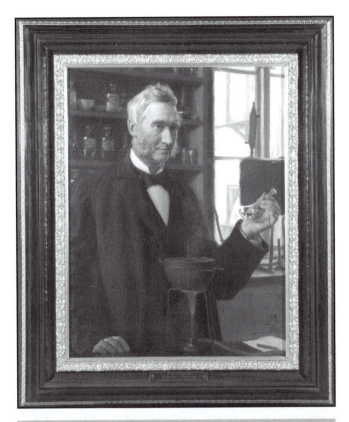

Panum in his laboratory. Oil painting by August Jerndorff, 1894. Used with permission of the Carsberg Laboratory, Copenhagen.

tory at the University of Copenhagen, where he served until his death in 1885.

Like other pioneers of experimental medicine, Panum's experimental contributions covered a wide range of problems within human physiology. He made small but original studies concerning embolism and the transfusion of blood. He investigated human vision and discovered 'Panum's area', a functional subdivision of the retina. Furthermore, his study on putrefaction was one of the first works investigating the nature of septicemia from a chemical point of view. In this study Panum injected different preparations of putrid material intravenously into five dogs, causing intoxication. He found a 'putrid poison', still active after boiling, arguing that the active agent was a chemical poison and neither a ferment nor a microorganism.

In the late 1870s the use of animals in medicine generated a public reaction in Denmark. By arguing against an unlimited use of vivisection and by publishing a Danish edition of the German Ernst von Weber's *The Torture Chambers of Science* (1879), the 'Society for the Protection of Animals' (1875) provoked a debate on vivisection. During this antivivisection campaign, in which Panum was criticized by colleagues, he argued that his experiments had saved more human lives than the number of animal lives he had taken. Panum explained that he had left practical medicine for the greatest benefit of the patients.

In his time, Panum primarily contributed to the development of medical science in Denmark and Scandinavia, where he co-edited the *Nordic Medical Archive* and was the chief organizer and president of the Eighth International Medical Congress convened at Copenhagen in 1884. His laboratory in the medical faculty in Copenhagen was the only place for conducting biological experiments in the 1860s and 1870s and was the starting point for the next generation of medical scientists in Denmark, including Christian Bohr and Carl Julius Salomonsen.

Bibliography

Primary: 1847. 'Observations made during the epidemic of measles on the Faroe Islands in the year 1846' (slightly abridged translation) *Curiosities of medicine* 1963: 210–236; 1865–69. *Haandbog I Menneskets Physiologi* (Copenhagen).

Secondary: Gjedde, A., 1971. *Peter Ludvig Panums videnskabelige indsats* (*Bibliotek for Læger*, supplement); Carstensen, J., 1967. *Peter Ludvig Panum. Professor der Physiologie in Kiel 1853–1864* (Neumünster); Gafafer, William F., 1934. 'Bibliographical biography of Peter Ludvig Panum (1820–1885), epidemiologist and physiologist.' *Bulletin of the Institute of the History of Medicine* 4: 258–280.

Morten A. Skydsgaard

PAPANICOLAOU, GEORGE NICHOLAS (b. Kymi, Greece, 13 May 1883, d. Miami, Florida, USA, 19 February 1962), *cytology.*

Papanicolaou was the son of doctor and politician Nikolaos Papanicolaou, who twice became Mayor of Kymi and four times was elected MP in the constituency of Evia (1875–79, 1881–85, 1887–90, and 1892–95). His mother's name was Maria Kritsouta. As a young boy, Papanicolaou loved nature and was curious about plants and animals. He also enjoyed the violin, his favorite instrument. Following medical studies at Athens University (1898–1904), he completed his military service in 1906, serving as an assistant surgeon.

Papanicolaou continued his postgraduate studies in Jena, Germany, despite his father's efforts to persuade him to stay in his birthplace and practice medicine with him. During this period, Papanicolaou's restless mind was diverted toward research and philosophy. He also became involved with several instigators of Dimotikismos (an early twentieth-century movement to establish the vernacular Greek as a formal language), including Manolis Triandafilidis, Alexandros Delmouzos, Dimitris Glynos, Ion Dragoumis, Georgios Skliros, Konstantinos Hatzopoulos, and Yiannis Psicharis. In 1907 he completed postgraduate studies in Jena and moved to the Zoological Institute in Munich, then the greatest research center of its kind in the world. His first teacher there was professor Ernst Haeckel (1834–1910), one of Europe's greatest early proponents of Darwinism. In 1910 Papanicolaou obtained his PhD in Zoology at the University of Munich, with a doctoral thesis

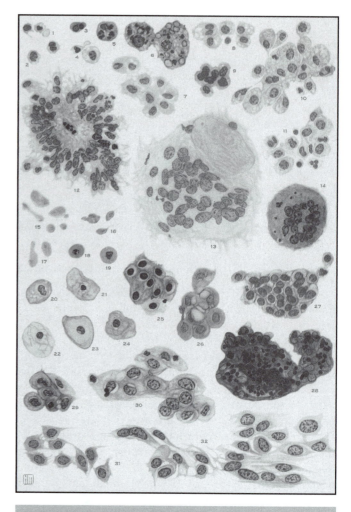

Vaginal and cervical cells showing pathological changes associated with infections and neoplasms taken using the 'pap' smear technique. Halftone reproduction from *Diagnosis of Uterine Cancer by the Vaginal Smear* (New York), 1943. Wellcome Library, London.

entitled, 'Über die Bedingungen der Sexuellen Differenzierung bei Daphniden'.

On 15 September 1910 Papanicolaou married Andromachi (Machi) Mavrogeni, daughter of a wealthy family and descendant of Mando Mavrogenous, heroine of the 1821 Hellenic Revolution. In 1911 he took the first step of his scientific career at the Oceanographic Institute of Monaco, where he participated in a mission on the oceanographic vessel *L'Hirondelle*, which belonged to Prince Albert the First. Later, Papanicolaou discontinued his stay abroad in order to become active in the Balkan wars against Ottoman sovereignty (1912–13), serving as first lieutenant in the Medical Corps of the Greek army.

During his time in the military, he met some Greek-American soldiers who told him of the opportunities in the United States. In 1913 he arrived in America with his wife and life-long research associate, 'Mrs Mary Pap', landing at Ellis Island on 19 October 1913 with just enough money for their visas and speaking no English. His first job in America was as a rug salesman. He later played the violin at restaurants, and served as a clerk for a Greek language newspaper, while Mary worked as a seamstress.

With the help of the famous geneticist Thomas Hunt Morgan at Columbia University, Papanicolaou was soon appointed as an assistant in the Pathology and Anatomy Department of the New York Hospital. In 1914 he became an assistant in anatomy at the Medical College of Cornell University, where he was to stay for forty-seven years. In 1927 he obtained American citizenship and was promoted to assistant professor of anatomy at Cornell University. In 1947 he became professor in the department of anatomy in the same university. Papanicolaou worked very hard for a half century at the Medical College of Cornell University, taking no vacations save for a scientific journey to Europe in 1957, which included a final stop at Kymi, Greece. In November 1961 Papanicolaou moved to Florida to become director of the Miami Cancer Institute, but died three months later of a heart attack at the age of seventy-nine. In November 1962 the Institute was renamed the Papanicolaou Cancer Research Institute in his honor.

Papanicolaou's research was devoted almost exclusively to the physiology of reproduction and exfoliative cytology. His experimental and clinical research work is represented in more than 160 original scientific publications, and condensed into five classic monographs. Papanicolaou is best known for his development of the 'Pap test' for cytological diagnosis of cancer, especially cancer of the uterus. In 1916, during his early work on the role of chromosomes in sex determination, he had noticed recurring cytological changes over a fifteen-sixteen day cycle in the vaginal discharge of the guinea pig. By correlating these changes with ovarian and uterine cycles, the scientists described a technique that in time became standard for measuring the sexual cycles in a variety of species. In 1923, applying his theory to humans, Papanicolaou began observing vaginal smear changes and discovered that women with uterine cancer presented abnormal cells, with enlarged, deformed or hyperchromatic nuclei. Later that year, he told an incredulous scientific audience of his technique of identifying cervical cancer by gathering cellular debris from the lining of the vaginal tract, and then smearing it on a glass slide for microscopic examination.

In the years that followed, Papanicolaou extended his technique to the respiratory, urinary, and upper gastrointestinal tracts, as well as the breast. His method has been used to screen for cancer in many organs and to evaluate the efficacy of radiotherapy. During his lifetime, Papanicolaou was the recipient of fifty-three awards. His face appeared on five postage stamps in three countries (Greece, Cyprus, and the United States), as well as on the 10,000 drachmas Greek banknote in 1995.

Bibliography

Primary: 1943. (with Traut, Herbert F.) *Diagnosis of Uterine Cancer by Vaginal Smear* (New York) 1948. (with Traut, Herbert F., and Andrew A. Marchetti) *The Epithelia of Woman's Reproductive Organs* (New York) 1954. *Atlas of Exfoliative Cytology* (Cambridge, MA); 1959. *Endometrial Cytology* (Cytology Laboratory Hahnemann Medical College); 1960. 'Exfoliative Cytology' (Symposium on Cancer), *Modern Medicine* 28(7): 89–96.

Secondary: Marketos, Spyros, 2000. *George N. Papanicolaou (1883–1962)* (Athens); Marketos, Spyros, 1996. *History of Medicine* (Athens); Barter, J. F., 1992. 'The life and contributions of Doctor George Nicholas Papanicolaou' *Surg. Gyn. Obst.* 174(6): 530–532; Kyle, R. A., and M. A. Shampo, 1983. 'George Papanicolaou', *JAMA* 21: 250; Carmichael, D. Erstine, 1973. *The Pap Smear: Life of George N. Papanicolaou* (Springfield, IL). (Contains a bibliography of his work); *DSB*; *DAMB*.

Maria Korasidou

PAPPWORTH, MAURICE HENRY (b. Liverpool, England, 9 January 1910; d. Hampstead, London, England, 12 October 1994), *medical ethics, medical education.*

Pappworth's father was a Russian immigrant master tailor, who changed the family's name from Papperovitch in the 1930s. After school at the Birkenhead Institute, Pappworth trained in medicine at Liverpool University, where he qualified with honors (1932) and obtained the MD and MRCP in 1936. After junior posts at the Liverpool Royal Infirmary, including a registrarship in the medical professorial unit under Henry Cohen (later Sir Henry and Lord Cohen of Birkenhead), he served in the Royal Army Medical Corps, finishing as a lieutenant colonel in charge of a British general hospital in India.

After demobilization Pappworth seemed set for a brilliant consultantship at a teaching hospital. However, in London, where he moved in 1946, he re-encountered the anti-Semitism that had been prevalent in prewar Liverpool, being told that no Jew could ever hold such a prestigious appointment. After working in locum jobs and rejecting offers of lackluster hospital appointments, Pappworth decided to become a freelance teacher for the membership examination of the RCP. Without passing this examination, taken a few years after qualification, physicians could not ascend to a senior registrar post and a subsequent consultant appointment. But the examination's pass rate was ludicrously low, sometimes only 12–15 percent. In part, this represented hidebound colleges' desire to control the entry of doctors into a limited number of posts. But it also represented the poor standards of undergraduate medical training and the total absence of postgraduate instruction. Pappworth determined to profit from these deficiencies. A brilliant teacher, he eschewed teaching the small print beloved of most candidates in favor of teaching the basic knowledge and methods that so many lacked. Junior doctors flooded to his courses, held in his consulting rooms in Harley Street or in public halls, and, though the cost was high (a pound note—then one-twentieth of a month's salary—dropped into a basket), his results were outstanding. On occasion, half of the successful candidates for a given examination had been to his classes.

Through his contact with junior doctors, Pappworth developed the other preoccupation of his career: medical research ethics. Coming from research centers, particularly the (Royal) Postgraduate Medical School in Hammersmith, many of his students were concerned with the legitimacy of research procedures. The concept of informed consent had not been introduced; most procedures were of no benefit to the patient, and some were even downright risky—to health or even to life—yet junior doctors were loath to hazard their careers by querying the details. Instead, they raised the issues with Pappworth, particularly when he drove them to his small clinical sessions in various peripheral hospitals. He wrote letters to the editors of the journals, querying articles that reported ethically doubtful research. His letters were often rejected for publication, so in 1962 Pappworth turned to the general press, describing fourteen cases with a commentary in *Twentieth Century*, an influential quarterly journal. He expanded these accounts into a book, *Human Guinea Pigs*, which took five years to appear, after encountering legal difficulties and reigniting the covert opposition of the medical establishment, which Pappworth had first encountered over his tuition for the MRCP examination. However, *Human Guinea Pigs*, which documented the cases and names of the experimenters, finally provoked the introduction of informed consent and scrutiny of projects by ethics committees.

Together with Henry Beecher (1904–76), his American counterpart, whose revelations were also taken up by the public media and aroused the fury of professional colleagues, Pappworth revolutionized research ethics, especially as he continued to scrutinize articles for possible infractions of official guidelines. Even the medical establishment finally forgave him: most physicians receive the Fellowship twelve to fifteen years after receiving their MRCP, but in Pappworth's case, the honor took fifty-seven years.

Bibliography

Primary: 1960. *A Primer of Medicine* (London); 1967. *Human Guinea Pigs* (London).

Secondary: Munk's Roll; Oxford DNB.

Stephen Lock

PARACELSUS (THEOPHRASTUS PHILIPPUS AUREOLUS BOMBASTUS VON HOHENHEIM)　(b. Near the Abbey, Einsiedeln, Switzerland, 1493/94?; d. Salzburg, Austria, 24 September 1541), *medicine, surgery, chemistry, medical theory.*

Life and Works

Theophrastus Bombast von Hohenheim was born at the end of 1493 or the beginning of 1494 at the Teufelsbrücke [Devil's bridge] near the abbey of Einsiedeln. His father, Wilhelm Bombast von Hohenheim (*c.* 1457–1534), came from a Swabian noble family and after his studies in Tübingen had taken the academic degree of a licentiate of medicine. His mother probably was a bondwoman of the Benedictine Abbey of Einsiedeln. Paracelsus therefore remained a bondman of the abbey for life. His school education is largely unknown. Following the death of his mother in 1502, father and son Hohenheim left Switzerland and moved to Villach. From 1513 to 1516 Theophrastus studied at the medical college of the University of Ferrara in Northern Italy, where he probably took the degree of Doctor utriusque medicinae. In 1529 Hohenheim wrote a 'Practica' under the name of Paracelsus. This name is either an adapted Greek-Latin version of Hohenheim or—quite unlikely—the allusion to a position equal to or even beyond the Roman physician Aulus Cornelius Celsus.

On his great travel he stayed at Salzburg in 1524–25, where he came into contact with the miners and workmen during a revolt. At this time Paracelsus wrote the 'Archidoxes' (a sort of 'master theory'), in which he put down his views on the 'Alchemia medica', as well as the 'Libellus de virgine sancta theotoca', a theological publication. In 1525 Paracelsus traveled to Baden Castle, where he successfully treated Margrave Philipp I of Baden and continued on to Strasbourg. In Strasbourg he was granted citizenship on 5 December 1526 and served in the 'Zur Luzerne' [The Lucerne], a guild of corn chandlers and millers, as well as surgeons. In the spring of 1527 the printer Johannes Froben, who suffered from a chronic leg disease, asked Paracelsus to treat him in his house, called The Front Chair, located in Totengässlein [Dead man's alley] in Basel. Through Froben Paracelsus came into contact with the intellectual elite of the city, such as the reformer of Basel, Johannes Oecolampadius; the legal scholar Bonifacius Amerbach; the painter Hans Holbein the Younger; and Erasmus of Rotterdam. Probably upon the recommendation of Oecolampadius, the protestant-aligned council named Paracelsus the official city surgeon of Basel in 1527 and at the same time, because the two positions were linked in personal union, professor—or Ordinarius—at the catholic medical college of the university.

Paracelsus gave sensational lectures to the medical students in Latin and also in German, trying to replace the classical medical authorities with his own New Medicine. His symbolic burning of a canonical instruction book on the Midsummer's Eve bonfire on 24 June 1527 led to his first disputes with the surgeons of Basel. In November of that same year, Paracelsus spent some days in Zurich, where he probably met the official surgeon of the city, Christoph Klauser, and the reformer Heinrich Bullinger.

On his return to Basel, Paracelsus heard of his well-wisher Froben's death; at the same time the dispute with the other surgeons in Basel arose again and culminated in an anonymous Latin lampoon poem, *Manes Galeni adversum Theophrastum sed potius Cacophrastum*, describing Paracelsus as a medical fake. In order to escape further struggles, Paracelsus was forced in February 1528 to flee Basel for Colmar, where he was offered hospitality by the physician Lorenz Fries. His attempt to publish two medical works, the 'Ten Books on pocks, palsy, teeth and French disease and similar diseases' and the 'Seven Books on all open diseases', however, was not successful.

In 1529 Paracelsus traveled via Esslingen to Nuremberg. His works on syphilis—'The complete recovery of Holtz Guaiaco' (1529) and 'Three books on the French disease' (1530)—were published here. In both publications Paracelsus attacked the Guaiacum wood praised by Ulrich von Hutten. He did not deny its efficiency as a remedy for syphilis, but instead recommended a moderate application mixed with mercury preparations. Since he had no success in Nuremberg in publishing another work on syphilis therapy, 'On the origin and issues of the French including the recipes of recovery, in eight books', and his 'Spital Book', focusing on surgery issues, he continued his travels to Beratzhausen an der Schwarzen Laber, where he worked on his 'Opus Paragranum' (which means 'beyond, next to, or corresponding to the seed'), dealing with the four pillars of medicine: philosophy, astronomy, alchemy, and virtue (of the surgeon).

At the same time he wrote the first prognostics (1529–30) as general astrological predictions. Other works written at this time also remained unpublished during his lifetime, such as the 'Interpretation of Several Figures of Johannes Liechtenberger' or the 'Interpretation of the Figures of Nuremberg'. After a short stay in Regensburg and Amberg, where he treated the citizen Sebastian Kastner, Paracelsus came to Horn Castle on Lake Constance. He might have met Bartholomäus Schobinger here, since he went to St Gallen in 1531 to treat Schobinger's father-in-law, the mayor Christian Studer. In St Gallen he also made contacts with the preacher Leo Jud from Zurich, to whom he dedicated his comet paper, 'Comet interpretation', in 1531. In the following years some other short treatises on natural events written by Hohenheim were published. In the treatises Paracelsus interpreted the events more theologically than astrologically, believing that he was able to perceive in them the visible will of God exhorting people to live better moral lives. After some disagreements with the established surgeons on his treatment methods, Paracelsus left St Gallen in 1535 and traveled to Meran via Innsbruck and Sterzing. In the summer of 1535 he stayed at Bad Pfäfers (near Ragaz), where he created a Consilium (consultation) for the prince-abbot Johann Jakob Russinger and published the spa paper 'Of Bad Pfeffers' in Zurich.

In 1536 Paracelsus stayed in Augsburg to supervise the printing of two books of the 'Grosse Wundartzney' [Great Surgery Book]. The first volume had been published, but without his consent, the same year in Zurich by the printer Hans Varnier. Annoyed about the anticipatory use of his manuscript, Paracelsus let the printer Heinrich Steiner from Augsburg, who had already published several prognostic papers of Hohenheim, print both volumes of the 'Great Surgery Book', completed on 28 July and on 11 August 1536. In the first volume Paracelsus published a letter to the official city surgeon of Augsburg, Wolfgang Talhauser, and included his answer in the second volume. Talhauser had lived in Augsburg since 1531 and received his first annual pay as a city surgeon in 1534. He probably met Paracelsus in 1536; this might have been a stimulant for the answer to Paracelsus's letter. In 1537, after having left Augsburg, Paracelsus, while at Eferding near Linz, was asked by Hans von Lotitz to travel to Mährisch-Kromau in order to treat the leading marshal of the Kingdom of Bohemia, Johann von Leipa. This treatment took place after 22 June 1537 at Znaim, von Leipa's country residence. However, on 28 September 1537 Paracelsus was invited to visit the district judge of Pressburg, Blasius Beham, and discontinued von Leipa's treatment. At the end of the year a legal dispute was carried out before King Ferdinand I of Bohemia, with von Leipa accusing Paracelsus of having abandoned the treatment too early. Despite the surgeon's petition to the King, both parties were ordered to come to Prague and later to Vienna. Paracelsus stayed in Vienna at the end of 1537; von Leipa, however, had to cancel his journey. King Ferdinand I suggested an arrangement between the parties, which Paracelsus followed by writing a 'Consilium', in which he described in detail his medical treatment.

After his stay in Vienna, Paracelsus continued his way through Villach and St Veit (Carinthia) to Klagenfurt. He hoped to get support from the Carinthian orders in printing his works 'Book of Tartarian Diseases', 'Labyrinthus medicorum', and 'The Seven Defenses' (therefore also called 'Carinthian Writings'). Despite their initial promises, the order did not finance the printing. In Klagenfurt he completed the 'Astronomia magna or the complete Philosophia sagax of the great and small world' as a summary of his cosmological and medical ideas. In this publication Paracelsus described the correspondence of the great (macrocosm) and the small world (microcosm) and designed an anthropology, which, despite his clinging to Christian tradition, places human beings in the center of the cosmos, suggesting a certain convergence with Florentine Neo-Platonism.

Between 1536 and 1539 Paracelsus published five more prognostics, four of them under the title of 'Practica Teütsch' [German Practica], which Paracelsus may have written for financial reasons. In 1541 he reached the bishop's town of Salzburg, perhaps to get employment from the alchemy-aligned archbishop Ernst of Bavaria. The last days of Paracelsus were elucidated by a testament published by the Paracelsian Michael Toxites in 1574. According to this document Paracelsus established his will on 21 September 1541 before the notary Hans Kalbsohr and seven witnesses; the former clerk of the royal court Michael Satznagel and the royal attorney Georg Teisenberger were designated to be the executors. Paracelsus died on 24 September 1541 and was buried at St Sebastian Cemetery in Salzburg. An inventory established by the notary Kalbsohr gives an indication on Paracelsus's financial situation, which can be described as moderate, but certainly not as poor. The ready money was given to friends and relatives, and a representative of the abbot of Einsiedeln came to pick up the most valuable piece of jewelry owed to the Abbey because of Hohenheim's bondage. The inventory of his books corresponded to those of other surgeons of this period.

With some self-consciousness Paracelsus had himself painted by a contemporary Conterfetter (a portrait artist), who remains anonymous to this day, known only by the monogram AH. The first copperplate was created in 1538 and shows Paracelsus in clay bust, with the face turned to the right. In 1540 AH created a half-length figure with the forty-seven-year-old turned three-quarters with a sword and a capsule pendant hanging from his neck. Both portraits have as an inscription the motto of Paracelsus: Alterius Non Sit, Qui Suus Esse Potest [No one should be another one's man, if he can be his own master]. Oil-paintings, drawings, etchings, copperplates or medals of Paracelsus created later follow either these copperplates or prove to be more or less original new creations.

Paracelsus's Patients

It remains debatable whether Paracelsus, who thought himself to be an extraordinary physician, really had success in healing diseases. His diatribes launched against the medical authorities, the physicians of his time, but also against the pharmacists, are well-known. He used his own medicine produced in alchemic processes. The few crumbs of information concerning his life clearly show that he was consulted, even before his stay in Basel, by Philipp of Baden, but also by Nikolaus Gerbel, a reputable secretary at the Strasbourg cathedral. In Basel, Johannes Froben was among his patients; Erasmus of Rotterdam, however, refused to be treated by Paracelsus. A dispute with the canon of Basel Cornelius von Lichtenfels, who refused to pay after being treated successfully, may be one of the reasons why Paracelsus fled to Colmar. At Amberg there was a dispute after the treatment of the citizen Sebastian Kastner, and in St Gallen, where Paracelsus carried out the medical treatment of the mayor Christian Studer, a conflict arose because after a surgery he wanted to heal the son of the bourgeois Caspar Tischmacher with alleged 'magic' remedies. The 'Consilium' for the abbot Russinger at Pfäfers

may have been preceded by a medical consultation; maybe the condition here was similar to the treatment of the Moravian Marshall Johann von Leipa, which ended in a court litigation in 1537. In 1540, however, Paracelsus refused to meet the demand for treatment of Hans Ungnad, baron of Sonneck, the leading captain of Lower Austria, because of the baron's physical weakness. It is striking that the majority of Paracelsus's patients were members of the aristocracy or the patriciate classes. This may be the result of the traditional problem of the sources, as reports on the treatment of the common people are unknown. However, this situation is different from the legends arising after Hohenheim's death. The historical collection 'Rhapsodia vitae Theophrasti Paracelsi' by the Danish royal chemist Peter Diderichsen Payngk referred to Paracelsus treating the lower classes.

Here and in other writings, such as a letter written by the Frankfort citizen Cyriacus Jacobus (d. 1551) to the Ottheinrich, Elector of Palatinate, Paracelsus was spoken of as a miracle man. Georg Joachim Rheticus also reports in a letter to Joachim Camerarius the Elder in 1558 that Paracelsus had successfully treated a person dangerously ill in St Veit. Further information on the miracle man Paracelsus is to be found in the pseudo-Paracelsian 'Secreta Secretorum', a collection of medical and chemical recipes handed down from the mid-sixteenth century. Paracelsus owes his reputation of having stepped down to the same level as the mob to his student, the later printer Johannes Oporinus from Basel. In a letter written in 1565, but only distributed in handwritten copies in 1570, Oporinus reported that his former teacher had been drunk quite often, but had nevertheless fulfilled his duties as a physician. This image of Paracelsus was adapted by the anti-Paracelsians in the following centuries and increased to an incredible extent. Thomas Erastus (1524–83), a determined adversary of Paracelsianism, reported only bad things about Paracelsus's life and work in his writing 'Disputationes de Medicina Nova Philippi Paracelsi' (1570–73), treating him as a drinker whose successful treatments were possible only with the power of Satan.

Paracelsus's 'Nova Medicina'

In his work 'Paragranum', written in 1529–30, Paracelsus for the first time explained his medical theories. These theories, detailed in the 'Opus Paramirum' (completed after 1531), neglected the traditional humoral pathology in favor of the three principles formulated by Paracelsus (Tria prima or Tria principia): Sal [salt], Sulfur, and Mercurius [mercury]. Furthermore Paracelsus assigned an archaeus (mixed Greek and Latin form that means vital force or spirit of the universe) to each organ, a force that controls the functions of the organs. Paracelsus thus established the ontological theory of disease, which presumed that the specific malfunction of a certain organ caused a disease, and not the imbalance of fluids related to the complete organism (Dyscrasia). Closely linked to these ideas was the theory of ens, stating that health is endangered by the ens naturale [constitution], the ens veneni [poisoning or infection], the ens astrorum [climate and environment], and the ens deale [divine providence]. Hohenheim's teaching that tartarian diseases arise when stones are created in the body by deposits and residues can be considered as independent of Tria prima and theory of ends. His monograph 'On miners' disease' (1522–23) is considered to be the earliest work on occupational disease of miners. The 'Astronomia magna' (or 'Philosophia sagax'), completed in 1537, remained unprinted and therefore was handed down only in handwritten copies. In this work Paracelsus explained his medical, cosmological, and anthropological theories.

In the field of surgery, to which he also dedicated one of his writings, he was not only an advocate of new ideas, but he also took over existing theories. However his repeated demands to read the 'book of nature' instead of interpreting the writings of the ancient and Arabian authorities, the emphasis on his own experience as a physician, and last but not least the use of the German language always placed him in great conflict with the established physicians.

Paracelsus's Theology

His writings on religion and theology were rarely published in the early modern times, although their circulation in circles of religious dissidents of Protestantism seems quite certain. Besides questions of Bible exegesis, the position of the Mother of God in God's plan for the world's salvation—a subject often treated in the Reformation—always played a major role in the work of Paracelsus. Furthermore, dogmatic and religious ethical texts can also be found in Paracelsus's bibliography, for example, 'Vita Beata', which called for a perfect Christian life. Paracelsus was a Catholic reformer who rejected the Mauerkirche [stone church] in favor of the Christian parish of the 'inner word' as well as the different 'sects' of Protestantism.

Paracelsus's Tria Principia and His Medicines

The Paracelsian alchemy centered around the Tria principia or Tria prima, which could mean, from the chemical point of view, the burning (sulfur), liquefaction (mercurius), and calcination (sal). Another central point in Paracelsus's ideas was distillation, the extraction of a volatile spiritus or spirit from a solid body. He described alchemy logically as the ars spagyrica, coming from the Greek words spao [separate] and ageiro [connect], which means to separate and to connect (in Latin 'solve et coagula'). The function of alchemy is to produce a subtle quinta essentia from the bodies. This leads to Chemiatrie: the extraction and production of medicines mostly from minerals or metals by use of fire. Some medicines of the early

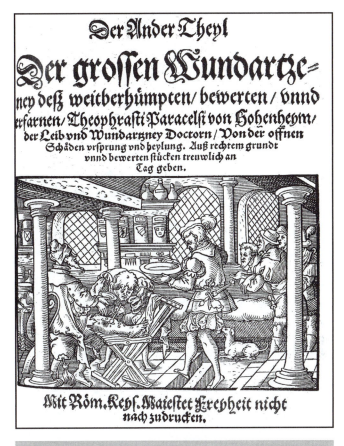

Treatment of a leg covered with sores. Woodcut from *The Grosse Wundartzney . . .*, Frankfurt, 1562. Rare Books, Wellcome Library, London.

modern era can be directly traced back to Paracelsus, for example the antimony preparations and his Laudanum, which became very famous later on. Antimony had already been used in surgery because of its blood-staunching and antiseptic effects before Paracelsus mentioned it in his 'Great Surgery Book', in which he describes the production of an antimony tincture by alchemic means. The first followers of Paracelsus already praised Laudanum, a preparation containing opium, which was considered to be a universal remedy. Nevertheless it has to be stated that Paracelsus clung to the traditional materia medica and also had herbal drugs in his pharmaceutical treasure.

Paracelsus the Alchemist

Although Paracelsus separated the Alchemia medica very strictly from the Alchemia transmutatoria, he did not deny in principle the possibility of metal transformation. But the objective of (al)chemical processes was for him the production of effective medicine rather than the transmutation of metals to gold. Still Paracelsus's use of alchemy for the production of medicine reinforced the imagination of posterity, which saw in him a German Hermes Trismegistos.

Legends also contributed to the idea of Hohenheim as an alchemist of transmutation who knew how to transform impure metals into gold. Fake letters he was supposed to have written to his father Wilhelm, an alleged travel companion Ulrich Poldörfer, Augustin Sattler, or Bartholomäus Korndorfer also increased Paracelsus's reputation as an authority on metal transformation.

Paracelsus the 'Magician'

During the review and reception of Paracelsus's writings by early Paracelsians since the 1560s, the essential features of Hohenheim's cosmological and ontological ideas became known only in shadows, but were not always understood by the editors and recipients. The 'Astronomia magna', taken from some unsecured drafts by Michael Toxites and published in 1571, showed that Astrologia and Magia were very significant in Hohenheim's theory of knowledge. Paracelsus was certainly aware of the danger resulting from the fact that he set up knowledge of the cosmos and God against religious doctrines. With the publication of the 'Paragranum' of 1539, he created fear in his contemporaries that he cured disease with the help of the devil. By 1580 he was mentioned on an Index for the first time before being moved, as an author and heresiarch [arch-heretic], to the first class of the Index published by Pope Clement VIII, where he remained until 1897. The unfavorable judgment of Oporinus was confirmed by another—alleged—student of Paracelsus: Georg Vetter, who worked as a priest at Beerfelden (Odenwald). In 1574 at Eberbach, he told Thomas Erastus that Paracelsus had called a cacodaemonum [evil demon], had joined the devil's movement when he was drunk, and had blasphemed God when he was sober.

History of the Reception of Paracelsus and His Works

There are no secured autographs of Hohenheim handed down, and a recipe sheet ascribed to him and kept in the Austrian National Library in Vienna can hardly have been issued by him. All the other texts—alleged autographs—have been proven to be transcriptions by scribes or students and published by early Paracelsians in the middle of the sixteenth century after being partially translated into Latin. Johannes Huser, a physician from Glogau, arranged the first collection (the so-called 'Baseler Quartausgabe') from 1589 to 1591 at the instigation of the archbishop of Cologne Ernst of Bavaria, although the manuscripts that he consulted are still missing today. A critical version of the medical and scientific writings of Hohenheim was published by the medical historian Karl Sudhoff from Leipzig in fourteen volumes from 1922 to 1933; the religious historian Kurt Goldammer from Marburg published a number of Theologica from 1955 to 1986. Karl Sudhoff also established the bibliographies still valid today of the manuscripts and printed writings of Paracelsus, completed with the 'Corpus Paracelsisticum' (2000–03) published by Jochim Telle and Wilhelm Kühlmann.

The history of the reception of Paracelsus has so far been recorded only partially. It is a fact that he strongly shaped generations of physicians and alchemists. Heterodox theologians from the sixteenth to the nineteenth century treated his social and religious ideas in their works, and his writings may have had a certain influence on the Rosicrucian movement and latter freemason organizations. Theosophists and anthroposophists of the nineteenth and twentieth century saw in Paracelsus a precursor of holistic thinking, trying to bring medicine, alchemy, anthropology, and religious ideas in line with one another. Even today his name is still recognized in esoteric circles.

Bibliography

Primary: 1922–1995. *Sämtliche Werke*, 1. Abt., Medizin., naturwiss. u. philosoph. Schriften (ed. Sudhoff, Karl) 14 vols. 1922–33, supp. vol. ed. Müller, M., and R. Blaser, 1960; 2. Abt., Theolog. u. religionsphilosoph. Schriften, vol. 1 (ed. Matthiessen, W.), 1923, vol. II–VII and Suppl. vol., with Index (ed. Goldammer, Kurt), 1955–95; 1989. *Grosse Wundartzney*. Augsburg 1536 (new edn. with afterword, Benzenhöfer, Udo) (Hannover); 2001–04. (Kühlmann, Wilhelm, and Joachim Telle, eds.) *Der Frühparacelsismus* 2 vol. (Corpus Paracelsisticum. Dokumente frühneuzeitlicher Naturphilosophie in Deutschland vols.1–2) (Tübingen); 2001/2004 (Frühe Neuzeit, 59/89).

Selected English Translations: 1941. (Sigerist, Henry E., ed.) *Four Treatises of Theophrastus von Hohenheim, called Paracelsus* (Baltimore); 1951. (Jacobi, Jolande, ed., Norbert Guterman, trans.) *Selected Writings* (London); 1990. (Goodrick-Clarke, Nicholas, ed. and trans.) *Paracelsus: Essential Readings* (Wellingborough, Northants).

Paracelsus Bibliographies: Sudhoff, Karl, 1894. *Bibliographia Paracelsica. Besprechung der unter Hohenheims Namen 1527–1893 erschienenen Druckschriften.* (Berlin) (rpt. 1958, Graz); Sudhoff, Karl, 1898. *Paracelsus-Handschriften.* (Berlin) (*Versuch einer Kritik der Echtheit der Paracelsischen Schriften*, vol. 2); Weimann, Karl-Heinz, 1963. *Paracelsus—Bibliographie 1932–60* (Wiesbaden); Paulus, Julian, 1997. *Paracelsus—Bibliographie 1961–96* (Heidelberg).

Secondary: Ball, Philip, 2006. *The Devil's Doctor: Paracelsus and the World of Renaissance Magic and Science* (London); Müller-Jahncke, Wolf-Dieter, 2001. *Paracelsus* NDB. vol. 20 (Berlin) pp. 61–64; Engelhardt, Dietrich von, 2001. 'Paracelsus im Urteil der Naturwissenschaften und Medizin des 18. und 19. Jahrhunderts' in *Darstellung, Quellen, Forschungsliteratur* (Halle) (Acta Historica Leopoldina vol. 35); Benzenhöfer, Udo, 1997. *Paracelsus* (Reinbeck); Telle, Joachim, 1994. 'Paracelsus als Alchemiker' in *Paracelsus in Salzburg* (Vorträge bei den Internationalen Kongressen in Salzburg und Badgastein anläßlich des Paracelsus-Jahres 1993), Dopsch, Heinz, and Peter Kramml, eds. (Salzburg), pp 157–172

(Mitteilungen der Gesellschaft für Salzburger Landeskunde vol. 14); Goldammer, Kurt, 1991. *Der göttliche Magier und die Magierin Natur. Religion, Naturmagie und die Anfänge der Naturwissenschaft vom Spätmittelalter bis zur Renaissance mit Beiträgen zum Magie-Verständnis des Paracelsus* (Stuttgart) (*Kosmosophie* vol. 5); Pagel, Walter, 1982. *Paracelsus. An Introduction to Philosophical Medicine in the Era of the Renaissance* 2nd edn. (Basel, Munich, and Paris); *DSB.*

Wolf-Dieter Müller-Jahncke

PARÉ, AMBROISE   (b. Laval, France, 1510; d. Paris, France, 20 December 1590), *surgery, anatomy.*

Humble Origins and Education as a Barber-Surgeon

Despite the humbleness of his origins, Ambroise Paré impressed almost everyone who knew him with his poise, courage, dignity, and compassion, qualities that helped him bring about significant changes in surgical practice and education. In addition to respecting his expertise in surgery, the beleaguered Valois kings of France seemed to appreciate his company as a reminder of what it was to be kingly. He was the most important European surgeon of the sixteenth century and a heroic figure in the history of French medicine.

Most accounts of his origins are unreliable, but from all indications it seems he was born about 1510 in the village of Bourg-Hersent, near the walled town of Laval in the ancient province of Mayenne. Little seems to have been discovered about his antecedents, but it has been conjectured that his father was either a cabinet maker or a barber-surgeon who served the Duke of Laval, Guy XVI, as a valet. The next Duke of Laval, Guy XVII, was to take Ambroise riding through Brittany to a campaign in 1543. Other family members were involved in the art of surgery as well. One of his brothers was a master barber-surgeon who practiced in the neighboring town of Vitre, and a sister, Catherine, married Gaspard Martin, a master surgeon who practiced in Paris.

Where Paré served his apprenticeship is unknown, but he describes an incident in 1525, when, with his brother Jean, the barber-surgeon, they unmasked a mendicant in Angers who was faking a gangrenous arm.

Paré went to Paris between 1530 and 1533, and very likely worked as an apprentice in a barber's shop. Soon he entered Paris's oldest hospital, the Hôtel Dieu, as a compagnon-chirurgien, something like a modern intern. If he arrived in Paris in 1533, he might have encountered Andreas Vesalius, who was there that year to study anatomy with Guinter von Andernach and Jacobus Sylvius. Paré probably assisted the physicians employed by the city to supervise this large hospital, duties which may have included performing dissections while physicians read from established texts and lectured to students. Paré remarked that as a worker at the hospital he had opportunities to examine a vast number of cadavers, many more than were available to medical students at the time. He finished his service at the Hôtel Dieu about 1536.

Shortly thereafter he began pursuing anatomical studies with friend and fellow surgeon Thierry de Hery. The two men passed the required examinations and were licensed together as master barber-surgeons in 1541.

Early Reputation as a Military Surgeon, Roles of Sylvius and Rohan

In 1537, even before he was licensed, Paré was on his way to Italy with the army as surgeon to René, Duke de Montejan. In the siege of Avigliana during the expedition to Turin, Paré, on his very first military expedition, discovered a greatly improved treatment for gunpowder wounds. Paré had been taught on the authority of Giovanni de Vigo, the eminent papal surgeon, and by others that gunshot wounds were poisoned and needed to be cauterized with boiling oil—a painful and destructive process. When the oil supply failed, Paré decided to treat the injuries like other penetrating wounds and applied the 'digestive' dressing of egg yolks, oil of roses, and turpentine. The young surgeon went to bed that night with a guilty conscience fearing for his patients who had been deprived of the horrible purifying process. He was surprised and pleased to find in the next few days that those spared the hot oil recovered more often and more rapidly. Relatively free of the deeply ingrained preference for precedent over observation that frequently prevailed in the healing arts of his day, Paré was able to learn from this finding, and he also listened to the local women healers, one of whom taught him that onion poultices prevented blistering in burn cases.

A Milanese physician called to treat Montejan for liver disease had occasion to observe Paré's work and told the duke that despite his youth, Paré had acquired experience and skill that would make him an invaluable asset to the nobleman and his household. But no one was able to cure Montejan's ailment, and he died at Turin in 1538.

By 1541 Paré was back practicing in Paris, where, using his official title of master barber-surgeon, he married Jeanne Mazelin. The witness to his marriage was a well-known anatomical illustrator of the time, Etienne de la Rivière, a friend who would be of service to Paré at many junctures in years to come.

During this same year, Jacobus Sylvius, the teacher of Vesalius, together with Paré's new military employer, the Vicomte de Rohan, who was greatly impressed by the young surgeon's practical knowledge and insight, began to urge him to write. While serving with the Vicomte at the siege of Perpignan in 1542, Paré devised a method of finding a bullet in the body of a patient after the physicians had failed. He asked the victim, Count Brissac, to assume the same position he was in when the bullet entered his back, and running his hand over the muscles of the shoulder blade felt the position of the ball. In 1543, during an expedition to Brittany, Paré was surgeon to the Duke of Laval, Guy XVII, successor of the nobleman that Paré's father had reputedly served. While on the Brittany campaign, Paré greatly impressed his employer as well as many others of the nobility.

Achievements as an Author in the Vernacular

On his return to Paris, Paré examined Vesalius's *De corporis humani fabrica* for the first time. Its folio-size pages and unforgettable illustrations set a stunning contrast to Paré's first publication which, delayed by his military duties, was not to appear for two more years. Small, simply printed and very solidly bound, *La Méthode de Taraicter les Playes faictes par Hacquebutes* (1545) was meant to be carried into the battlefield. In its preface, addressed to 'young surgeons of good will', Paré expressed the hope that his readers would be able to make use of its sixty-four text pages and twenty-three woodcut illustrations.

Paré's complete rejection of the accepted method of treating gunshot wounds was a more direct confrontation with traditional medical authority than were Vesalius's polite revisions of classical anatomy. Moreover, Paré's findings were expressed not in elegant academic Latin, but in the common tongue. He dedicated the work to his friend, patron, and former military commander, Vicomte de Rohan. Published at Paris in 1545, a Dutch edition appeared two years later in 1547. A second edition of this seminal work appeared in 1552 (dated 1551). Revised and better illustrated, it was later absorbed into Paré's *Dix Livres* and then into the collected works.

In 1549 Paré published his first treatise on anatomy (*Brève Collection de L'administration Anatomique*), which was based on dissections he conducted with other skilled surgeons at the École de médecine. A solid but simply printed work without illustrations, it was intended to improve the background and expertise of barber-surgeon apprentices. Remarkably, it included an obstetrical innovation, the first account since the ancients of podalic version.

Twelve years later, Paré completely revised his anatomy, under the title *Anatomie Universelle du Corps Humain* (1561). While still in a small, convenient format, it included forty-nine woodcuts, many modeled on those of Vesalius, with full credit given to the Belgian anatomist. Paré also included original surgical illustrations. This work was absorbed almost unchanged into his collected *Oeuvres*, and remained in use well into the 1600s.

A tragic tournament accident in 1559 resulted in a serious head wound which, after an agonizing decline, ultimately ended the life of Henri II. Among the medical practitioners who were called from France and the Holy Roman Empire to attend the royal patient were Paré and Vesalius. Both later wrote accounts of the case, and the two skilled practitioners appear together in a well known print depicting the king's final hours. This notable occurrence prompted the king's physician, Chapelain, to request a treatise by Paré on this type of injury. *La Méthode Curative des Plays & Fractures de La Teste Humaine* appeared in 1562. Two years later Paré combined a thorough revision of the latter work with material on urology, largely derivative, and more importantly his first detailed account of how he used ligatures instead of cautery in amputations, in a work entitled *Dix Livres de la Chirurgie* (1564). It also included an interesting analysis of the recent increase of battlefield mortalities, as well as a harrowing personal account of the compound fracture the author himself sustained and from which, against considerable odds, he recovered.

The 1567 plague epidemic in Paris prompted the royal family to request a treatment on that subject by Paré which appeared in 1568, *Traité de la Peste*. The plague treatise was reissued in 1580. Eloquent but almost entirely derived from traditional authorities, the work included an endorsement of the use of antimony for which Paré was later to be attacked. Another of Paré's less original works, *Deux Livres de Chirurgie* (1573), consisted mostly of traditional lore on sexual reproduction, obstetrics and monsters.

In 1574 *Cinq Livres de Chirurgie* included more information on fractures and Paré's response to attacks by the surgeon, Le Paulmier, but scarcely a year later Paré assembled the results of more than forty years of practice and thirty years of diligent study and writing into a comprehensive text which Malgaigne, a surgeon and the great nineteenth-century authority on Paré, termed the first complete surgical treatise since Guy de Chauliac over two hundred years before. Paré devoted much care and considerable funds to its illustrations. *Les Oeuvres* was reedited with minor additions in 1579, published in Latin in 1582, and improved and amplified with pertinent memoirs by Paré in 1585.

Among Paré's lesser works, but of interest in the light they shed on the opposition he faced, are his *Réponse de M. Amboise Paré, premier Chirurgien du Roi, aux calumnies d'aucuns Médecins & Chirurgiens, touchant ses Oeuvres* (1575), defending his collected works, *Discours de la Mumie* (1582), attacking popular beliefs on the efficacy of ground mummy and unicorn's horn, and his 1584, *Réplique d'Ambroise Paré, etc. à la Réponse faîte contre son Discours de la Licorne Réplique*, further rebutting the proponents of these distasteful and dubious nostrums.

Resentment and Criticism from Established Authorities

In 1562 Paré's career hit a high point when, on New Year's Day, as a great family friend and favorite of long standing, he was sworn in as Premier Surgeon to Charles IX. This position gave him a certain amount of authority over surgery in France. It also made him the target of jealousy and resentment from many with more impressive sounding academic credentials.

In about 1568, a regent-physician of the Faculté de Médecine, Julien Le Paulmier, produced a work which on two counts serves as a tribute to Paré's achievements. First, this treatise, covering the same material as Paré's work almost twenty years earlier, casually repeats Paré's doctrines on the treatment of gunshot wounds and amputations without attribution, as if it were accepted wisdom. Second, though a learned physician and not a lowly surgeon, Le Paulmier wrote not in Latin but, like Paré, in the common tongue.

Despite his quiet reliance on Paré's innovations, Le Paulmier attacked Paré (whom he nevertheless disdained to name) for supposed errors in wound treatment that he believed increased mortality among the wounded in the terrible battles of Dreux, St Denis and Rouen. Paré was deeply offended, and wrote a measured reply which is in the *Cinq Livres* [Five Books]. Almost immediately, Le Paulmier arranged for the publication of a venomous counterattack supposedly authored by an anonymous barber-surgeon. As intemperate as this attack might seem, it was only a sample of what was to come.

The death of his patron and friend Charles IX, in 1574, left Paré more vulnerable to attacks from his professional opponents. Two weeks after the printing of Paré's collected works was completed in April 1575, the officials of the Faculté de Médecine led by its dean, Etienne Gourmelen, launched an all-out attack on Paré. They declared this compendium could not be published without their permission and dismissed Paré as an uneducated barber-surgeon unfit to belong to the college of surgeons. Paré campaigned for and gained the right to offer a defense, but a few months later the dean condemned the book as immoral and against the best interests of France. The famous surgeon was accused of lying about his experience, misquoting the medical classics, and including obscene details about sexual reproduction.

Today it seems quite transparent that the physicians were resorting to slander in order to protect themselves against competition from the more competent corps of surgeons that Paré was working to enlarge. It must have been fairly clear to officials at the time as well, because shortly after the case was taken to court, a settlement was made, the book appeared, and it sold out rapidly.

In 1581, at about the same time he was leaving Paris to avoid the inconvenience of the plague, Etienne Gourmelen published his own surgery, which included criticism of Paré's use of the ligature in amputation. It was this final assault which goaded Paré to write his *Apologia*, validating the breadth and richness of his surgical experience, which he contrasts to Gourmelen's medical innocence and theoretical arrogance, and in which he addressed the eminent former dean as the 'little master'. These memoirs appeared in the fourth edition of his *Oeuvres*, published in 1582, when Paré was seventy-two years old.

Clinical Genius

Paré demonstrated amazing boldness and ingenuity in tackling cases that seemed hopeless, some of which were among common soldiers, others among eminent members of the nobility. On his first expedition in 1537–38, an ordinary soldier presented an arm which had been shredded by a musket ball and become gangrenous. Inflammation had traveled down to the elbow. No other surgeons would take the case. Paré was prevailed upon by the man's friends to make the attempt to cure him and consented only reluctantly. Amputating at the elbow, Paré cauterized the wound, made incisions to drain the stump, and urged the patient to exercise as much as possible to increase his strength. However, the patient developed 'convulsions', the descriptions of which suggest tetanus.

Paré had the man taken from the drafty shed in which he was lodged to a stable steaming with fresh manure. After massaging the patient's neck and back with traditional lineaments, he had him wrapped in sheets and straw and buried to the neck in manure. After three days, the patient's rigidity decreased, and Paré pried his jaws open with a screw dilator and fed him raw eggs, milk, and broth. Convulsions finally ceased, the patient's arm healed, and Paré, in a phrase that was to become his trademark formula, concluded that he had treated him, but 'Dieu le guérit' [God healed him]. Paré urged young surgeons not to abandon difficult cases too lightly.

Thirty years later, Charles IX sent Paré to attend the Marquis d'Auret who had suffered for seven months from a gunshot wound in the thigh. Upon his arrival, Paré was discouraged to find the Marquis suffering with high fever, a jaundiced face with sunken eyes, a dry and rough tongue, and a weak, low voice. His thigh was purulent and festering and was presenting symptoms that we would consider evidence of osteomyelitis. The leg was flexed almost to the buttock, which displayed a decubitus ulcer which extended more than three inches wide.

The committee of physicians and surgeons who attended the Marquis were so fearful of his reaction to pain that they had not ordered his bed changed for almost two months. Paré indicated that the patient's young age was a source of hope, and he outlined and obtained endorsement for a plan of treatment. Within hours, the Marquis's thigh had been drained and dressed; he was in a clean bed and for the first time in weeks was sleeping peacefully. Paré's physical treatment of the wound was traditional, but his ingenuity in maintaining his patient's morale through the course of a painful recovery was brilliant. He employed massage, soothing lotions, and calming sounds such as simulated rain, all the while carefully maintaining grooming. He used positive stimuli from musicians and jesters.

The Marquis's recovery was celebrated by his subjects, as he was both generous and much beloved.

Paré and 'Religion'

Academic disagreements were not the only conflicts to beset Paré. He lived in a time of great religious turmoil, and this unrest took the lives of many around him. When he was sent by Charles IX to treat Admiral Coligny (a Protestant and close friend of the king) after an attempt on Coligny's life, Paré barely survived the beginning of the St Bartholomew's Day Massacre by fleeing across the rooftops and hiding in the King's bedroom. Throughout his life Paré was always a moderate, critical of fanatics in both the Catholic and Protestant factions. In 1562, shortly after his appointment as Premier Surgeon, Paré barely survived an assassination attempt by poison which was made 'because of religion', as he put it. The word *religion* was taken by most nineteenth-century historians to mean 'my Protestant convictions'. This opinion is sometimes regarded as established fact, and Paré is still sometimes referred to as 'the Huguenot surgeon in the Catholic court', but as several recent historians (Dumaitre, 1986; Hamby, 1967) point out, the weight of evidence is on the other side. Paré stood as godfather to many children, thus publicly asserting his loyalty to the Roman church before congregations and clergy in his own Paris neighborhood. Clerical authorities would not have allowed a suspected Huguenot to serve this function and it is hard to imagine a man of Paré's integrity taking such a role falsely. Paré's own parish church was presided over by a notorious heresy-hunter who would scarcely have ignored even rumors to this effect.

The 'religion' Paré refers to thus seems to be the fanaticism of his would-be murderers and their resentment of his moderation. The last historical image we have of Paré comes from the journal of an eyewitness who saw Paré in 1590, in the midst of a long hard siege, confront the military governor of Paris, the Archbishop of Lyons. The journal-writer quotes Paré as saying, 'Monseigneur, these poor people whom you see here about you are dying of the cruel rage of hunger, and demand pity of you. For God's sake Monsieur, give it to them, if you would have God countenance you.' The keeper of the journal further describes the astonishment of the Archbishop and the lasting effect of the old man's words on the hardened politician.

Ambroise Paré was beloved in his day as much for his compassion as for his insight and competence. He served as a valuable role model for many in the next two generations of surgeons, striking a new balance between tradition and innovation in surgery. He left a highly skilled surgical faculty behind him, including Jacques Guillemeau, Antoine Portail, Pierre Pigray, and Severin Pinceau. After Paré's clinical advances, following upon Vesalius' achievements in renewing anatomical investigation, one would have expected that it would be easier for surgeons and physicians to argue from experience as well as authority.

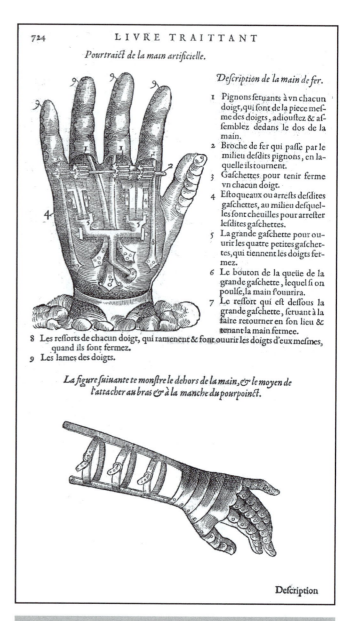

Prosthetic hand designed by Ambroise Paré. Woodcut from *Les oeuvres de M. Ambroise Paré . . .*, Paris, 1575. Rare Books, Wellcome Library, London.

On the contrary, the pettiness, jealousy, and greed that marked most of Paré's enemies in life gradually prevailed after his death in the institutions most important to surgical practice. Due to the avarice and short-sightedness in the College of St Côme, and the quiet sabotage by the physicians of the Faculté de Médecine who tended to despise all surgeons, standards were sacrificed in the interest of profit until a new revival slowly began late in the seventeenth century.

Bibliography

Primary: 1585. *Les Oeuvres*, 4th edn. (Paris); 1665. Johnson, Thomas. *The Works of that famous Chirurgon, Ambroise Parey,*

Translated out of the Latin and Compared with the French (London); 1840–1841. *Oeuvres complete d'Ambroise Paré, edited by Malgaigne, J.F.,* 3 vols. (Paris); 1960. (Hamby, Wallace B., ed.) *Case Reports and Autopsy Records of Ambroise Paré* (Springfield, IL).

Secondary: Berriot-Salvadore, Evelyne, 2003. *Ambroise Paré (1510–1590): pratique et écriture de la science à la renaissance* (Paris); Crenn, Bernard, 1990. *Actes du Colloque Internationale: 'Ambroise Paré et son temps'* (Laval, France); Dumaitre, Paule, 1986. *Ambroise Paré Chirurgien de Quatre Rois de France* (Paris); Hamby, Wallace B., 1967. *Ambroise Paré Surgeon of the Renaissance* (St Louis); Le Paulmier, Stephen, 1887. *Ambroise Paré d'après de nouveaux documents* (Paris); Malgaigne, J. F., 1840. Introduction in *Oeuvres complètes d'Ambroise Paré* (Paris) pp. I–CCCLI; *DSB*.

Ynez Violé O'Neill

PARENT-DUCHÂTELET, ALEXANDRE-JEAN-BAPTISTE

(b. Paris, France, 29 September 1790; d. Paris, 7 March 1836), *public health.*

Parent-Duchâtelet was born into a Parisian family that had been rich before 1789. Stripped of their seigneurial rights during the Revolution, the Parent family left Paris for Châtelet, a country house near Montargis. The oldest of six children, Parent-Duchâtelet spent his childhood there and was educated by his parents. When he was sixteen, his father sent him to Paris to continue his studies, and he pursued medicine.

Parent-Duchâtelet received his MD from the Paris Faculty of Medicine in 1814 at the age of twenty-four. Although he continued to practice medicine at the Pitié Hospital, after 1821 he devoted himself to public health. His principal publications were the two-volume *De la prostitution dans la ville de Paris* (1836) and twenty-nine articles on public health, most of which were first published in the *Annales d'hygiène publique et de médecine légale.* After his death they appeared in two volumes as *Hygiène publique* [Public Hygiene] (1836). Colleagues praised his early sociohygienic studies on ships carrying fertilizer on the Bièvre river, which was the site of many industries, and on the sewers of Paris, and by 1827 recognized him as one of the leading French public hygienists. That same year Parent-Duchâtelet competed for the chair of hygiene at the Paris Faculty of Medicine, but the position went to proto-hematologist Gabriel Andral.

Along with his friend and colleague Louis-René Villermé, Parent-Duchâtelet was one of the leaders of the French public health movement. He was a founding editor of the of the movement's organ, the *Annales d'hygiène publique et de médecine légale,* and was a frequent contributor. He was a member of the Royal Academy of Medicine and served on the Paris Health Council [Conseil de salubrité de la ville de Paris et du département de la Seine], an advisory board of health to the Prefect of Police, who was the administrator in charge of public health for Paris.

Parent-Duchâtelet developed an international reputation as the leading French urban and occupational hygienist, and he published major studies of sewers and sewer workers, dock workers, tobacco workers, the horse butchering industry, and prostitution. He was also the theorist of the new interdisciplinary specialty of public hygiene and the main spokesman for the professionalization of the discipline. His goal was to make public hygiene scientific, by which he meant studied rigorously and supported by numerical data, employing onsite interviews, observations, and use of surveys. All his studies illustrated these methodologies. He also emphasized the interdisciplinary nature of public hygiene as being reliant on the knowledge of physicians, veterinarians, engineers, architects, statisticians, and administrators. A variety of experts was necessary to investigate and manage complicated public health problems, he believed.

The work for which Parent-Duchâtelet is best known is his study of prostitution in Paris, which earned him the sobriquet of 'the Newton of the bawdy house'. After eight years of research he concluded that prostitution was an 'industry against hunger', suggesting that prostitutes themselves were blameless. He did blame prostitutes for spreading disease but exonerated the men who visited them. A realist, Parent-Duchâtelet did not believe men would change their habits, nor would women abandon the trade. Therefore, he proposed the registration and regular medical inspection and treatment of prostitutes to manage the spread of venereal diseases. Historians have criticized him for helping institute a draconian surveillance system of the women involved in prostitution while liberating men from responsibility for their actions.

Just as his study of prostitution was on the verge of publication, Parent-Duchâtelet suddenly became ill with pneumonia and died.

Bibliography

Primary: 1836. *De la prostitution dans la ville de Paris* 2 vols. (Paris); 1836; *Hygiène publique* 2 vols. (Paris).

Secondary: La Berge, Ann, 1992. *The Early Nineteenth-Century French Public Health Movement* (New York); Harsin, Jill, 1985. *Policing Prostitution in Nineteenth-Century Paris* (Princeton); Leuret, François, 1836. 'Notice historique sur A. J. B. Parent-Duchâtelet.' *Annales d'hygiène publique et de médecine légale* 16: v–xxiv.

Ann F. La Berge

PARK, WILLIAM HALLOCK

(b. New York, New York, USA, 30 December 1863; d. New York, 6 April 1939), *medicine, bacteriology, epidemiology.*

Park, son of Rufus Park, a businessman, and Harriet Joanna Hallock, graduated from City College of New York (1883). In that year, he entered Columbia University, College of Physicians and Surgeons, graduating in 1886. After an internship and a two-year surgical residency, in 1889 he undertook a year of postgraduate study in Vienna. Returning to New York City (1890), Park established a part-time medical practice and accepted a scholarship to study bacteriology in Prudden's laboratory at Columbia. Park's clinical and bacteriological studies of diphtheria drew the attention of Hermann Biggs, director of the laboratory of the New York Board of Health (first municipal laboratory in the United States), who appointed him associate director (1893). When Biggs became health officer of the City, Park became director of the laboratory, remaining for forty-three years. Concurrently, from 1900, Park was professor and chairman of the department of bacteriology of the Bellevue Hospital Medical College, later New York University's College of Medicine. In 1933 he was named the first Hermann M. Biggs professor of preventive medicine.

When Park joined the staff of the laboratory, and well into the twentieth century, diphtheria was a major cause of morbidity and mortality in the United States. Park made major contributions to its control: by demonstrating the role of healthy carriers in its transmission and the importance of identifying and isolating them in the households of cases (1893), by providing diphtheria antitoxin free of charge for the treatment of cases (1894), and by promoting the use of the Schick Test followed by active immunization with toxin-antitoxin of those testing positive (1915–20). In 1900 his laboratory undertook studies of the bacterial contamination of milk, fundamental to the control of infantile diarrhea, a major cause of childhood mortality. Park was also concerned with the possibility of contamination of milk by healthy typhoid carriers. These studies provided the justification for strict regulation of New York City's milk supply.

In 1907 and for years afterward, Park's laboratory monitored typhoid carrier Mary Mallon ('Typhoid Mary') who had infected scores of people for whom she cooked (Park, 1916). Park also made major contributions to the control of highly prevalent bovine tuberculosis in children by demonstrating the presence of the organism in milk. Over the years, his laboratory expanded to investigate the full range of bacterial infections, combining research with service, made possible by contributions from private sources to augment funding by the municipal administration.

Park's textbook, *Pathogenic Microorganisms*, was the 'bible of bacteriology' for medical students and bacteriologists throughout the publication of its eleven editions between 1899 and 1939.

Park was active in many professional organizations. He was a charter member and, subsequently, president of the Society of American Bacteriologists and the American Epidemiological Society. He was president of the Society of Experimental Pathologists, vice president of the New York Academy of Medicine, and president of the American Public Health Association. Among his many honors were the prestigious Sedgwick Memorial Medal from the American Public Health Association and the Public Welfare Medal of the National Academy of Sciences.

At the dedication in 1936 of a new laboratory building named for Park, a letter from President Roosevelt was read: 'Your contribution to medical progress will continue to benefit the people of New York, and of the Nation, and of the World long after this splendid laboratory has crumbled into dust' (Schaeffer, 1985, p. 1302). Indeed, so it is, as the laboratory building was demolished years ago.

Bibliography

Primary: 1916. 'Typhoid Bacilli Carriers.' *Journal of the American Medical Association* 51: 981–982.

Secondary: Leavitt, Judith W., 1996. *Typhoid Mary: Captive to the Public's Health* (Boston); Schaeffer, Morris, 1985. 'William H Park (1863–1939): His Laboratory and His Legacy.' *American Journal of Public Health* 75: 1296–1302; Oliver, Wade W., 1941. *The Man Who Lived for Tomorrow. A Biography of William Hallock Park, M.D.* (New York); *DAMB*.

Warren Winkelstein, Jr.

PARK ROSS, GEORGE ARCHIBALD

PARK ROSS, GEORGE ARCHIBALD (b. Dingwall, Scotland, 19 January 1879; d. Hilton, Natal, South Africa, 19 May 1958), *public health, malariology.*

Park Ross achieved distinction as a public health official in the Province of Natal, South Africa. Born in the Scottish highlands, he was the son of a merchant, George Ross, and an Edinburgh-bred mother, Catherine Park, to whose family the eminent explorer-physician Mungo Park had belonged. In about 1901, Park Ross attached his third given name, Park, to his surname.

Park Ross entered medical studies at the University of Edinburgh in 1895 and graduated in 1901, having served for a year (1900–01) with the Lovat Scouts during the Boer War. His medical qualifications included the Diploma of Public Health (RCS Edinburgh) and the Diploma of Tropical Medicine (Liverpool). In late 1903, he joined the staff of the Seamen's Hospital, Albert Docks, attached to the London School of Tropical Medicine. He thus worked under both Ronald Ross and Patrick Manson, and it was Manson who facilitated his appointment as Medical Officer on the Anglo-Portuguese Boundary Commission, which surveyed in the Zambezia regions in 1904–05. On leave from the Commission in early 1905, Park Ross visited Durban, where his skills were drafted for microscopy amidst an epidemic of malaria. Natal and malaria were to subsequently become the chief geographical and medical concerns of his career, which focused especially on the ecology and epidemiology of disease in lowland, semitropical areas. Reports of his early investigations include one on hookworm (1906) which became his MD thesis (Edinburgh, 1908), and on complex causation that required differential diagnosis (1906, 1910).

After Union in 1910, public health fell to the central government. Within the Union department, Park Ross advanced from a toehold as government bacteriologist and pathologist and assistant port health officer at Durban, to become assistant and ultimately deputy chief health officer in Natal. Meanwhile, with enhanced authority as a major in the South African Medical Corps, he conducted a vigilant sleeping sickness prevention program, to screen and treat all military personnel returning from German East Africa to tsetse-infested portions of Zululand. The program also entailed demarcation of a tsetse zone to which unlicensed entry by veterans was proscribed. Such draconian measures could not be sustained after 1918, but were echoed in Park Ross's later insistence, based upon high incidences of mortality among labor recruits brought from non-malarial areas to work on lowland railway construction and sugar estates in the mid-1920s. He advocated, unsuccessfully, that men from endemic areas not be recruited for the gold fields, but reserved for employment in the Natal lowlands.

Park Ross won international acclaim in the mid-1930s for the anti-malaria campaign in Natal. Locally he gave a strong face and voice to public health, sometimes outrunning his superiors and the colonial mentality with his foresight and increasing sense of the necessity of a comprehensive approach. Popular suspicion among African people was gradually overcome through the activities of African Malaria Assistants. The peak of success occurred in 1933–34, with demonstrations that the spraying of interiors of African dwellings with a pyrethrum-based insecticide dramatically reduced incidences of malaria. When malaria subsided, he deployed the Health Assistants in tuberculosis surveys and education. Some joined Sydney Kark, pioneer of community health care. Park Ross's achievements in disease control and prevention were thus equaled by a human legacy—the invaluable cohort of health workers he had nurtured.

Bibliography

Primary: 1913. 'A Fictitious Native Disease (*Isigwebedhla*).' *Annals of Tropical Medicine and Parasitology* 7: 371-376; 1923. 'Control of Malaria in the Union.' *Medical Journal of South Africa* 18: 134-146; 1936. 'Insecticide as a Major Measure of Control of Malaria: being an account of methods and organisation put into place in Natal and Zululand during the past 6 years.' *Quarterly Bulletin of the Health Organisation of the League of Nations* 51: 114–132.

Secondary: Jeeves, Alan, 1997. 'Migrant Workers and Epidemic Malaria on the South African Estates, 1906–1948' in Jeeves, Alan, and Jonathan Crush, eds., *White Farms, Black Labor: The State and Agrarian Change in Southern Africa, 1910–1950* (Portsmouth, NH) pp. 114–136, 305–312; LeSueur, David, Brian Sharp, and Christopher Appleton, 1993. 'Historical Perspective of the Malaria Problem in Natal with Emphasis on the Period 1928–1932.' *South African Journal of Science* 89: 232–238.

Marcia Wright

PARKER, PETER (b. Framingham, Massachusetts, USA, 18 June 1804; d. Washington, D.C., USA, 10 January 1888), *surgery, missionary medicine.*

Parker was the fifth child of Nathan, a farmer of modest means, and Catherine Murdock. He grew up in an atmosphere of stern Calvinism. He attended Day's Academy at Wrentham (1826) and Amherst College (1827–30); in 1830 he transferred to Yale, where he completed his undergraduate study. In 1831 he commenced graduate studies in theology and medicine at Yale. The American Board of Commissioners for Foreign Missions accepted his application for the post of medical missionary to China in October 1833. Parker received his MD from Yale in March 1834 and was ordained by the Presbyterian Church in Philadelphia in May. He sailed for China in June and arrived at Canton on 26 October 1834. Due to illness, Parker went to Singapore to recuperate in December 1834. There he studied local languages and opened a dispensary.

Parker returned to Canton in autumn 1835 to open the Canton Ophthalmic Hospital in the foreign factory district, which could accommodate forty patients. Besides treating diseases of the eyes, Parker also performed lithotomy and surgical removal of tumors. Lamqua, a local artist specializing in Western-style art, vividly portrayed patients suffering from large tumors, and the stark contrast of their condition before and after treatment. The hospital attracted a large number of Chinese patients, whose endurance of pain Parker praised. He was sufficiently overburdened with clinical demands that he was unable to engage in proselytizing activities. In his diaries, Parker described the anxiety and sense of guilt caused by the situation. Together with the American missionary Elijah C. Bridgman and the English surgeon Thomas R. Colledge, Parker founded the Medical Missionary Society in China in February 1838. In July Parker went to Macao to open a hospital while the Canton hospital was refurbished, returning to Canton three months later.

Delegates from the Imperial Commissioner Lin Ze-xu, who was in charge of stamping out the opium trade, visited Parker several times on the eve of the first Opium War. Lin inquired about geographical matters and cures for opium addiction, and he asked Parker to translate some passages from Vattel's *Law of the Nations*. Lin, who had a hernia, also acquired trusses from Parker, although he would not allow the doctor to examine him, as the two never actually met. The outbreak of war forced Parker to leave China in July 1840. In January 1841 Parker delivered a sermon in Congress and met politicians and dignitaries. Soon after his marriage with Harriet Webster in March, Parker undertook a fundraising tour to England and France.

Parker went to Canton again in June 1842. He served as a translator in Caleb Cushing's diplomatic mission, which negotiated the first treaty between China and the United States. The American Board disapproved of Parker's foray into diplomacy at the expense of missionary work and severed its relationship with him in 1845. Parker nevertheless continued his medical practice at Canton, and he introduced anesthesia to China, using ether on a Chinese patient in 1847 and chloroform the next year. He was, however, increasingly drawn to diplomatic work and served as chargé d'affaires for the American legation to China (1846–55). Parker was appointed Commissioner to China in 1856, but the American government did not support his proposals of aggressive action against China. He was discharged in 1857 and returned to the United States (1858), spending his retirement in Washington.

Bibliography

Primary: 1846. 'Notes of surgical practice amongst the Chinese.' *Monthly Journal of Medical Science* 66: 393–398.

Secondary: Gulick, Edward V., 1973. *Peter Parker and the Opening of China* (Cambridge, MA); Stevens, George B., 1972. *The Life, Letters, and Journals of the Rev. and Hon. Peter Parker* (Wilmington, DE); Spence, Jonathan, 1969. *To Change China: Western Advisers in China 1620–1960* (Boston); *DAMB.*

Shang-Jen Li

PARKES, EDMUND ALEXANDER (b. Bloxham, Oxfordshire, England, 29 March 1819; d. Bitterne, Hampshire, England, 15 March 1876), *hygiene.*

The son of a textile manufacturer, William Parkes and his wife Frances Parkes (née Byerley), Parkes was raised a Non-Conformist, his parents being prominent Unitarians. He was educated at the Blue Coat School in Warwick and at Christ's Hospital in London and University College, London, graduating MB in 1841; he was made an MRCS in 1840.

In 1841 Parkes entered the Army Medical Service and spent three years as an assistant surgeon in India and Burma. He then left the Army to take a position at University College Hospital, London, but his brief military career provided him with valuable experience of a range of diseases and formed the basis of his early publications, *The Dysentery and Hepatitis of India* (1846) and *Researches into the Pathology and Treatment of Asiatic or Algide Cholera* (1847). These works drew upon contemporary theories of physiology and highlighted the role of respiratory and blood disorders.

Parkes's expertise led to his being employed by the newly formed General Board of Health, in 1849, to consider the vexed question of the contagiousness of cholera. The recent epidemic in London confirmed his view that cholera was contagious only in certain circumstances, an opinion which was broadly in line with that of the Board of Health. In the same year, Parkes was promoted first physician of University College Hospital and professor of clinical medicine. His editorship of the *British and Foreign Medico-Chirurgical Review* between 1852 and 1855 is also indicative of his elevated status within the profession. Amidst these duties, Parkes found time to write on diseases of the heart and skin and the effects of alcohol upon health. In August 1850, he married Mary Jane Chattock; they had no children.

The Crimean War of 1854–56 saw Parkes return to military medicine. During the war he was involved in several aspects of medical planning, including assisting the engineer Isambard Kingdom Brunel (1769–1849) in the preparation of a prefabricated hospital. Afterward, he became the first professor of hygiene at the newly formed Army Medical College, at which he became a popular teacher and a renowned researcher. His work on human excretion earned him an FRS in 1861.

During his time at the Army Medical College Parkes wrote his most famous work, the *Manual of Practical Hygiene* (1864). This book became indispensable to all military medical officers and was extensively used by civilians. The *Manual* was notable not only for its sound practical advice but for being based on the most up-to-date theories of pathology and physiology, including human nutrition.

The holistic nature of military hygiene, which encompassed everything from diet and personal habits to sanitary engineering, is evident throughout Parkes's later work and reflected his religious beliefs. One of his last works was a pamphlet written for the Society for the Promotion of Christian Knowledge, *On Personal Care of Health* (1876), which followed an old tradition of providing sanitary advice for persons at various stages in their life. As in his other writings, Parkes stressed the desirability of maintaining a healthy balance between body, soul, and environment. His last book, *Public Health* (1876), dealt with the burgeoning field of 'state medicine' and is notable for its call for more action in rural sanitation, which he felt had been neglected.

Parkes's remaining years were dogged by ill health and his early death from tuberculosis was the cause of much sorrow. He and his wife had no children of their own, but their nephew, Louis Coltman Parkes, followed in his uncle's footsteps as a writer on hygiene and public health. Parkes's name also lives on in a prize awarded annually by the Army Medical Service for the best dissertation on hygiene.

Bibliography

Primary: 1847. *Researches into the Pathology and Treatment of Asian or Algide Cholera* (London); 1864. *Manual of Practical Hygiene* (London); 1876. *On Personal Care of Health* (London).

Secondary: Harrison, Mark, 1994. *Public Health in British India* (Cambridge); Cantlie, Neil, 1974. *A History of the Army Medical Department* (Edinburgh); *Oxford DNB.*

Mark Harrison

PARKINSON, JAMES (b. Shoreditch, London, England, 11 April 1755; d. Hoxton, London, 21 December 1824), *general practice, neurology.*

The son of an apothecary and surgeon, Parkinson apprenticed with his father for his medical training and took over his practice following his death. We know little of his early education, but from his slim volume—*The Hospital Pupil*—we can assume that his recommendations for the proper grounding of a physician in Latin, Greek, natural philosophy, and shorthand were his grounding as well. He attended John Hunter's (1728–93) lectures on surgery and anatomy, making notes in shorthand, which were published by his son a century later. It is thought that he may have been a founding member of the London Medical and Chirurgical Society as well as a founding member of the Geological Society.

Parkinson married Mary Dale when he was twenty-six, and they had five children, one of whom became a doctor and later published some cases with his father. During the political scandals in England following the American and French revolutions, Parkinson became a quiet revolutionary, reformer, and pamphleteer and was a member of the reform groups, the Society for Constitutional Information and the London Corresponding Society. He wrote pamphlets in favor of revolution without bloodshed, restoration of the rights of the disenfranchised, equitable taxation, the amendment of the poor laws that imposed prison for those who sought employment in other parishes, abolition of the game laws that allowed the rich to hunt on the lands of the poor (but not vice versa), and proper remuneration of the clergy from the vast revenues of the bishops. Under suspicion of being involved in the Pop-Gun Plot to assassinate King George III, he was called to account to the Privy Council, where he admitted only that he was a member of the societies and that he was 'Old Hubert', the *nom de plume* of an anonymous writer of political tracts.

He was a prolific writer on many subjects, most aimed at the lay public rather than at the medical profession. His first paper was a critical view of the medical teaching of Hugh Smith. He also wrote on the importance of sport and healthy lifestyle, advice on self-medication, and the improvement of trusses. He published a home medical advice book, a chemical pocketbook, a book of advice to parents who wanted their children to enter the medical profession, and a monograph on gout, which explained how a substance in the blood must have precipitated in the joints and how an alkaline agent of soda could be beneficial to the condition. Always pursuing the interests of the public, he spent his Sundays opening Sunday schools for the poor.

His lasting fame is associated with a small, sixty-six-page volume that described six cases of a disorder that he called the shaking palsy or paralysis agitans, published in 1817, when he was sixty-two. He noted that Galen, Sylvius, Juncker, Cullen, and others had recorded an illness of shaking palsy, but he described it in such detail that others could confidently diagnose it. His description was a very full one but did not note the masklike facies (even though it is now called Parkinsonian facies) and did not accurately define rigidity. Parkinson was unable to observe any postmortem material and encouraged others to seek a cause, which he postulated might be in the cervical cord or medulla. His suggestions for therapy included bleeding, blistering, vesicatories, and creating a draining issue with a caustic. In an age of large randomized clinical trials it is sobering to note that Parkinson described an important syndrome and made a major contribution to medicine by the simple observation of a few patients, some just seen passing in the street.

In his later years he was more interested in geology but did publish with his son the first postmortem description of ruptured appendix and a case of trismus that was treated successfully.

It is likely that Parkinson would have been forgotten, as there was little attention paid to his description of shaking palsy, particularly in England. Upon his death, there was no obituary, no portrait of him exists, and his grave in Hoxton Parish burial ground has no marker. A photograph that accompanies some reprints of his book is obviously incorrect, as he died before the birth of photography. When his name was raised in a discussion in Paris in 1850, he was referred to as 'Patterson'.

Jean-Martin Charcot (1825–93), who was interested in separating the tremor of multiple sclerosis from that described by Parkinson, first started calling the disorder Parkinson's disease, as he didn't like the term paralysis agitans, noting that there was rigidity but not paralysis. The English still ignored Parkinson, but the endocrinologist Leonard Rowntree, visiting England from the United States, noted the lack of attention and in 1912 wrote a paper for the *Johns Hopkins Hospital Reports*, subsequently published as a book. The increasing interest in the disease during the twentieth century brought Parkinson's name to the fore, and he is now one of the best-known eponymous figures in medicine.

Bibliography

Primary: 1800. *The Hospital Pupil* (London); 1805. *Observations on the Nature and Care of Gout* (London); 1817. *An Essay on the Shaking Palsy* (London); 1822. *Outlines of Oryctology: An Introduction to the Study of Fossil Organic Remains* (London).

Secondary: Morris, A. D., 1989. *James Parkinson: His Life and Times*, Rose, F. Clifford, ed. (Boston); Kelly, Emerson C., 1971. 'James Parkinson' in Kelly, E. C., ed., *Classics of Neurology* (Huntington, NY); Critchley, Macdonald, ed., 1955. *James Parkinson (1755–1824): A Bicentennial Volume of Papers Dealing with Parkinson's Disease. Incorporating the Original, "Essay on the Shaking Palsy"* (London); Rowntree, L., 1912. *James Parkinson* (Baltimore); *DSB*; *Oxford DNB*.

Jock Murray

PARRAN, THOMAS, Jr. (b. near St Leonard, Maryland, USA, 28 September 1892; d. Pittsburgh, Pennsylvania, USA, 16 February 1968), *public health, venereal disease.*

Parran was born and raised on his father's tobacco farm near St Leonard in southern Maryland. His early education was at home. He graduated from St John's College in Annapolis with a bachelor's degree in 1911. He obtained his medical degree from Georgetown University Medical School in 1915 and served his residency at Sibley Memorial Hospital in Washington, D.C. His lifelong interest in public health and medical research was piqued by two summers spent working in the District of Columbia Health Department laboratory of Joseph J. Kinyoun, who had been the first director of the Hygienic Laboratory, the predecessor of the National Institutes of Health (NIH). Kinyoun recruited Parran to join a field team of young U.S. Public Health Service (PHS) physicians who were building privies and surveying rural sanitary conditions in the American South and Midwest.

In September 1917 Parran qualified for an assistant surgeon's commission in the PHS. This led to a series of field assignments in rural health services administration, sanitation, and the control of communicable diseases, during which he became very knowledgeable about the role of local health departments. He recognized the need for their reorganization and better funding for more effective provision of services. Between assignments he held administrative positions in Washington. In 1923 he took the six-month laboratory methods course at the Hygienic Laboratory.

In September 1926 Parran was appointed assistant surgeon general in charge of the division of venereal diseases in the PHS. In this capacity, Parran worked to remove the moral stigma from venereal diseases. For him, syphilis was a serious medical condition and needed to be treated as such. In 1930 Franklin Roosevelt, then governor of New York, recruited Parran on a leave of absence from the PHS to become State Health Commissioner for New York. When Roosevelt was elected president in 1932, Parran became one of his chief advisors on questions of national health priorities and medical research and was very active in New Deal politics. He was appointed to the Committee on Economic Security involved in drafting the Social Security Act of 1935. Title VI of the Act authorized $8 million dollars for state and city public health departments and $2 million dollars for scientific research into disease.

In April 1936 Parran was appointed Surgeon General of the United States, a position he held with distinction until 1948. In the late 1930s and 1940s he pursued his syphilis control campaign through research, the development of treatment centers, and public education. He sought to increase public awareness of the threat that syphilis posed to the health of the nation and its economic cost. His best known publication is his book on this topic, *Shadow on the Land: Syphilis* (1937). Parran also set about expanding the presence of the U.S. federal government in public health matters. World War II offered opportunities for new initiatives, including the transformation of malaria control programs into the establishment of the Communicable Disease Center (forerunner of the Centers for Disease Control) and widespread screening for tuberculosis. With adroit political maneuvering by Parran, the PHS became the primary federal health agency. In addition, the research capacity of the NIH was increased and its ability to award research grants to universities and other institutions was engineered.

Parran was also a leader in international health issues. His work was instrumental in the development of the World Health Organization as part of the United Nations and he traveled widely on fact finding missions for this organization. In October 1948 he left the PHS and became the first dean of a new school of public health at the University of Pittsburgh, which was endowed by the Mellon family. After ten years of academic administration, he retired in July 1958 and became involved with Mellon family philanthropy. He was appointed president of the Avalon Foundation and continued as trustee of the A. W. Mellon Educational and Charitable Trust. His many philanthropic and public health activities continued until his death in February 1968.

Bibliography

Primary: 1937. *Shadow on the Land: Syphilis* (New York).

Secondary: Brandt, Allan M., 1985. *No Magic Bullet: A Social History of Venereal Disease in the United States since 1880* (New York), chap. 4; Furman, Bess, 1973. *A Profile of the United States Public Health Service, 1798–1948* (Washington, DC). chaps. 16, 17, and 18; *DAMB*.

Caroline Hannaway

PASTEUR, LOUIS (b. Dole, France, 27 December 1822; d. Villeneuve l'Etang, France, 28 September 1895), *crystallography, chemistry, microbiology, immunology.*

Pasteur was born in Dole and grew up in Arbois, towns in the Jura. Pasteur's father, a veteran of the Napoleonic wars and a tanner by occupation, believed in the importance of education. After a ruthlessly classical and scientific secondary education, Pasteur entered the sciences section of the Ecole normale supérieure (Normale sup), whose function was to produce high quality lycée teachers (*agrégés*). After passing the *agrégation*, Pasteur, though recognized for his pedagogical skills, contrived to stay in Paris and work in the laboratory of Jérôme Balard, whose fleeting fame came from his discovery of bromine in 1826. In 1849, with the help of leading Parisian scientists, he got a position in chemistry at the University of Strasbourg and subsequently married the rector's daughter.

In 1854 Pasteur became professor of chemistry and the first dean of the faculty of sciences in Lille. He stayed there until 1857, when he was appointed administrator and director of scientific studies at Normale sup. Although Pasteur's administrative career at Normale sup ended as a result of a student *fronde* against his 'cruel and unusual' discipline, he succeeded in whipping the sciences section into superb shape, making its research efforts scientifically competitive with the Ecole polytechnique. Pasteur stayed in Paris: Normale sup, including directorship of the laboratory of physiological chemistry, the Sorbonne (1867–74), and director of the Institut Pasteur. A stroke in 1868 left him with a non-disabling hemiplegia, and he steadily weakened after a second stroke in October 1887. Between 1889 and 1895 he lived in a splendid apartment in the Institut Pasteur, an institution privately funded but also publicly supported, which was the nucleus of the future medical empire with the greater French empire it supported.

Crystallography

Partly influenced by Auguste Laurent, Pasteur became interested in crystallography (optical activity and crystalline asymmetry). His research on chirality earned him his doctorate (1847) and established his scientific reputation. Pasteur's work on the crystals of tartaric acid, the chief organic acid in wine, adumbrated his famous future. His work on these crystals led to the study of fermentation, which, like crystallography, was a hot research topic with a number of high-stake issues to be resolved. In studying wine and, at governmental request, its diseases, Pasteur, the man with the microscope, approached the liquid from a new point of view: that of microbiology. His brilliant, original research led to the development of a new science, enology, and a controversial preventive cure (heating) for wine's bacterial diseases. Several scholars have noted that Pasteur's scientific work often proceeded by analogy. The analogy he found in organic processes between fermentation and putrefaction because of the growth and action of microorganisms revolutionized biological science and medical thought and eventually surgery.

From crystallography to rabies, or to put a conceptual spin on things, from fermentation to pathology: the journey appears discontinuous, but commentators usually follow Pasteur in seeing a logical thread running through his research life. The trick seems to be to associate asymmetry and optical activity with life, to note that various fermentations require the intervention of a living organism, then to leap by analogy from fermentation to putrefaction and disease. This idea was important to Pasteur but seems far-fetched to us, and seeing his accomplishment as some sort of Aristotelian *Gesamtkunstwerk* hardly matters to the history of medicine.

Fermentation and Spontaneous Generation

When Pasteur began research on fermentation, two clashing views existed: the dominant chemical theory, according to which living yeast cells are irrelevant because dying yeast cells and putrefying substances cause the process; the second, the weaker germ, or vitalistic, theory, in which a living yeast cell converts sugar into alcohol and carbonic acid. Two of the big guns of chemistry, Wöhler and Liebig, supported the chemical theory, but Pasteur's classic paper on lactic fermentation (1857) was a serious blow against the quasi-monopoly of the chemical theory in explaining fermentation. Pasteur went on producing study after study brilliantly demonstrating experimentally that the process is an organic one carried out by 'living' ferments or microorganisms, particularly in his famous memoir on alcoholic fermentation in 1860. (Eduard Buchner's discovery of cell free fermentation was announced two years after Pasteur's death.) Pasteur was interested in the practical implications of this research as well as in the molecular structure and optical activity of industrial products such as amyl alcohol. His linking of asymmetry and optical activity with life, that will-o'-the-wisp of science, might also have inspired him.

Pasteur enjoyed controversy. Entering the debate over spontaneous generation or heterogenesis gave him the public scientific stage on which he so expertly performed. He rightly insisted that the issue was related to his work on fermentation. He was also on the side of the angels ('official science'), who believed that living organisms are unable to develop without the agency of preexisting living matter. Pasteur's position might have been experimentally weak, but it was concordant with all his scientific work up to that time and would continue to be with his future work; the origin of life was not a subject amenable to science as he practiced it. His five years of first rate work on fermentation and the applications of that research made him the most likely person to be correct on the issue of the origin of ferments. As the debate about spontaneous generation spluttered on, Pasteur's interests shifted to 'the pathological implications of the germ theory' to explain infectious diseases (Geison, *DSB*, 10: 374). He had found his future research passion, the pathological as a form of life.

Silkworm Diseases

One of the minor disadvantages of being a successful scientist with powerful political friends is that they expect you to come up with solutions to problems that pose political danger for them. So the old chemist and politician Jean-Baptiste Dumas asked Pasteur to take on the disease that was killing silkworms and destroying the important silk production industry in southern France. Knowing nothing about silkworms, Pasteur was seduced into the project by a governmental assignment with its modest perks, by his love of traveling on a scientific adventure, by the possibility of fighting a disease and saving an industry, and above all by 'the prospect of investigating the possible impact of the microbe on living matter' (Debré, 1998, pp. 178–179). No doubt he was also made overconfident about solving the problem because of his great success in identifying wine diseases and coming up with a panacea.

The silkworm adventure occupied Pasteur for over five years, though the stroke he suffered in 1868 and deaths in his family must have slowed his progress. It also took him a while to accept the idea of a new kind of microbe (a corpuscular parasite) longer than it took his assistants, who included Emile Duclaux. Though Pasteur and his team eventually diagnosed two diseases, it was easier to understand *pébrine* than *flacherie* with its complex etiology. To conquer the diseases, Pasteur became an egg man, selecting uninfected eggs to distribute to breeders with detailed hygienic instructions on procedures; he 'became a practical sericulturist' (Geison, *DSB*, 10: 376). Commentators struggle to see a unity in Pasteur's scientific work with the object of relating it to human diseases. Patrice Debré is most cryptic and most enlightening: 'the caterpillar led to man'; in disciplinary terms, Pasteur went 'from microbiology to veterinary science and to medicine' (Debré, 1998, pp. 179, 218). As with his work on wine, Pasteur's work on silkworm diseases led to a classic monograph, *Studies on Silkworm Diseases* (1870), which was dedicated to the Empress Eugénie—he was keenly aware of the importance of politics to science. Anyone wishing to study contagious diseases, including budding physicians, could find in that study the basics on 'the interaction of parasite, host, and environment in the production of disease' (Geison, *DSB*, 10: 376). A confident Pasteur often gave this advice.

The debates over fermentation continued into the 1870s, causing Pasteur to refine and even modify his view on the role of oxygen in the process. His *Studies on Beer* (1876) explicitly recognized the importance of oxygen in brewing beer, a popular liquid in the north and east of France. He also did original but far from definitive work on yeast, a complex subject of key importance in the wine and beer industries. Pasteur finally recognized that the chemical theory was not entirely wrong yet insisted that his biological or physiological theory was correct. The debate had fallen victim to the academic disease of logomachy. Pasteur, bored with the squabbles over fermentation and spontaneous generation, turned to new scientific and medical challenges.

Like others, Pasteur thought that both fermentation and disease could be explained by 'germ theory'. An analogy is not a proof, he maintained; there is no scientific proof without experimentation. Yet analogy led to medical change, perhaps even revolution in therapy. Joseph Lister's reading of Pasteur's paper on lactic fermentation encouraged him to accept the role of bacteria in postoperative infections. Lister generously gave Pasteur credit 'for having provided in the germ theory of fermentation "the sole principle" upon which the antiseptic system' was founded (Geison, *DSB*, 10: 384). Pasteur's paper on butyric acid led Casimir Davaine to theorize that the rodlike organism he had seen in anthrax-infected blood years before was similar to the butyric ferment, and analogy established a possible etiology for the disease. Pasteur followed this work but did not get around to publishing his first paper on anthrax until 1877, four years after he was elected, by a margin of one vote, as a member at large to the Academy of Medicine.

The Academy of Medicine; The Medical Connection

The entry of Pasteur into the Academy of Medicine was a turning point in his relationship with medicine as well as in conflictual and cooperative relations with doctors, who were often his collaborators. As a famous scientist, a winner of top prizes, and a member of leading scientific societies, he brought more prestige to the doctors' society than it did to him. His work had been important for medicine for a long time before his election. In 1863 he told General Favé, the emperor's aide-de-camp, that he was 'ready to approach that great mystery of the putrid diseases, which constantly occupy my mind' (Debré, 1998, p. 260). One of his reasons for requesting the construction of a laboratory of physiological chemistry at Normale sup in 1867 was the economic importance of doing work on common rural, economically devastating infectious diseases. Intellectually curious medical students and physicians had always been attracted to Pasteur's lectures, and some of them certainly recognized the relevance of his work to their profession. Many doctors and veterinarians were on his side. Pasteur had no difficulty in getting access to hospitals to collect samples or to speculate on the efficacy of cotton wool dressings in preventing wounds from becoming infected. And it is difficult to conceive of Pasteur's experiments without the cooperation of his supporters in veterinary medicine.

Of course, many prominent physicians and surgeons criticized and opposed the germ theory of disease and especially Pasteur's imperial advocacy of it. They had learned and practiced medicine within an intellectually coherent medical paradigm that ensured professional success and even cured some patients. It was not clear how acceptance of germ theory would improve the practice of medicine until some powerful practitioners led the way in introducing sanitary practices and antiseptic and aseptic surgery. Pasteur, short of temper and big of ego, grew tired of questions and criticisms by people from another paradigm and stopped going to meetings of the Academy of Medicine.

Determined to extend germ theory to all diseases, Pasteur plunged into the medical quarrel over the etiology of disease. The two main theories of causation were based on the conflicting and interacting phenomena of miasmas and contagion, but by the late nineteenth century a new version of germ theory was coming to prevail in the medical community, one that we would hail as the triumph of bacteriology. Studies of fermentation, putrefaction, and infection provided the observational basis on which the concept of germ theory was founded. Pasteur's experimental work on diseases in wine, silkworms, poultry, livestock, and, finally, human disease was largely responsible for establishing the scientific foundation of germ theory and for making it an essential part of medical education and practice.

In most of the iconic accounts of Pasteur's work, his collaborators get relegated to the role of simply carrying out the master's orders. We now know that this is nonsense and that members of his teams, including Joseph Grancher and Emile Roux, were key figures in the success of Pasteur's work and that this in no way detracts from the originality and brilliance of Pasteur's achievements. It is often noted—indeed, he drew attention to it himself—that Pasteur was not a physician but merely a chemist, as he might say with the false modesty of a superior person. Somehow all of the physicians and veterinarians who played such an important role in Pasteur's work rarely get the credit they deserve, though Pasteur was often generous in giving them their due. The anthrax research team included Auguste Vinsot, a young veterinarian, who was a graduate of Maisons-Alfort, and Roux, a young physician who had imbibed the maestro's sermons at the Academy of Medicine and was even admitted to the famous laboratory at Normale sup. Grancher and Isidore Straus worked in the annex facility on rue Vauquelin, seen by hierarchically minded writers as a less prestigious position than one in the *sancta sanctorum* of Normale sup, though it would be difficult to conceive of the success of the 'rabies project' without Grancher. The success of the rabies treatment led Pasteur to add three more doctors to the team: Albert Chantemesse, Albert Charrin, and Octave Terrillon, a surgeon. Pasteur himself said that the facility was a real clinic and should be called one.

Nor did Pasteur lack friends and supporters among surgeons in the debate over the importance of aseptic and antiseptic procedures in surgery. Edouard Nicaise, Félix Terrier, Just-Lucas Champonnière, and Samuel Pozzi became supporters of the application of the germ theory in medicine after making a pilgrimage across the channel to see Listerism in action. Stéphane Tarnier, Ulysse Trélat, and Alphonse Guérin (not to be confused with the hostile Jules Guérin) must also be counted in the ranks of Pasteurians in medicine. Parisian hospitals provided an inexhaustible supply of a variety of microbes, and Pasteur's powerful friends and even some germ-theory agnostics invited him with Roux and Chamberland to visit their clinics in the Lariboisière, Necker, and Cochin hospitals, where they collected samples of pus, blood, and lochia to analyze back in the laboratory. Often the Pasteurians identified the microbes, sometimes even discovered them, and then recommended aseptic or antiseptic procedures. Debré enthuses that 'by the end of the 1870s the hospital loomed almost as large as the laboratory in Pasteur's life' (Debré, 1998, p. 336).

The impact of Pasteurism, translated into medicine as Listerism, must be carefully defined. In 1854–56 Florence Nightingale reduced mortality in the barrack hospital at Scutari from about 40 percent to 2 percent; she knew nothing about germ theory but a lot about the importance of cleanliness (personal and institutional), ventilation, light, clean water, and efficient administration. Add germ theory and you get a Pasteurian program. Lister reduced his post-amputation death rate from 16 percent to 6 percent in practicing antiseptic surgery. His French disciples got similar good results. So far, so good. Yet as Lewis Thomas argues, little 'beyond bed rest and good nursing care' could be done in hospitals to treat infectious diseases. For Thomas, an observer of the scene at the Boston City Hospital, 'the start of the real revolution in medicine' came in 1937 with the use of sulfanilamide in treating pneumococcal and streptococcal septicemia. It seemed 'beyond belief' that patients under a death sentence were cured in a day or so (Thomas, 1983, p. 35).

Chicken Cholera

Pasteur is a medical hero. A *Heldenleben* can also be constructed for Robert Koch, the major figure in the creation of scientific bacteriology. Koch revealed the life cycle of the anthrax bacillus and its eternal spores; Pasteur took up its study and definitively established the fact that this major animal and minor human disease is caused by a live micro-organism. At the same time, Pasteur was working on chicken or fowl cholera, now called infectious pasteurellosis of fowls, which is unrelated to the cause of human cholera, the *Vibrio comma*. In a clever experiment in 1878 Pasteur showed that chickens, which were usually not susceptible, could be infected with the disease if their body temperature were lowered a few degrees. Raising the temperature of rabbits, which were usually susceptible, kept them immune. The environment as well as the germ was shown to be a factor in disease.

Pasteur's investigation of anthrax began as a result of a request by the worried minister of agriculture. Pasteur's team included Charles Chamberland, his official laboratory assistant; Vinsot; and Roux. As often occurred, the investigation was 'displaced', in this case to a farm near Chartres. The team used large domestic animals in a feeding experiment to confirm Koch's idea that the infection came from spores in the food. Pasteur revealed that the spores from buried infected corpses were brought to the soil by earthworms, 'a vector of death' (Debré, 1998, p. 317). Almost as a footnote to this research Pasteur discovered the 'septic vibrio', and so explained death from septicemia while refuting critics of the stature of the physiologist Paul Bert, who thought that he had shown that anthrax blood could kill after its 'bacteridia' had been killed. (In his experiment Bert had killed the anthrax bacilli but not the pathogens causing septicemia.) This incident provides an example of how an ongoing, even friendly exchange with other people could provoke Pasteur into a new discovery. His 'prepared mind' was often ready to seize what for others was lost opportunity.

Chicken Cholera, Anthrax, and Vaccination

Anthrax bacilli were ideal for microscopic examination because of their relatively large size, so the disease provided a good model for the germ theory. Like some physicians and veterinarians (Davaine and Henri Toussaint, for example), Pasteur pondered the achievement of Edward Jenner (1749–1823) in using cowpox material as a smallpox vaccine. It seemed a unique achievement, an 'accident' seized by Jenner's 'prepared mind', the smallpox agent being a real virus invisible to researchers did not help. In his work on chicken cholera Pasteur came up with perhaps his greatest idea: the attenuation or weakening of the microbe that causes a disease and then using it as a vaccine. The novelty was not that a disease could be its own preventive, as Pasteur recognized, but that he had identified the causative microorganism and used as a vaccine the organism cultivated in broth outside a living organism. Once the technical problems had been overcome, perhaps infectious diseases could be prevented.

Not that chicken cholera was all that important. The big test was in bringing anthrax under the control of the Pasteurian mini-empire. Whether or not the discovery that the oxygen-exposed and therefore weakened chicken cholera germ as an effective vaccine was, like the discovery of penicillin, a happy accident or the result of a deliberate experiment by Roux is debatable. But there is no doubt that Pasteur beat his competitors (Chaveau and Toussaint) in the search for an effective anthrax vaccine and ensured, at least temporarily, the triumph of his biological theory of vaccination with the difficult-to-explain immunity it conferred. Creating the anthrax vaccine was difficult because of the need to weaken the microbes while preventing the development of the bacilli's notorious spores. Pasteur succeeded in producing a vaccine, and in the process showed how a microbe could be attenuated and even returned through culture in animals to its original virulence.

Pasteur's public demonstration (what Latour calls the 'theater of proof') at Pouilly-le-Fort of the efficacy of the anthrax vaccine, a product of the laboratory, was the prelude to the successful vaccination of hundreds of thousands of animals (Latour, 1988, pp. 85, 87). Controversies swirled round the new 'Apollo', hostile salvos were fired from the big guns of German bacteriology and from Italian veterinary medicine; many of the criticisms were fair, but French microbiology proved to be right in the sense that by 1894 millions of sheep and nearly half a million cattle were vaccinated, with a clear drop in the mortality rate from anthrax. A vaccine against swine erysipelas proved equally effective in the late 1880s and 1890s. The role of germ theory in explaining infectious disease was now established on a solid experimental basis and generally accepted by veterinarian, medical, and hygienist communities. The relevance to human medicine of all these triumphs in veterinary medicine was not so clear.

Rabies

No more dramatic demonstration of the importance of Pasteurism for human medicine could have been imagined than Pasteur's decision to take on the disease of rabies, of great mythic significance though a minor health threat compared to any number of big killers of humans. The horrors of a death from rabies encouraged Pasteur to pursue the difficult research on this viral disease. There was also the distinguishing fact that the person being vaccinated already had the disease, which fortunately had a long-enough incubation period to allow successively virulent abdominal injections to confer what remained a mysterious immunity. In the creation of a rabies vaccine Pasteur and his team took several steps different from the work on vaccines for fowl cholera and anthrax, chiefly in the use of animals to cultivate the unseen agent. (Eventually, the monkey was found best for weakening the virus.) This process was not completely new to Pasteur, given his use of living media in experimenting with the two bacterial diseases. Using a series of increasingly virulent inoculations, he succeeded in making dogs immune to rabies. As in the case of the anthrax vaccine, he used unvaccinated control animals, in this case dogs made rabid by injection.

At the second international hygiene conference (Copenhagen, 1884) Pasteur noted the legal and ethical problems involved in extending vaccination from animals to humans but argued that the treatment of rabies, a fatal disease in animals and humans, offered a solution. The medical opinions of Alfred Vulpian and Joseph Grancher convinced Pasteur to treat the young Joseph Meister, badly bitten by a rabid dog. The success of that treatment was followed by other successes. Pasteur's statistics were often justly criticized, but in large part he ended up in the right. Of people bitten by rabid animals less than 0.5 percent of those vaccinated die; for the unvaccinated victims, the percentage reported as dying has varied historically from 5 percent to 50 percent; so a 16 percent mortality rate arrived at by a ten-year study (1915) seems like a reasonable conservative compromise.

Pasteur's enterprise itself was transformed by 'the rabies project', which 'moved from laboratory experiments [200 or so] to clinical applications' (Gelfand, 2002, p. 716). No one was more important in that shift than Grancher, professor and prominent Parisian physician, politician, and leader of the Pastorians in the defense of their treatment for rabies against the attacks of fellow professionals and the press, which were both eager to exploit the few inevitable deaths occurring among those treated. What is puzzling is not the death of patients but the fact that a distinguished clinician like Michel Peter would not recognize and accept these deaths as 'normal' for any therapeutic procedure. More than being consumed by envy, he was probably still suffering from a residual hostility to germ theory. In medicine there is always the probability that over time a ferocious opposition to novelty will cause the doctor to begin to resemble a character out of Molière.

Throughout his work on germ theory Pasteur thought a great deal about an explanation for how a vaccine confers immunity—and we are still thinking about it now. The 'rabies project' caused him to radically modify his opinion as he was lured away from his biological theory, which assumed a loss of the nutrients required by the microbe, to a modified chemical theory of immunity dependent on the manufacture of a dead substance by the microbe. Others, including Chauveau, Davaine, and Toussaint, had entertained similar unfruitful speculations. Pasteur was clever enough to know that it was better to go with what he knew, namely the manufacture of vaccine that works, though we know not how. And soon he had Elie Mechnikov's phagocytic theory to remind him of the biological theory he had jilted. Anthrax made Pasteur into 'Apollo' but rabies put him on 'the front page of the newspapers' and made possible his most famous creation, the Institut Pasteur (Debré, 1998, p. 461).

Institut Pasteur

Fighting rabies was expensive. Just the creation of facilities for the experimental dogs was a major project requiring governmental support. His laboratory with annex at Normale sup could not accommodate dozens of dogs in addition to resident chickens, rabbits, and guinea pigs. So in 1885 Pasteur helped establish a major facility in the park of Saint-Cloud, where a rundown state domain was transformed to give him a new complex of kennel, laboratory, and living quarters. (He still had his apartment at Normale sup.) There was no shortage of stray dogs, rabid or not, delivered from the streets of Paris. This facility became the Villeneuve-l'Etang branch of the Institut Pasteur. The success of the rabies clinic at Normale sup soon overwhelmed it. Pasteur came up with the idea of setting up a private establishment to vaccinate patients against rabies. A private scientific institution was an unusual idea in France and for Pasteur. The success of the project was amazing, with French and foreign subscriptions totaling over 2.5 million francs. The czar and Pasteur made large contributions, and Madame Boucicaut (owner of the Bon Marché department store) an even larger gift.

When the 'Rabies Palace' opened in November 1888 in the rural suburb of Grenelle, it had a trinitarian mission: treating rabies according to the Pasteurian dogma, studying virulent and contagious diseases, and providing advanced studies for young scientists. The institute was also intimately entwined with the political, social, and financial powers of the French state. It was clear from the beginning that the institute, with its laboratories and departments for medical biology, rabies, and vaccine production and sales, was to be an empire of medical science and commerce. Apollo and Hermes in tandem: the double-edged alliance pushing medical research and care—no wonder their staffs are often confused in medical iconography. Pasteur, weakened by age and disease, lived on for seven years at the institute. He now molders in Napoleonic glory in a crypt in the institute.

Bibliography

Primary: 1922–1939. (Pasteur, Vallery-Radot, ed.) *Oeuvres de Pasteur* 7 vols. (Paris); 1940–1951. (Pasteur, Vallery-Radot, ed.) *Correspondance* 4 vols. (Paris).

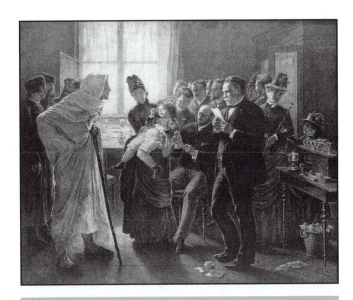

Rabies vaccination in Pasteur's clinic, Paris. Pasteur stands in the foreground reading from a paper, 1887. Lithograph by F. Pirodon after Laurent-Lucien Gsell. Iconographic Collection, Wellcome Library, London.

Secondary: Gelfand, Toby, 2002. '11 January 1887, the Day Medicine Changed: Joseph Grancher's Defense of Pasteur's Treatment for Rabies.' *Bulletin of the History of Medicine* 76: 698–718; Debré, Patrice, 1998. *Louis Pasteur* (trans. Forster, Elborg) (Baltimore); Geison, Gerald L., 1995. *The Private Science of Louis Pasteur* (Princeton); Morange, Michel, ed., 1991. *L'Institut Pasteur. Contributions à son histoire* (Paris); Latour, Bruno, 1988. *The Pasteurization of France* (trans. Sheridan, Alan, and John Law) (Cambridge, MA); Thomas, Lewis, 1983. *The Youngest Science. Notes of a Medicine Watcher* (New York); *DSB*.

Harry W. Paul

PATIN, GUY   (b. Houdan [now Hodenc-en-Bray], France, 31 August 1601; d. Paris, France, 30 March 1672), *medical philosophy, literature, Galenism, medical polemics.*

Patin was born into a family whose members had been bourgeois for several generations. His father studied law at Orleans and Bourges, but his Huguenot sympathies during the French wars of religion (1562–98) prevented him from practicing in Paris. He was greatly concerned with his young son's education so that his ambitions would not be similarly frustrated. After early studies at the College at Beauvais and later at the College of Boncourt, Patin studied medicine in Paris from 1622 to 1627. On 10 October 1628 he married Jeanne de Jeanson, the daughter of a wealthy Parisian wine merchant. They had ten children, of whom four sons survived to adulthood, two of them following their father into the medical profession. By 1630 Patin had established a comfortable life in Paris and a successful medical practice among the wealthy.

Intellectual Interests

Patin's modern renown rests on his extensive, lively correspondence with his contemporaries about their shared intellectual interests in the latest works of law, theology, philosophy, literature, history, and medicine. Patin described himself not as a bibliophile but as a bibliomaniac. His correspondents included distinguished seventeenth-century intellectuals such as Gabriel Naudé, a close personal friend and Mazarin's librarian, and Pierre Gassendi, the prominent philosopher. Other noteworthy correspondents included preeminent physicians of the day. Written between 1640 and 1670, Patin's correspondence offers a window into medical issues of the seventeenth century and into his views on medical theory and practice. Never intended for publication (the first edition appeared eleven years after his death), Patin's correspondence attests to the forthright, even intemperate expression of views for which he was well known. These qualities made him an effective polemicist for the causes he espoused. Much of his correspondence details Patin's extensive book collecting; he was especially interested in the history and literature of medicine. In the 1630s, he began to collect medical theses written at the University of Paris. He was a great advocate of the publication of medical works and new editions of hard-to-obtain works, and he also edited medical works of his contemporaries, including those of Jean Fernel, physician to Henry II, and Jean Riolan the younger, his fellow Parisian physician. His correspondence also reveals his support for dissident religious views. He was sympathetic to the Huguenots and admired John Calvin. In the famous religious battle of his day, he sympathized with the Jansenists and was antagonistic towards the Jesuits. His correspondence corroborates his seventeenth-century reputation as the staunchest proponent of classical medicine and the most committed advocate of the Faculty of Medicine.

Faculty Advocate

Patin became a member of the Faculty of Medicine shortly after receiving his degree—a status of which he was inordinately proud. (In the seventeenth century, the Faculty of Medicine was a corporate body of physicians with control over the teaching of medicine at the university and the practice of medicine in Paris.) From the time of his admittance, the Faculty of Medicine became Patin's central interest. He was greatly concerned with the preservation of its rights, the admission of those he considered worthy to its ranks, the expulsion of those he considered unworthy, the election of good officers, and the augmentation of the authority and wealth of its members. One of the staunchest defenders of the privileges and prerogatives of the Faculty, Patin praised those contemporaries who aided him in this cause and attacked those who undermined the Faculty. The highest office in the Faculty was the dean; Patin was elected to the position and held it for several terms.

Patin received other significant recognition from the academic medical community. He succeeded Jean Riolan the younger as a chaired professor in the Collège Royal in 1654. In that capacity, Patin taught botany, pharmacy, and anatomy. In 1655 he was offered a position at the University of Bologna, and in 1658 the Venetian Ambassador tried to persuade him to take up a lucrative position there. But Patin resisted all inducements to leave Paris.

Galenism vs. Chemical Medicine

Patin is best known as one of the staunchest seventeenth-century advocates of Galenism. For Patin, Galenism was the most credible source of medical theory and practice. He insisted on a return to genuinely classical medicine denuded of the innovations of Arab physicians such as Avicenna (Ibn Sīnā); he endorsed the publication of new editions of Galen and Hippocrates to serve this end. Patin fought with great fury against the innovation of his contemporaries, especially those associated with the followers of Paracelsus.

Paracelsians were inclined to challenge Galenism as too theoretical and too divorced from practical experience. They instead introduced chemical remedies; they also looked to new ways to explain diseases, applying chemical explanations to physiological processes and invoking causes of disease that were more hidden or 'occult' than the Galenic imbalance of the four humors. Patin was a leading advocate for the Paris Faculty of Medicine at a time when Paracelsianism was trying to make inroads into the practice of medicine in France. He led a campaign to cleanse the pharmacopoeia of all chemical remedies or any other remedy deemed irrational for failing to subscribe to Galenist principles of the way disease and health worked. His crusade was so vehement in part because he believed chemical remedies were lethal; he explicitly denounced the prescription of laudanum, antimony, opium, and quinine.

Patin insisted that only herbal remedies were effective and that doctors could morally prescribe only those medicaments that could be explained in Galenic terms. His adherence to Galen also led Patin to be the seventeenth century's most vehement defender of phlebotomy (bleeding) as the medical therapy best reflecting Galenic medicine's quest to balance bodily humors. Throughout his medical career, Patin recommended bleeding for many diseases, among them apoplexy, epilepsy, and any inflammation, and unlike many of his contemporaries who were beginning to question the practice, he advocated it for patients of all ages and conditions of health. This therapeutic recommendation was also consistent with Patin's desire to maintain a simple, consistent pharmacopoeia and therapy, and this simplicity he defended against all newcomers. He also was a vehement critic of new theories in medicine; he was the leading opponent of William Harvey in France. He defended the Faculty against provincial physicians, especially those from Montpellier who were much more sympathetic to innovations, including Paracelsianism.

Medical Polemicist

Patin is renowned for his contentiousness and he engaged in many vehement disputes with his contemporaries; he was well known for a no-holds-barred style of medical disputation in pamphlets. One of his longest running and most vociferous pamphlet campaigns was the one he fought against Théophraste Renaudot, who had the support of Cardinal Richelieu for his medical institutions, among them plans to build a teaching hospital in Paris, which Patin quite rightly saw as a threat to the preeminence of the Faculty of Medicine over the teaching and practice of medicine. A Montpellier-trained physician, Renaudot was also sympathetic to chemical medications. (Their dispute was featured in Molière's play *L'amour médecin*.) The death of Richelieu paved the way for the Faculty to triumph in its suit against Renaudot. After defeating Renaudot, the Faculty urged the Parlement of Paris to enforce its claim that no one who was not a doctor or licentiate of the Faculty of Paris could practice medicine in Paris. This claim was sustained by an order of 1 March 1644 that was directed in large part against all those who had practiced with Renaudot, many of them credentialed by the University of Montpellier.

Patin insisted on the pre-eminence of the Faculty of Medicine of Paris over its more progressive rival, the Faculty of Montpellier, which also favored the use of chemical remedies like antimony. As dean of the Paris faculty, Patin went so far as to remove the name of a colleague, Jean Chartier, from the list of the Faculty because he published a work in favor of the antimony remedy. Patin's letters include mention of many of his contemporaries who he believed had been poisoned by the use of antimony, including Cardinal Mazarin. Patin again battled the apothecaries in his position as dean of the Faculty; the apothecaries not only favored chemical medicines but also sided with Renaudot against the Faculty. Patin condemned them for their avarice, and in 1647 the Faculty published a new pharmacopoeia with simpler remedies designed to allow doctors to prescribe without the services of apothecaries.

But Patin and the Faculty of Medicine eventually suffered significant setbacks. In 1657 the barber-surgeons decided to combine with the academically trained surgeons of Saint-Côme, a union that removed the barber-surgeons from the control of the Faculty. And despite all the sharp invective Patin had produced to denounce its use, the Faculty approved the use of antimony in 1660. At this point, Patin became disaffected from the Faculty; he had dedicated his life to preventing the introduction of chemical remedies into the pharmacopoeia and targeted antimony as a dangerous poison. The letters of the last years of his life became even more embittered. Ultimately the chemical physicians against whom Patin battled so relentlessly have received more credit for their chemical understanding of

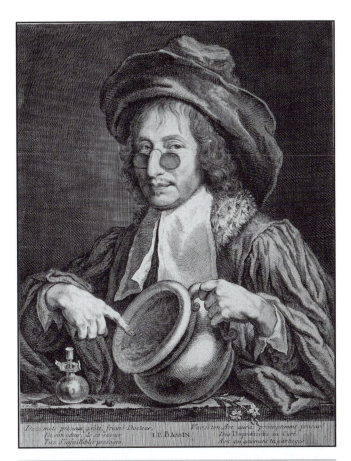

Guy Patin with herbs and medicines. Line engraving by R. Nanteuil, Iconographic Collection, Wellcome Library, London.

physiological processes than Patin has for his opposition to that understanding and their practices. Patin remains known by modern physicians as the first physician to describe, *fibrodysplasia ossificans progressivo*.

Bibliography

Primary: 1632. *Traité de la conservations de santé, par un bon regime et légitime usage des choses requises pour bien et sainement vivre* (Paris); 1683. *Lettres choisis de feu M. Guy Patin* (Frankfort); 1718. *Nouvelles lettres de feu M. Guy Patin, tirées du cabinet de M. Charles Splon* (La Haye).

Secondary: Packard, Francis R., 1925. *Guy Patin and the Medical Profession in Paris in the Seventeenth Century* (New York); Pic, Pierre, 1911. *Guy Patin* (Paris).

Kathleen Wellman

PAUL OF AEGINA (aka PAULUS AEGINETA, PAUL D'EGINE) (b. Aegina, Greece; fl. Alexandria, *c.* 640), *medicine, surgery.*

An encyclopedic medical writer born in Aegina, Paul lived, studied, and practiced in Alexandria and remained there even after its Arabic conquest. Very little is known of his life. Like Oribasius, whose work he used and continued, Paul mainly summarized, selected, and excerpted the views of medical authorities of the past on various subjects. In this way he preserved and transmitted material that would not have survived otherwise, which is the chief merit of all authors of his kind.

Paul's main work, *Epitome*, a compilation in seven books based on Oribasius, was intended as a short but compendious summary of earlier medical thought and practice for the convenient use of doctors. Its strength lies in Paul's capacity to select the best classical traditions on each subject and to present the material in a systematic and conceptually clear way. His account of the elimination of stones in the kidneys, liver, and spleen was a classic, and that of ophthalmic surgery the most detailed one surviving from antiquity. In pharmacology he used mainly Dioscorides as a source and achieved the most complete synthesis of ancient traditions on drugs and materia medica.

But Paul was also a remarkable surgeon, and his input in this field in book VI of the *Epitome* also contained much original material. The book was structured by a division into manual operations and treatment of fractures and dislocations; it discussed procedures like tracheotomy, tonsillectomy, paracentesis, cauterization, venesection, and cupping. This book exerted a strong influence on Arabic medical literature.

Book I developed a complex humoralism, which constituted the basis for Paul's pathology and therapy. The theory of four elements and temperaments was a digest of Galenism interpreted through Oribasius's perspective. The crucial factor in maintaining the good balance of humors was diet. The best temperament was the mean between many pairs of extremes. This formula provided Paul with a mode of explaining individual features, including those of internal organs and their components, as variations from an ideal mean.

Book II dealt with acute and chronic fevers and the pulse as a basis for prognosis; Book III with diseases and their therapies, reviewed in the traditional order of the affected parts, from head to feet (hair, eye, ear, nose, throat, heart, and so on); Book IV with incurable skin diseases like leprosy and elephantiasis; Book V with poisonous bites and their antidotes; and Book VII with a summary of simple and compound medicines. Two other works of Paul, on gynecology and on poisons, are mentioned in the Arabic sources but are now completely lost.

Bibliography

Primary: Adams, Fr., trans., 1844–1847. *The Seven Books of Paulus Aegineta* I–III (London); Brian, R., ed. and trans., 1855. *Le chirurgie de Paul d'Egine* (Paris); Heiberg, J. L., ed., 1921–1924. *Paulus Aegineta*, CMG 9 (Berlin).

Secondary: Andorlini, I., 2004. *Medicina, medico e società nel mondo antico* (Florence) pp. 59–61, 231; Salazar, C., 1998. 'Getting the Point: Paul of Aegina on Arrow Wounds.' *Sudhoffs Archiv* 82: 170–187; Signorelli, R., 1967. 'Ostetrica e ginecologia nel bizantino Paulo d'Egina e nell' arabo Albucasi.' *Minerva medica* 58: 4118–4131; Tabanelli, M., 1964. *Studi sulla chirurgia bizantina, Paolo di Egina* (Florence); Straubel, K., 1922. *Zahn- und Mundleiden und deren Behandlung bei Paulos von Aigina*. Dissertation, University of Leipzig; Heiberg, J. L., 1919. 'De codicibus Pauli Aeginetae observations.' *Revue des Etudes Grecques* 32: 268–277; Garlt, E., 1898. 'Paul von Aegina' in Garlt, E., *Geschichte der Chirurgie* I (Berlin) pp. 558–590; *DSB*.

Manuela Tecusan

PAUL, JOHN RODMAN (b. Philadelphia, Pennsylvania, USA, 18 April 1893; d. New Haven, Connecticut, USA, 6 May 1971) *epidemiology, preventive medicine, poliomyelitis, serological diagnosis.*

Paul, the son of a lawyer, received an undergraduate degree from Princeton University (1915) and a medical degree from Johns Hopkins (1919). He directed the Ayer Clinical Laboratory of the Pennsylvania Hospital until recruited to the faculty of the department of medicine of Yale University School of Medicine (1928). In 1931, with James Trask, he established the Yale Poliomyelitis Study Unit. In 1940 he was appointed head of the section of epidemiology and preventive medicine at Yale. He remained active, as emeritus professor of epidemiology, after his retirement in 1961. From 1961 until 1966 he directed the Serum Reference Bank of the WHO and from 1966 until his death he held the post of lecturer in the history of science and medicine. Paul was elected to the National Academy of Sciences (1945) and inducted into the Poliomyelitis Hall of Fame of the National Foundation for Infantile Paralysis (1958).

Paul's research was wide-ranging in the realm of infectious disease epidemiology. He studied, among other conditions, rheumatic fever, infectious mononucleosis, hepatitis, and, most intently, poliomyelitis. His *History of Poliomyelitis* (1971), chronicling the development of knowledge regarding the clinical, epidemiological, natural history, and control of the disease from antiquity to modern times, continues to be recognized as a 'classic' and authoritative source. His study demonstrating that the decreasing attack rate from the disease with increasing age was attributable to immunity acquired during infancy from nonparalytic, or unrecognized, cases was cited seventy years after publication as a landmark (Comstock, 2003). Further evidence regarding the importance of early infection and its effect on the age distribution of poliomyelitis was provided by a study of neutralizing antibody patterns in population samples studied in eight widely separated populations. Paul's research and participation on advisory committees to the National Foundation for Infantile Paralysis played a role in the successful development and testing of the inactivated poliovirus vaccine in 1953–54.

In 1969 Paul was invited to prepare a history of the first fifty years of the American Epidemiological Society. The Society had been established in 1927 as the first forum for the presentation and discussion of epidemiological science in the United States. The resulting 148-page book provides important insights into the development of epidemiology in mid-twentieth century America. Significantly, it contains detailed biographical sketches of seven of the most important practitioners of the period who had been charter members of the Society, namely, Charles V. Chapin, Haven Emerson, Wade Hampton Frost, Leslie T. Webster, Lloyd Aycock, Hans Zinsser, and Eugen L. Opie (Paul, 1973).

In his teaching, Paul emphasized the importance of epidemiology as the basic science of public health. His participation on innumerable committees, commissions, and advisory boards—locally, nationally, and internationally—was always informed by this philosophy.

Bibliography

Primary: 1933. (with Salinger, R., and J. D. Trask) 'Studies on the Epedemiology of Poliomyelitis I and II.' *American Journal Hygiene* 17: 587–600, 601–612; 1958. *Clinical Epidemiology* (Chicago); 1971. *A History of Poliomyelitis* (New Haven); 1973. *An Account of the American Epidemiological Society* (New York).

Secondary: Comstock, G. W., 2003. 'Snippets from the Past: Seventy Years Ago in the Journal.' *American Journal of Epidemiology* 158: 1210–1212; *DAMB*.

Warren Winkelstein, Jr.

PAUL, MILROY ASERAPPA (b. Colombo, Ceylon, 20 January 1900; d. Colombo, Sri Lanka, 8 October 1988), *surgery, anatomy, medical administration.*

A pronounced feature of Western medicine in colonial Sri Lanka that lasted well into the mid-twentieth century was the color bar, which ensured the highest ranks remained almost exclusively the domain of British personnel. Against such a backdrop, Paul was exceptional, one of the very few Sri Lankans admitted into the medical profession's elite.

Paul inherited both medicine and wealth. An obituary noted that 'Milroy Paul, although having the advantage of distinguished medical forbears on both sides of his family, was a man who, by sheer hard work and brilliance, achieved great distinction in his own country and became widely known outside Sri Lanka'. He was the eldest son of Samuel Chelliah Paul, MD, FRCS (England), surgeon, obstetrician, and physician, the first Ceylonese FRCS, and the first Senior Surgeon, General Hospital, Colombo. S. C. Samuel Paul, son of Dr William Paul, graduated with a first class, from Presidency College, Madras, India, winning the Johnstone Medal and the George Smith Prize for Pathology. Paul's mother was Dora Eleanor Paul (née Aserappa), a daughter of S. de M. Aserappa, MD (Edin.) and heiress to a large estate and the founder of the Women's International Club, Colombo.

Paul had five brothers. One died young but the others included a lawyer in the Indian Civil Service, a deputy director of industries (Ceylon), a deputy director of agriculture (Ceylon), and a surgeon, A. T. S. Paul, the first cardiothoracic surgical specialist at the General Hospital, Colombo.

Paul began his primary schooling in 1906 at the CMS Ladies College and then attended the Government Training College, both at Colombo. His secondary education was at Royal College, also at Colombo. He began with the classics but later turned to science. He was listed second in the world in geography at the Cambridge senior examination, which included Latin, history, and English literature. He won several prestigious prizes, including the Rajapakse prize (for best junior student), the senior mathematics, and the de Soysa science prize.

He commenced his medical studies at the Ceylon Medical College (later the Faculty of Medicine, University of Ceylon (1942)) but after the first year he transferred to King's College Hospital, London, where his surgical teacher was Sir Cecil Wakeley. He won a medal for best student and a prize for surgery.

He graduated MBBS from King's College (1925), having won the Self Medal. At King's College Hospital he gained prizes in surgery, orthopedic surgery, hygiene, psychological medicine, and forensic medicine. He obtained the MRCP (London) (1926) and the FRCS (England) (1927). He was casualty officer (1926) and Surgical Registrar (1927) at King's College Hospital.

He returned to Ceylon in 1927 and was surgeon at Jaffna Hospital (1930–33) and was then at the General Hospital, department of medical and sanitary services, Colombo. He was acting professor of anatomy at the Ceylon Medical College. He joined the Ceylon Army's Medical Corps (CMC) (1930). During World War II he was a major and honorary surgeon to the British Military Hospital. He was honorary surgeon to the Royal Air Force in Ceylon until the RAF left (1960) and acted as the medical referee for pilots. He was also commander of the Ceylonese St John's Ambulance Brigade, Colombo.

In 1936 he was appointed the first professor of surgery in the Medical College, a post he held until his retirement (1965). He also served as consultant surgeon to the General Hospital, and consultant surgeon to the Children's Hospital, both in Colombo. He served the Ceylon Medical Council as registrar (1933–82). He was founder president (1963–64) of the Ceylon Association of Surgeons (now College of Surgeons, Sri Lanka). He was a founding member of the Sri Lanka Association for the Advancement of Science (1944) and the association's general president (1954). The Sri Lanka National Academy of Sciences elected him general president (1977–79). He was also president of the Ceylon Medical Association.

Paul maintained international links in surgery, especially with the RCS (England). He was appointed Hunterian professor and delivered three Hunterian Lectures: *The surgical anatomy of the spermatic cord* (1950), *Congenital abnormalities of the midline abdominal wall* (1953), and *Haemorrhages from head injuries* (1955). He was elected an honorary fellow of the Association of Surgeons of Great Britain & Ireland in 1982 and was a founder fellow of the International College of Surgeons.

His eighty-one publications over fifty-five years in journals in the UK, Australia-New Zealand, United States, and India covered a wide range of topics in general surgery, surgical techniques, parasitic diseases, congenital abnormalities, anatomy, orthopedics, trauma surgery, ophthalmology, general surgery, urology, cutaneous and liver amoebic abscesses, aneurysms, appendicitis, cleft palate and harelip, and intra-abdominal cysts of congenital and parasitic origins. He authored numerous case reports and contributed a chapter on 'Amoebiasis' to *Tropical Surgery*.

His distinctive characteristics as a teacher and researcher greatly influenced and molded young students. His versatility and capacity for innovative thinking were illustrated in papers and lectures: e.g., he discussed new concepts in hepatic amoebic liver abscess, movements of the worm *Ascaris lumbricoides* inside the abdomen—a lecture that enthralled his audiences—and the development of new surgical techniques. He remained unimpressed with students who merely regurgitated factual knowledge ('theoretical Johnnies'), and his hallmark as a teacher was to stimulate original thinking. His lasting contribution to medical education was encouraging students to use innovation to solve the many and sometimes unique clinical problems that beset his country and South Asia. In research his career record is a model inspiring many in Sri Lanka, but matched by only a very few. The 'razor-sharp pungency of his wit' endeared him to students and junior staff as 'one of the best known and best loved medical personalities' in Sri Lanka (Editorial, 1985, pp. 1–2), and a biographer regarded him as 'A legend in his lifetime' (Gunaratne, 1992, p. 85).

Paul married Winifred Hanah Ponmany (daughter of Dr B. Canagasabai) in 1927, and their son, lawyer Wakeley W. Paul, was named for Sir Cecil Wakeley. After Winifred's death (1944), he married (1945) Irma Maheswari Tampoe Philips. They had four children: the eldest son became a psychiatrist, their daughter became a geriatrician, the second son was a dentist, and the youngest son worked as an accountant. Paul's leisure activities were tennis, dancing, reading, mathematics, and English literature.

Bibliography

Primary: 1950. 'The Blood and Lymph Pathways in the Spermatic Cord (with Particular Reference to Their Applied Anatomy and Physiology).' *Annals of the Royal College of Surgeons* 7: 128—150; 1953. 'The Surgery of the Congenital Anomalies of the Midline Ventral Abdominal Wall.' *Annals of the Royal College of Surgeons* 313: 313–335; 1955. 'Haemorrhages from Head Injuries.' *Annals of the Royal College of Surgeons* 17: 69–101; 1965. "Amoebiasis" in Basu, A. K., ed., *Tropical Surgery* (London).

Secondary: 1985. (Editorial) 'Prof. Milroy A. Paul.' *Ceylon Medical Journal* 30: 1–2; Wickramasinghe, S. Y. D. C., 1985. 'Prof. Milroy A. Paul. A Tribute.' *Ceylon Medical Journal* 30: 3–6; Gunaratne, Mahasara, 1992. *Five Dons* (Colombo) pp. 85–102.

S. N. Arseculeratne

PAVLOV, IVAN PETROVICH
(b. Riazan' [now Ryazan], Russia, 14 September [26 September] 1849; d. Leningrad [now Petersburg], Russia, 27 February 1936), *physiology.*

The son of a priest in the provincial city of Riazan', Pavlov began his studies in the local seminary, but left in 1870 to enroll in the University of St Petersburg, where he studied natural sciences. After graduating in 1875, he pursued a medical degree at the Military Medical Academy where he remained to write his doctorate, a study of the nerves of the heart, which he defended in 1884.

After struggling for years to get by on a meager salary, Pavlov was made a professor at the Military Medical Academy in 1890, first in pharmacology and then physiology. In the same year Pavlov also became the director of the physiology laboratory at the Institute of Experimental Medicine, where he undertook an ambitious project to understand the way that nerves regulate the digestive system. Pavlov wanted to test the effect that stimulation of individual nerve fibers had on the production of digestive juices, and this led him to invent a new method of surgically creating 'fistulas' in his laboratory dogs, apertures which could be used to study the physiology of digestion in live animals rather than in dead specimens.

Pavlov's study of the digestive system earned him the Nobel Prize in 1904, the first won by a physiologist, and many of his findings proved to be of lasting importance, particularly his discovery that the vagus nerve is the secretory nerve of the gastric glands. By 1904, however, Pavlov had begun a new and much more ambitious research project, an attempt to analyze the physiological structures which underlie the processes of cognition. Pavlov had noticed that his laboratory dogs salivated at the sight of food, and sought to understand the physiology of this reaction. Involuntary physical responses, he concluded, were not just inborn: they could be created through repeated association. These 'conditioned reflexes', he hypothesized, were caused by structures in the nervous system, and the behavior of animals (and perhaps humans) could ultimately be explained solely with reference to the physiological actions produced when these reflex structures responded to external stimuli. There would be no need to resort to 'subjective psychology' to explain the mind.

In an era of Russian history that was notorious for its political upheavals, Pavlov was a proponent of moderate liberalism, remarking in 1918 that he would 'not have sacrificed even one laboratory frog' for the sake of the Bolshevik revolution. Such a statement could have meant exile or worse, but Pavlov enjoyed the special status of Russia's only Nobel laureate, and the Bolshevik regime used their support of his research as a symbol of their commitment to scientific

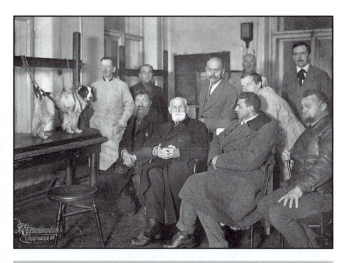

Pavlov (center) seated in his laboratory with colleagues and visiting delegates of the American Relief Association, 1922. Photograph, Archives and Manuscripts, Wellcome Library, London.

progress. In the last years of his life, however, Pavlov publicly announced his desire to see the outcome of the USSR's 'historic social experiment'. One biographer has speculated that the regime's unstinting financial support finally produced a change of heart, or that, as a patriot, Pavlov may have been moved by the resurgence of Germany. Whatever the case, the Soviet government repaid him by making his 'doctrine' of higher nervous activity the official line in Soviet physiology, establishing Pavlov as an authority in materialist science who was quoted alongside Marx and Lenin for decades.

In the United States Pavlov's theories of the conditioned reflex were embraced by pioneering behaviorist psychologists like John Watson (1878–1958), but the American behaviorists preferred not to speculate about what structures might cause the behaviors they observed. Thus they did not pursue Pavlov's primary project, uncovering the elemental physiological structures underlying cognition.

Bibliography

Primary: 1951–1954. *Polnoe sobranie sochinenii* [Complete Collected Works] 6 vols. (Moscow); 1897. *Lektsii o rabote glavnykh pishchevaritelnykh zhelez* [Lectures about the work of the main digestive glands] (St Petersburg); 1982. (trans. Thompson, W. H.) *The Work of the Digestive Glands: A Facsimile of the First Russian Edition of 1897, Together with the First English Translation of 1902* (Birmingham, AL); 1927. (ed. and trans. Anrep, G. V.) *Conditioned Reflexes: An Investigation of the Physiological Activity of the Cerebral Cortex* (Oxford) [rept. 2003 (New York)].

Secondary: Todes, Daniel P., 2002. *Pavlov's Physiology Factory: Experiment, Interpretation, Laboratory Enterprise* (Baltimore); Joravsky, David, 1989. *Russian Psychology: A Critical History* (Oxford); Babkin, Boris P., 1949. *Pavlov: A Biography* (Chicago); *DSB*.

Benjamin Zajicek

PAVLOVSKII, EVGENII NIKANOROVICH (b. Biriuch, Russia, 5 March [22 February] 1884; d. Leningrad? [now Petersburg], Russia, 27 May 1965), *parasitology*.

Pavlovskii, the son of a school director, was born in the southern Russian province of Voronezh, the only one of six siblings to survive childhood. He graduated from the Borisoglebsk gymnasium (1895–1903) in Tambov Province. He entered the prestigious Military Medical Academy in St Petersburg and studied medicine, zoology, and comparative anatomy (1903–09). After briefly working as a military doctor (1909–11), he continued his earlier studies of scorpions and their toxins, defending his doctoral dissertation on this topic at the Academy (1913).

After the 1917 Revolution, Pavlovskii was appointed professor and head of the department of biology and parasitology of the Military Medical Academy (1921–56) and soon established himself as the leading parasitologist in the Soviet Union, a position he retained for over forty years. He held many other academic and administrative offices, including head of the department of parasitology of the All-Union Institute for Experimental Medicine (1933–53), head of the department of parasitology and microbiology of the Gamaleia Institute of Epidemiology and Microbiology (starting in 1953), and director of both the Tadzhik Base (later Division) (1940–51) and the Crimean Division of the USSR Academy of Sciences (1951–54). He became a member of the Academy of Sciences (1939) and of the Academy of Medical Sciences (1944). He joined the Communist Party in 1941.

Pavlovskii wrote or edited over 1,200 scientific works on parasitology, entomology, and zoology. He directed over 180 interdisciplinary expeditions to Central Asia, the Russian Far East, the Crimea, and many other regions of the USSR to study a host of pathogens, many transmitted by insect and arthropod vectors. Among these diseases were plague, typhus, amebiasis, the tick-borne encephalidites, cutaneous leishmaniasis, helminth infections, malaria, brucellosis, and tularemia.

To elucidate the life cycles of pathogens in order to devise methods to curtail human infection, he systematically described parasitic biocenoses, which are ecological systems in which parasites, disease vectors, and primary and secondary hosts interact in specific climatic zones (e.g., taiga, forest, steppes, or deserts). He determined the physical boundaries delimiting the area of distribution of animal reservoirs harboring a host of human pathogens. He then used the observed patterns to support his theory of 'geographic landscapes' which were capable of maintaining parasitic biocenoses. As an example of such a system, in the 1930s Pavlovskii and his collaborators discovered that great gerbils (*Rhombomys opimus*) served as a reservoir for the parasites of the desert form of cutaneous leishmaniasis (*Leishmania major*) in Turkmenistan. He and his colleagues decreased the incidence of human cases by decimating the population of great gerbils in the region using poisons and plowing their burrows (1946, vol. 1, p. 122).

After 1948, in addition to his major field of work, Pavlovskii began to perform experiments in rabbits and hens to support the theory of the inheritance of acquired traits propounded by the now discredited theorists of Soviet biology, Michurin and Lysenko (1961, pp. 371–387).

Pavlovskii's painstaking studies contributed to the local control of parasites and provided a model for the epidemiologic investigation of natural reservoirs elsewhere in the world. Pavlovskii believed that with his theory of geographic landscapes, he could predict the most likely infectious threats in any region newly colonized by people. The impact of his work was limited outside of the Soviet Union by the intellectual barriers of the Cold War, but it was carried on by his twenty-five doctoral students, many of whom went on to direct departments, institutes, and laboratories of parasitology in the Soviet Union.

Bibiolography

Primary: 1946–48. *Rukovodstvo po parazitologii cheloveka* [Manual of Human Parasitology] 2 vols., 5th edn. (Moscow); 1961. *Obshchie problemy parazitologiii i zoologii* [General Problems of Parasitology and Zoology] (Moscow); 1964. *Prirodnaia ochagovost' transmissivnykh boleznei v sviazi s landshaftnoi epidemiologiei zooantroponozov* [The Natural Nidality of Transmissible Diseases in Relation to the Landscape Epidemiology of Zooanthroponoses] (Moscow).

Secondary: Prokhorova, Ninel Pavlovna, 1972. *Akademik E. N. Pavlovskii* (Moscow); Strelkov, A. A., ed., 1956. *Evgenii Nikanorovich Pavlovskii*, 2nd edn. (Moscow).

Michael Z. David

PAZ SOLDÁN, CARLOS ENRIQUE (b. Lima, Peru, 17 April 1885; d. Lima, 30 November 1972), *social medicine, public health.*

Paz Soldán was the tenth child of a prominent family of intellectuals and politicians that could trace its origins to the colonial period. He attended Lima's prestigious high school, Guadalupe, and later studied medicine at San Marcos University School of Medicine. After graduation, Paz Soldán worked in the Peruvian military under a French medical officer with experience in Africa and who participated in the reorganization of the Peruvian Army. Although he never studied abroad, Paz Soldán would travel frequently to Europe, the United States, and Latin America. In 1915 he founded and supported a publication that would last decades: *La Reforma Médica* (mimicking Rudolf Virchow's periodical). It was a combination of an academic journal and a magazine that published news and articles of interest to physicians. The subtitle of the journal was comprehensive: 'medical chronicles, hygiene, legal medicine, and sanitary policies'.

Only in the early 1920s did Paz Soldán occupy the coveted post of *catedrático*, holding the chair of hygiene in San Marcos's Medical School, a position he would retain until 1958. His course combined environmental sanitation, pub-

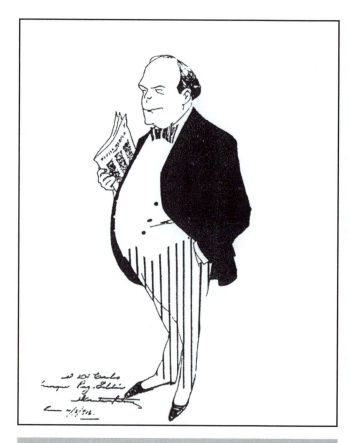

Carlos Enrique Paz Soldán. Cartoon dated 4 March 1916 from a Lima newspaper. Image supplied by Marcos Cueto.

lic health administration, and community education and prevention, and was taught in the last year of medical studies. For years he was also the permanent secretary of the prestigious National Academy of Medicine. He was an early and strong advocate for the creation of a Health Ministry, something that only occurred in Peru in 1935. During the 1920s Paz Soldán consolidated a versatile and distinguished career. He became an officer of the Peruvian Red Cross, created the Institute of Social Medicine in San Marcos, and organized in Lima the Eighth Pan American Conference of the Pan American Sanitary Bureau (the agency that in time would be known as the Pan American Health Organization). In later years he was considered an expert in international health and was on the organizing committee of the World Health Organization.

Paz Soldán's understanding of social medicine meant the elaboration of modern legislation on public health, local sociomedical studies, and hygienic education for all social classes. He believed in the Incan tradition of social medicine and said that although this valuable tradition was lost because of the violent Spanish conquest, it should be recovered by modern Western medical doctors. He was also a supporter of positive eugenics, defined as the hope that better sanitation and education would lift up the indigenous race. During the 1940s the Institute, Paz Soldán, and the German refugee Max Kuckzynski conducted remarkable studies in the Peruvian Amazon.

A prolific writer and an eloquent speaker, he was a master of combining his diverse activities. He was the author of a number of studies on the history of Peruvian medicine and participated actively in an ephemeral society and journal on this discipline. For years he was an advisor to different Peruvian ministers of health. He met and maintained correspondence with the historian of medicine Henry Sigerist, and with the Belgian René Sand, considered the father of European social medicine.

Bibliography

Primary: 1916. *La medicina social (ensayo de sistematización)* (Lima); 1918. *Las bases medico-sociales de legislación sanitaria el Perú* 3 vols. (Lima); 1939. (with Kuczynski, Max) *La Selva Peruana, sus pobladores, y su colonización sanitaria en seguridad sanitaria* (Lima); 1954. *Himnos a Hipólito Unanue* (Lima).

Secondary: Cueto, Marcos, 2002. 'Social Medicine in the Andes, 1920–1950' in Rodríguez-Ocaña, Esteban, ed., *The Politics of the Healthy Life: An International Perspective* (Sheffield) pp. 181–197. Mendoza, Walter, and Oscar Martínez, 1999. 'Las Ideas Eugenésicas en la Creación del Instituto de Medicina Social.' *Anales de la Facultad de Medicina* 60(1): 61–65.

Marcos Cueto

PÉAN, JULES-ÉMILE (b. Marboué (Eure-et-Loir), France, 30 November 1830; d. Paris, France, 30 January 1898), *surgery.*

Born in a small village, Péan was the only son among seven children. Although he liked to portray himself as rising from humble peasant origins to become a famous and, by all accounts, the wealthiest French surgeon of his time, his family circumstances were comfortable. Supposedly, Jean-Pierre Péan, a miller, wanted his son to become a notary. However, after following a country practitioner, the young man opted for medicine. According to the story, the father, shocked by his bill from a Paris surgeon for a minor procedure, remarked on the lucrative prospects that career offered.

Péan arrived in Paris at age twenty-one. During his internship (1855–59), he served under the leading surgeon, Auguste Nélaton (1807–73). He completed his MD in 1860, sustaining a thesis on resection of the shoulder joint. In 1873 Péan became chief surgeon to the Saint-Louis hospital where he remained until reaching obligatory retirement age in 1892. Still in full vigor, he then founded his own institution for foreign patients, *l'Hôpital International* (renamed *Hôpital Péan* after his death). There he worked for another six years, performing his final operation only days before he died.

Péan owed his reputation (and his colossal fortune) to an extensive private practice. His patients, he declared, came first, then his circle of students, and last, scholarship. He never became a Faculty professor. But he did gain wide international recognition as a member of surgical societies in cities around the world—with the notable exception of Paris, where he was met with envy and hostility from rivals. He was awarded the highest rank of commander of the Legion of Honor and finally, in 1887, was received into the Academy of Medicine.

Péan achieved remarkably good results despite never adopting Listerian antisepsis. A strictly empirical surgeon, he never acknowledged the practical relevance of Pasteur's germ theory. Operative speed, combined with superior manual dexterity and scrupulous attention to cleanliness above all seemed to favor his success. Péan departed from surgical custom in two significant ways: he minimized direct hand contact with the operative field, and he did not practice on cadavers. Both these measures he adopted following a dangerous dissection wound he had received while a prosector. When operating in the patient's home, as he usually did, he was able to implement sanitary measures. He also paid careful attention to postoperative nutrition.

Péan was deemed by many to be an audacious and reckless surgeon. Taking advantage of the introduction of anesthesia, he performed radical, high-risk, often mutilating operations on virtually every organ. He believed all cancers were operable. Best known for innovative abdominal surgery and in particular for gynecological operations, Péan astonished contemporaries in 1864 when, still at the beginning of his career, he performed the first successful ovariectomy in Paris, removing a cyst weighing ten kilograms. (The Strasbourg surgeon Koeberlé and several British and American surgeons preceded him.) Péan eventually reduced the mortality for this customarily lethal intervention to less than five per cent, and he claimed to be the only surgeon in Paris to do the procedure routinely during the next fifteen years. He devised new procedures for hysterectomies, introducing the practice of breaking up the tumor (*morcellement*) so as to remove fragments via the vagina. He was among the first to demonstrate the feasibility of extirpating cancers of the spleen and the stomach.

Péan displayed extraordinary sangfroid during operations. In a group portrait that now hangs in the Musée d'Orsay in Paris, Péan appears towering above onlookers as he explains the surgery he is about to begin on the unclothed female patient. In his hand is the hemostat, an instrument he helped to perfect, used to clamp blood vessels before dividing them. Péan declared the 'art of taming [blood vessels] without getting them angry' (1898, p. 1390) to be the key to his success, initially in surgery of the peritoneal cavity and subsequently in controlling bleeding of the membranes covering the lungs, the brain, and the joints. A man of imposing height and powerful build, Péan remained in robust health into his late sixties. To the shock and disbelief of his colleagues and the public, he fell victim to a common cold contracted while hunting which rapidly evolved into a fatal bronchopneumonia.

Bibliography

Primary: 1867. *L'ovariotomie peut-elle être faite à Paris avec des chances favorables de succès? Observation pour servir à la solution de cette question présentée à l'Académie des Sciences le 7 janvier 1867* (Paris); 1875–92. *Leçons de clinique chirurgicale professes a l'Hôpital Saint-Louis* 7 vols. (Paris); 1892. [Farewell address at Hôpital Saint-Louis] *Gazette des hôpitaux* 65: 1389–1390.

Secondary: Faure, Jean-Louis, 1930. 'L'oeuvre de Péan.' *Bulletin et mémoires de l'Académie de médecine* 104: 367–392.

Toby Gelfand

PEDRO-PONS, AGUSTI (b. Barcelona, Spain, 9 May 1898; d. Barcelona, 27 March 1971), *medicine.*

Pedro-Pons was born in the bosom of a middle-class family. He attended the Faculty of Medicine in Barcelona (1914–19) and spent the following years learning and working as an assistant at Santa Creu Hospital. While trying to obtain a university position, he took his doctor's degree in 1925 with a thesis on Banti's disease. In 1927 he won a chair of Medicine at the Barcelona Medical Faculty, and started a brilliant career.

As the subject was then divided into two chairs, Pedro-Pons shared its teaching with Francesc Ferrer Solervicens. These university chairs had the hospital wards known as A and B Medical Clinics annexed, and due to a distinctive hospital organization and also to the disciplinary strength of Internal Medicine, those medical units sheltered all subspecialties and their correspondent laboratories.

Pedro-Pons had a great talent as an organizer, and this resulted in the creation of true cooperation. In a first stage, his clinical training stimulated notable scientific research that was collected in two volumes, *Anales de la Clinica Medica A* (1932–33, 1934–35). These works proved how he and his team succeeded in benefiting from caring for hundreds of patients despite the slender resources available. Pedro-Pons's clinical gifts shone out in this period, excelling in clinical semiology and as a bedside teacher.

A new stage started in 1939 with his appointment as president of the Catalan Academy of Medical Sciences, which office he held until 1958. That position, along with his intensive medical work, consolidated his public renown. In 1943 Pedro-Pons and psychiatrist Ramon Sarró (1899–1993) created a new medical journal, *Medicina Clínica*, which became and still is a useful tool to discuss medical research and is an authoritative reference in the Spanish medical world. That year also marked the death of Ferrer Solervicens and was the beginning of Pedro-Pons's tenure as head of internal medicine in Catalonia, when he became the most famous internist and private consultant in the country. He reorganized the entire internal medicine department at the hospital by adapting new wards according to several subspecialties, extending the dispensary premises, and creating laboratories to back clinical needs and

an emerging research agenda. It was during these years that Pedro-Pons consolidated a true medical school of internal medicine. As a result, more than a dozen of his disciples became university professors in the following years and many people who trained in that school obtained relevant hospital posts throughout the country.

Pedro-Pons, with the helpful assistance of Pere Farreras Valenti (1919–68), his most conspicuous disciple and a highly reputed internist and hematologist, made possible the publication of *Tratado de Patología y Clínica Medicas.* This work marked a milestone in the Spanish medical world. Heir to a distinctive Western tradition of medical textbooks, the treatise was the result of Pedro-Pons' teamwork experience in medical pathology and became a reference for Spanish and Latin American students and physicians.

Pedro-Pons secured a public profile thanks to his social and medical reputation. He was appointed dean of the Barcelona Medical Faculty (1954–57) and president of the Barcelona Royal Academy of Medicine (1957–71). He also chaired a number of national and international medical congresses and directed several Spanish medical journals.

Pedro-Pons retired from his chair in 1968, but he went on working as chief of internal medicine at the recently created *Vall d'Hebron* Hospital of the Public Insurance Scheme, where he kept up his program of medical education, care, and research until his death.

Bibliography

Primary: 1950. *Tratado de Patología y Clínica Médicas* 6 vols. (Barcelona).

Secondary: Corbella, Jacint, and Jaume Roige, 2000. *Dr. Pedro-Pons (1898–1971), en homenatge* (Barcelona); Cid, Felip, 1981. *Pedro-Pons, l'home i l'obra* (Barcelona); Lloveras, Gonçal, 1964. *Dr. A. Pedro Pons* (Barcelona).

Alfons Zarzoso

PEN (b. ?, ?; d. Kompong Cham, Cambodia, 1919), *Cambodian traditional medicine, botany.*

Kru Pen's personal biography remains a mystery, and the precise form of training that he received is not known. It can be supposed that it resembled that of most 'krus', or traditional Cambodian healers ('kru' derives from the Sanskrit 'guru'). This training involves the study of Theravadin Buddhist texts and prayers, often at the side of a monk, and an apprenticeship with a master, either a monk or a layperson. The apprenticeship deals with medicinal plants and other medicinal substances of the Cambodian pharmacopoeia, the techniques for preparing medicines, and the formulas that are to be murmured in order to make the medicine active. Kru Pen's master was Jru Pok, a half-caste Khmer (the dominant ethnic group in Cambodia) and Phnong (a minority ethnic group). Pok was a famous healer known to have cured himself of leprosy.

Kru Pen specialized in the treatment of leprosy as well. He used a treatment he learned from his master that combined a particular diet with a medicine made of the seeds of a tree named *krabao phlae thom* (*Hydnocarpus anthelmintica Pierre*). The seeds were roasted, crushed, and mixed with charcoal for an oral treatment. This technique was called 'Pen's method' by French colonial sources. In 1881 Pen founded a village fifteen kilometers from Kompong Cham city (Eastern Center) and established a leprosarium there that sheltered twenty-eight patients from all regions of Cambodia according to data for 1907. Kru Pen's reputation was so impressive that he was appointed the leprosy specialist at the palace of King Norodom of Cambodia, according to one French colonial source.

At that time, health care policy in the French colonial empire had two main goals: profit and minimizing the expense of running the colonial administration ('*mise en valeur coloniale*'). This was the social and economic context in which Kru Pen was asked to collaborate with the French health administration, a request that initially made him ill at ease because French doctors often viewed traditional healers as quacks. B. Menaut, Inspecteur de l'Hygiène [Public Health Inspector] in Cambodia, discovered Pen's health center by chance as he traveled around the countryside dispensing vaccinations. A sense of trust developed between the two men (Menaut, 1930). In 1908 Pen gave his French colleague the secret for making his medicine.

Menaut then began research on *krabao* seeds and developed, together with the pharmacien-major [pharmacist-in-chief] Alexis, chemist at the Laboratory of Phnom Penh, a new, efficient, and cheap method for extracting the ethers from the *krabao*. These ethers were used in the production of injections and creams for indigenous lepers. The method was inspired by the one used for the production of ethers of chaulmoogra (*taraktogenos*). The ethylic oils proved to be successful in improving the patients' appetite as well as their general health; they also worked well on the ulcers and perforating sores which were not curable until this discovery. Thanks to the abundance of *Hydnocarpus anthelmintica Pierre* trees in Cambodia, the chemistry laboratory of Phnom Penh was able to cover the needs of the mother country and the entire French colonial empire from 1925 onward.

The Résident de France [provincial governor] in Kompong Cham put a large house made of bamboo at Kru Pen's disposal to use in his work with lepers. In 1915 he was appointed director of the first leprosarium of Cambodia by the Gouverneur Général de l'Indochine [Governor-general of Indochina, the highest authority in the colony]. By then, however, his activity began to decline because his prosperity made people suspect that he was exploiting the lepers' misfortune, according to a colonial source.

After he died of cholera in 1919, his sons kept up his work, but separated their own private leprosarium from the official colonial one close by. At that time, the French leprosarium welcomed eighty Hansenians. The leprosarium at Troeng still exists today.

Bibliography

Primary: Gaide, Laurent, and Bodet, 1930. *La prévention et le traitement de la lèpre en Indochine* (Hanoi); Menaut, Bernard, 1930. *Matière médicale cambodgienne* (Hanoi); Petelot, Alfred, 1952. *Les plantes médicinales du Cambodge, du Laos et du Viêtnam* (Saigon).

Anne Y. Guillou

PENFIELD, WILDER GRAVES (b. Spokane, Washington, USA, 26 January 1891; d. Montreal, Canada, 5 April 1976), *neurosurgery.*

Penfield was born in Spokane, Washington, but had his early schooling in Hudson, Wisconsin. His father, Charles Samuel Penfield, was an unsuccessful and disinterested physician who took to the outdoors to revive his health and eventually spent much of his life wandering in the frontier wilderness. His mother, Jean Jefferson Penfield, encouraged Wilder to succeed academically and early in his schooling laid plans for him to win a Rhodes Scholarship, which he did on his second attempt while attending Princeton, the university he selected because it was in a small state where competition for the scholarship would be less. At Princeton he demonstrated his leadership and athletic skills. At Oxford he came in contact with William Osler and Charles Sherrington, who had a great influence on him and became his lifetime heroes.

During a summer break he left for a Red Cross Hospital in France, but his ship, the *SS Sussex*, was torpedoed. He was initially reported as dead, but survived with a serious leg injury. He convalesced back at Oxford in Osler's home at 13 Norham Gardens, 'The Open Arms'.

After his BA at Merton College he began his medical studies at Johns Hopkins in Baltimore, and in 1917 married Helen Katherine Kermott. In the summer of 1917 they traveled to Paris to work at a Red Cross Hospital before returning for his last year of medical studies; he graduated with his MD in 1918. He undertook postgraduate work at the Peter Bent Brigham Hospital in Boston under Harvey Cushing and returned for his final scholarship year at Oxford under Sherrington and a further year at the National Hospital, Queen Square, in London.

He returned to New York for training in general surgery and neurosurgery at the Presbyterian Hospital under Allan Whipple. He turned down a lucrative offer from the Henry Ford Hospital in Detroit, which would not allow him research time, and instead stayed in New York, accepting an appointment at Presbyterian Hospital. With support from Whipple he spent some months with Don Pio del Rio Hortega in Madrid and made some important observations on microglia and their ability to transform into scavenger cells in the presence of brain damage. Back in New York in 1924, he founded the Laboratory of Neurocytology and remained on the staff as an attending associate surgeon until 1928. He had responsibilities for developing the neurosurgical services and there was joined by a research fellow from Iowa, William Cone.

Edward Archibald, professor of surgery at McGill University, was looking for a surgeon to specialize in neurosurgery and recruited Penfield in 1928. Before taking up his appointments at McGill and the Royal Victoria Hospital he traveled to Europe to work with Offrid Forester in Breslau, working on epilepsy caused by head injury.

Back in Montreal one of his first patients was his sister, Ruth, and in an unusual act of bravado he operated on her, partially removing a malignant brain tumor that allowed her to live a further three years. He worked on perfecting his surgery of severe epilepsy. He was inspired by the work of his teacher, Sherrington, and also Hughlings Jackson, who felt that epilepsy was an experiment of nature that could reveal the functional organization of the brain. He used the new neurosurgical techniques to operate on epileptic brains while the patients were still awake and able to relate what they were experiencing as he stimulated the cerebral cortex with electrodes, initiating a controlled seizure.

At this point in his career Penfield had gained experience in neurology, general surgery, neurosurgery, laboratory and cytological procedures, physiology, and experimental surgery. He had made effective contacts with world leaders in neurophysiology, neurocytology, and neurosurgery and was gaining a reputation as a leader himself. He embarked on the idea of writing a textbook of the cytology and cellular pathology of the brain, but with contributions from many disciplines of neuroscience. This cooperative effort further interested him in the idea of a collaborative institute of neurology with colleagues from various disciplines working on an equal footing. His initial drawing for the building, scribbled on a napkin, still exists. He was encouraged in this venture by Charles Martin, dean of McGill, Sir Arthur Currie, principal of McGill, and Alan Gregg of the Rockefeller Foundation. After an initial refusal, Martin and Currie were successful in obtaining $1,232,652 from the Rockefeller Foundation and commitments of support for building and endowment from McGill, the city of Montreal, the Province of Quebec, and the public. Always an accomplished diplomat, Penfield smoothed the way by developing good relationships with the French neurological and academic communities in Quebec.

A cornerstone for the Montreal Neurological Institute (MNI) was laid in October 1933, and the doors officially opened on 27 September 1934, a model for units that combined clinical care, research, and postgraduate medical education. Penfield was director from 1934 to 1960.

To assure success he fostered support from many organizations, foundations, and private donors, and he attracted outstanding clinicians and scientists to build a broad base in clinical care and neuroscience. William Cone

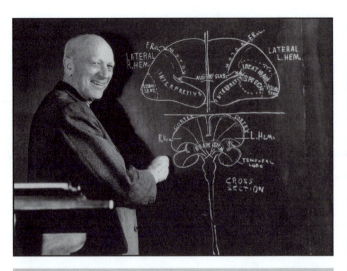

Wilder Penfield teaching at the blackboard, Montreal Neurological Institute, 1963. From the Wilder Penfield Archive, Montreal Neurological Institute.

came with him from New York and he enlisted the cooperation of the faculty at McGill and associated hospitals. He later attracted Herbert Jasper in electroencephalography, K. A. C. Elliott in neurochemistry, and outstanding clinicians such as Francis McNaughton, William Feindel, Preston Robb, and Brenda Milner. In 1948, recognizing that Canadian neurologists and neurosurgeons did not have a voice or recognition internationally, he called together a group to form the Canadian Neurology Society.

Although he was building a world-renowned neurological institute, he worked hard at his own research, which centered on the surgery of epilepsy. He developed techniques to map the brain of epileptics, determining the site of the epileptic discharge, and made remarkable observations of the reactions of his patients who were having their temporal lobes stimulated and excised while awake. Although it was developed as a technique to pinpoint the focus of seizure activity so that it could be removed, the memory experiences experienced by the patients when their temporal lobes were being stimulated also revealed how the brain held memories. The memories that were relived by the patient while the temporal lobe was being stimulated became the basis of many studies of human memory. He accumulated a vast amount of experimental data over two decades, which he revealed in the 1954 Maudsley Lecture. He indicated that there was a rich stream of memory and consciousness that could be elicited in some people by an epileptic seizure and by experimental cortical stimulation. The memories would continue to run forward like a movie, and they were so real that it seemed as if his subjects were experiencing them again. These vivid memories resided in the temporal lobes and needed only some means of recall. The memories continued until he withdrew the electrode from the temporal lobe cortex. Stimulating other areas of the brain cortex did not get this effect. He developed the techniques further to map areas of the brain, demonstrating a supplementary motor area, a second sensory area, and four areas of the cortex involved in speech. He evolved the controversial concept of the centrencephalon, an area in the brainstem that served as a subcortical control and integration region for the cortex, allowing the brain to act as a single functioning organ.

Although the memory experiments of his epileptic surgery received a great deal of attention, it should not be forgotten that he was also getting dramatic results in the control of seizures in the patients that underwent cortical resection, remarkable because most of these patients had uncontrolled seizures and had failed to respond to medical therapy. It is now recognized that this is not just a last resort therapy, but one now to be offered early in the management of patients with complex partial epilepsy, a major contribution to epilepsy management.

Penfield had become a Canadian citizen in 1934 and during World War II was a colonel in the Canadian Army Medical Corps, heading projects on motion sickness, decompression sickness, and air transportation of head injuries.

After stepping down as director of the MNI in 1960 he entered what he called his second career of writing, traveling, and lecturing. He was given awards, including the Order of Merit from Queen Elizabeth and membership in both the Canadian and British Royal Societies.

He helped found and was the first president of the Vanier Institute of the Family and served on the board of governors of McGill, as an officer of the Rockefeller Foundation, and as curator of the Osler Library. He wrote a biography of Alan Gregg and a history of the MNI. He completed a Biblical novel drafted by his mother and wrote many books on the mind and brain. Using the letters he wrote to his mother each week, he wrote of his life, completing *No Man Alone: A Surgeon's Life* in the third draft three weeks before he died of cancer, which brought his life story up to the establishment of the MNI, his great legacy.

Bibliography

Primary: 1941. (with Erickson, T. C.) *Epilepsy and Cerebral Localization: A Study of the Mechanism, Treatment and Prevention of Epileptic Seizures* (London); 1950. (with Rasmussen, T.) *The Cerebral Cortex of Man: A Clinical Study of Localization of Function* (New York); 1954. *Epilepsy and the Functional Anatomy of the Human Brain* (London); 1975. *The Mystery of the Mind: A Critical Study of Consciousness and the Human Brain* (London); 1977. *No Man Alone: A Surgeon's Life* (Montreal).

Secondary: Lewis, J., 1981. *Something Hidden: A Biography of Wilder Penfield* (Toronto); Eccles, John, and W. Feindel, 1978. 'Wilder Graves Penfield.' *Biographical Memoirs of Fellows of the Royal Society* 24: 473–513.

Jock Murray

PENNA, BELISÁRIO   (b. Barbacena, Brazil, 29 November 1868; d. Sacra Família, Brazil, 4 November 1939), *public health, hygiene.*

Penna was born into a noble family of the Brazilian Empire. He initiated his medical studies in 1886 in Rio de Janeiro and finished them at the School of Medicine of Bahia in 1890, one year after the establishment of the republican regime. He returned to his birthplace and worked as a physician with Italian immigrants. He also worked in towns in the Brazilian state of Minas Gerais. In 1904 he returned to Rio as a sanitary inspector and participated in Oswaldo Cruz's campaign to control yellow fever. This experience inspired him to devote his life to public health and the population's hygienic education. Up to 1911 Penna participated in campaigns to combat smallpox, yellow fever, and malaria, sometimes accompanying Oswaldo Cruz and Carlos Chagas.

In 1912 Penna and the physician Arthur Neiva led a medical expedition to study the poverty- and drought-stricken areas in Brazil's inland. The human misery, abandonment, and disease in the area made a great impression on Penna. The following year he traveled throughout Brazil to learn more about its sanitary conditions. The 1916 publication of a report illustrated with photographs from the expedition, which appeared in the journal *Memoirs of Oswaldo Cruz Institute*, had a great impact in the newspapers and among the public. Of special importance were its dramatic descriptions of social and health conditions in rural Brazil, where illiteracy, ancylostomiasis, goiter, Chagas' disease, schistosomiasis, and malaria reigned.

Between 1914 and 1918 Penna worked in suburban Rio de Janeiro creating rural prophylaxis health posts. In 1916 he started a crusade for rural sanitation by way of newspaper articles, pamphlets, and public lectures. These activities emphasized teaching hygienic principles to the population and making the elites aware of the urgency of national sanitary problems. In January 1918 he created the Pro-Sanitation League of Brazil, a nationalistic movement for public health reform. Penna criticized the autonomy of the states regarding sanitation matters, the oligarchic local interests that blocked Federal sanitary interventions, and the disregard for the country's rural inhabitants. Rural endemic diseases were, for Penna, the main obstacles to national development and integration of Brazil's hinterland, and he discarded race and tropical climate as an explanation for the country's backwardness. He proposed that the central government assume the country's sanitation with a new and truly national sanitary organization.

The political mobilization for rural sanitation was successful. In late 1919 the National Congress created the National Department for Public Health, which enlarged to a national level the authority of the federal sanitary services, until then restricted to the country's capital and ports. The department included a board of sanitation and rural prophylaxis, of which Penna was placed in charge from 1920 to 1922. During this

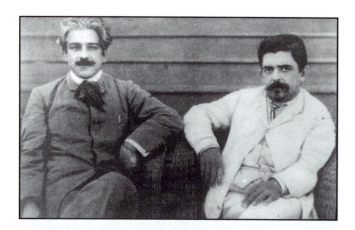

Penna (right) and Oswaldo Cruz during the campaign against malaria in the Amazon region, 1910. Photograph, Oswaldo Cruz Foundation Historical Archives.

period he traveled through the country for the installation of preventive health posts and the control against rural endemic diseases in several states.

Due to his problems with political interferences and bureaucratic obstacles to his work, Penna left his post and turned to educating the populace. Between 1925 and 1926 Penna was the protagonist of a public debate at the National Academy of Medicine concerning leprosy, in his opinion the main national sanitary problem.

Penna supported the emergence of Getúlio Vargas's authoritarian regime in 1930 and became director of national sanitary services, believing that conditions existed to implement his ideas. In 1932 he was Minister of Education and Public Health for a few months. A lack of resources due to the world's economic crisis and continuing political interference led Penna to leave the post and retire from civil service in 1933. Disappointed with Vargas, he became a leader in the nationalist and fascist-like movements that were repressed after a coup d'état attempt in 1938.

Bibliography

Primary: 1916. (with Neiva, Arthur) 'Viagem científica pelo Norte da Bahia, Sudoeste de Pernambuco, sul do Piauí e de norte a sul de Goiás.' *Memórias do Instituto Oswaldo Cruz* 30: 74–224; 1918. *O saneamento do Brasil* (Rio de Janeiro).

Secondary: Hochman, Gilberto, 1998. *A Era do Saneamento* (São Paulo).

Gilberto Hochman

PEPPER, WILLIAM (b. Philadelphia, Pennsylvania, USA, 21 August 1843; d. Pleasanton, California, USA, 28 July 1898), *medicine, medical education, philanthropy.*

Pepper's parents were William Pepper, professor of medicine at the University of Pennsylvania (Penn), and Sarah Platt Pepper. He completed his AB at Penn in 1862 and his

MD in 1864, and by the end of 1865 he had an attending appointment at the Pennsylvania Hospital. Between 1866 and 1868 he served as pathologist at Pennsylvania Hospital, curator at Philadelphia General Hospital, and lecturer in morbid anatomy at Penn. In 1870 he became lecturer in clinical medicine; he was appointed clinical professor of medicine in 1876; and in 1883 he acceded to the chair of the theory and practice of medicine at the University of Pennsylvania medical school. He married Frances Sergeant Perry in 1873; they had three children.

Pepper was a prolific writer on clinical matters. In 1870 he helped prepare the fourth edition of Meigs's *Diseases of Children,* and he founded the *Philadelphia Medical Times.* In 1886–87 he edited a multivolume *System of Medicine by American Authors.*

In 1871 Pepper initiated a drive to raise funds for a university-owned hospital, a component of a new and useful strategy for medical education reform in the United States. When the Hospital of the University of Pennsylvania opened in 1874, Pepper emerged as the leading force behind Penn's new momentum. By 1877, his advocacy helped lead to stricter admission requirements, a three-year graded course, formal clinical teaching, and fixed salaries for professors. Early in his tenure as university provost, the medical school's academic year was extended, and in 1893 Penn implemented a four-year medical course.

As provost (a position he held from 1881 to 1894, while retaining his professorship and his private practice), Pepper undertook the modernization of the entire university, starting with a change in governance rules intended to make his office more effective. Among other achievements, he was responsible for Penn establishing a graduate school—the Wharton School of Business—a veterinary school, a school of nursing, and the university museum of archaeology.

Upon his resignation as provost he established at Penn the William Pepper Clinical Laboratory in memory of his father. While the Pepper Laboratory never became a major research facility, it did set a precedent for research-based medical schools.

Pepper was a public figure of local, national, and international standing. The most enduring of his many projects for Philadelphia is the public library, which opened in 1891 with a bequest left by his uncle. On a national level, Pepper devoted much effort—in vain—toward establishing a national university in Washington, D.C. His work as President of the first Pan-American Medical Congress in 1893 resulted in his lionization by medical and political leaders in Latin America.

Despite chronic illness Pepper led a very active life, but increasingly took advantage of his personal wealth to travel to good climates for some rest. He died at a friend's home in California shortly after saying that, at age fifty-four, he felt like a 'worn-out old man'.

Pepper felt obliged to use his inherited fortune and his professional prestige to the advantage of society. His civic schemes for Philadelphia reminded associates of Benjamin Franklin's activities a century earlier. And although Pepper's clinical work was marginal to the development of scientific medicine, the changes he brought to the University of Pennsylvania and its medical school remain central to the modernization of the university and of medical education in the United States.

Bibliography

Primary: 1869. *Descriptive Catalogue of the Pathological Museum of the Pennsylvania Hospital* (Philadelphia); 1877. *Higher Medical Education, the True Interest of the Public and of the Profession* (Philadelphia); 1887. *Contribution to the Climatological Study of Phthisis in Pennsylvania* (New York).

Secondary: Corner, George W., 1965. *Two Centuries of Medicine: A History of the School of Medicine, University of Pennsylvania* (Philadelphia); Thorpe, Francis Newton, 1904. *William Pepper, M.D., LL.D.* (Philadelphia); *DAMB*.

Edward T. Morman

PERCIVAL, THOMAS (b. Warrington, Lancashire, England, 29 September 1740, d. Manchester, England, 30 August 1804), *medicine, medical ethics*.

Percival was the son of Joseph Percival, a merchant, and his wife Margaret Orred. His parents died when he was three, and his older sister raised him. He received the education of the middling classes, beginning with private seminary and then moving on to Boteler Grammar School in Warrington and Manchester Grammar School. He may have been the first student at the Warrington Academy, famous for educating many Dissenting scientists. Percival's grandfather, Peter Percival, had practiced medicine in Warrington, as did his uncle, Thomas, and when the latter died (1750) he left his nephew his valuable library, some private means, and the determination to study medicine.

Around 1761, Percival began attending lectures in medicine at the University of Edinburgh. In 1764 a dispute with the medical faculty led him, as well as other students, to leave Edinburgh and go first to London, where he was elected FRS (March 1765), and then to Leiden, where he received his MD (July 1765). He set up practice in Warrington, where he married Elizabeth Bassnett (1766). Five of their offspring were still living in 1804.

In 1767 Percival moved to Manchester. Though already notorious for the pollution caused by industrial use of soft coal, the city was also known for its flourishing intellectual and cultural life. Percival, together with other members of the city's professional and business elite, founded the Manchester Literary and Philosophical Society. He was elected president for all but one year between 1782 and 1804. Other prominent early members were the chemists Thomas Henry (1734–1816) and John Dalton (1766–1844), the surgeon and obstetrician Charles White (1728–1813), and the reforming physician John Ferriar (1761–1815). Percival and Ferriar became allies in the effort to improve public hygiene, and they were among the earliest advocates of public health legislation to ameliorate the impact of factories. In 1773 Percival published *Essays Medical and Experimental*. Among the essays were 'Proposals for Establishing More Accurate and Comprehensive Bills of Mortality in Manchester', an early contribution to the growing body of research in medical demography and epidemiology. It was translated into Italian (1774).

Percival was briefly involved in the Manchester Infirmary in the 1780s, and he helped to found the Manchester Fever Hospital (1796). The code of regulations he drew up for the Infirmary (1792) led to the publication of his best-known work, *Medical Ethics; or, a Code of Institutes and Precepts, adapted to the Professional Conduct of Physicians and Surgeons* (1803). Part of the work deals with the relationship between physicians and patients in private practice, and scholars have noted the extent to which Percival drew upon the Hippocratic corpus and its many commentators from classical antiquity to the eighteenth century. Even more important were the ethical relationships Percival sought to establish in public hospitals and infirmaries, which treated charity patients. His *Medical Ethics* set standards of humane behavior, arguing that, wherever practicable and consonant with proper medical treatment, poor patients should be allowed the same choice of medical attendant and regimen as would be allowed the rich. His work formed the basis for the code of ethics adopted by the American Medical Association in 1847.

Percival's book for young people, *A Father's Instructions; Consisting of Moral Tales, Fables, Reflections*, was published between 1775 and 1800.

Bibliography

Primary: 1807. Percival, E. C., ed. *The Works, Literary, Moral, and Medical, of Thomas Percival* 4 vols. (London); 1773. *Essays, Medical and Experimental* (London); 1975. (Leake, Chauncey D., ed.) *Percival's Medical Ethics* (Huntington, NY).

Secondary: Baker, Robert, Dorothy Porter, and Roy Porter, eds., 1993–95. *The Codification of Medical Morality* (Dordrecht); Sheehan, Donal, 1941. 'The Manchester Literary and Philosophical Society.' *Isis* 33(4): 519–523; *Oxford DNB*.

Lisa Rosner

PERCY, PIERRE FRANÇOIS (b. Montagney, France, 20 October 1754; d. Paris, France, 18 February 1825), *surgery, military medicine, medical literature*.

Born the son of a military surgeon, Percy first studied mathematics with the aim of joining the artillery. A good classical education made him an accomplished Latinist and a fine writer, skills that stood him in good stead as a lifelong author of essays and books on military medicine. Trained in surgery at Besançon, Percy perfected his skills under the guidance of the surgeon Antoine Louis in Paris.

In 1776 he joined the army as an assistant military surgeon and his entire career would focus on the fate of wounded men. Since France was at war with Europe almost continually during the Revolution and Empire, Percy's services were much in demand. He excelled in battle surgery (his term) and became famous for his attempt to preserve limbs by resection, rather than resorting to amputation.

In the Rhine army in 1792, Percy was first to organize *brancardiers* [stretcher-bearers], assigning soldiers to transport casualties to a field hospital (confusingly called *ambulance*). The stretchers were constructed so that the shafts could be used as defensive weapons. During the German campaign of 1799–1800, he devised a vehicle to transport surgical supplies and first aid to the battlefield. This carriage imitated a German model of a long, round vehicle, so the French dubbed it '*wurst*': up to ten surgeons could ride on its back. Though welcome, the *wurst* was cumbersome and was soon replaced by Larrey's two-wheeled 'flying ambulance'.

These were important technical advances to help wounded soldiers promptly. Even more imaginative was Percy's proposal, made to the French general Jean-Victor Moreau and to the Austrian general Paul von Kray in 1800, that field hospitals and the wounded should be respected by opposing armies. Percy even asked that drums and musical instruments be stilled near hospitals. Unfortunately, the world would have to wait sixty years for these ideas to be enacted by what became the Red Cross.

While a champion of humane military medicine, Percy never reached his goal of seeing a French army medical corps established. Napoleon, wary of doctors, denied his physicians and surgeons the independence that organized military medicine requires, and they remained subordinated to the quartermaster. But Napoleon valued Percy, raising him to inspector general of the armies, decorating him with the Legion of Honor, and awarding him a baronetcy in 1809.

In addition to achieving a full military career, Percy also remained active in civilian life. In 1794, when the new Paris Health School was created, he became professor of surgery ('external pathology'), teaching there as his military duties allowed until the Bourbons destituted him in 1815.

After the battle of Waterloo, at which he was present, Percy evidently hoped for a representative government, for he was elected a deputy. The restored Bourbons would not tolerate such independence and deprived him of his professorship and his military post.

Percy retired to his country house at Mongey and spent his remaining ten years administering his domain, collecting ancient arms, and writing numerous essays for dictionaries and encyclopedias. He was elected to the Academy of Sciences in 1807, defeating Napoleon's physician Corvisart, elected in 1811, and to the Academy of Medicine. His campaign journals have remained a classic.

Bibliography

Primary: 1792. *Manuel du chirurgien d'armée* (Paris) (2nd edn., 1830); 1794. *Pyrotechnie chirurgicale pratique, ou l'art d'appliquer le feu en chirurgie* (Strasbourg) (2nd edn., 1810); 1904. *Journal des campagnes du baron Percy, chirurgien-en-chef de la grande armée* (Paris).

Secondary: Weiner, Dora B., 1993. *The Citizen-Patient in Revolutionary and Imperial Paris* (Baltimore); Weiner, Dora B., 1969. 'French Doctors Face War: 1792–1815' in Warner, Charles E., ed., *From the Ancien Régime to the Popular Front: Essays in the History of Modern France in Honor of Shepard B. Clough* (New York); Bergounioux, J., 1904. 'Le baron P. F. Percy, chirurgien-en-chef de la Grande Armée, et son *Journal de campagne*.' *La France médicale*, 51ème année: 343–349, 362–372; Laurent, 1827. *Histoire de la vie et des ouvrages de Percy* (Paris).

Dora B. Weiner

PERDOMO NEIRA, MIGUEL (b. La Plata, Colombia, 29 September 1833; d. Guayaquil, Ecuador, 24 December 1874), *popular medicine.*

Perdomo Neira gained a reputation as the 'people's doctor' during his travels throughout Colombia and Ecuador in the 1860s and 1870s. As a lay healer (*curandero*), Perdomo performed minor surgery and dispensed drugs according to their humoral qualities while maintaining a devoutly Catholic approach to healing. These patterns of treatment fit squarely within the Hispanic medical spectrum that dominated most of the northern Andes. Perdomo's broad popular following contributed to legal and social conflicts with authorities in Quito and Bogotá, confrontations that illustrate the professionalization of biomedical practitioners in this region.

The manners by which curanderos acquire medical knowledge are seldom documented. Born in a small rural town, Perdomo likely apprenticed with a barber (lay surgeon) in that he was drafted as a surgeon into the Conservative army of Julio Arboleda in the late 1850s during one of Colombia's many civil wars that spawned social and political instability throughout the century. Toward the end of the war, Perdomo took refuge in an indigenous community and learned of drugs with analgesic, coagulative, and anti-inflammatory properties. His favorite drug, a powerful purgative he called 'El Toro', speaks to the humoral nature of his healing. It is quite likely that Perdomo learned about healing from a priest, perhaps one associated with a San Juan de Dios hospital. He formed a hospital near Popayán in the late 1860s that served scores of people from the Cauca Valley and beyond. His devout Catholicism was evident in his adoration of an image of the Sacred Heart of Jesus and his charitable approach to healing; he sold the drugs but did not charge for his procedures.

Perdomo traveled southward into Ecuador in 1867, where he earned public acclaim but also provoked political controversy. The Quito Municipal Council imprisoned Perdomo for practicing medicine without a license. This first conflict with biomedical physicians took place within the transformation of the colonial *protomedicato* (regulatory board) into an agency that would monitor public health and the licensing of physicians. Scores of his supporters, including the Governor of the province, petitioned for his release, granted only upon payment of a hefty fine and an agreement that he would leave the country.

After a year at the hospital in the Cauca Valley, Perdomo traveled north into the Department of Antioquia in 1869. Testimonials increasingly focused on his surgical abilities and his charitable healings. While in Medellín he penned a revealing account of his approach to healing, much of which is a partisan Catholic criticism of contemporary affairs. He criticized physicians who were motivated by money and who sought to distance themselves from the population that God intended them to treat. This fusion of 'miraculous' healing, Catholic beliefs, and Conservative political affiliation made him a danger to the dominant Liberal government in Bogotá.

Perdomo arrived in Bogotá in April 1872, just as biomedical physicians had succeeded in establishing a Faculty of Medicine at the newly founded National University. Weeks before he set foot in the city, Liberal newspapers blasted his ardent Conservatism, while more moderate papers heralded his popular approach to healing. Liberal physicians demanded that he demonstrate his skills at the University, critiquing his 'ignorance' of scientific medicine. The death of one of his patients sparked a riot between his supporters, medical students, and the local police. Although Perdomo left the city, he continued to travel through Colombia and Ecuador before his death in Guayaquil in December 1874.

Bibliography

Primary: 1867. *Un ultraje inmerecido* (Quito); 1872. *La iglesia católica en presencia del siglo XIX* (Bogotá).

Secondary: Sowell, David, 2001. *The Tale of Miguel Perdomo Neira: Medicine, Ideologies, and Power in the Nineteenth-Century Andes* (Wilmington, DE); Abel, Christopher, 1994. *Health Care in Colombia, c. 1920–c. 1950: A Preliminary Analysis* (London).

David Sowell

PERRONCITO, EDOARDO BELLARMINO (b. Viale d'Asti, Italy, 1 March 1847; d. Pavia, Italy, 4 November 1936), *parasitology, veterinary medicine.*

Perroncito was the second son of Luigi, a shoemaker, and Lucia Pastrone, a dressmaker. He went to school at Asti, won a scholarship, and was thus able to enroll in the Regia Scuola Superiore di Medicina Veterinaria at Turin, the oldest such institution in Italy. In 1867 he obtained his degree in veterinary medicine. After a short period as municipal veterinarian he became the assistant of Sebastiano Rivolta and in 1873 his successor as professor of veterinary pathological anatomy. Perroncito soon developed a strong interest in parasitology. In 1875 the Italian government sent him to visit Louis Pasteur in Paris. In 1881 he began to teach courses in parasitology at the Medical Faculty of Turin, and four years later the first official chair was created for him. He retired in 1923. Perroncito's private life was filled with affliction. He first married Arminia Aletti, becoming closely related to Giulio Bizzozero and Camillo Golgi, and then Mirte. Both wives died prematurely. His two sons, Mario and Aldo, died of tuberculosis.

Perroncito's scientific production ranged from the microbiological analysis of water to pathological anatomy, from the study of the diseases of animals to those of humans and even plants, from the problems of apiculture and silkworm breeding to public health. His first studies concerned *Echinococcus* and were exemplary in their methodology: he investigated the pathological agent in vivo and in vitro and described its appearance and forms in animals for slaughter, the reproductive cycle, and the lesions provoked. Finally, he subjected it to various treatments to develop countermeasures. Thus, Perroncito confirmed that humans infected by the beef tapeworm had received it from eating raw meat. In the same way he investigated several other parasitic infections. After 1868 he differentiated various types of bovine tuberculosis and showed the histological identity of the typical lesions provoked by this disease in bovines and in humans. Other merits concern intestinal trichinosis and avian fever. Based on these experiences he strongly advocated a strict supervision of meat, the construction of slaughterhouses, and the adoption of refrigeration. Later, he was also engaged to apply Pasteur's studies on prophylaxis and the cure of rabies. In 1887 he founded in Turin a 'Laboratorio Pasteur' for the production of vaccines against anthrax.

Perroncito's name is mainly linked to the demonstration that the anemia of miners is directly connected with the presence of *Ancylostoma duodenale*. In 1879 he was engaged to investigate the disease that struck thousands of miners working in the Mount St Gotthard Tunnel. Perroncito's postmortem examination of a miner revealed the presence of 1,500 tiny worms in the mucous membrane. He demonstrated that these nematodes, first described by Angelo Dubini in 1843, fed on the blood of the vessels of the intestine. He developed a method to study their complete reproductive cycle in vitro and experimented with a series of possible remedies. Finally, he developed the ethereal extract of male fern to act as an effective vermicide. Perroncito's treatment of hookworm disease was a great success and was applied likewise to other categories of workers exposed to great humidity. After years of quarrels about the priority of this discovery, he was awarded the Prix Montyon of the Institute de France (1931) in recognition. He received honorary degrees from the universities of London, Vienna, Strasbourg, and Manchester; was nominated three times honorary president of the International Congresses of Hygiene and Demography; and was appointed a member of the medical and scientific societies and academies of Paris, Lyon, Brussels, Tokyo, Moscow, Buenos Aires, La Plata, and Boston, as well as many international committees. He was also elected mayor of his hometown and town councilor of Turin.

Bibliography

Primary: 1882. *I parassiti dell'uomo e degli animali utili* (Milan); 1886. *L'anemia dei minatori in Ungheria* (Turin).

Secondary: Ghisleni, P., 1937. 'Edoardo Perroncito.' *Giornale dell'Accademia di Medicina di Torino* 100: 39–47; *DSB*.

Ariane Dröscher

PETER OF ABANO (aka PETRUS APONICUS, APONENSIS, PETRUS DE APONE, PETRUS DE EBANO, PIETRO D'ABANO, PIETRO DE SCLAVIONE, PADUANUS, PATAVINUS, RECONCILIATOR, CONCILIATOR) (b. Abano, Italy, *c.* 1250; d. Padua, Italy, *c.* 1316), *medicine, astronomy, astrology, philosophy.*

Peter was born in Abano, a village near Padua in northern Italy, the son of Constantius de Sclavione, a notary. He studied at Paris, graduating as a doctor of philosophy and physic. He practiced medicine in Padua between 1303 and 1307 after his graduation and returned there from Paris, where he had taught since 1299. He was a papal physician for Honorius IV (1285–87) and perhaps also Benedict XI (1303–04) and John XXII (1316–34); to one of these he dedicated his manuscript, *De venenis.* Peter traveled extensively, reaching Constantinople in search of a copy of the *Problemata* of Aristotle, which he translated and commented upon; he supposedly visited Spain, England, and Scotland as well. There is evidence that he lived and possibly taught in Bologna. Peter most likely died in Padua in 1316, after his second trial for heresy, but some evidence suggests he died later.

Peter was an extremely prolific writer. His medical works include the *Conciliator differentiarum philosophorum et precipue medicorum,* often simply referred to as the *Conciliator* and titled *Conciliator controversiarum . . .* in some editions (1310); the *Liber compilationis physionomiae* (1295) on physiognomy; and the *Liber de venenis* (1310?), on poisons. His other works focused on astronomy, astrology, and philosophy and were imbued with Peter's medical references. These works include the *Lucidator dubitabilium astronomiae* (1316), also referred to simply as the *Lucidator,* and a commentary and translation of Aristotle's *Problemata* (1310). Peter was also an active translator; he certainly knew Greek and might have had a reading knowledge of Hebrew. Among his translations are the *Problemata* of Alexander of Aphrodisias, six Galenic treatises, an alphabetized version of Dioscorides' work (a Greek version of which he found in Constantinople), and some minor works of Hippocrates. A comprehensive bibliography of Peter's own writings is included in Thorndike's work and remains today the most complete account of Peter's life available in English.

Peter was educated in accordance with the medieval scholastic tradition of the thirteenth and fourteenth cen-

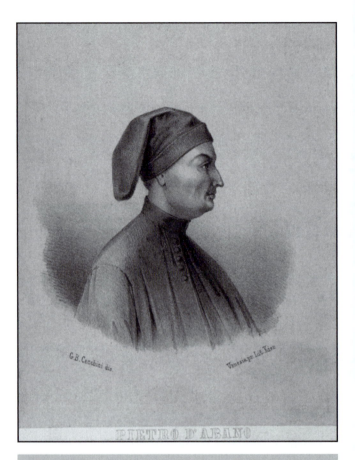

Peter of Abano. Lithograph by G. B. Cecchini. Iconographic Collection, Wellcome Library, London.

tury, as his citations of Arabic physicians and astronomers in his works clearly indicate. However, his attitude toward medical science, and indeed knowledge in general, was more radical than the approach adopted by many of his contemporaries. Peter stressed on more than one occasion his disdain for 'men who are ignorant of the causes of things [and] immediately want to reduce everything to the divine' (*Expos. Prob. Arist.*, 25, 2, and Siraisi, 1970, p. 337). As Nancy Siraisi indicated, Peter preferred physical and determinable causes, rather than divine ones, to explain the functioning of the world, and this might be a result of his medical and astrological training. In fact, Peter identified astrology and medicine as inseparable sciences, as he illustrated in *differentiae* 10 and 113 of the *Conciliator*: '[. . .] astronomy is not only useful but essential to medicine.' According to his contemporaries, it was in fact because of his belief in astrology that Peter administered drugs at what he considered the most propitious moments while advising against surgical procedures and phlebotomy when the stars were not favorable. Indeed, the role of the stars and the moon in medicine is central to an understanding of Peter's thought and conflicts that resulted from it.

Tradition ascribed to Peter the founding of Averroism in northern Italy, but recent historiographers agree that Peter was not the first Averroist and was not as central in the promulgation of heterodox Aristotelism in Padua or Paris as previous historians and philosophers had asserted. Peter did acknowledge Averroes (Ibn Rushd) in his works, preferring, for instance, the views of Averroes over Avicenna's (Ibn Sīnā,) on the origin of the human species. The Averroes view, which argued for the origin of the soul and life uniquely from matter, was the reason the inquisitors tried Peter in Paris the first time, according to what he wrote in the forty-eighth *differentia* of the *Conciliator*. According to Michele Savonarola and other sources, he escaped that trial by convincing the University of Paris's faculty of theology that he was innocent and by stating that the Dominican friars accusing him were the real heretics. However, he was unable to persuade the inquisitors in his second trial in Padua in 1315. According to the most reliable sources uncovered so far, he died in prison while waiting for his execution.

Peter of Abano is renowned for his most influential treatise, the *Conciliator*. This work attempted to solve a number of contradictions and problems arising from different medical sources such as Aristotle, Galen, Avicenna, and other philosophers included in the medical curriculum of most European universities at the time Peter wrote. The work is a collection of 210 *differentiae* or problems. For each one, Peter first defined the problem and the terminology used to explain it; second, he mentioned what other philosophers and medical commentators had written on the subject. Third, Peter provided the real solution to the problem, and finally he answered possible criticisms and observations which might arise from his elucidation. The first ten *differentiae* are concerned with simple questions regarding the nature of medicine and the physician himself. The next 100 *differentiae* treat medical theoretical problems in which the opinions of previous philosophers and physicians had conflicted. The remaining problems concern more practical medical matters as well as simple concepts of hygiene. The most common edition of this work was printed in Venice in 1565 in numerous copies and is the basis for recent reprints of the *Conciliator*. However, this 1565 edition, despite being the most frequently cited and widely distributed, included some omissions, as pointed out by Vescovini; the 1476 edition did not present the same shortcomings.

The *Liber de venenis* [On Poisons] is the other principal medical work composed by Peter. The six chapters examine the subject of poisons: they are listed and classified, their action described, and their remedies illustrated. An appendix to this work examined the concept of a remedy against all poisons, or *bezoar*, which in some editions of the manuscript was described as a divine stone. However, in the rest of the work, Peter stated his preference for a specific remedy for each poison. He recognized that theriac could be used universally but understood it was less effective in this panacean function.

Another extensive treatise authored by Peter, abbreviated as *Expositio Problematum Aristotelis*, is a commentary on the *Problemata* of Aristotle, which Peter had brought back from Constantinople. Although not uniquely medical, this text presented a wealth of references to medicine and physiological notions. It is divided into thirty-eight chapters or *particulae*, each dealing with a different and specific topic. In this, as in his other works, Peter could hardly discuss medical topics without a connection to astrological and astronomical notions. As Siraisi and Lynn Thorndike have noted, in chapter eighteen of the *Expositio* Peter's distinction between astrology and astronomy was very similar to the modern definition of the terms.

A fourth work, of predominantly astrological focus and containing several references and metaphors dealing with medical science, was the *Lucidator dubitabilium astronomiae*. This text followed mainly the same organization of the *Conciliator* in the exposition of its subject. The citations were very precise, as in the larger works, and drew from a vast library, including Arab, Greek, Hebrew, and Latin sources.

Peter of Abano's reputation in the Middle Ages was as remarkable as other famous physicians of the period, such as Taddeo Alderotti at Bologna or Jean de Saint-Amand in Paris. Evidence shows that Peter commanded respect both in literary and archival records. His friendships with individuals of the caliber of Dante, Marco Polo, and the Dondi family constitute evidence of his social and intellectual high standing. Apologetic biographies and references to Peter by illustrious physicians, scientists, and historians of later centuries, such as Michele Savonarola and Champier, illustrate the great reputation Peter had made for himself and the seemingly unattainable erudition he had demonstrated in the composition of his works. Even more eloquent were the exceptions made for him by the government of the city of Padua, where he returned in order to teach in the university at the beginning of the fourteenth century. Despite a ban for all citizens of the city to teach in the studio, the government made an exception and modified the law specifically so that Peter was allowed to be hired. The stipend he received from the commune represented an exorbitant amount for the period and could hardly have been matched in other cities in northern Italy and indeed in all of Europe. In addition, his vicissitudes with the inquisitors showed that he not only upset the clerics because of his rationalist beliefs but also angered other physicians envious of Peter's success and fame; this latter aspect was evident in the accusations that led to his second trial for heresy. Even though Peter was ultimately condemned by the inquisitors, his works became some of the cornerstones of Renaissance academic education, and his heretical tendencies resulted in all sorts of legends about his powers as a magician and a necromancer, which fueled even more interest in his writings.

Bibliography

Primary: 1475. *Aristotelis Stagirite philosophorum summi problemata atque divi Petri Apponi Patavini eorundem expositions . . .* (Mantua);

1565. *Conciliator controversiarum, quae inter philosophos et medicos versantur* (Venice) (This edition includes his treatise *De venenis, On poisons*). Also edited by E. Riondato and L. Olivieri (Padua, 1985); 1988. *Lucidator dubitabilium astronomiae*, in Federici-Vescovini, Graziella, ed., *Il 'Lucidator dubitabilium astronomiae' di Pietro d'Abano: opere scientifiche inedite* (Padua).

Secondary: Olivieri, Luigi, 1988. *Pietro d'Abano e il pensiero neolatino. Filosofia, scienza e ricerca dell'Aristotele greco tra i secoli XIII e XIV* (Padua); Tognolo, Anotonio, ed., 1985. 'Pietro d'Abano' *Medioevo: Rivista di Storia della Filosofia Medievale* 11: 1–219; Paschetto, Eugenia, 1984. *Pietro d'Abano: Medico e Filosofo* (Florence); Siraisi, Nancy G., 1970. 'The Expositio Problematum Aristotelis of Peter of Abano.' *Isis* 61: 321–339; Thorndike, Lynn, 1923. *A History of Magic and Experimental Science*, vol. 2 (New York) pp. 874–947 (contains a comprehensive bibliography of Peter's work); Ferrari, Sante, 1900. 'I Tempi, la Vita, le Dottrine di Pietro d'Abano' in *Atti della R. Università di Genova*, vol. 14 (Genoa); *DSB*.

Alessandro Medico and
Walton O. Schalick III

PETER OF SPAIN   (aka PETRUS HISPANUS, PEDRO JULIÃO, PETRUS JULIANI, JOHN XXI) (b. Lisbon, Portugal, c. 1205; d. Viterbo, Italy, 1277), *medicine, theology.*

Considered by some the most important physician-philosopher of the thirteenth century, Peter was born in Portugal to one Julianus, perhaps a physician himself. Known as Pedro Julião (Petrus Juliani) prior to his university training, Peter undoubtedly received his early education in Lisbon before attending the University of Paris, c. 1220. From then on he is referred to as Peter of Spain (Petrus Hispanus), sometimes with confusing homonyms.

Peter appears to have studied the arts, philosophy (likely with Albertus Magnus), medicine, and perhaps theology at Paris. It is likely he also had some training at Montpellier, but evidence does not support that he spent any time at the School of Salerno or the court of Frederick II (purportedly with Master Theodore, astrologer to the Emperor) as some have previously suggested. He taught at the University of Siena (c. 1245–50), and he may also have taught in Lisbon from 1250 to 1264, during which time he probably advised Alfonso III of Portugal.

We know that at the end of 1262 he attended the Genoese cardinal Ottobono Fieschi (the future Pope Adrian V) at Viterbo. Following his affiliation with the papal court, he received a series of benefices, beginning with the deanship of Lisbon. About 1271, Peter became the physician to Gregory X and assumed a new deanship in Vermuy (Braga), where he was elected archbishop. Since the pope wished to keep him in close attendance as his physician, Peter's position was changed to that of cardinal-bishop of Tusculum. It is possible he attended Innocent V and more likely Adrian V in their rapid successions of 1276. Following a prolonged conclave and the ensuing popular unrest, Peter himself was elected Pope that same year and chose the name John XXI.

Pope John's papacy was notable for efforts to broker peace among the western Christian princes, particularly those of Sicily, France, the Hapsburgs, Castile/Leon, and England, and between the Greek and Roman churches, following the Second Council of Lyons (1274). Despite the demands of the papacy, Peter continued his medical and scientific studies, allocating new space in the palace for that purpose. Unfortunately, John died six days after a building accident at one of his private apartments in Viterbo, the site of his entry into the papal court. He had been pope for less than a year and was buried in the Cathedral of Saint-Laurent. After his death, some suggested his medical and scientific learning seduced him into the magical arts.

While Peter's written output includes numerous bureaucratic, pontifical documents, and sermons, he penned a philosophical text, *Summule logicales*, which received the praise of Dante (*Paradise* XII, 134–135) as well as influential commentaries on Aristotle's *Book on the Principles of Nature* and the pseudo-Aristotelian *Physiognomy*.

Peter's medical works are at once theoretical and practical. Straddling the period in which the universities absorbed large volumes of both philosophical and medical translations, Peter carefully navigated the contemporary views of the relationship between philosophy and medicine, allowing medicine's subordination to philosophy and yet asserting its particularities as a field. His medical works probably included *Book on the Eye, Anatomy, On the Parts of the Human Body, On the Formation of Man, On Coitus*, and *On Good and Bad Women*. The work on ophthalmology, in particular, has received a great deal of attention in modern times. Several other works on regimens or diets included *On the Conservation of Health, On Surgical Diets, Regimen of Health, Letter to Emperor Frederick on the Regimen of Health*, and *Regimen of Health for All Months*. His texts on medical interventions are *On Phlebotomy, Experiments, On the Natures of Certain Herbs*, and *Questions on Laxative Medicines*. His writings about particular conditions included *On Maturing Apostemes, On the Bite of a Rabid Dog*, and a treatise on gout.

Importantly, he wrote commentaries on Johannitius's *Introduction to Galen's Ars parva*, Hippocrates' *Prognostics* and *Aphorisms*, Philaretus's *On Pulses*, and Theophilus's *On Urines*—in short, on the *Articella*. It is possible that Peter introduced the *Articella* to northern Italy, although this may have also been accomplished by Taddeo Alderotti in Bologna. Peter's commentaries extended beyond the *Articella* to include Constantine's *Viaticus*; Isaac's *On Fevers, On Universal and Particular Diets*, and *On Urines, A Little Text on the Regimen of Acute Diseases, The Tegni*; Hippocrates' *On the Nature of Children*, and *On the Fevers from Hippocrates*; and Mesue's (Ibn Māsawayh's) *On Fevers*.

Peter is best known for the wildly popular *Thesaurus pauperum*, later translated from Latin into Italian, English,

Spanish, and Portuguese. The nature of the treatise is at variance with Peter's more securely known works because it is less philosophical and more pragmatic. Nevertheless, a large number of the text's more than sixty-six manuscript witnesses identify Peter as *Thesaurus*'s author. The work appeared in numerous early printed versions dating from 1497. Its practical nature invited many additions and interpolations in later copies, thus rendering the recreation of the urtext somewhat challenging. Nevertheless, the work represents a compelling amalgam of sources, linguistic influences, and ideas on diseases from head to foot.

Bibliography

Primary: 1972. *Tractatus called afterwards Summule logicales* (First Critical Edition from the Manuscripts with an Introduction by de Rijk, L. M) (Assen); 1973. (Periera, Maria Helena da Rocha, ed. and trans.) *Obras médicas de Pedro Hispano* (Coimbra).

Secondary: de Asúa, Miguel, 1998. 'The Relationship between Medicine and Philosophy in Peter of Spain's Commentary on the *Articella*' in *Papers of the Articella Project Meeting, Cambridge, December 1995* vol. 3 (Cambridge and Barcelona) pp. 13–27; Salmón, Fernando, 1998. *Medical Classroom Practice: Petrus Hispanus' Questions on* Isagoge, Tegni, Regimen Acutorum, *and* Prognostica *(c. 1245–50)* (Cambridge and Barcelona); Schipperges, Heinrich. 1994. *Arzt im Purpur: Grundzüge einer Krankheitslehre bei Petrus Hispanus (ca. 1210 bis 1277)* (Berlin); De Rijk, L. M., 1970. 'On the Life of Peter of Spain, The Author of the Tractatus, Called Afterwards Summule Logicales.' *Vivarium* 8: 123–154.

Walton O. Schalick III

PETIT, JEAN-LOUIS (b. Paris, France, 13 March 1674; d. Paris, 20 April 1750), *surgery*.

The son of a merchant of comfortable means, Petit displayed an early aptitude for anatomical dissection. At age sixteen he began a two-year surgical apprenticeship, during which he frequented Paris hospitals, and after that he served as an army surgeon for five years. Returning to Paris in 1698, Petit completed the requirements to become a master of the surgeons' company in 1700.

He soon gained a reputation for his private instruction in anatomy and surgery. Elected provost to the surgical company, he presented innovative lessons on the use of surgical instruments in various procedures. Admission to the Royal Academy of Sciences in 1715 represented unusual recognition for a surgeon at that time. He performed operations on royal personages, including the king of Poland and a future king of Spain, and his advice was sought throughout Europe.

Petit introduced several methods for controlling hemorrhage during and following amputations. Best known was his 'screw tourniquet', a vise-like instrument used to compress major arteries. Pressure could be adjusted as needed, and the surgeon no longer depended upon an assistant to maintain the tourniquet. Petit improved the operation for fistula of the lachrymal (tear) duct, and he devised procedures for surgical treatment of adhesions of the tongue and imperforate anus in newborn infants. His bandage for tears of the Achilles tendon produced better healing with less pain than the standard surgical intervention. Petit's revised edition of his *Traité sur les maladies des os* (1723) became the definitive text on orthopedic surgery and was translated into many languages. His comprehensive richly-illustrated *Traité général des opérations de chirurgie* (3 vols., 1776 and 1790) appeared posthumously.

In 1724 Petit was named to the chair of surgical 'principles' at the new Paris College of Surgery, and in 1731 he became one of the founding members of the Academy of Surgery. He wrote several articles for the Academy's first volume of *Mémoires* (1743). In his essay on differential diagnosis between biliary cysts of the gallbladder and abscesses of the liver, Petit urged surgeons not to be afraid to perform punctures of the gallbladder provided there were adhesions to the abdominal wall. He also pointed out that gallbladder stones might be extracted in a manner comparable to lithotomies for stones of the urinary bladder. Petit advised, 'Do not expect nature always to perform miracles; the clever surgeon should observe nature, not intervening as long as things are progressing, and then take advantage of the favorable moment to act' (Petit, 1743, p. 175). This statement summed up his cautious but not timid approach to surgical intervention in an era before 'heroic operations' were possible. He won wide recognition as the most skilled surgeon of the first half of the eighteenth century.

Petit was said to have a serene temperament. He avoided the recurring professional feuds between physicians and surgeons. Toward the end of his career he studied Latin in an effort to compensate for his lack of a university education and to demonstrate his respect for this new requirement for surgeons. Petit had the misfortune to lose his son, Jean-Baptiste, who had embarked on a brilliant surgical career of his own when he succumbed at the age of twenty-seven.

Bibliography

Primary: 1723. *Traité sur les maladies des os* 2nd edn. rev. (Paris); 1743. 'Remarques sur les tumeurs formées par la bile retenue dans la vésicule du fiel, et qu'on a souvent prises pour des abcès au fiel.' *Mémoires de l'Académie royale de Chirurgie* 1: 155–187; 1776, 1790. *Traité général des opérations de chirurgie* 3 vols. (Paris).

Secondary: Gelfand, Toby, 1980. *Professionalizing Modern Medicine: Paris Surgeons, Medical Science and Institutions in the 18th Century* (Westport, CT); [Grandjohn de Fouchy, Jean-Paul] 1750. 'Eloge de J.-L. Petit.' *Histoire de l'Académie royale des sciences* 1754: 192; Louis Antoine, 1750. 'Eloge de J.-L. Petit' in Dubois, E.-F., d'Amiens, ed., *Eloges lus dans les séances de l'Académie royale de chirurgie* 1859: 1–19.

Toby Gelfand

PETTENKOFER, MAX VON (b. Neuburg, Germany, 3 December 1818; d. Munich, Germany, 10 February 1901), *hygiene.*

Pettenkofer is chiefly remembered for his contributions to hygiene, a discipline that he helped to promote to the rank of an experimental science in the nineteenth century. His accomplishments in general chemistry and the physiology of nutrition were equally important.

Pettenkofer, the son of a farmer, was given the chance of a better education thanks to an uncle who happened to be apothecary to the Bavarian court. After finishing the gymnasium he initially enrolled as a student of philology at Munich University, but had to give in to his uncle's insistence he concentrate on studies of a more practical direction. As a result, the young man enrolled for natural sciences and philosophy and was also an apprentice to the court pharmacy. After a short and rebellious interlude as an actor at a provincial theatre, which was met with similar dislike by his uncle and his future wife, Pettenkofer resumed his university studies, now in pharmacy and medicine, and graduated in 1843.

Subsequently he showed little inclination to practice either of these fields. Instead he completed his education in chemistry in Würzburg with Josef Scherer and in Giessen with Justus Liebig. In 1845 he became an assistant in the royal mint, where he made his reputation as a versatile chemist, and he became a professor of medical chemistry in 1847.

Pettenkofer mastered experimental investigations into the physical and chemical qualities of earth, soil, and human bodies. Together with Carl Voit, he experimentally studied basic metabolic laws such as dietary requirements or gaseous exchange. Investigations undertaken in 1850 into the heating of the royal palace with hot air laid the foundation of a lifelong obsession with the physical properties of buildings and soils. He identified the desiccation of the palace's walls as being a result of the hot air, and he would later develop a theory of infectious diseases that explained the occurrence of a given disease as a function of an alteration of the soil, especially the lowering of groundwater levels that facilitated the dissemination of miasmas into the air.

After 1854, when Pettenkofer became a member of the royal cholera commission, he further developed his views on infectious diseases. By pointing to the soil as the most important source of infection, he found himself in opposition to hygienists such as John Snow, who was advocating drinking water as the main source. According to Pettenkofer a pathogen in the soil (which could be called X) required a certain alteration of the soil's physical qualities (Y) to result in the disease (Z). Although his views were never undisputed, Pettenkofer became the leading German hygienist during the 1860s. He was offered the headship of the newly founded Imperial Health Office in Berlin in 1876, but preferred the directorship of a newly created

Institute for Hygiene at Munich University, which he began in 1879. Pettenkofer, who had been co-editor of the *Zeitschrift für Biologie* since 1865, also founded the influential *Zeitschrift für Hygiene* in 1872.

When Robert Koch in 1884 identified the *Vibrio cholerae* as the pathogen of cholera, Pettenkofer demanded that this bacterium constituted the X in his theory. Koch and others insisted that the Y was unnecessary for the explanation and that a bacterial etiology was sufficient to explain cholera epidemics, which were spread via drinking water and not soil. Despite a heroic self-experiment during the 1892 Hamburg epidemic in which Pettenkofer demonstrated that the ingestion of pure cultures of the bacterium did not always cause cholera, contemporaries adhered more and more to the competing Berlin Koch school of hygiene.

Pettenkofer, who had been ennobled in 1883, continued to be the doyen of German experimental hygiene. After finding he was suffering from an incurable disease, he committed suicide in 1901.

Bibliography

Primary: 1848. *Ueber Chemie in Ihrem Verhältnisse zur Physiologie und Pathologie* (Munich); 1855. *Untersuchungen und Beobachtungen über die Verbreitungsart der Cholera* (Munich); 1886. 'Zum Gegenwärtigen Stand der Cholerafrage.' *Archiv für Hygiene,* 4 (et cont).

Secondary: Weyer-von Schoultz, Martin, 1998. '"Hygiène et assainissement des villess": Zur wissenschaftlichen Begründung der "Stadthygiene" des 19. Jahrhunderts und deren Konsequenzen.' *Berichte zur Wissenschaftsgeschichte* 21: 231–236; Jahn, Ellen, 1994. *Die Cholera in Medizin und Pharmazie im Zeitalter des Hygienikers Max von Pettenkofer* (Stuttgart); Evans, Richard J., 1990. *Death in Hamburg: Society and Politics in the Cholera Years, 1830–1910* (Harmondsworth); Kisskalt, Karl, 1948. *Max von Pettenkofer* (Stuttgart); *DSB.*

Christoph Gradmann

PHILISTION OF LOCRI (fl. 350 BCE), *medicine.*

Doctor to the tyrant Dionysius II of Sicily, Philistion became acquainted with Plato, who met him in Sicily during one of his visits in 387, 364, or 362 BCE. He may then have moved to Athens, where he may have taught the great mathematician-astronomer and Plato's collaborator, Eudoxus of Cnidus. But neither the authenticity of Plato's letter nor the biographical tradition, mainly reported by Diogenes Laertius, is entirely reliable.

Philistion represents a phenomenon labeled 'Sicilian' (as opposed to 'Cnidian') medicine, which was characterized by a blend of Empedoclean ideas (notably the theory of the four primary elements—earth, water, air, and fire) and physiological views such as the concept of innate heat or of the primacy of the heart as site of life and consciousness. Yet sharp distinctions into 'schools', especially at this early date, are artificial and must be taken with a large pinch of salt.

Philistion held that the body was composed of the four Empedoclean stuffs, an idea he combined with a theory of the four qualities (hot, cold, dry, and wet). A variant of this combination was to become the cornerstone of Aristotle's physics. It also exerted an influence on Plato's views on the generation of disease, where the elements featured more prominently than the humors (*Timaeus* 81e–86a). Philistion's ideas in physiology were equally notable. Like Aristotle later, he held that the function of respiration was the cooling of innate heat, and he entertained a notion of cutaneous respiration that, again, stretches back (perhaps) to Empedocles and forward (certainly) to Plato. Through this lineage, leading from Empedocles to Plato and Aristotle, Philistion's theories demonstrated the strong links between philosophy and medicine in fourth-century BCE Greek thought. But he is only one among the physicians known to have shared in one or another of these mainstream ideas of the future. His degree of originality is difficult to assess.

Philistion maintained a cardiocentric physiology, in which the blood vessels (not yet separated into veins and arteries) started from the heart and carried not only blood but also air (*pneuma*). Probably inspired by Alcmaeon of Croton and Diogenes of Apollonia, he attached great importance to *pneuma* and to respiratory exchanges in general, and ranked the perturbation of those exchanges among the main causes of disease. According to the Anonymus Londinensis papyrus, a work produced in Aristotle's school, he offered a general etiology in which pathological states were caused by three factors: the imbalance of the four primary element qualities, a conception he shared with many, including Polybus of Cos and Petronas of Aegina; external agents like climate, diet, and wounds; and internal blockages resulting from the miscarriage of *pneuma* (20.20 – 25 = fragment 4 Wellmann).

Philistion wrote on regimen, pharmacology, and surgery. His treatments for various ailments were influential, as proved by their survival in later reports from Athenaeus, Galen, and Oribasius.

It has been claimed that Philistion performed human dissections long before the great Alexandrians, but this is a matter of speculation and there is no evidence to support it.

Bibliography

Primary: Wellmann, M., 1901. *Fragmentsammlung der griechischen Ärzte, I: Die Fragmente der sikelischen Ärzte Akron, Philistion und des Diokles von Karystos* (Berlin) pp. 109–116, 68–71.

Secondary: Nutton, V., 2004. *Ancient Medicine* (London) pp. 46, 72–73, 82, 115; Longrigg, J., 1998. *Greek Medicine. From the Heroic to the Hellenistic Age. A Source Book* (London); Staden, Heinrich von, 1989. *Herophilus. The Art of Medicine in Early Alexandria* (Cambridge) p. 388; Harris, C. R. S., 1973. *The Heart and the Vascular System in Ancient Greek Medicine* (Oxford) esp. pp. 19–20, 37–8, 116–19; Bidez, J., and G. Lebouc, 1944. 'Une anatomie antique du coeur humain. Philistion de Locres et le "Timée de Platon.' *Revue des Etudes Grecques* 57: 7–40; Taylor, A. E., 1928. *A Commentary on Plato's Timaeus* (Oxford) p. 599.

Manuela Tecusan

PICKERING, GEORGE WHITE (b. Whalton, Northumberland, England, 26 June 1904; d. Oxford, England, 3 September 1980), *clinical science, education.*

The youngest child and only son of the Elsdon school master George Pickering and his wife, Ann Hall, Pickering was born at Whalton in rural Northumberland. His father died when Pickering was three, and the family moved to Newcastle upon Tyne. Initially educated by his mother, Pickering went to school when he was seven and entered the Royal Grammar School at Newcastle aged nine. When he was fourteen, he became the youngest member of the Newcastle Literary and Philosophical Society, in whose library he developed an omnivorous reading habit and a strong interest in natural history and archaeology. He transferred to Dulwich College, where he was top of his class, and won a scholarship to Pembroke College, Cambridge. In 1925 and 1926 he obtained firsts in both parts of the Natural Science Tripos, coming top of the whole university in his first year. In the third year he decided to do physiology and was greatly influenced by his teachers Joseph Barcroft (1872–1947), E. K. Rideal (1890–1974), and E. D. Adrian (1889–1977). His strong performance won him both an entrance scholarship to St Thomas's Hospital and a fellowship of Pembroke College. Increasingly interested in clinical medicine, he declined the fellowship after much deliberation. He qualified (1928), was house physician to the cardiologist Sir Maurice Cassidy (1880–1949), and passed his MRCP examination (1930). In the same year he married Carola Seward, daughter of the paleobotanist Sir Charles Seward.

With his Cambridge training and his interest in science, Pickering was ideally suited to join Thomas Lewis's (1881–1945) department of clinical science at University College Hospital. He was appointed assistant and lecturer in cardiovascular physiology. Along with T. R. Elliott's (1877–1961) neighboring department of medicine, Lewis's unit was part of a new infrastructure that the Medical Research Council had established for the full-time pursuit of clinical research. Pickering's contemporaries at UCL included John McMichael (1904–93), F. H. Smirk (1902–91), and Harold Himsworth (1905–93). During his eight years with Lewis, Pickering worked on blood circulation and temperature regulation, and he started his studies of high blood pressure. The MRC had also created full-time chairs at other London medical schools, and when F. S. Langmead (1879–1969) retired from St Mary's Hospital in 1939, Pickering succeeded him. As a wartime evacuation measure, Pickering's unit was transferred to Harefield Hospital, where under less-than-advantageous conditions they worked on the natural history of constrictive pericarditis and on peptic ulcer. After the war, they returned to the St Mary's site, where the conditions for clinical research were not optimal either (their laboratory was located in a small converted shop). Nevertheless, many of Pickering's assistants subsequently had distinguished careers in vascular and renal research. At St Mary's, Pickering undertook his groundbreaking studies on the etiology of high blood pressure, in collaboration with the medical statistician and geneticist Alexander Fraser Roberts, which led to a drawn-out controversy with the Manchester clinician Robert Platt (1900–78) over the nature of essential hypertension. In Oxford as a visiting professor in 1954, Pickering was not impressed by the conditions. There were considerable funds from the Nuffield Foundation, but great differences between the parties involved in medical training and research over the directions that should be taken. Thus, when offered the regius chair of medicine in the following year, he hesitated. His considerable demands were met, however (they included an inpatient and an outpatient service, a staff of assistants and technicians, and a large laboratory), and he moved to Oxford in 1956.

Pickering developed a growing interest in education and its reform, in medicine as well as other subjects. He was a member of the University Grants Committee from 1944 to 1954 and during this time visited all universities and medical schools in the country. In 1968 he retired from the regius chair and became Master of Pembroke College. He continued to publish and lecture on medical science, education, and other matters until his death. Pickering's many honors included a knighthood (1957) and FRS (1960). He was a member of the Medical Research Council and the Clinical Research Board from 1954 to 1958, a trustee of several foundations, and President of the British Medical Association in 1963.

Bibliography

Primary: 1955. *High Blood Pressure* (London); 1961. *The Nature of Essential Hypertension* (London); 1967. *The Challenge to Education* (London); 1974. *Creative Malady* (London); 1978. *Quest for Excellence in Medical Education* (Oxford).

Secondary: Swales, J. D., ed., 1985. *Platt versus Pickering* (London); McMichael, Sir John, and W. S. Peart, 1982. 'George White Pickering.' *Biographical Memoirs of Fellows of the Royal Society* 28: 431–449; *Oxford DNB*.

Carsten Timmermann

PICKLES, WILLIAM NORMAN (b. Leeds, Yorkshire, England, 6 March 1885; d. Aysgarth, Yorkshire, England, 2 March 1969), *general practice, epidemiology.*

From a medical family, 'Will' Pickles's father was a general practitioner in central Leeds and four of his five brothers also entered general practice (the youngest trained in medicine, but failed to qualify). Studying at Yorkshire College (subsequently the University of Leeds), Pickles qualified in 1909 with the lesser diploma of the Society of Apothecaries; he had failed the final examination of the London MB BS but passed a year later. As a student he worked as a locum tenens in general practice, and after qualification continued this practice, but returned to Leeds

for a short-term appointment as resident obstetric officer, and then served as a ship's doctor for one voyage to India. In 1912 Pickles went as a locum to Aysgarth, Wensleydale, in North Yorkshire, returning the following year. Save for four years in the Royal Navy during World War I (when he traveled widely and saw active service), he remained there for fifty-three years. At that time the Dales were remote, with scattered farmsteads, no affordable transport, and many unmetaled tracks that became quagmires in the winter. Pickles did many house calls on horseback or with a pony and trap, subsequently graduating to a bicycle and a motorcycle before buying a car.

In 1928 he took up epidemiology, inspired by an epidemic of infective hepatitis and by reading *The Principles of Diagnosis and Treatment in Heart Affections* by James Mackenzie (1853–1925). Himself a general practitioner, Mackenzie had emphasized the opportunity for research in general practice, claiming that 'medicine will make little progress . . . until the general practitioner takes his place as an investigator'. The conditions in Wensleydale were highly conducive to epidemiological research: poor communications meant that the inhabitants rarely left home, but their rare trips away often resulted in the importation of infections, such as hepatitis or influenza. And Pickles knew his patients well, writing subsequently: 'As I watched the evening train creeping up the valley with its pauses at our three stations, a quaint thought came into my head . . . that there was hardly a man, woman, or child in all three villages of whom I did not know the Christian name and with whom I was not on terms of intimate friendship.'

His initial study was on hepatitis A; of the 250 known cases of jaundice in Wensleydale (population 5,700), the Aysgarth practice had attended 118. Pickles traced the whole epidemic to a girl he had seen on the morning of the village fete and who he had not believed would be able to get up that day. His paper, published in 1930, established the long incubation period of hepatitis A with great accuracy (twenty-six to thirty-five days), and the next year he began to chart other epidemics. He or his wife, and subsequently daughter, transcribed data from a pocket diary onto blue-lined graph paper, with each disease having its own colored symbol (e.g., influenza as a red square, measles a blue one) and each village being treated separately. Thus Pickles showed again that the incubation periods of other diseases—rubella, mumps, and pertussis—were different from those given in the textbooks. He also gave a classic account of Bornholm disease (epidemic myalgia) and coined the name 'Farmer's lung', because it was caused by the repeated inhalation of moldy hay. Another concept entailed asking patients for their views—they well appreciated the connection between chicken pox and shingles at a time when this was little recognized by professionals.

Pickles's writings attracted the attention of epidemiologists, such as Major Greenwood (1880–1949) and Austin Bradford Hill (1897–1991), who invited him to London, where he gave an influential lecture, and to write *Epidemiology in Country Practice*. Dedicated to the people of Wensleydale, this book finally appeared in 1939 and became a classic after being rejected by several major publishers. Although Pickles continued as an active general practitioner up to the late 1930s, campaigned for diphtheria immunization as soon as it became available, and returned to medical school once a year for a refresher course, increasingly his life became concerned with giving evidence to and serving on influential committees, lecturing, and receiving awards and honors. After the war he traveled extensively and cultivated a wide circle of friends. Thus in 1948 he gave the prestigious Cutler Lecture at Harvard, while in 1953–56 he served as founder-president of the College of General Practitioners. A firm believer in a state health service, which removed medicine from the marketplace and freed doctors from debt, he looked forward to the creation of health centers with their diagnostic facilities and teams of ancillaries. Not only does his work illustrate Louis Pasteur's contention that chance favors the prepared mind, but it also led to the reinvigoration of research in general practice, started by William Budd (1811–80) and James Mackenzie (1853–1925) and flourishing today.

Bibliography

Primary: 1939. *Epidemiology in Country Practice* (London).

Secondary: Pemberton, J., 1952. *Will Pickles of Wensleydale* (London); *Oxford DNB*.

Stephen Lock

PINARD, ADOLPHE   (b. Méry-sur-Seine, France, 4 February 1844; d. Méry-sur-Seine, 1 March 1934), *obstetrics, prenatal care, eugenics.*

Pinard was born in a village in the Champagne region, the son of a small-scale farmer. Inspired by the local schoolteacher and doctor, Pinard first studied pharmacy in Paris and then entered medical school. The Franco-Prussian War interrupted his studies and delayed his internship. He received his MD at age thirty, but his work with the surgeon Alfred Richet and the prominent obstetrician Stéphane Tarnier helped his rapid advancement. He became *accoucheur* at Lariboisière Hospital in 1882 and professor of clinical obstetrics at the Paris Medical School in 1889, with additional responsibilities as head of the Baudelocque [maternity] Clinic when it was established the following year.

Pinard's work in obstetrics focused primarily on difficult pregnancies and prenatal care to increase the chances of healthy newborns. His most important clinical contribution was replacing vaginal examination with abdominal palpation in order to minimize puerperal infection. Pinard showed how palpation permitted determination of the presentation of the fetus. The Pinard maneuver is named for his technique of external version, in which the fetal feet are brought within reach of the obstetrician in a breech delivery.

Another problem that concerned Pinard was the treatment of hemorrhage resulting from *placenta previa*. Rather than using extreme measures to induce premature delivery, Pinard advocated breaking the amniotic membrane and using an intrauterine balloon to stop bleeding. In the case of women with contracted pelvises, Pinard revived the use of symphysiotomy (cutting the cartilage to spread the pubic bone) and other measures to temporarily enlarge the birth canal for safe delivery, instead of using forceps.

An example of Pinard's renown was his invitation for a consultation in January 1904 with the Czarina of Russia, during her difficult pregnancy before the birth of her son Alexis. In gratitude, the House of Romanov made a generous donation to Pinard's Baudelocque Clinic.

The poor condition of pregnant women whom Pinard saw at Baudelocque Clinic drew his attention to the relationship between prenatal care and healthy births. In 1892 he joined with Marie Bequet de Vienne to open a new *maison maternelle* to serve as 'a refuge or asylum for pregnant women'. Pinard noted that birth weights of newborns at Beaudelocque were higher than average, even though the infants came from the lower classes. After a three-year study, he found that the birth weights of 500 children born to women who had spent at least ten days at the refuge were, on average, 280 grams higher than those of 500 children born to women who came directly to Baudelocque and who had worked until the onset of labor. Pinard concluded that rest before delivery was crucial to the health of the newborn. Pinard's work influenced a whole generation of reform legislation to protect newborns and provide assistance to expectant mothers.

Pinard revived the term 'puericulture', initially coined in 1860 by Charles-Alfred Caron, to refer to all measures favoring the health of newborns. As he put it, 'puericulture is the science that has as its goal research, study, and application of all knowledge about the reproduction, preservation, and improvement of the human species' (1912, p. 1123). By extending the notion of prenatal care to 'puericulture before conception', Pinard's ideas helped justify the establishment of a eugenics movement that had a particularly French perspective.

Pinard was a founding member of the French Eugenics Society, serving initially as vice president and then as president. Although he had retired from the medical faculty in 1914, Pinard was persuaded to run for the Chamber of Deputies in 1919 because of the extreme concern in France about population losses and the low French birth rate following World War I. He won easily, and by virtue of his seniority at age seventy-five, he became the Chamber's president. In 1926 Pinard introduced a bill requiring a premarital examination. Although his bill failed to win approval, premarital examination became a main campaign issue of the French Eugenics movement between the wars, and it eventually became law in 1942.

Pinard retired from the Chamber in 1928 and died six years later at the age of ninety. His most influential legacy was the legislation and practice to protect the health of newborns in France.

Bibliography

Primary: 1878. *Traité du palper abdominal au pointe de vue obstetrical et de la version par manoeuvres externes* (Paris); 1895. 'Note pour servir á l'histoire de la puericulture intra-uterine.' *Bulletin de l'Academie de Médecine,* 3e sér., 34: 593–597; 1899. 'De la conservation et l'amélioration de l'espèce.' *Bulletin Médical* 13: 141–146; 1912. 'De l'eugénnetique.' *Bulletin Médical* 26: 1123–1127.

Secondary: Dumont, M., 1994. 'Sesquicentenaire de la naissance d'Adolphe Pinard (1844–1934).' *Journal de Gynécologie Obstétrique et Biologie de la Reproduction* 23: 351–357; Schneider, W. H., 1986. 'Puericulture and the Style of French Eugenics.' *History and Philosophy of the Life Sciences* 8: 265–277.

William H. Schneider

PINDBORG, JENS JØRGEN (b. Copenhagen, Denmark, 17 August 1921; d. Gentofte, Denmark, 6 August 1995), *odontology.*

Pindborg was the oldest child of merchant Marius Pindborg and Sigrid Waaben Pindborg. He displayed an early interest in both literature and science, but decided to keep the former as a hobby. He began odontological studies at the Danish School of Dentistry in Copenhagen in 1940, mainly because the course took only three years and Pindborg did not want to burden his parents for too long. Upon graduation in 1943, he worked as a clinical assistant at the School of Dentistry, but spent most of his time in a small histological laboratory. Beginning in 1945 he also served as a dentist in the Danish navy, which allowed him to conduct extensive studies of the epidemiology of gingivitis necroticans among the servicemen. In 1948 Pindborg was made the director of a newly established histological department at the school of dentistry, and he defended his thesis on the effects of chronic fluorine and cadmium poisoning on rat incisors (1950).

During a postdoctoral stay at the University of Illinois College of Dentistry (1951–52), Pindborg was further introduced to the emerging field of oral pathology. He was determined to promote research in that field in Denmark, and he returned to the histological laboratory at the School of Dentistry in Copenhagen, where he served as professor of oral histopathology from 1959 to 1991. He held that position alongside his post as director of the dental clinic at Rigshospitalet (1953–91).

Through the 1950s Pindborg conducted research into the basics of oral histopathology, often in close cooperation with medical doctors. His attention focused on pathology of the oral mucous membranes, especially oral cancer, and in 1955 he described the calcifying epithelial odontogenic tumor (now known as the Pindborg tumor), while also working on the classification of odontogenic tumors. In 1966 Pindborg became the director of the newly established WHO International Reference Center for Odontogenic Tumors. By that time, he had also begun extensive epidemiological studies of precancerous conditions, especially leukoplakias caused by reverse smoking and betel nut chewing in India, Thailand, and Burma. Pindborg was the obvious choice to head the WHO center for oral precancerous conditions set up in 1967. In 1981 he reacted to the first reports on AIDS and was especially interested in the information that most patients displayed oral fungus infections. Research in that field at Pindborg's histopathology department in Copenhagen showed that most HIV infections are accompanied by oral changes that often precede other symptoms, thus allowing an earlier diagnosis and a more rapid onset of treatment.

Pindborg received much international recognition for his contribution to the field of oral pathology. He held several honorary doctorates and conducted a busy lecturing program across the world during his last decades. Beginning quite early in his career, he worked to establish oral pathology as an independent research field—one in which dentists should participate on an equal footing with medical doctors. Pindborg was the first dentist in Denmark to receive the right to diagnose patients on the basis of laboratory tests, which provoked strong reactions from Danish pathologists. Also, he was instrumental in establishing dentistry as an integral part of the Danish hospital system.

Pindborg published a range of odontological textbooks and served as editor of the Danish Dental Journal from 1962 to 1995. He served on the board of the Danish Medical Research Board (1972–77 and 1984–87) and on the Danish Council of Ethics (1988–90). He married three times, the last time just over a year before his death.

Bibliography

Primary: 1970. *Pathology of the Dental Hard Tissues* (Copenhagen); 1992. *Atlas of the Diseases of the Oral Mucosa* 5th edn. (Copenhagen).

Secondary: 1995. 'Pindborg, Jens Jørgen.' *Kraks Blå Bog* (Copenhagen); Mikkelsen, Otto, 1991. 'J. J. Pindborgs erindringer om sit odontologiske liv.' *Tandlægebladet* 95: 389–452; Snorrason, Egill, 1982. 'Pindborg, Jens Jørgen.' *Dansk biografisk leksikon* (Copenhagen).

Søren Bak-Jensen

PINEL, PHILIPPE (b. Roques, France, 20 April 1745; d. Paris, France, 25 October 1826), *psychiatry, clinical nosography.*

Pinel was born in a farmhouse at Roques in southwestern France—the son, grandson, and nephew of master barber-surgeons, the doctors of the peasantry and of the urban poor under the old regime. He owed mastery of Latin and a lifelong passion for learning to Jean Pierre Gorsse, a student of the Jesuits and the village teacher at St Paul Cap-de-Joux, where Pinel grew up. Chosen as a scholarship student by the Fathers of the Christian Doctrine, a Catholic teaching order with humanist and Gallican leanings, the young man progressed to a master's degree in the humanities at Toulouse and studied for two and a half years toward a doctorate in theology. At the time of his twenty-fifth birthday, he abruptly changed to medicine and obtained an MD degree from the Toulouse faculty in 1773. He did not write a thesis, contrary to what is often asserted, because none was required at that time.

Why exchange the cross for the scalpel? We have so few personal documents that an answer must be inferred. The pull of the family tradition and the presence in Toulouse of his three young brothers, all apprentice surgeons, surely influenced his decision. So did his intensive study of mathematics with Jean Baptiste Gardeil, a doctor and friend of the Paris encyclopedists. Also, theology must have seemed increasingly irrelevant in a world where the philosophy, literature, and polemics of the Enlightenment inspired so many brilliant publications. And finally, the memory of the Protestant Jean Calas, broken on the wheel at Toulouse in 1762, may have raised lasting doubts and been ultimately responsible for the absence of the Catholic religion from the teaching and practice of psychiatry by its founder in France.

In 1774 Pinel moved to Montpellier, seat of the oldest and most prestigious French medical school. There the discussion in medical circles focused on Boissier de Sauvages's nosology, since classification in natural history, including the classification of diseases, had been made fashionable by Linnaeus. At the same time, Montpellierains reacted strongly against the dualism of Descartes and the mechanism of Boerhaave. They toyed with the animism of Georg Stahl, but widely adopted vitalism, as championed by Théophile de Bordeu and Paul Joseph Barthez. Pinel was strongly influenced by both Bordeu and Barthez. A chief attraction was the private Haguenot library, recently made available to students, which contained the Western world's medical heritage in 853 volumes. Pinel spent four years reading most of them, as the references in his published works indicate. Most of the books were in Latin, but quite a few were in English, a language that Pinel decided to learn. That was a significant move toward his future career; he translated William Cullen's *First Lines of the Practice of Physic* in 1785. But not all his time was spent reading; his medical degree entitled him to attend clinical rounds at the Hôtel Dieu St Eloi. That was his first exposure to hospitalized patients, and in a rare autobiographical remark he recorded his surprise at how favorably patients reacted to his concern and empathy with their suffering. He also formed a friendship with another postgraduate student, Jean-Antoine Chaptal, whom he helped recover from a serious depression. Chaptal introduced Pinel to the Montpellier Academy of Sciences, where Pinel presented three papers, all on mathematics. Twenty-five years later, when Chaptal was Minister of Internal Affairs under the Consu-

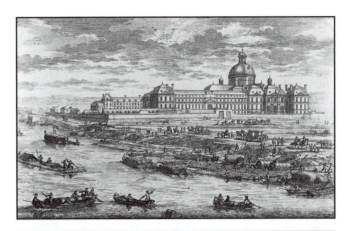

Hôpital de la Salpêtrière, Paris, where Philippe Pinel symbolically unchained the lunatics. Line engraving by Adam Perelle, *c.* 1680. Iconographic Collection, Wellcome Library, London.

late, his prompt and decisive intervention empowered Pinel to launch his most ambitious experiment.

But in the 1770s and 1780s a successful career in medicine seemed beyond Pinel's reach. He moved to Paris in 1778 and eked out a living as a translator; as editor of the *Gazette de santé* and of several volumes of selections from the *Transactions of the Royal Society*; as contributor to the *Journal de Physique* and to *La médecine éclairée par les sciences physiques*; and occasionally as a medical consultant, especially at Jacques Belhomme's *maison de santé* for mental patients.

The center of Pinel's professional involvement at that time was the Royal Gardens, open to qualified amateur investigators and teachers. There he pursued and published work in comparative anatomy, such as studies of the animal skull (later adapted to human skulls and published as section three of his *Traité*), chemical experiments concerning the injection and preservation of specimens captured by hunters (enabling him later to draw up instructions for naturalists on global voyages), and observations on animal behavior (he later coauthored a successful proposal to add a menagerie to the *Musée*). He also taught a course in 'zootomy' that was open to the public.

Thus, when the Revolution finally opened a career to his talents, Pinel was a physician who conceived of the health and illness of living beings as part of natural history, and subject to its laws. He made new connections when a friend—probably the physician-philosopher P. J. G. Cabanis—introduced him into the salon of Madame Helvtius at Auteuil. There he met Benjamin Franklin (who tried to lure him to America) and Michel Augustin Thouret, soon to become dean of the Paris Health School. A few years later, Cabanis and Thouret, who were members of the hospital committee of the National Assembly, procured for Pinel the position of 'physician of the infirmaries' at Bicêtre Hospice. That was the beginning of his career, on 11 September 1793.

The hospices of Bicêtre and the Salpêtrière formed part of the *Hôpital Général* to which Louis XIV had, in the mid-seventeenth century, relegated beggars, vagabonds, and other undesirables. By the time of the Revolution the addition of sections for prisoners, the 'deserving poor', stray children, and (at the Salpêtrière) prostitutes, retired nurses, and even a school, swelled the number of inmates to about 4,000 and 8,000, respectively. Surgeons cared for the physical ailments of those people; the seriously ill were carried to the Hôtel Dieu. The appointment of a physician was a humanitarian novelty.

Pinel's attention was immediately captured by a group of about 200 deranged men milling about in one of the courtyards. He observed them intently, talked with them, and listened carefully, and then he attempted an overall classification he called the 'Table of 200 Madmen', which has been preserved. It outlined the precipitating events of their illnesses, the specific types of illness, and the manner in which their minds and personalities were affected. Soon afterward he gave a talk to the Society for Natural History titled 'Memoir on Madness: A Contribution to the Natural History of Man'. This is a fundamental text for modern psychiatry.

In the fall of 1794, when the Jacobin fury had been spent, the Revolutionaries founded the Paris Health School and appointed twelve full and twelve associate professors. Pinel, at first chosen as associate professor of medical physics and hygiene, exchanged chairs and emerged in 1796 as professor of internal medicine. A textbook in French was called for, and Pinel responded with *Nosographie philosophique ou Méthode de l'analyse appliquée á la médecine*, which was based largely on Cullen's precedent. In its six successive editions (1798–1818), a whole generation of French doctors learned medicine according to Pinel's classification of diseases. His appointment as physician-in-chief of Salpêtrière hospice in 1795 allowed him to add his personal clinical experience to his theoretical teaching.

Two aspects of the *Nosographie* deserve our attention. One involves Pinel's choice of 'essential fevers' as the first of five classes of diseases. That choice turned out to be a mistake, because fever is a symptom and not a disease. Critics, especially among the young generation of Pinel's students, soon began attacking his concept, but he was unconvinced and clung to his choice.

The other innovation of the *Nosographie* is positive and lasting. It concerns the mental maladies, or *insaniae*, that Pinel grouped in his fourth class—the nervous illnesses, or 'neuroses', a term borrowed from Cullen. By including mental maladies in his classification of diseases, Pinel reconceptualized madmen and madwomen as mentally ill patients. He argued that physicians—not healers, priests, or assorted practitioners—should care for the mentally ill.

In the meantime, his 'Memoir on Madness' had become known, and the most selective of the newly formed student societies, the Society for Medical Emulation, invited him to lecture about his recent observations of the mentally ill. He obliged on three occasions. His first conference, 'On Periodic or Intermittent Madness', already contained the ideas elaborated in the second edition of the *Traité*, published in 1809. Pinel was aware of the rich content of that chapter when he wrote that 'one attack of madness comprehends all the varieties one might investigate in the abstract' (1798, p. 21). He pointed out that manic episodes often showed an observable onset, course, and decline, with a precipitating cause that can be ascertained so that precautionary measures can be taken. Accordingly, mental disease often resembled other diseases. He analyzed various mental functions that might be impaired, or intact—most shockingly as when a homicidal maniac pursues his purpose with perfect logic. Pinel's most original observation impressed the philosopher Hegel and has been analyzed by the late Gladys Swain. It concerned the importance of lucid intervals between irrational episodes. These moments can allow a skilled therapist access to the remainder of the approachable personality and, hopefully, involve the patient in his or her own recovery.

Pinel's feeling of professional and intellectual fraternity with the students prompted him to offer them a second memoir, 'On the Moral Treatment of the Insane'. The term 'moral treatment' has caused rivers of ink to flow, because the French word *moral* should be translated as 'psychologic' and not as 'moral', which has a judgmental connotation. Pinel is partly to blame for this fundamental misunderstanding, because he repeatedly described the treatment but never defined it precisely. Consequently, this second memoir remains the least understood—though the best known—of all of Pinel's writings on mental alienation.

Pinel's conception of moral treatment for the mentally ill emerged from an Enlightenment movement that rejected the traditional notion of the mad as being totally devoid of reason and thus requiring coercive, physical modes of treatment directed against a somatic derangement. With roots in eighteenth-century English private asylums, moral treatment found expression at the turn of the eighteenth century in the Retreat at York founded by William Tuke, a Quaker layman, and in the work of Chiarugi in Florence and Benjamin Rush in Philadelphia. But Pinel's version, which included theoretical as well as practical components, was more comprehensive, and it was securely anchored to hospital medicine.

Moral treatment requires, first of all, that the physician respect the patient as a person; value judgments are not pertinent to a physician's function. But respect and patience are not sufficient, for the doctor must decide which therapeutic interventions may be helpful, even if they inflict physical pain. Pinel at times prescribed the straitjacket, prolonged baths, or even cold showers on the head that might be painful, but he insisted that threats or restraint be brief, and that they always be followed by expressions of 'pure philanthropy and by a friendly reconciliation'. He was obviously describing the traits and methods of Jean-Baptiste Pussin, the 'governor' of the insane at Bicêtre and Pinel's mentor in asylum management. In Pinel's first memoir we already find a description of that ideal administrator: he showed dedication and good judgment, as well as an appropriate mix of natural authority and compassion, of firmness and sensitivity, and of enlightened experience and constant vigilance.

Indeed, the most controversial issue in the first memoir concerns the authority of the asylum's director. It is worth remembering that in our own day, in Michel Foucault's version of this method, the asylum director becomes a tyrannical 'medical personage' who imposes silence, generates a feeling of guilt, and demands from the patient total submission to the director's will. (This important critique is discussed below.) Pinel would not have recognized Foucault's analysis, nor would he have shared his opinion. In fact, Pinel described a mental hospital as a large family composed of turbulent and impetuous persons who need to be curbed rather than exasperated; restrained whenever possible by feelings of respect and appreciation, rather than through abject fear; and guided gently, though with unbending firmness.

Pinel here argues that many mentally ill persons need structure and rules that they are not—or are no longer—able to impose on their own behavior. Their uncooperative or disruptive actions compel the physician to apply a wide range of measures that would induce or force them to comply. Pinel did not perceive the danger involved in thus granting asylum directors so much power, nor could he imagine the inhumane excesses to which such uncontrolled license could lead.

The third memoir that Pinel presented to the Society for Medical Emulation in 1798 seems at first sight rather confused, and he reworked it thoroughly into chapter four of the second edition of the *Traité*. It is entitled 'Observations on the Insane and their Classification into Distinct Species'. Essentially, he aimed at defining an order of diseases—the mental derangements, or *insaniae*—as part of his fourth class: nervous diseases, or 'neuroses'. Having already devoted chapter one to periodic insanity, he did not have much more to say about continuing 'mania', or madness. Therefore he mainly discussed melancholia, his first 'species' seen as a variation of mania, which sometimes presented in bipolar alternation. There was a rich tradition of writings on that topic—at least since Celsus, Soranus, Rufus, and Aretaeus—and Pinel knew them well. Melancholia is often characterized by the patient's focus on one issue, and the consequent loss of interest in any unrelated person, event, or activity. Pinel here offered a good definition of what Esquirol would call 'monomania', a concept that had a short vogue in the 1820s and 1830s. As for the other two main species of mental alienation, dementia and idiocy, even the lively descriptions and dramatic histories provided by Pinel could do little to excite the students' interest. Those afflictions were known to be incurable, and therefore they held little fascination for the future doctors in Pinel's audience.

This third memoir shows that in 1798 Pinel was struggling to arrive at a definitive classification of all varieties of mental alienation, to be listed in his *Nosographie*. That proved to be a difficult task, and he made many adjustments in the course of the book's six editions.

The success of the *Nosographie* undoubtedly engendered a wish to publish the three lectures on mental alienation, but three essays do not make a book. So Pinel added the memoir on deformed human skulls that he had just presented to the Academy of Sciences, as well as two sketchy chapters on medical treatment and on the management of the asylum that he would develop fully in the second edition (1809). The *Traité* made Pinel world-famous. It was translated into German, Spanish, English, and Italian, but the wretched 1806 English translation by a young obstetrician from Sheffield was a disaster. This uninformed doctor freely substituted his own text, opinions, notes, and references for the author's. Unfortunately, this antiquated and mangled version remains the only text of Pinel's *Traité* available to the English-speaking world, and it is still widely quoted (Davis, 1806; Weiner, 2000).

By the time the *Traité* appeared in the fall of 1800, Pinel was deeply involved in caring for the sick at the Salpêtrière, where he had lived since 1795. The Paris hospital authorities had in the meantime reduced the number of inmates to about 4,000—mainly elderly women, many of whom were chronically ill. Pinel cared for acutely ill patients in the general infirmary. He gradually asserted his authority over a group of powerful nurses who had administered the inmates of the Salpêtrière under the old regime. But more important than harnessing the nurses was Pinel's creation of a clinical teaching service—bedside instruction for the medical students was a prime objective at that time. Pinel and Corvisart were, by all accounts, the most accomplished and inspiring clinicians in early nineteenth-century Paris. Pinel published hundreds of case histories in *La médecine clinique rendue plus précise et plus exacte par l'application de l'analyse*, which was issued in three editions (1802, 1804, 1815).

But his heart was set on finding a way to help the large numbers of mentally ill women—about three hundred in his special infirmary, the 'fifth section'. He felt that his most urgent need was to make order, and for that he needed Pussin—his trusted assistant at Bicêtre—and Pussin's wife, Marguerite Jubline. Pinel asked for their transfer to the Salpêtrière as early as 1798, but the ministers of internal affairs, first François de Neufchâteau and then Lucien Bonaparte, turned a deaf ear. Their successor Chaptal, in contrast, responded within days, and the Pussins arrived at the Salpêtrière in May 1802. In the meantime, Chaptal had also decreed that the treatment of all hospitalized mentally ill women in the Paris region be transferred to Pinel's hospice.

Pinel's experiment of 1802–05 consisted of three phases. First, he and his assistant, Augustin Jacob Landré-Beauvais, examined each of the 569 women already hospitalized in order to verify the diagnosis and change the therapy, if necessary. They found that 91 percent of them were too sick to be treated, but 9 percent—fifty-two women—were potentially curable, and Pinel transferred them to special quarters.

The second part of the experiment involved taking a careful history of each new arrival and assigning her to the appropriate ward. We have succinct case histories for all of these women—more than one thousand—written in often minuscule script in the margin of each entry of the folios titled '*Mutations des folles*'. These entries are of extraordinary interest because they document the diagnostic acumen and empathy of this physician.

The third part of Pinel's project is of general relevance to the history of psychiatry because it details his concept of the asylum, particularly the section where the convalescents were lodged. They were to have clean and pleasant accommodations, gardens to walk in, and most importantly, regular work—all under skilled supervision. Pinel had unbounded faith in the therapeutic value of a meaningful occupation, pursued during regular hours with like-minded companions, and for pay—even if the pay was minimal. On 24 June 1805 he submitted his results to the Academy of Sciences, and the academy was so impressed that it ordered publication of Pinel's report in the official congressional journal, the *Moniteur universel*. The contents of that report reappear as section four of the second edition of the *Traité*.

Pinel's career had reached its apogee. The remaining twenty years of his life were sad, but he lived them stoically. He died at the Salpêtrière in 1826 and was buried in the Père Lachaise cemetery.

How do we evaluate Pinel's passionate and erudite legacy? To his colleagues and students, the author of the *Nosographie of Clinical Medicine* and the *Traité* was a learned guide and outstanding clinician. For posterity he has remained a philanthropic innovator. But several of the contemporary generation of young investigators, such as G. L. Bayle, questioned his nosographic categories. In fact, nosology died at the turn of the nineteenth century because new knowledge about the etiology of diseases made an all-inclusive nosologic chart impossible. G. L. Bayle was Pinel's first, but not his only, major critic. F. J. V. Broussais ridiculed his theory of 'essential' fevers, and most important, A. L. J. Bayle's thesis of 1822 proved that general paresis can be diagnosed in the brain. The road to biological psychiatry had been opened.

Worse was in store for Pinel's image, and that attack came from his own son, Dr Scipion Pinel. In 1823, while his father was still alive, Scipion published a fictitious tale that showed Pinel facing the rabid Jacobin Couthon and fearlessly freeing the insane from their shackles. The myth of Pinel the Chainbreaker was thus created. It is immortalized in two enormous paintings—on the walls of the National Academy of Medicine and in front of the Charcot Library at the Salpêtrière—that are known all over the world and reprinted in textbooks again and again. The 'chainbreaker' myth prevailed for more than 100 years.

Scipion was not alone in wanting to hide Pinel the thinker, clinician, and teacher behind the veil of a myth. Pinel's intellectual son and heir, J. E. D. Esquirol, became his star student, the first well-trained psychiatrist, and his successful rival. He opened a small *maison de santé* under Pinel's sponsorship, succeeded Pussin at the Salpêtrière as supervisor of the mentally ill women, and taught the first course on psychiatry at the hospice. His monarchist politics paid off under the Restoration. He undertook several inspection tours of the nation's asylums, became the medical director of Charenton Hospice, and eventually was the main architect of the Law of 1838 that still regulates the hospitalization of mental patients in France. But he did not succeed Pinel as physician-in-chief of the Salpêtrière, as he may have hoped, nor did he rise to a professorship, nor to membership in the Academy of Sciences. Did the teacher block his student's ambitions? We have no evidence. Rather, Esquirol built on Pinel's ideas and wrote excellent analyses and clinical descriptions collected in an influential book, *Des maladies mentales*. Taking his cue from Scipion, Esquirol paid ample homage to Pinel the philanthropist while obscuring the thinker and innovative clinician, the founder of psychiatry in France.

In the 1960s, the so-called antipsychiatry movement called into question the epistemological basis of confinement, in particular its efficacy and its problematic ethical status. The horrifying discovery of the concentration camps and the gulag had contributed to a mistrust of all 'total' institutions, including mental hospitals, where, it was said, autocratic physician-directors regimented patients' bodies in order to control their minds. The original notion of the asylum as cure was inverted to portray it as the *cause* of mental illness. Close supervision, mandatory and exacting physical work, and strictly regulated hours for meals, exercise, and prayer degraded the inmates into automatons. Worse, the powerful bourgeois psychiatrists used the patients for research, extracting valuable knowledge from hapless proletarians. Led by the brilliant philosopher Michel Foucault, this assault on psychiatry spread, with authors such as Klaus Dörner, Thomas Szasz, and Andrew Scull adding fuel to the fire. Antipsychiatry, along with the advent of psychotrophic medications in the previous decade, contributed to the de-institutionalization of hundreds of thousands of mental patients throughout the Western world.

The establishment of psychiatry in French academic life was long delayed. It was not until 1877 that a Faculty chair for *maladies mentales* was created, for Benjamin Ball, at Ste Anne Hospital in Paris. Pinel's message remains pertinent today: society owes decent care to all of its mentally ill people, including the destitute. His important professional legacy lies in the theoretical realm; his exploration of periodic insanity, with a likely bipolar variation, remains seminal. So does his conviction that a patient does not 'lose his mind' or 'go out of his mind', but that certain mental faculties can be impaired while others may remain intact. The importance he attached to a carefully taken detailed personal history, as well as a history of the illness, cannot be overemphasized. Pinel was, first of all, a fine clinician who continues to teach by example. He was instrumental in bringing psychiatry into the purview of modern medicine.

Bibliography

Primary: 1798. *Nosographie philosophique ou Méthode de l'analyse appliquée á la médecine* 2 vols. [3 vols. 1803, 1807, 1810, 1813, 1818] (Paris); 1800. *Traité médico-philosophique de l'aliénation mentale* (2nd edn., 1809) (Paris); 1806. (Davis, D. D., Eng. trans.) *A Treatise on Insanity* (Sheffield); 1802, 1804, 1815. *La médecine clinique rendue plus précise et plus exacte par l'application de l'analyse* (Paris).

Secondary: Pigaud, Jackie, 2001. *Aux portes de la psychiatrie: Pinel, l'ancien et le moderne* (Paris); Weiner, Dora B., 1999. *Comprendre et soigner: Philippe Pinel et la médecine de l'esprit* (Paris) (Contains a 14-page detailed bibliography of Pinel's writings) [trans. Spanish 2002, trans. English, *Observe and Heal: Philippe Pinel and the Birth of Psychiatry in the French Revolution* (Aldershot, forthcoming)]; Postel, Jacques, 1981. *Genèse de la psychiatrie: Les premiers écrits de Philippe Pinel* (Paris); Weiner, Dora B., 1979. 'The Apprenticeship of Philippe Pinel, A New Document: Observations of Citizen Pussin on the Insane.' *Amer. J. Psychiat.* 136: 1128–1134; Swain, Gladys, 1977. *Le sujet de la folie: Naissance de la psychiatrie* (Toulouse); *DSB*.

Dora B. Weiner

PINOTTI, MÁRIO (b. Brotas, Brazil, 21 January 1894; d. Rio de Janeiro, Brazil, 3 March 1972), *public health, malariology.*

Pinotti was born in Brotas, a small town in the State of São Paulo, where his father, an Italian immigrant, had a pharmacy. In 1914 he graduated from the School of Pharmacology of Ouro Preto, and in 1918 from the School of Medicine of Rio de Janeiro, in what was then the capital of Brazil. In 1919 he entered the national public heath service.

In 1924 and 1925, thanks to a fellowship from the Rockefeller Foundation's International Health Board (IHB), he studied at the Italian Malaria School, located in Netuno, where he became acquainted with leading malariologists such as Alberto Missirolli, Bartolomeo Gosio, and Lewis W. Hackett and learned modern control methods. Upon his return from Italy, Pinotti worked in several national Brazilian organizations involved in the fight against yellow fever. He even became assistant to the director of the yellow fever services that were under the command of the IHB.

In April 1941 the National Service for Malaria was created to coordinate all actions taken against malaria. Pinotti was appointed its director in August 1942, a position he held until 1956, when the services in charge of malaria, bubonic plague, and yellow fever were merged with the National Department for Rural Endemic Diseases. Pinotti was appointed director of the new department and remained in the position until 1958. During the sixteen years (1942–58) in which he conducted antimalaria work, Pinotti provided remarkable technical and scientific skills to the sanitary services that dealt with endemic diseases. He gave them a national and international projection and consolidated the popular and political belief that malaria was one of the main problems of Brazil.

In 1952 Pinotti and his team at the Institute for Malariology, a department of research and teaching within the National Service for Malaria, started to test alternative therapies for malaria. In 1953 he published an article with a proposal for mixing chloroquine (the main drug used to treat malaria) with cooking salt, producing it by the government, and distributing it free to the population of the endemic areas, using all means of transport. The proposal was conceived as an innovative and autochthonous response to the challenge of the traditional method of periodically administering antimalaria drugs in a country such as Brazil, with vast and isolated rural areas of low habitational density where the use of insecticides of residual action was inefficacious—especially in the Amazon.

The chloroquinated salt, which became known as 'Pinotti's Method', reached international visibility and was used outside Brazil. It was widely distributed throughout Brazil's inland areas until the mid-1960s, having been tested in Africa and Asia and even recommended by the World Health Organization. Such prestige led Pinotti to preside twice over the Brazilian Society of Hygiene, to be accepted in 1959 at the National Academy of Medicine, and to belong to many other prestigious academic associations.

The climax of his public life was reached when he was appointed Minister of Health in 1958, during the government of Juscelino Kubitscheck (1956–60). Pinotti wrote the health program of the Kubitscheck campaign, emphasizing the fight against diseases as a strategy for national integration and economic development. In 1960 Pinotti left his ministerial post after becoming involved in political turmoil. He would not occupy any other public position for the rest of his life.

Pinotti's path is exemplary for Brazilian public health during the period beginning with World War II and ending in the early 1960s. It was characterized by his conviction that coordinated and vertical governmental interventions were needed at the national level and that health played an essential role in the modernization and integration of the country, and by his firm belief that new drugs and insecticides would defeat infectious diseases.

Bibliography

Primary: 1953. 'Novo Método de Controle da Malária pelo emprego de medicamentos misturados ao sal de cozinha utilizado na alimentação diária.' *Revista Brasileira de Medicina* 10: 241–246.

Secondary: Moraes, Hélbio F., 1990. 'Biografia do Professor Dr. Mário Pinotti' in Moraes, Hélbio F., *Sucam: sua origem, sua história* (Brasília) pp. 257–264.

Gilberto Hochman

PIQUER ARRUFAT, ANDRÉS (b. Fórnoles, Aragón, Spain, 6 November 1711; d. Madrid, Spain, 3 February 1772), *medicine.*

Piquer was the son of farmers and started his studies thanks to an ecclesiastic fellowship, moving to larger and larger cities in order to further develop his professional career. He studied philosophy and medicine at the University of Valencia (1727–34), where he became a professor of anatomy and assistant physician of the General Hospital (1743), and a physician of the Royal Court in Madrid (1751). Ferdinand VI made him vice president of the Royal Academy of Medicine and a member of the Protomedicato Court—the high state court of Spain for the assessment, control, and reform of the health professions. Piquer became First Doctor to the king in 1758, increasing his salary from 8,000 to 21,000 *reales* per year, and he held the same office under Charles III. Several manuscripts edited by his son in 1785 show us his medical practice style and his most famous clinical records.

Piquer helped reform the teaching of medicine, writing on a wide range of medical topics. Many of his thirty-three books reached large audiences, such as his clinical semiology and pharmacology work first published in 1735 (revised in 1743, 1758, 1768, 1776, and 1791); his *Treatise on fevers,* which had five editions (Madrid, Montpellier, Amsterdam, Paris, and Mexico); and his *Treatise on medical practice,* which was edited in Amsterdam and in Venice.

As a nosologist, Piquer searched for specific clinical signs as a way to catalog illnesses. Some of his disease definitions were controversial, relevant, or pioneering such as those for malaria, epilepsy, and bipolar disease (mania-melancholy), respectively. During his life, he changed his criteria for classifying fevers and explaining etiological factors. In therapeutics, he explained from an essentialist or qualitative theory (e.g., heat and coldness) what in his youth he had supported in an iatrochemical way (e.g., cephalics—remedies for the head cure by the action of the volatile salt over the thick lymph retained in the fibers, canals, and brain glands). In general, teleology, anthropocentrism, and antimaterialism are the key presuppositions in Piquer's scientific explanations.

As a practitioner, Piquer was a careful observer of symptoms, yet he was critical of the popular prejudices of his patients. Throughout his life, he avoided polypharmacy and complex preparations—mainly those coming from the 'chemical oven'—prescribing instead the soft and harmless remedies that favored the patient's education on self-care. He was a pioneer propagator of Peruvian bark to cure intermittent fevers (malaria), but he rejected other specific remedies. Because Piquer considered the doctor to be Nature's assistant, his motto was double-edged: avoid iatrogenesis and do not mask the natural history of diseases.

As a teacher and philosopher, Andrés Piquer criticized sensualism and the doctrine of common sense, defending medical knowledge based on clinical experiences and inductive-deductive reasoning. Even though it was not an explicit topic of his *Modern Logic* (1747, 1771), therapeutic effects had the epistemological value of counter-proof, a method of diagnosis verification. He advised against two key dangers of his time: the lack of skill in the use of logical explanation, and the transfer to patients of data based on nonclinical experiences, such as certain anatomical observations or animal vivisection.

Known as the Spanish Hippocrates, Piquer epitomized the enlightened, yet Catholic, doctor sought by the Spanish Crown. All of his writings—medical and philosophical alike—show his desire to provide an intellectual, moral, and technical education for doctors.

Bibliography

Primary: 1735. *Medicina vetus et nova* (Valencia); 1751. *Tratado de calenturas según la observación y el mecanismo* (Valencia); 1764. *Praxis Medica* (Madrid).

Secondary: Frías Núñez, Marcelo, 2003. 'El discurso médico a propósito de las fiebres y de la quina en el tratado de las calenturas (1751) de Andrés Piquer.' *Asclepio* 50: 215–233; Miqueo, Consuelo, 1998. 'Empirismo clínico y tratamiento de las enfermedades mentales' in Barcia, Demetrio, ed., *Historia de la psicofarmacología* (Madrid) pp. 299–332; Mindán Manero, Manuel, 1991. *Andrés Piquer. Filosofía y medicina en la España del siglo XVIII* (Zaragoza); López Piñero, José María, 1987. 'Andrés Piquer y el hipocratismo en la España de la Ilustración' in Piquer, Andrés, *Las epidemias de Hippócrates* (Madrid) pp. 9–37.

Consuelo Miqueo

PIROGOV, NIKOLAI IVANOVICH (b. Moscow, Russia, 13 November 1810; d. Vishnia [now Pirogovo], Vinnitsa oblast', Ukraine, 23 November 1881), *surgery, pedagogy, military medicine.*

The thirteenth child in the family of a Moscow bursar, Pirogov studied for two years in a private boarding house. Beginning at the age of fourteen, he studied at the medical faculty of Moscow University from 1824–28. Among his teachers were the anatomist Kh. I. Loder and the clinicians M. Ia. Mudrov and E. O. Mukhin. Pirogov specialized in surgery at the Professorial Institute in Derpt (now Tartu, Estonia). In 1829 he received the gold medal for carrying out an assignment on the dressing of large arteries in the surgical clinic of I. F. Moier. In 1832 he defended his dissertation, Iavliaetsia li pereviazka briushnoi aorty pri aneurizme pakhovoi oblasti legko vypolnimym i bezopasnym vmeshatel'stvom [On the dressing of the abdominal aorta during an aneurism of the inguinal area by practical and safe intervention], in which he generalized the results of the experimental study of collateral blood flow after an operation, and the reduced surgical risk.

From 1833 to 1835 he trained in anatomy and surgery with B. Langenbeck, in Göttingen, and became a professor of Derpt University in 1836. He was the founder and head of the hospital surgical clinic of the Medical-Surgical Academy in Petersburg (1841–56). He was simultaneously head doctor of the surgical department of the second military land forces hospital and director of the technical section of the Saint Petersburg Instrument Factory, and in 1846 he was named director at the Medical-Surgical Academy of the Institute of Practical Anatomy.

The classic works of Pirogov laid the foundations of operational surgery, topographic anatomy, and plastic surgery on bones. He was the founder of military field surgery and the anatomical-experimental orientation of surgery in Russia. Pirogov is rightly named 'the Father of Russian Surgery'. His scientific school was not limited to his immediate students; all Russian surgeons of the second half of the nineteenth century were heirs of his attitudes and methods. The greatest scientists among those Pirogov personally taught were L. A. Bekkers, A. P. Val'ter, A. P. Zablotskii-Desiatovskii, V. A. Karavaev, A. A. Kiter, P. Iu. Nemmert, P. S. Platonov, M. A. Favorskii, and K. K. Shtraukh.

Among his classic works are *Khirurgicheskaia anatomiia arterial'nykh stvolov i fastsii* [Surgical anatomy of arterial vessels and facets] (1837); *Polnyi kurs prikladnoi anatomii chelovecheskogo tela, s risunkami* [A full course for the applied anatomy of the human body, with drawings (of descriptive-physiological and surgical anatomy] (1843–48), *Illiustrirovannaia topograficheskaia anatomiia raspilov, provedennykh v trekh napravleniiakh cherez zamorozhennoe chelovecheskoe telo* [The illustrated topographic anatomy of saw cuts, conducted in three axes through a frozen human body] (1852–59), each of which was awarded the Demidov Prize of the St Petersburg Academy of Science, and served as the basis for topographic anatomy and operational surgery. These works were founded on applied human anatomy, leading to original methods for making anatomical preparations. In this case, the method involved the sawing up of frozen corpses, or 'ice-cold anatomy', the basis of which had been laid in 1836 by Buial'skii.

Generalizing from the results of 800 autopsies at the time of the outbreak of cholera in St Petersburg in 1848, Pirogov argued that cholera strikes primarily the gastrointestinal tract, an indication that the cause of the disease is an organism from food. The results of that research were reported in his monograph *Patologicheskaia anatomia aziatskoi kholery* [The pathological anatomy of Asiatic cholera], published in 1849 in French and the following year in Russian. It was awarded the Demidov Prize.

The first in Russia to speak for the development of plastic surgery, Pirogov gave a lecture in 1835 at the St Petersburg Academy of Sciences titled 'O plasticheskikh operatsiiakh voobshche i o rinoplastike v osobennosti' [About plastic operations in general and about rhinoplastics in particular]. He did the pioneering work in the area of osseous plastics, publishing 'Osseous-plastic lengthening of the shin bones by removal of the foot' in 1854. The method of joining the supporting stump by the amputation of the shin at the expense of the fifth bone is well-

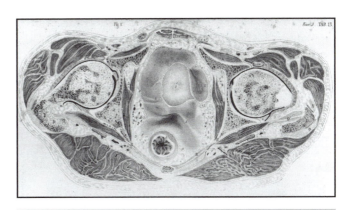

Cross-section of the torso of the human body from *Anatome topographica sectionibus per corpus humanum congelatum . . .* Petropoli, 1852. Rare Books, Wellcome Library, London.

known as Pirogov's operation. Pirogov's name is also known for his broadly applied proposition regarding abdominal access to the exterior iliac artery and the lower third of the ureter.

Even before the discoveries of Louis Pasteur and Joseph Lister in the area of antisepsis and asepsis, Pirogov conjectured in his clinical lectures that the festering of wounds was due to live stimuli, which he named 'hospital miasmas'. He set aside a special ward in his hospital for infectious 'miasmas', which required separate personnel in the gangrene division and the use of special instruments and dressing material for such patients. In several of his subsequent works, Pirogov spoke as an upholder of the preventive orientation in medicine and public health.

Pirogov played an exceptional role in the development of anesthesia. At the beginning of 1847, he conducted broad experimental and clinical investigation of the anesthetic properties of ether, and he was one of the first in Russia (14 February 1847) to perform a tonsillectomy under ether anesthesia. He was the first in the world to complete an operation under direct intestinal anesthetic, using an apparatus of special construction. In May–June 1847, Pirogov published three monographs in St Petersburg on the subject of ether, and they had the greatest significance in publicizing the new method in Russia.

In July–August 1847, Pirogov was assigned to the Caucasus. At the siege by Russian forces of the fortified mountain village of Salta, he became the first in world practice to successfully apply ether in wartime.

He was a participant in the defense of Sebastopol during the Crimean War (1854–55), where he used women as nurses to tend the wounded at the front. He also served as a consultant–surgeon in military theaters during the Franco-Prussian (1870–71) and Russo-Turkish (1877–78) wars. Pirogov generalized the results of that work in 'Nachala obshchei voenno-polevoi khirurgii, vziatye iz nabliudenii voenno-polevoi praktiki i vospominanii o Krymskoi voine i Kavkazskoi ekspeditsii' (1865–66) [The principles of general military field surgery, taken from the observation of military-hospital practice and reminiscences about the Crimean war and the Caucasian expedition]; 'Otchet o poseshchenii voenno-sanitarnykh uchrezhdenii v Germanii, Lotaringii i El'zase v 1870 g.' (1871) [Report about visits to military-sanitary institutions in Germany, Lorraine, and Alsace in 1870]; and 'Voenno-vrachebnoe delo i chastnaia pomoshch' na teatre voiny v Bolgarii i v tylu deistvuiushchei armii' (1879) [Military-medical affairs and private care in the theater of war in Bulgaria and in the rear of the active army in 1877–78].

Pirogov formulated a series of positions that became the basis of the organizational, methodological, and tactical principles of military medicine. His definition that 'war is a traumatic epidemic' entered the literature. It reflected the great significance he attached to the unfavorable factors of the military environment, which enabled the growth of complications from wounds and a series of diseases among soldiers. Pirogov's opinions on conducting surgical interventions at dressing stations and in field lazarettos changed over the span of his career, but to the end of his life he supported the active–preventive path of military field surgery. He is the founder of studies about sorting wounded personnel according to their medical condition.

The works of Pirogov have great significance for military field surgery in regard to the problems of immobilization and shock. He was the first to employ the practice of using rigid plaster casts for complex breakages of limbs (1847), and he applied a plaster cast under field conditions (1854). Pirogov's clinical picture of shock from wounds is a classic, and he is also responsible for detailed characterizations of the pathogenesis, prevention, and treatment of shock, concussion of the brain, gaseous edema of tissues, and other conditions.

Pirogov was the first to speak out against complications in the medical security system of the Russian Army, pointing out that multiple chains of command and the exclusion of doctors from the management of military medical institutions were the main stumbling blocks hindering the rational care of the wounded.

In 1840 he was one of the first to initiate reform of the higher medical schools. Pirogov stressed the need to create hospital clinics, and he formulated the tasks involved in implementing them. In 1841 the principle of hospital-based clinics was established in Russia at Pirogov's surgical clinic in the Medical–Surgical Academy, and in 1842 the first medical was opened. Hospital clinics followed at Moscow University in 1846 and then at the universities of Kazan, Derpt, and Kiev.

Pirogov was an internationally known authority, as attested to by his invitation for a medical consultation with future German chancellor Otto von Bismarck (1859) and the Italian revolutionary, Giuseppe Garibaldi.

Shortly after the publication of Pirogov's pedagogical article 'Voprosy zhizni' [Problems of Life] in the journal *Morskoi sbornik*, he was invited to serve at the Ministry of Education. He held the office of warden of the Odessa (1856–58) and Kiev (1858–61) educational districts and was a spokesman for the autonomy of universities, for general primary education, and against class and ethnic restrictions in the area of education. He repeatedly put together plans to transform Jewish schools, aiming to end their caste exclusion. As a pedagogue, Pirogov considered it most important of all to foster in students and teachers a 'respect for human dignity, [and] truth'.

Beginning in 1862, Pirogov audited the foreign training of young Russian scientists (in Germany), and in that capacity he served at more than twenty universities and published a series of articles in the newspaper *Golos*.

He was a corresponding member of the Petersburg Academy of Sciences (1847), an academician of the Medical–Surgical Academy (1846), and a privy counselor (1859).

Pirogov examined general philosophical problems in his article titled 'Problems of Life' and in his unfinished memoirs, *Dnevnik starogo vracha* [Diary of an Old Doctor] (1879–81). 'Problems of Life' summarized the author's opinions on education and is well-known in two different editions that reflect the evolution of his religious and philosophical ideas. The first edition (1856) was published four times during his lifetime and translated into German and French; the second edition (1887) was printed in his posthumous collected works. The second edition of the article is of particular interest because Pirogov anticipated the appearance of psychoanalysis. He called for the analysis of each thought separately and elucidation of its genesis.

A characteristic trait of Pirogov as a doctor and pedagogue was his strongly expressed self-criticism. For instance, his 1854 article in the *Voenno-meditsinskii zhurnal*—'O trudnostiakh paspoznavaniia khirurgicheskikh boleznei i o schast'e v khirurgii' [About the difficulties of the identification of surgical illnesses and about luck in surgery]—was based on the analysis of personal medical mistakes.

The significance of the figure of Pirogov and the originality of his opinions drew the interest of diverse researchers, including L. D. Trotsky, who published a 'political portrait' of Pirogov in 1913.

The Society of Russian Doctors was founded (1892) in his memory, and it regularly called 'Pirogov congresses' of doctors until 1919 (the tradition was revived in 1995). In 1897 a monument to Pirogov, sculpted by V. O. Sherwood, was erected in Moscow with funds collected by an all-Russian subscription among doctors.

In 1897 the Russian Surgical Society of Pirogov opened a separate, three-floor Pirogov Museum in St Petersburg, with a significant display of exhibits, regularly conducted congresses of surgeons, and so forth. In 1930 the museum lost its status as an independent institution, and the section of exhibits was destroyed. Nearly 150 lithographic plates on marble that were used in the publication of Pirogov's *Ice-cold Anatomy* were barbarically crushed for ballast. In 1947

Pirogov's museum–estate was opened in the village of Pirogovo, not far from the city of Vinnitsa. The museum includes a house and pharmacy, as well as a burial vault where the embalmed body of Pirogov is preserved in a sarcophagus.

Pirogov is the eponym for the osseous plastic amputation of the shin, methods of making anatomical preparations from frozen corpses, and surgery in the area of the inguinal ligament.

Bibliography

Primary: Rossiiskaia gosudarstvennaia biblioteka [Russian State Library], Nauchno-issledovatel'skii otdel rukopisei [Scientific-research department for manuscripts]. Tikh/III, 2, 4 (birth certificate); Tikh/II, 6, 48; M, 3735, 4; 169, 72, 87; 417, 3, 46 (Letters from Pirogov to various people); Tikh/III, 3, 1–2 (Materials relating to the jubilee of 1881); 358, 388, 12 (The excision of articles about Pirogov); 580, 2, 5 (Materials of S. S. Iudin on the biography of Pirogov, 1950) (Moscow).

Secondary: Kozovenko, M. N., 2004. 'Pervyi Pirogovskii muzei v Rossii.' ['The First Pirogov Museum in Russia'] *Voenno-meditsinskii zhurnal* 6: 68–74; 1992. 'N. I. Pirogov—uchenyi, chelovek, grazhdanin.' ['N. I. Pirogov—scientist, man, citizen'] *Sbornik nauchnykh trudov Nauchno-issledovatel'skogo tsentra 'Meditsinskii muzei'* [Collection of scientific works of the Scientific-research center 'Medical Museum'] RAMN (Moscow); 1991. (Zarechnak, Galina V., ed. and intro.) *Questions of Life: Diary of an Old Physician* (Canton, MA); Geselevich, A. M., 1976. *Letopis' zhizni N.I. Pirogova (1810–1881)* [Chronicle of the Life of N. I. Pirogov (1810-1881)] (Moscow); 'Zhizn' i deiatel'nost' N. I. Pirogova' ['Life and Activity of N. I. Pirogov], 1957. *Sobranie sochinenii N. I. Pirogova v 8 tomakh* [Collected Works of N. I. Pirogov in 8 Volumes] I: 7–56; Bertenson, I. V., 1881. *Nikolai Ivanovich Pirogov, ocherk ego obshchestvennoi deiatel'nosti kak professora, vracha-khirurga, pisatelia i pedagoga* [Nikolai Ivanovich Pirogov, the Study of His Public Actions as a Professor, Surgeon, Writer, and Pedagogue] (St Petersburg).

Mikhail Poddubnyi

PISO, WILLEM (b. Leiden, the Netherlands, 1611; d. Amsterdam, the Netherlands, 24 November 1678), *natural history, tropical medicine, pharmacy.*

Piso was born in Leiden. He matriculated at the university there in 1623 and received his MD in Caen (France) in 1633. He established a medical practice in Amsterdam and was involved in the flourishing cultural life of the Dutch Republic. Leading humanists and poets such as Caspar Barlaeus and Joost van den Vondel were among his friends. In 1637 Piso was sent to the Dutch settlement in Recife, Brazil, where he was appointed personal physician to Governor Johan Maurits van Nassau, who had a great interest in science. Piso was appointed head of the medical service, and accompanied Johan Maurits on his campaigns. Under the governor's authority, Piso was also sent out to gather data on the natural history and medical customs of Brazil. He collaborated with the young and brilliant Georg Marcgraf. The results of their joint efforts were published in 1648 as *Historia naturalis Brasilae*, which is still considered to be a pioneering book.

Piso sailed back to Holland in 1644, and after some peregrinations he settled in Amsterdam in 1648, where he resumed his medical practice. Until his death in 1678, Piso played an important role in Amsterdam's scientific and cultural life. Specimens of exotic creatures that Piso had brought from Brazil found their way to the cabinets of Amsterdam naturalists. In addition, he reworked the notes he wrote in Brazil and added an edition of the partly unpublished books that the VOC (Dutch East India Company) physician Jacob Bontius (1592–1631) had written on the East Indies. Both works were published as *De Indiae utriusque re naturali et medica* (1658). Moreover, Piso was an influential member of the municipal Collegium Medicum, serving as its *decanus* from 1656 to 1660, and again in 1670.

Piso is mostly remembered for his pioneering work on tropical medicine. His mind was more that of an anthropologist than of a classic intellectual. One of the most striking features of the *Historia naturalis Brasilae* is its matter-of-fact approach, which contrasts sharply with contemporary works. Both in the part written by Margraf on natural history and in the contribution by Piso on medicine, ancient sources and concepts are treated with reservation. Both researchers were much aware of the fact that they were describing something new and, as a consequence, that the traditional European perspective was not sufficient. Piso was one of the first to point out that the health of Europeans in the tropics was preserved by adopting the native way. For example, Dutch soldiers arrived in Brazil in baroque attire, and Dutch women wore heavy, dark woolen clothing, swaddling their children as they did in the Netherlands. Piso emphasized the beneficial role of unhindered perspiration and light clothing. On several expeditions to the interior of Brazil, Piso had gathered much information from the natives. He described not only endemic tropical diseases (and their remedies), but poisonous animals and toxic plants as well. For example, he was the first European to prescribe ipecacuanha as a cure for various forms of dysentery. Likewise, he described various American specifics such as sarsaparilla, sassafras, and guaiacum. According to Piso, intestinal parasites were best treated with tobacco syrup, which is highly toxic but extremely effective.

Bibliography

Primary: 1648. *De medicina Brasiliensi libri quator* in *Historia naturalis Brasiliae* (Leiden and Amsterdam); 1658. *De Indiae utriusque re naturali et medica libri quatuordecim* (Amsterdam).

Secondary: Pies, Eike, 1981. *Willem Piso (1611–1678). Begründer der kolonialen Medizin und Leibarzt des Grafen Johann Moritz von Nassau-Siegen in Brasilien* (Düsseldorf); Guerra, F., 1979. 'Medicine in Dutch Brazil' in Boogaart, E. van den, ed., *Johan Maurits van Nassau-Siegen 1604–1679. A Humanist Prince in Europe and*

Brazil (the Hague) pp. 472–493; Andel, M. A., 1937. 'Introduction' to *Gulielmus Piso. Capita nonnulla de ventris fluxibus, de dysenteria, de lue indica, de ipecacuánha* in *Opuscula selecta Neerlandicorum de arte medica* vol. XIV (Amsterdam) pp. xii–xxxviii.

Eric Jorink

PITTALUGA FATTORINI, GUSTAVO (b. Florence, Italy, 10 October 1876; d. Havana, Cuba, 27 April 1956), *parasitology, hematology.*

A renowned speaker and compulsive writer, this Italian-born physician from a ruined aristocratic lineage spent most of his adult life in Spain, where he became one of the leading figures in laboratory medicine. He contributed to establishing the modern concept of medicine as applied biology. His primary interest in parasitic diseases led him to the study of hematopathology. An understanding of blood as the 'internal milieu' allowed him to become aware of the links between blood changes and endocrinal and metabolic disorders, all on a hereditary or congenital, constitutional basis. Pittaluga displayed a forceful presence among the ranks of the committed intelligentsia reformers that led Spain to its flourishing during the Second Republic. His exile stands as an example of the unfortunate fate of true liberal personalities at times of extremely powerful political statism on either the right or the left.

Climates, Diseases, and Promotion

Pittaluga obtained his MD and PhD degrees at the University of Rome, where he excelled in pathology and psychiatry. While a resident at Guido Bacelli's clinic, he contributed to the experiments on chemical prophylaxis against malaria led by Giovanni Battista Grassi in Ostia, in the summer and autumn of 1901. Other experiments were undertaken in several parts of Italy, and as soon as he obtained his PhD, Pittaluga traveled to Spain to develop similar field trials, backed by the Milanese firm that produced the drug. Between August 1902 and April 1903, when he presented his findings at the International Medical Congress held in Madrid and Barcelona, he succeeded in launching an experiment in Baix Llobregat, a marshy region south of Barcelona. More significantly, he became acquainted with a number of medical personalities who were to be crucial to his future. Paramount among his new friends was Francisco Huertas, personal physician to Santiago Ramón y Cajal and coauthor with Antonio Mendoza of the first official field experiment on the prevention of malaria in Navalmoral, Spain's most stricken area. Huertas served as vice-president of the International Medical Congress and, together with Pittaluga, presented the conclusions of the session on malaria.

Pittaluga obtained Spanish citizenship in 1904 and married María Victoria González del Campillo, Huertas's sister-in-law. Obliged to renew his medical qualifications,

he gained his MD degree in 1905 and a few months later was awarded a new PhD for a thesis on the pathogenesis of serotherapeutic syndromes—an experimental study that he carried out at Ramón y Cajal's Laboratory for Biological Research. Those two years were full of experimental work and yielded some celebrated results on the embryology of dog and human *Filaria*. In 1906 he was appointed staff member of the National Institute of Hygiene (NIH), also under the direction of the Spanish Nobel Prize winner, where he set up a parasitology section that remained under his guidance until his resignation in 1924. In 1909 he led an NIH mission to the Spanish colony in the Gulf of Guinea, pursuing the same goal as that of British, German, and French expeditions to West and East Africa from 1903 to 1908—the quest for clues to combat 'sleeping sickness'. He contributed to entomology by describing a species of hematophagous diptera that he designated *Clemmys africana haemoproteus Cajali*, in homage to his scientific mentor.

The trip itself served as a test of the prophylaxis against malaria, a condition that affected only one of the white members of the expedition (whose carelessness was mentioned by Pittaluga), whereas it took a heavy toll among the native carriers. The social importance of that mission helped Pittaluga easily win the chair of parasitology and tropical diseases at the Faculty of Medicine of the Central University in 1911, a position he held until the Civil War. He enhanced the teaching facilities with two laboratories at the San Carlos Hospital and the *Residencia de Estudiantes*, an institution of excellence founded in 1910 by the Board for Advanced Studies and Scientific Research. Thanks to his work, child leishmaniasis was described for the first time in Spain in 1912. He became director of the newly founded Catalonian Health Service, which initially targeted two prevalent endemic diseases: tuberculosis (urban) and malaria (rural). In addition, from 1920 to 1924 he was president of the Spanish Anti-Malaria Commission, which was the expression of official plans to fight that parasitic disease in rural areas. Between November 1920 and July 1922, the campaign was launched in the small village of Talayuela (Cáceres) under the direction of Pittaluga. It was developed by some of his disciples, particularly Sadi de Buen (who was to become the chief field officer of the anti-malaria struggle after 1924) and two experienced Italian Red Cross collaborators, the physician Massimo Sella and the nurse Bianca Marcosanti. A distinctive trait of the Spanish campaign was that only trained physicians and health assistants were given a place in its ranks, which meant that rural physicians became involved in mastering microscopy and laboratory techniques. In 1922 Pittaluga produced a handbook on tropical diseases based on his contribution and experience, and those of his followers. Finally, in 1928 he founded the journal *Medicina de los países cálidos*, the leading vehicle for Spanish medical parasitology, which he edited until 1936. However, after winning his chair at the University of Madrid, he directed his efforts primarily toward another aim: the study of blood diseases.

Hematology: A Way of Developing Laboratory Medicine

Shortly after securing his academic position, Pittaluga focused on the morphological and physiological study of blood disorders. In 1916 he started to organize postgraduate courses on hematology, and he established an outpatient clinic at the University in 1918. He contributed a chapter on blood diseases to the *Handbook of Internal Medicine* (1916) edited by Teófilo Hernando and Gregorio Marañón, the book that heralded the triumphant arrival of the pathophysiological approach on the Spanish medical scene. He was also called to serve the heir of the crown, the Prince of Asturia, who suffered from hemophilia. Another outstanding undertaking was the launching of the journal *Archivos de Cardiología y Hematología* (1920–36), which Pittaluga co-edited with Luis Calandre. He published his own handbook on blood diseases in 1922 and, in 1934, an ambitious monographic study of diseases of the reticuloendothelial system, a systematic essay illustrated by the clinical work of Pittaluga and his team. Notably, the concept of 'hemodystrophy' (first formulated in 1915) was applied to a group of disorders that required diagnosis by a mixture of morphopathology, endocrinal and metabolic pathophysiology, and constitutional analysis. This proposal was supported by evidence from other Spanish colleagues of the time, including Marañón and Nóvoa Santos.

In 1930 Pittaluga opened a laboratory for clinical research at the Faculty of Medicine, leading to a clash with the younger and no less ambitious Professor Carlos Jiménez Díaz, who strove for his own Medical Research Institute. There is no doubt that Latin American medicine was strongly influenced by Pittaluga's doctrines. He was rewarded with an honorary professorship in histology at the National University of Mexico (1935) and membership in the Medical Academies of Buenos Aires, Rio de Janeiro, Mexico, and Cuba, among others.

Medical Science and Politics

Besides his scientific work, Pittaluga used his social skills and ample network of acquaintances among the better-off classes to earn himself a central position on the managerial side of science. He joined the Liberal faction, led by Melquiades Álvarez, that was known as the Reform party, which kept out of the government-forming game during the first decade of Alfonso XIII's reign. A close friend of the philosopher José Ortega y Gasset, Pittaluga helped develop several of Ortega's political initiatives between 1915 and 1923, such as the League for Political Education and the weekly *España*. He also collaborated

with Gregorio Marañón and others in forming the Institute (later, the League) for Social Medicine in 1917–20. He became a private adviser to José Castillejo, the strong man—permanent Secretary—at the Board for Advanced Studies. Pittaluga was one of the very few physicians to join the first Manifesto of the Spanish League for Human Rights in 1922. He participated as the Spanish representative to the Health Organization of the League of Nations from its birth, and he repeatedly served as vice-president of its Scientific Committee. In 1923 he was elected to the Parliament that was ended by the coup d'état led by General Primo de Rivera. He was elected again when the Second Republic was formed in 1931, although he left Alvarez's faction and politics altogether shortly afterward. Later, in 1935, he joined Manuel Azaña's party. In 1930 Pittaluga was appointed director of the National School for Public Health, which was founded on paper in 1926 but only became a reality under his direction. Under his guidance, the (medicalized) concept of 'public health' expanded to include such problems as sanitary engineering and architecture. He left that post in 1932 to become editor-in-chief of the official journal of the National Public Health Department, *Revista de Sanidad e Higiene pública*, where he remained until the beginning of the Civil War. He contributed to the design and running of the Permanent Board for Health Research that was created to foster experimental research and training, and he led the newly created (1934) National Institute of Health, which took over all central public facilities concerned with public health matters.

Ill-Fated Period of Exile

Pittaluga belonged to the mildly progressive wing of the Republican movement and was in no way a Bolshevik. A workers committee, born from the disorders of the first days of the military Fascist uprising, forced him to abandon the direction of the National Health Institute, and in October 1936 he left for France. There he managed to continue working and publishing on blood disorders, in association with the Center for Hematological Research led by Arnault Tzanck, at the Saint Antoine Hospital in Paris. In 1938 Editorial Hachette in Argentina published his handbook on blood, *La Sangre*. He displayed his commitment to the defeated ideals of the Spanish Republic in his decisive contribution to organizing the first two meetings of the Union of Spanish University Professors Abroad, in Paris (1939) and in Cuba (1944). The German invasion of France forced him to escape again, and after a long and painful process during which the Rockefeller Foundation refused to help him enter the United States, he settled in Cuba in 1942. He again had to produce new qualifications to be able to work as a physician. Friends obtained a position for him as researcher at the Medical Hydrologic Institute for a couple of years. This difficult situation probably spurred his compulsive publication activity in the general press in his final year there (articles that were later compiled as books) and the updating of materials from previous books. He published two new handbooks on hematology (1943, 1945), with an updated selection of readings, and he died while finishing a *Treatise on the Pathological Physiology of Blood.*

Pittaluga had tried to return to Spain under cover of the 1953 law that allowed Republicans not subject to criminal prosecution to rejoin Spanish civil life. But although he was officially reappointed to his chair at the University of Madrid in 1955, he died before he could make his last dream come true.

Bibliography

Primary: 1903. *Investigaciones y estudios sobre el paludismo en España. Études et recherches sur le paludisme en Espagne (1901–1903)* (Barcelona); 1905. *Estudios acerca de los dípteros y de los parásitos que transmiten al hombre y a los animales domésticos* (Madrid); 1912. *La enfermedad del sueño (Tripanosomiasis humana) en la Colonia española del Golfo de Guinea* (Madrid); 1934. *Las enfermedades del sistema retículo-endotelial* (Madrid); 1945. *Diagnóstico y tratamiento de las hemodistrofias* (Havana).

Secondary: Rodríguez Ocaña, Esteban, Rosa Ballester, Enrique Perdiguero, Rosa María Medina, and Jorge Molero, 2003. *La acción médico-social contra el paludismo en la España metropolitana y colonial del siglo XX* (Madrid); Barona, Josep Lluis, 2001. 'El tortuoso camino hacia el exilio de Gustavo Pittaluga' in Mancebo, María Fernanda, Marc Baldó, and Cecilio Alonso, eds., *L'exili cultural de 1939. Seixanta anys després* (Valencia) pp. 425–434; Giral, Francisco, 1994. *Ciencia española en el exilio (1939–1989): el exilio de los científicos españoles* (Barcelona); Martín Gómez, Silvestre, 1988. *Vida y obra de D. Gustavo Pittaluga Fattorini* (Madrid).

Esteban Rodríguez-Ocaña

PLATO (b. Athens, Greece, 427 BCE; d. Athens, 348/347 BCE), *philosophy, mathematics, astronomy, medicine.*

Life

Plato began his philosophical work as a regular member of the circle of Socrates. The son of Ariston and Perictione, he was a man of high social standing, descended from a line that related him perhaps to Solon, and certainly to reactionary extremists such as his uncle Critias, one of the leaders of the short-lived oligarchic regime of the Thirty Tyrants (404 BCE). These connections are sometimes brought to bear on Plato's criticism of democracy and on his philo-Spartan ideals in politics, but such a view is oversimplistic. In 404 BCE Plato, just like his teacher, refused to collaborate with the oligarchy at home—despite his family ties. Yet in 399 BCE, he watched the restored democracy try Socrates for impiety and condemn him to death. Plato's political views and his shocking pessimism about democracy are more credibly attributed to the disturbed period through which he lived, rather than to his social background.

At Socrates' death, many of his followers fled Athens. Plato withdrew to Megara, where an offshoot of the Socratic circle, led by Euclid, set up the foundations of Megarian logic. He probably completed his military service in campaigns at Tanagra and Corinth, then embarked on his first visit to Syracuse. There he may have met the tyrant's physician, Philistion of Locri, and established contacts with Archytas of Tarentum and the circle of Pythagoreans. Plato's two subsequent returns to Sicily were made infamous by his role in the aborted rebellion and coup organized by the tyrant's brother-in-law, Dion, on whom Plato had a strong influence. After returning to Athens, some time around 380 BCE, Plato founded the Academy, which became a great center for the exploration of philosophy, as well as mathematics, astronomy, and scientific ideas in general. Plato's circle of friends, collaborators, and pupils included Theodore of Cyrene, Archytas of Tarentum, Eudoxus of Cnidus, Theaetetus, and Menaechmus. After his death the Academy was headed by Speusippus, the son of Plato's sister, Potone.

Although Plato is one of the greatest names of the Western tradition and his works have for the most part survived, both his personal profile and his philosophical views are shrouded in mystery. The biographical tradition, especially regarding Plato's relationship with Socrates, is extremely insecure—fact is irremediably contaminated with fiction from fanatics and detractors alike. Scraps of information come from Plato's own works, where members of his family, such as his brothers Adeimantus and Glaucon, are featured among the characters. One valuable source is formed by the seven letters attributed to Plato, but these must be used with extreme care. Most (if not all) are spurious, although they were written by someone with inside knowledge.

Works

Plato's views cannot be recovered with certainty because he chose to write dialogues, a literary form shared with other members of Socrates' circle. The dialogue form allowed him never to have to speak *in propria persona.* He could develop the views of various interlocutors (of which Socrates was the main one) in an unsystematic way, shifting perspectives according to characters and topics. These dialogue conventions, together with some remarks (especially in the *Phaedrus* and *Republic*) that seem to devalue written records at the expense of living dialogue and debate, and a few anecdotes in the biographical tradition have given rise to the controversial but influential belief that there was an 'unwritten doctrine' that Plato developed orally in his teaching at the Academy. Supposedly it went far beyond what we can read now in the surviving dialogues, surpassing them in importance.

The chronology of Plato's works involves the problem of development in his thought and is something of a minefield. Neither content nor form (as revealed, in particular, by stylometric analysis) has yielded conclusive results for a strict chronology. One of the difficulties comes from the fact that Plato was in the habit of returning to the same work and (re)writing it over a long period of time, probably involving others in the work. The dialogues divide roughly into three large groups: early (Socratic) (e.g., *Charmides, The Apology, Crito*), middle (*Meno, Phaedo, Symposium, Republic*), and late (*Theaetetus, Parmenides, The Sophist, The Statesman, Philebus, Timaeus, Critias, The Laws*).

The early dialogues depicted Socrates in conversation, pursuing the 'true definition' of some ethical notion such as courage or friendship through questions of the 'what–is–X?' type and always ending in uncertainty and impasse (*aporia*). From the middle period onward, Plato distanced himself from Socrates and developed a positive metaphysics of Forms. These were abstract entities, corresponding to predications such as 'equal' or 'just', which Plato posited as having separate existence and absolute reality (in contrast to the physical objects they were realized in) and as being the only source of knowledge, including perceptual knowledge. According to Aristotle, Plato's theory of Forms was born mainly in response to the extreme relativism of Cratylus the Heraclitean, who conceived that everything, including personal identity, was in a state of permanent flux. The late dialogues were predominantly concerned with epistemological problems such as the possibility of true knowledge and certainty, which deepened the old themes: the difference between knowledge and opinion; knowledge as knowledge of Forms; and the Good as the ultimate source of the Forms' truth, intelligibility, and existence. At this stage, Plato was aware of great difficulties within his metaphysics of Forms (typically, how do separate Forms 'participate in', or relate to, each other?), and (arguably) there were signs of revisionism. Plato's entire philosophy was permeated by old ethical and political questions inherited from Socrates, such as the relation between pleasure and excellence, or 'virtue' [*arête*], or the nature of justice and other excellences—which prompted a famous analogy between the state and the individual soul.

Science and Medicine

Plato's attitude toward science was deeply influenced by his metaphysics. His theory of Forms not only assumed the reality of universals and abstract standards, but also made them objects of knowledge over and above the sensibles. Mathematical objects lay halfway between Forms and sensibles, so mathematics had a privileged status for Plato. The *Republic* offered a scheme in which all sciences were subordinated to dialectics (the study of 'what is good'), and it proposed an ideal program of education leading from geometry, mathematics, and astronomy to the acquisition of that supreme science. Plato was also interested in natural phenomena, and his idealism did not rule out the possibility of an empirical science. The extent to which Plato can be seen as an empiricist remains debatable, however.

Plato had a sound knowledge of and interest in contemporary medicine. Throughout his dialogues he employed

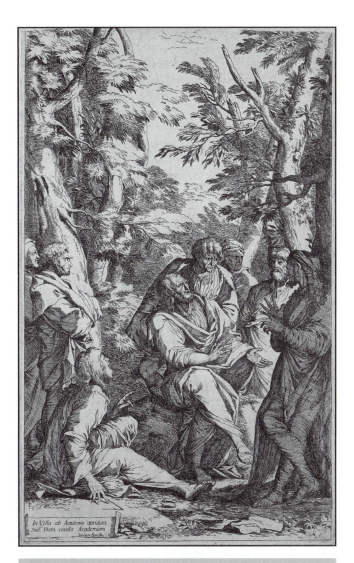

Plato teaching students at his Academy. Engraving after Salvatore Rosa, *c.* 1650. Iconographic Collection, Wellcome Library, London.

medical language and displayed great familiarity with Hippocratic and other medical theories. He put them to various uses, especially in ethics, combining the sources in ingenious ways and extracting original conclusions for his own, nonmedical, purposes. Most notably, he developed in the *Timaeus* a theory of diseases that dominated the medieval West for many centuries.

The reason why medicine received so much attention in Plato's work can be gleaned from a famous passage in the *Phaedrus*. He saw in medicine a discipline that, although empirical by nature, was not confined to empirical method but also employed 'true reason'. According to Plato, medicine applied the logical method of division to states of affairs in the body, taking the whole (body?) as its starting point. In other words, it considered relations between the whole body and its parts (although scholars are not agreed about the meaning of 'whole'). This capacity to master an empirical domain through reason was evinced in prognosis, and because of it, medicine worked for Plato as a symbol of the most desirable virtues an 'art' [techne] could possess—the powers of prediction and control. Medicine offered a paradigm of proper procedure to all other professions, from rhetoric to statesmanship, and Hippocrates emerged as the champion of that universally valid procedure.

The main advantage of Plato's position was that it allowed him to use medicine in support of the thesis that values like 'the Good' in subjective domains such as ethics, psychology, and politics had an objective reality, being the kinds of thing in which one acquired an expertise equivalent to that of the doctor. Hence the predilection, in Plato, for language that featured the doctor as a paradigm for the statesman and where notions such as health, disease, therapy, drugs, and the like were transferred from body to soul, and to state. More generally, the conceptual status of medicine as construed by Plato explained both his attraction to it as a permanent source of inspiration and the extensive use of Hippocratic material throughout his work.

Plato's use of medical material was extremely original and creative. In *Laws* i–ii, for instance, he explored a 'homoeopathic' conception of pharmaceutical action advocated by some Hippocratics and sought to apply it to ethics and psychology. He thereby arrived at the notion that one could be treated against dangerous emotions, desires, or tendencies through controlled exposure to them. The process he described is one of self-discovery, exposure, and cure—and the drug envisaged for it was wine. This theory had an impact on Aristotle, whose celebrated views on the cathartic function of tragedy were inspired by Plato's comments on the putative function of wine and symposia in the *Laws*.

In various dialogues, Plato developed enormously influential views (although not systematic and not always consistent with each other) on the nature of soul and its relation to the body. What is widely known as the 'tripartition of soul' was the Platonic theory that soul consisted of three 'parts' (*mere*) or 'powers', 'functions', 'capacities' (*dynameis*), each one having its own seat in a particular part of the body. The rational soul (*logistikon*) resided in the head or brain, the passionate soul (*thymooeides*) in the heart, and the desiderative soul (*epithymetikon*) in the liver.

Plato was chiefly interested in the analysis of psychological processes (thinking, desire, and emotions such as anger), but unlike Aristotle he paid less attention to their biological aspects. Nevertheless, his *Timaeus* contained incipient accounts of respiration, nutrition, and digestion, and functional descriptions of various bodily organs, including the vessels. Above all, Plato was the first to assert that the system of blood vessels originated in the heart. All his predecessors, including those who attached functions to the heart, thought that the blood vessels originated in the brain. Plato instead described the heart as the fountain and 'knot of the veins'. The meaning of that rather poetic phrase is disputed; it certainly

does not imply that Plato saw the heart as initiating the movement of blood, and he ignored the heart's structure and chambers. But it is remarkable that, while attributing a leading role to the brain and regarding the head as the most divine part of man—the shelter of reason and of the immortal part of the soul—Plato also described the heart as the origin of the vascular system, an idea with rich consequences for Aristotle.

Plato gave a fairly clear account of the relative position of the lungs and of their connection to the heart through the blood vessels. Perhaps inspired by Empedocles, he conceived of respiration as consisting of two simultaneous and circular movements of air—through the lungs and through the skin. In his view, these exchanges were governed by the mechanics of air moving in a continuum, with no contribution from internal organs such as the thorax, muscles, and so on. Expiration through the lungs had a double and contradictory role. On the one hand it cooled the heat of the heart, moderating passions such as anger, fear, or excitement; on the other hand it fed the heat or fire within—a conception also encountered in some Hippocratic treatises (*Fleshes, Nature of the Child*). This contradiction is typical of ancient attempts to understand the function of air in the organism, in the absence of any notion about oxygen and combustion.

In physiology, Plato presented a nebulous image of all bodily functions, which he regarded as being clustered together. Blood and *pneuma* traveled through the same channels and irrigated the body, ensuring the distribution of nutritious and sensory material simultaneously with respiration. This primitive scheme was common to all early Greek thinkers, for whom functions were not yet properly distinguished because the digestive tract was the only tract known to them.

At the basis of Plato's physiology, as presented in the *Timaeus*, were the four elements—earth, water, air, fire—each one endowed with a specific 'power' and shaped by various geometrical figures. The first constituent in the generation of the body was marrow: the spherical marrow of the brain, containing the divine and immortal soul, and the elongated marrow containing the mortal parts. The rest of the body was framed around the marrow, beginning with bone, which was made from earth kneaded and soaked in marrow. Flesh was made from water, fire, earth, and a saline ferment; sinews, from bone and unfermented flesh; and so on.

Plato's nosology and medical etiology in the *Timaeus* were influenced by Philistion, in that he attached less importance to the humors. Instead, Philistion accorded greater causal relevance to air and breathing on the one hand, and to the elements and their balance on the other. However, Plato made some room for the humors in his etiology and developed an interesting theory about the humoral generation of disease from a process of reversal, which led to the decomposition of tissue. His 'diseases of decomposition' probably constituted an original category.

Bibliography

Primary: 1900–1907. Burnet, John, ed., *Platonis Opera* vols. I–V (Oxford) [new edition in progress, 1995–]; 1937. (Cornford, F., trans. and commentary). *Plato's Cosmology. The Timaeus of Plato* (London); 1953. Jowett, B., ed. and trans. *The Dialogues of Plato* vols. I–III (Oxford).

Secondary: Nutton, V., 2004. *Ancient Medicine* (London) pp. 115–118; Lloyd, G. E. R., 2003. *In the Grip of Disease. Studies in the Greek Imagination* (Oxford); Kraut, R., ed., 1992. *The Cambridge Companion to Plato* (Cambridge); Owen, G. E. L., 1986. *Logic, Science and Dialectic. Collected Papers in Greek Philosophy* (Ithaca, NY); Vlastos, G., 1981. *Platonic Studies* (Princeton); Vlastos, G., ed., 1970–71. *Plato. A Collection of Critical Essays* vol. I (*Metaphysics and Epistemology*), vol. II (*Ethics, Politics and Philosophy of Art and Religion*) (New York); Riginois, A., 1976. *Platonica. The Anecdotes Concerning the Life and Writings of Plato* (Leiden); Lloyd, G. E. R., 1968. 'Plato as a Natural Scientist.' *Journal of Hellenic Studies* 88: 68–92.

Manuela Tecusan

PLATTER, FELIX (b. Basel, Switzerland, October 1536; d. Basel, 28 July 1614), *medicine, anatomy.*

Platter was the son of Thomas Platter, then school rector in Basel, and his wife Anna. He enjoyed an excellent education and also became a very accomplished lute player, a skill for which he was to be known throughout his life. In 1551 he began to attend medical lectures at Basel University. A year later he moved to Montpellier, where he spent the next four and a half years studying medicine. The methodological and practical approach that Platter later developed was profoundly shaped by the kind of medicine he encountered at Montpellier University, which was then a leading center of Hippocratic medicine. Students were offered extensive opportunities to acquire practical experience and surgical skills, and they were able to attend anatomical dissections at fairly regular intervals. Platter studied in particular with Saporta, Rondelet, and Du Chastel, who also took him along on his patient rounds. Platter left Montpellier in 1556 as a graduate and returned to Basel, where he received his doctoral degree in 1557. As had been agreed years before, he then married Margaretha Jeckelmann, the daughter of a well-known barber-surgeon in Basel. For several years the couple did not have a household of their own, and lived with Felix's father. They had no children.

Platter began to practice as a physician. Having overcome the initial difficulties that awaited any young, new physician who tried to establish a practice of his own at that time, Platter was quickly able to make a name for himself among the more affluent, upper-class patients. He began to teach at Basel University, and in 1570 he became its rector. In 1571 he succeeded his first medical teacher, Johannes Huber, as a town physician and professor of medicine. Platter held both positions until his death in 1614. As

a town physician he was, among other things, responsible for the organization of public measures against the plague and was frequently consulted as a medical expert in forensic matters. As a professor, Platter entertained a close network of epistolary correspondents. Thanks to his published works and his very accommodating behavior toward students from other universities, he contributed decisively to the Basel medical faculty's rapid growth of prestige and popularity among medical students and the scientific community in late-sixteenth-century Europe.

Platter's contemporary fame as a physician and scientist rested primarily on his knowledge and skills as an anatomist. He had witnessed various autopsies at Montpellier, and in Basel he personally dissected numerous corpses, in public demonstrations as well as privately. He published the results of that anatomical work in his first major treatise, *De corporis humani structura et usu libri III* (1583). The title alludes to Andreas Vesalius's *De humani corporis fabrica* of 1543, and Platter became one of the most influential propagators of Vesalian anatomy. In some instances, however, he also produced new findings of his own. Among them we find the first known illustration of the specific characteristics of the female skeleton as compared to that of the male: distinguishing differences in the cranial sutures, the ossification of the rib cage, the shape of the pelvis, and the mobility of the coccyx. The book was a milestone in the history of Western medical ideas about the natural, bodily foundations of sexual difference. It went through several editions and was in turn, together with Vesalius's work, the major source for one of the most successful anatomical treatises of the early seventeenth century—the *Theatrum anatomicum*, which Platter's younger colleague in Basel, Caspar Bauhin, published in 1605. Platter's account of female genital anatomy and menstrual physiology found a prominent place in Israel Spachius's 1597 edition of the *Gynaecia*, the major gynecological compendium of the time.

Platter's sustained interest in anatomy was not driven only by his scientific curiosity and his desire to demonstrate the miracles of divine creation in its most perfect specimen, the human body. He also considered detailed anatomical knowledge indispensable for the practical work of a physician, because it provided the empirical basis for a thorough understanding of what happened deep inside the body in different types of disease. Platter strove for a systematic correlation of signs and symptoms in the living patient with the changes that could be observed postmortem in the corpse, which made him one of the founding fathers of a scientific pathological anatomy.

Platter's works on practical medicine, his 1597 book on fevers, and above all, his *Praxeos, seu de cognoscendis, praedicendis, praecavendis, curandisque affectibus homini incommodantibus tractatus* were, in hindsight, not nearly as innovative. Published between 1602 and 1608, the three volumes of the *Practice* were devoted to damaged functions—to pain and to diseases (*vitia*) of the body and its excretions. They offered a solid and systematic account of the whole of medicine, however, and became one of the most successful medical textbooks of the period. New editions continued to appear until the eighteenth century. Platter's textbook of practical medicine was complemented in 1614 by his famous *Observationes medicae*, a collection of some 700 case reports based on notes that Platter had taken over the many years of his work as a practical physician. The *Observations* ranks among the best and most detailed examples of this popular genre of the sixteenth and seventeenth centuries, offering very lively, personal, and illuminating glimpses of everyday medical practice. Some of the reports were supplemented by a summary of the postmortem findings in autopsy, in an attempt to arrive at a truly causal account of different disease processes. His extensive and detailed accounts of various 'psychiatric' anomalies, altered states of consciousness, and sensory disturbances have rightly attracted the attention and admiration of generations of psychiatrists. Platter also made a point of providing all the necessary information about the kind and quantity of the various ingredients used in his treatments, thus countering the widespread tendency to keep secret the composition of specific remedies that, supposedly, were unusually effective.

Platter's nephew, Thomas Platter the younger, published the *Quaestionum medicarum paradoxarum et endoxarum centuria posthuma* in 1625, but the degree to which this work was a fruit of Platter's own pen remains somewhat dubious. Further works by the elder Platter have come down to us in manuscript and are extant in modern editions only. Among them is a very detailed account of an outbreak of the plague in Basel, with a street-by-street and house-by-house report of the number and names of those who had died—one of the earliest examples of epidemiological statistics. Platter had no doubts that the plague was spread by corrupt air, as well as by contagion.

Platter's autobiography ranks among the most personal and vivid ego-documents of the early modern period. It describes his upbringing, medical training, and practice, as well as many aspects of ordinary life such as wedding preparations and matrimonial relationships.

Bibliography

Primary: 1583. *De corporis humani structura et usu libri III* (Basel); 1597. *De febribus libri III* (Frankfurt); 1602–08. *Praxeos seu de cognoscendis, praedicendis, praecavendis curandisque affectibus homini incommodantibus tractatus,* 5 books, 3 vols. (Basel); 1614. *Observationum in hominis affectibus plerisque corpore et animo. . . incommodantibus libri tres* (Basel); 1625. (Platter, Thomas, ed.) *Quaestionum medicarum paradoxarum & endoxarum, iuxta partes medicinae dispositarum centuria posthuma* (Basel); 1976. (Lötscher, Valentin, ed.) *Tagebuch (Lebensbeschreibung) 1536–1567* (Basel and Stuttgart); 1987. (Lötscher, Valentin, ed.) *Beschreibung der Stadt Basel 1610 und Pestbericht 1610/11* (Basel and Stuttgart).

Secondary: Huber, Katharina, 2003. *Felix Platters 'Observationes'. Studien zum frühneuzeitlichen Gesundheitswesen in Basel* (Basel); Hochlenert, Dieter, 1996. 'Das 'Tagebuch' des Felix Platter. Die Autobiographie eines Arztes und Humanisten' (Dissertation, University of Tübingen); Lötscher, Valentin, 1975. *Felix Platter und seine Familie* (Basel); Karcher, Johannes, 1949. *Felix Platter. Lebensbild des Basler Stadtarztes* (Basel).

Michael Stolberg

PLETNEV, DMITRII DMITRIEVICH (b. Bobrik-Moskovskii, Khar'kov *guberniia* [province], Russia, 25 November [7 December] 1871; d. Orel, Russia, 11 September 1941), *therapy, cardiology.*

Pletnev was born into a noble family. His father was a landowner and distinguished justice of the peace in Lebedinskii *uezd* (district), Khar'kov *guberniia* (province). He graduated from the First Khar'kov gymnasium in 1890, then studied at the medical faculties of Khar'kov (1890–92) and Moscow (1892–95) universities. In 1895–96 he worked at the University of Vienna, and from 1896 he was a house surgeon in the therapeutic department of the Catherine Hospital in Moscow. In 1906 he defended his dissertation, carrying out classic research into heart arrhythmia, and then was sent abroad by Moscow University in preparation for the rank of professor. He interned on that basis at the clinic of F. Kraus in Germany, and from 1907 he was a sessional lecturer in the department of individual pathology and therapy.

In 1911, as a mark of protest against the infringement of the rights of universities by L. A. Kasso, the Russian Minister of Education, Pletnev and a group of professors and teachers left the university and moved to the Geneva Medical Institute, where he was elected professor in the department of the introductory therapeutic clinic.

In 1917 he returned to Moscow University, where he headed the departments of faculty (until 1924) and hospital therapy (1924–29). Beginning in 1928 he headed the therapeutic clinic of the Moscow Region Clinical Institute. In 1932 the jubilee of Pletnev's professional activities was broadly celebrated, and the building in which his clinic was located was named for him. Here in 1930 Pletnev organized and headed the second department of therapy at the Central Institute for the Refinement of Doctors. Simultaneously, from 1929 he was consultant for the First Communist (now the Main) Hospital for the Armed Forces, and from 1932 he occupied the post of director of the Institute of Functional Diagnostics and Experimental Therapy.

In 1929 Pletnev was dismissed from Moscow University for nonappearance at the commission for the reelection of instructors. It was characteristic of his personality to present himself as a leading scientist, sharp-tongued and often clashing with colleagues and superiors. In June 1937 he was arrested after articles inspired by the secret police about his sadistic violence with patients appeared in the newspaper *Pravda*, and he received a two-year conditional sentence. In the same year he was again arrested and accused of collaboration in the killing of the writer M. Gor'kii and party leader V. V. Kuibyshev. In the 1938 trial over the so-called Right Trotskyist bloc of N. I. Bukharin and A. I. Rykov affair, Pletnev was sentenced to twenty-five years in prison. In the course of the following decades, evidence and rumors repeatedly appeared in the press from eyewitnesses claiming to have met him in places of confinement in the districts of Vorkuta, Magadan, and elsewhere.

After the declassification of part of the archives in the magazine *Izvestiia TsK KPSS* (1990, no. 11, pp. 124–131), material was published explaining the secret of Pletnev's death. On 11 September 1941, as German forces approached the Orel prison, he was shot along with other prisoners (including the prominent political activists M. A. Spiridonova and Kh. G. Rakovskii).

Pletnev's role as one of the founders of the clinic for internal illnesses in the USSR is generally recognized. His approach to the patient was distinguished by the high professionalism of a many-sided doctor. During his lifetime his mastery of the diagnosis of coronary thrombosis was well-known, as was his talent as a lecturer—always presented in auditoriums overflowing with doctors. The circle of his interests encompassed problems of general pathology, clinical medicine, and the history of medicine. Even before the advent of ECG research he formulated criteria for the differential diagnosis of heart attacks, which contributed to the diagnosis of heart aneurisms, and independently from R. Lersh he developed the theory of extracardiac pathogenesis of attacks of angina pectoris. Pletnev was one of the pioneers of x-ray study and the psychosomatic approach to internal illness in the USSR.

Pletnev's main work, *Bolezni serdtsa* [Illnesses of the Heart] (1936), along with G. F. Lang's manual titled *Bolezni sistemy krovoobrashcheniia* [Illnesses of the System of Blood Circulation] (1938), should be seen as the product of a great phase of research by Soviet therapists into the problems of the physiology and pathology of the heart. Pletnev's *Osnovi terapii khronicheskoi nedostatochnosti serdtsa* [The Bases of Therapy for Deficiencies of the Heart] (1932) had a widely applicable character. He wrote classic monographs on clinics for typhus (1922) and acquired cardiovascular syphilis (1928). His book *Russkie terapevticheskie shkoly* [Russian Therapeutic Schools] (1923)—studies in the history of ideas, with examples of prominent medical activists—has not lost its significance. He was also the editor of the journal *Klinicheskaia meditsina* and many manuals for doctors discussing, for example, the use of x-rays, infectious illnesses, and other subjects.

Bibliography

Primary: Tsentral'nyi istoricheskii arkhiv g. Moskvy [The Central Historical Archive of the City of Moscow]. F. 418, op. 65, d. 510, l. 24, 32, 58, 62, 86–98, 124; op. 306, d. 601, l. 13; op. 403, d. 16, l. 12; op. 413, d. 62, l. 1–5, 6; op. 413, d. 101, l. 1–7 (Moscow).

Secondary: Topolianskii, V. D., 1993. 'Dmitrii Dmitrievich Pletnev i psikhosomatika' ['Dmitrii Dmitrievich Pletnev and Psychosomatics']. *Istoricheskii vestnik Moskovskoi meditsinskoi akademii imeni I.M. Sechenova* II: 66–77; Borodulin, V. I., and V. D. Topolianskii, 1989. 'Dmitrii Dmitrievich Pletnev'. *Voprosy istorii* 9: 36–54; Borodulin, V. I., 1988. *Ocherki istorii otechestvennoi kardiologii* [Studies of the History of Russian Cardiology] (Moscow).

Mikhail Poddubnyi

PLINY THE ELDER (b. Novum Comum, Cisalpine Gaul [now Como, Italy], 23/24; d. Stabiae, near Pompeii, Italy, 24 August 79), *botany, history of medicine, medicine, natural science, pharmacology.*

Gaius Plinius Secundus was born into the municipal ruling class and took his place as a member of the Equestrian Order, the second tier in Roman society. Pliny's parents gave him a good education, and in keeping with the Augustan ideals of the Equestrian Order, he served as a military officer, holding several posts in Germany. In 47 he took part in a campaign under the governor of Upper Germany, Domitius Corbulo. He served with Titus, son of Vespasian (Pliny would dedicate his *Natural History* to him), in another post. Returning to civilian life, Pliny divided his time between Rome, where he was occasionally an advocate in the courts, and his estates. During that time, he laid the foundations of his *Natural History* (*Historia Naturalis*).

Pliny seems to have worked quietly during the reign of Nero. It was only with the establishment of the Flavian dynasty under Vespasian that he was able to enjoy the patronage of the emperor's elder son, Titus. He held several equestrian administrative posts, including procurator of Hispania Tarraconensis and prefect of the fleet at Misenum—the office he held at the time of his death. Pliny was also an official 'friend of the Emperor' and a member of the imperial council. Although he was busy in imperial service, Pliny nevertheless found time to compose a (lost) *History of Rome* and to complete the *Natural History*. The questing spirit of the author is illustrated by the manner of his death. Pliny the Younger, his nephew and adopted son, states that his uncle put to sea in command of a naval detachment from Misenum on 24 August 79. He was drawn both by duty and by curiosity concerning a strange cloud visible in the mountains near Pompeii. After rescuing a friend from the sea, Pliny continued to sail inshore, taking copious notes. He landed at Stabiae, but the eruption of Vesuvius eventually made retreat impossible and he succumbed, either to the effects of the gas cloud or from volcanic ash—the most famous victim of the cataclysm.

Pliny, like Cornelius Celsus, was an encyclopedist—an educated layman. But Pliny's *Natural History* was more wide-ranging and uncritical than Celsus's *On Medicine*, and in its listing of the products of the natural world, Pliny's work sought to encompass all that was known (as well as previously unknown) within and beyond the boundaries of the Empire. The Plinian pharmacopoeia could therefore draw from a great number of sources. According to Pliny, the *Pax Romana* made such an undertaking possible, enabling him and others similarly inclined to examine people and nations, mountains and plants. Pliny's vision of nature was firmly ethnocentric. Unlike Aristotle, he did not engage in the study of the natural world for its own sake, but rather sought out its secrets to benefit man. From those utilitarian concerns arose the thirty-seven books that compose the *Natural History*.

Twelve books (XX to XXXII) concerned medicine, including the use of animal and plant products in the treatment of disease and what Pliny regarded as magical and superstitious practices derived from the East. Books XX–XXVII documented the uses of plants and plant products for the treatment of—among other conditions—epilepsy, malaria, tuberculosis (phthisis), eye diseases (including cataract), gastrointestinal afflictions, and diseases of the skin. In Book XXV Pliny discussed plants that were specifically used for medicinal purposes, noting that such knowledge was gained by the effort of 'the ancients', principally Roman, whose diligence and industry contrasted favorably with most of those in Pliny's time. Pliny's predecessors in this field included Cato the Elder and Gaius Valgius (who left Augustus an unfinished work on plant medicines). He also discussed Mithridates of Pontus, whom he regarded, not without reason, as an expert on plant toxicology (although Pliny condemned *theriac*, the Mithridatic antidote composed of fifty-four ingredients, as reflecting the desire for polypharmaceutical treatment as well as the boastful nature of the physicians who prepared and endorsed it). After Mithridates' defeat, his library was taken to Rome and the medical works translated by Pompey's freedman, the grammarian Lenaeus.

Pliny also mentioned Greek writers, such as Crateuas, Dionysius, and Metrodorus, on the subject of plant medicines. Although he did not cite him by name, Pliny probably drew on Dioscorides as well. But their work is nevertheless viewed unfavorably compared to that of the 'greatest botanical authority of our time', Antonius Castor, whose garden Pliny himself visited. Castor was living proof of his own ministrations, having passed his hundredth year in excellent health. The lesson to be drawn was that Roman usage of medicinal plants was superior to that of the Greeks and those who used them in conjunction with spells, charms, and amulets—the Magi, or magicians, of Eastern origin. For Pliny, medicine was primarily *materia medica*, derived and cultivated from a bountiful nature that was known to Romans and used by Romans. Accordingly, in Book XXXI Pliny examined remedies derived from aquatic animals; the nature of various waters, both fresh and salty; medicinal bathing; and the use of salt, garum, and soda ash. Information on the medicinal uses of sea creatures concluded in Book XXXII.

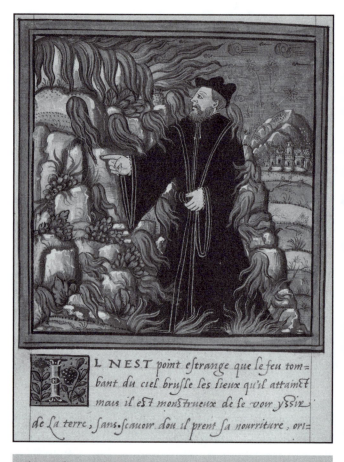

The prodigious death of Pliny, in which his body was reduced to ash by the flames of Vesuvius. Quarter-page miniature in gold and colors from Pierre Boaistuau, *Histoires prodigieuses*, 1560. Archives and Manuscripts, Wellcome Library, London.

Contemporary Greek medical practice in Rome found no favor in Pliny's eyes. In Book XXVI, he used the success of Asclepiades of Bithynia to draw a moral lesson. Whereas Hippocrates, Diocles of Carystus, Praxagoras, Chrysippus, Herophilus, and Erasistratus were praised for their knowledge of medical herbs, Asclepiades, by contrast, represented an age in which people had forgotten the injunctions of the ancient authorities. Asclepiades' fivefold treatment regimen—which Pliny described as fasting, occasional abstinence from wine, massage, walking, and carriage rides—was simple common sense to Pliny, yet people flocked to Asclepiades as though he were heaven-sent. But a significant part of Asclepiades' success, which Pliny acknowledged, derived from the fact that his treatments were pleasant. By contrast, much of ancient medicine insisted on emesis, purgation, venesection, and surgical procedures that caused great pain but had dubious effect, such as operating for peritonsillar abscess (quinsy), which Asclepiades expressly forbade, to Pliny's endorsement.

Pliny's attack on Asclepiades was unfair. But he condemned Asclepiades in particular, and Greek medicine generally, on the flimsy grounds that they had abandoned the use of medicinal plants and endorsed Eastern practices of superstition. Those practices were discussed in Book XXX, which examined the origins of magic among the Zoroastrians of Persia and its spread to Greece, as well as Pliny's description of their treatments for various diseases. One such treatment involved using puppies to relieve pain by transference. The animal was placed close to the afflicted part and took up the affliction. Examination of the dog's internal organs determined the source of the pain, and the remains were buried to ensure a cure.

Book XXVIII discussed medicines derived from animals (ranging from elephants to chameleons) and also from man, such as gladiator's blood drunk by epileptics (which could involve sucking on wounds inflicted in the arena), and consumption of the leg bone marrow and brains of infants. To Pliny, these cannibalistic practices were of Greek and Persian origin. He provided remedies using human urine, however, including men's urine for gout, a mixture of urine with the ash of burnt oyster shells to treat baby rash, and one's own urine to treat dog bite. There were also treatments based on menstrual fluid, women's milk (good for nausea, fevers, and toad bites), saliva from a fasting woman (for bloodshot eyes), and—from Pliny's own experience—a woman's breast-band tied around the head for the relief of headache.

Book XXIX continued the descriptions of animal products in healing (especially eye remedies), but its chief feature was a sustained and vitriolic attack on Greek medicine. According to Pliny, Greek medicine lay in darkness until the Peloponnesian War and was brought to the light by Hippocrates (although in an earlier chapter Pliny appeared to countenance medicine's origins in Egypt). But Hippocrates and the other ancient authorities were not presented favorably. Hippocrates was depicted as a plagiarist who copied accounts, inscribed on the walls, of the assistance patients believed they had received in the temple of Aesculapius on Cos. After the temple burned down, Hippocrates founded the clinical (*clinice*) branch of medicine. That opened the floodgates to profiteers, beginning with one of Hippocrates' pupils, Prodicus of Selymria, who devised treatment using ointment. Internecine disputes followed, with torrents of verbiage by Chrysippus, and the greed of his pupil Erasistratus, who received 100 talents for curing King Antiochus.

To Pliny, it was avarice above all else that condemned Greek doctors. Physicians, especially in imperial service, commanded figures of up to 600,000 sesterces. Crinas of Massilia combined medicine with astrology and was successful to the extent that his estate amounted to 10 million sesterces, and he spent a similar sum on rebuilding his native city. Thessalus was prominent during the reign of Nero, whose monument on the Appian Way was inscribed 'champion doctor', but for Pliny it was symptomatic of a corrupted (and corrupting) discipline. He saw medical practice in daily flux, and each Greek newcomer with the power of speech was able to attract a new clientele that could be slaughtered with impunity. After twenty-eight books recounting nature's bounty, which anyone could use, it seems that Pliny had finally lost patience with foreign—that is to say, Greek—medical practices and practitioners. The fear of a foreigner's power over a Roman is best seen in Pliny's account of the coming of surgery to Rome. Pliny, unlike Celsus, did not discuss surgery, and his reasons reinforced the Roman nature of Plinian medicine. According to Pliny, citing the historian Cassius Hemina writing two centuries earlier, Rome imported its medicine from Greece in the person of Archagathus (a name meaning 'good beginning'), who was from Laconia in the Peloponnese. Archagathus may have come at the behest of the Senate in 219 BCE. Initially well received, he was soon condemned because his surgical practices and the use of cautery had begun to merit the appellation 'executioner' (although those skills had probably helped him gain employment in the first place). Pliny also cited Cato the Elder's words to his son to beware of all things Greek—especially their physicians, who conspired to kill all foreigners and charged for it into the bargain. Pliny endorsed Cato's opinion by adding that only doctors, immune from legal retribution, could kill with impunity.

The sheer range of Pliny's medical and pharmacological writings—from the commonplace to the exotic, from recipes that impressed to those that repelled, from folk medicine to magico-religious treatments, all woven together with an agreeable prose style—ensured their popularity throughout late antiquity and the Middle Ages. Excerpts titled the *Medicine of Pliny* and the *Physic of Pliny* were produced, and their value would not be seriously questioned until the Renaissance. But whereas Celsus provided a more nuanced view of Greek medicine, Pliny, writing less than fifty years later, offered a caricature. He was willing to ignore the distinctions between Greek medical theories and practices, and he kept silent on the undoubted abuses of Roman medical practices. That approach reflected Pliny's desire not only to return to an idealized Roman world of the household and kitchen garden, governed by the virtues of self-reliance and the medical knowledge imparted by a beneficent *paterfamilias*, but also to place Greek medical knowledge, exemplified by his lists of diseases and their treatment derived from Greek sources, in stable Roman hands.

Bibliography

Primary: 1892–98, 1906–09. (Mayhoff, Carolus, ed.) *C. Plini Secundi Naturalis Historiæ libri XXXVII* (Leipzig) [Reprinted 1967–70 (Stuttgart)]; 1967–71. (Rackham, H., W. H. S. Jones, and D. E. Eicholz, eds.) *Pliny. Natural History*, 10 vols. (London).

Secondary: Murphy, Trevor, 2004. *Pliny the Elder's* Natural History. *The Empire in the Encyclopedia* (Oxford); French, Roger, 1994. *Ancient Natural History: Histories of Nature* (London and New York); Beagon, Mary, 1992. *Roman Nature. The Thought of Pliny* the Elder (Oxford); French, Roger, and Frank Greenaway, eds., 1986. *Science in the Early Roman Empire: Pliny the Elder, His Sources and Influence* (London and Sydney); *DSB*.

Julius Rocca

PODALIRIUS   (see under MACHAON).

POKROVSKAIA, MARIIA   (b. Province in Penza, Russia, 1852; d. ?, 1921?), *public health, hygiene.*

Pokrovskaia, a graduate of the St Petersburg Women's Medical Courses in 1881, practiced medicine in St Petersburg and in several *zemstvo* (elective institutions of local self-government) positions. In addition, she edited and published a journal, *Zhenskii Vestnik* (1901–06), and published numerous articles on medical issues. She worked as a teacher at a girls' school until she enrolled in the medical courses in 1876. After working as a *zemstvo* doctor for several years, she returned to St Petersburg to work as a *Duma* (city government institution) physician. Pokrovskaia wrote numerous articles on medicine, hygiene, public health, health care for women, and child care. She published them in medical journals such as *Vrach* and *Russkaia Meditsina*; in the so-called 'thick journals' such as *Vestnik Evropy* and *Russkaia Mysl'*; and in her own journal, *Zhenskii Vestnik*. As editor of *Zhenskii Vestnik* she wrote frequent editorials about the necessity of better education for women, universal suffrage, and the importance of improved health care for the poor.

Pokrovskaia's work in public health centered on hygiene and individual health. In one of her earliest articles she explored the relationship between smoke in peasant huts and the incidence of cataracts. Her research on this issue was inconclusive. Later, she studied the living conditions of urban workers, discussing overcrowding, lack of basic sanitation, and poor ventilation. That article recommended funding for inexpensive housing to alleviate overcrowding, and also advocated hygiene education in schools and communities. Pokrovskaia wrote a fictional book, *How I Was a City Doctor for the Poor*, which has generally been considered a thinly veiled autobiography. The story describes the living conditions of the urban poor, their lack of access to health care, and their unique health problems.

Pokrovskaia became quite well-known for her work on prostitution. At a time when society expected chastity in women, Pokrovskaia advocated chastity for both sexes. In 'On the Cultivation of Chastity' she wrote, 'We find ourselves hearing the opinion more and more often that men, just as women, must be equally pure before marriage'. Pokrovskaia urged mothers to teach their sons to respect women and abstain from sex, saying, 'It should be particularly valuable to mothers to develop in their sons a respect for people, for women'. She saw that approach as the only way to end the prostitution problem.

Pokrovskaia also believed there was a connection between prostitution and alcoholism. Because the brothels profited from alcohol sales, both clients and prostitutes were encouraged to drink, and she believed that the system of monitoring prostitutes led to alcoholism. She asked, 'can a system that creates outcasts in modern society, that reduces a woman to total degradation and drives her to alcoholism, that compels her to become debauched and get men drunk, really be protecting the nation's health?' ('Prostitution and Alcoholism', 1905).

Pokrovskaia attended and spoke at the Congress on the Struggle Against Trade in Women and worked with the Society for the Protection of Women.

Pokrovskaia, like many of her contemporaries, saw her medical training as a means to help the less fortunate in society. Her medical articles centered on issues such as the unhealthy living conditions of St Petersburg workers, treatment of tuberculosis, and health and sanitation. She used her journal, *Zhenskii Vestnik,* to advocate women's education, universal suffrage, and the importance of improved health care for the poor. In addition, she frequently participated in meetings of the Pirogov Society (a medical society concerned with public health and hygiene) and appeared at government hearings on issues such as prostitution, housing, and public health.

Bibliography

Primary: 1900. 'The Struggle with Prostitution' (St Petersburg); 1901. 'On the Cultivation of Chastity in Boys' in *For the Assistance of Mothers* No. 3. Partially translated in 2002, Bisha, Robin, Jehanne Gheith, et al., eds., *Russian Women 1698–1917: An Anthology of Sources* (Bloomington, IN); 1902. 'Women and Diet' (St Petersburg); 1905. 'Prostitution and Alcoholism'. *Journal of the Russian Society for the Protection of Public Health* 5–6 [Partially translated in Bisha et al., 2002.]

Secondary: DenBeste-Barnett, Michelle, 2002. 'Emerging Professionalism: Women Physicians in Late Imperial Russia'. *Review Journal of Philosophy and Social Science* 27(1–2): 275–294; Norton, Barbara, and Jehanne Gheith, eds., 2001. *An Improper Profession: Women, Gender and Journalism in Late Imperial Russia* (Durham, NC, and London); DenBeste-Barnett, Michelle, 1999. 'Publish or Perish: The Scientific Publication of Women Physicians in Late Imperial Russia'. *Dynamis* 19: 215–240; Clyman, Toby W., and Judith Vowles, eds., 1996. *Russia through Women's Eyes: Autobiographies from Tsarist Russia* (New Haven); Johanson, Christine, 1987. *Women's Struggle for Higher Education in Russia: 1855–1900* (Kingston, Ont.).

Michelle DenBeste and
Denise Best

POMPE VAN MEERDERVOORT, JOHANNES LIJDIUS CATHARINUS   (b. Bruges, Belgium, 5 May 1829; d. Brussels, Belgium, 3 October 1908), *military surgery, medical education.*

Pompe van Meerdervoort was born in Bruges, which was then under Dutch rule, the third son of Johan, a Dutch army officer, and his wife Johanna. In 1845 Pompe (as he was called in Japan) entered the Dutch National School of Army Medicine in Utrecht, graduating in 1849. In the same year, he started his service with the Dutch navy and worked on board ship until 1855. He was then asked by Willem J. C. Huyssen van Kattendijke (1816–66), an officer of the Dutch navy, to join his team for teaching modern naval science and technology in Japan.

Arriving in Nagasaki in 1856, Pompe started his teaching course the following year. He was greatly assisted by one of the students, Matsumoto Ryōjun (1832–1907), who was a junior court physician to the Shōgun and who would later become the Surgeon General of the Japanese army. Matsumoto's attendance signaled the Shogunate's recognition of the need to study Western medicine, and he helped Pompe attract more medical students who had been sent to Nagasaki by their domains. On numerous occasions, Matsumoto also helped negotiate with Japanese officers at Nagasaki and Edo to obtain various permissions, most notably to dissect human cadavers.

Pompe had to start from scratch. Many students had learned virtually nothing about basic sciences such as physics, chemistry, anatomy, and physiology. Their skill in the Dutch language lay in reading texts, not listening and speaking. Such initial difficulties were quickly overcome, however, and his teaching progressed smoothly. Permission to dissect an executed criminal was granted in 1859. Pompe's most crucial achievement was the establishment of a teaching hospital, the first of its kind in Japan. After lengthy negotiations, he finally convinced the Shogunate to build such a hospital (Nagasaki Yōjōsho), equipped with 124 beds and other facilities for medical education. Between its completion in 1861 and Pompe's departure the following year, the hospital treated about 930 patients (the cadavers of two of them were dissected at the school). To Pompe's surprise, the hospital's major clients were not the poor, but the wealthy—a pattern repeatedly observed in early hospitals in Japan. Apart from medical teaching, Pompe was remarkably active in the treatment of cholera. When cholera hit Nagasaki for the second time in 1858, he and his students treated patients in the city.

Pompe left Japan for the Netherlands in 1862. He retired from the navy's medical service and married Henriette Johanna Louise in 1864. In 1866 he settled in the Hague, where he opened a private medical practice and involved himself in the activities of the Dutch Red Cross. He continued to help the Japanese medical students in Europe when occasion arose.

Pompe's memoir of his activities and observations in Japan, published in two volumes in 1867–68, is a first-rate source for medical historians. He was not the first European doctor to teach medicine in Japan, nor is he the most famous. However, unlike his more famous predecessors such as von Siebold (1796–1866), who taught medicine privately and in an ad hoc manner, Pompe taught medicine as systematically and comprehensively as possible under the circumstances. Moreover, his teaching was an official duty commissioned by the government of Japan, signaling the close alliance between that country and Western medicine after the Meiji Revolution in 1868.

Bibliography

Primary: 1867–1868. *Vijf Jaren in Japan* [Five Years in Japan] (Leiden). [Abridged in Japanese translation as *Pompe Nihon Taizaiki*, trans. Numata Jirō and Arase Susumu (Kyoto), 1968. Abridged in English translation as *Doctor on Desima*, trans. and annotated Wittermans, Elizabeth P., and John Z. Bowers (Tokyo) 1970]; 1980. (Teizō, Ogawa, and Sakai Shizu, eds.) *Matsumoto Jun Jiden; Nagasyo Sensai Jiden* [Autobiographies of Matsumoto Jun and Nagayo Sensai] (Tokyo).

Secondary: Miyanaga, Takashi, 1985. *Pompe: NihoniIgaku no chichi* [Pompe: The Father of Japanese Medicine] (Tokyo).

Akihito Suzuki

PORTAL, ANTOINE (b. Gaillac, France, 5 January 1742; d. Paris, France, 23 July 1832), *medicine, anatomy, medical history.*

The eldest son of an apothecary, Portal spent his childhood in a town on the Tarn River, in an old wine-producing region of southwestern France. At eighteen, he went to Montpellier to study medicine and developed an interest in surgery. He devoted his doctoral thesis to dislocations and developed a new traction device for treating them. After defending the thesis in 1765, he left for Paris to continue his medical studies. He never received the Paris doctorate, which was ordinarily a prerequisite for practice in the capital. Through a family connection, however, he won appointments in 1766 as anatomy teacher to the young Dauphin (heir to the throne—the future Louis XVI) and in 1769 as physician to the Dauphin's brother, the Count of Provence. Such positions conferred the right to practice medicine in Paris. Portal remained close to the royal family, and in 1785 letters of nobility from Louis XVI made him a chevalier.

Portal opened a private anatomy amphitheater and worked energetically to win a socially prominent clientele for his medical practice. The first in a long series of official positions soon followed. In 1769 he joined the anatomy section of the Academy of Sciences and won appointment to the chair of medicine at the Collège de France, a royal establishment. At the College he taught anatomy, surgery, operative medicine, and pathological anatomy. In 1778 he was appointed to the chair of anatomy at the Jardin du Roy, the royal center for natural history. Despite his ties to the old court, Portal weathered the Revolution and the rule of Napoleon well, continuing his teaching at the Collège de France and at the Jardin du Roy, now called the Museum of Natural History. The radical revolution abolished the royal academies, but in 1795 a more moderate government created a National Institute of Sciences and Arts (later the Institut de France). Portal was among the initial members. With the restoration of the Bourbon monarchy, Portal returned to favor. He won appointment in 1815 as first medical consultant to Louis XVIII, the former Count of Provence. In 1818, at the age of eighty, he attained the long-coveted office of royal first physician, a position he retained under Louis's successor, Charles X, who made him a baron and commander of the Legion of Honor. Portal used his authority to bring about the creation of a Royal Academy of Medicine in 1820, thereby filling the void left by the abolition of the old Royal Society of Medicine in 1793. He was named honorary president of the Royal Academy for life.

Portal published extensively over his long career; a book on epilepsy appeared in 1827, when he was eighty-five. Other works included a practical surgical handbook (1768); a seven-volume history of surgery and anatomy since Noah's Flood, which mingled narrative with critical observations on surgical procedures; a work on pulmonary phthisis, which argued that the disease is not contagious; and a five-volume textbook on medical anatomy (1805). At the instigation of the government, he published 'instructions' for the general public on topics in public health, such as first aid for victims of drowning, asphyxia from mephitic vapors, and the bites of rabid animals. Portal produced no major innovations or discoveries, though he was among the first in France to correlate lesions observed in the organs postmortem with symptoms of disease in the living patient.

Portal's career illustrates the important role of the French royal court in shaping the medical elite under the Bourbon dynasty.

Bibliography

Primary: 1770–73. *Histoire de l'anatomie et de la chirurgie . . .* (Paris); 1792. *Observations sur la nature et sur le traitement de la phthisie pulmonaire* (Paris).

Secondary: Weisz, George, 1986. 'Constructing the Medical Elite in France: The Creation of the Royal Academy of Medicine 1814–20.' *Medical History* 30: 419–443; DSB.

Matthew Ramsey

POTT, PERCIVALL   (b. City of London, England, 6 January 1714; d. Hanover Square, London, England, 22 December 1788), *surgery.*

Pott, the only son of Percivall Pott (1681–1717), a notary and scrivener, and his wife, Elizabeth Symonds (d. 1745), was born in Threadneedle Street. Pott was educated at a private school at Darenth in Kent. In 1729 he was bound surgical apprentice to Edward Nourse, assistant surgeon at St Bartholomew's Hospital, for a premium of 200 guineas. Pott's duties included preparing dissections for demonstration in Nourse's lectures on anatomy and surgery. Even as an apprentice Pott gained a reputation for

surgical skill and, obviously, collegiality. On 7 September 1736, because of attendance at a surgical case, he was unable to present himself to the court of examiners of the Barber-Surgeons' Company. Nonetheless he received the freedom of the company and was granted the grand diploma, usually acquired with difficulty. He took the livery of the company in 1739. In the same year that the Company of Surgeons was formed (1745) Pott was appointed assistant surgeon at St Bartholomew's Hospital and in 1749, full surgeon. In 1753 Pott and William Hunter (1718–83) were elected the first lecturers in anatomy to the new company. He became a member of the court of examiners (1763) and master of the company (1765). Pott married Sarah Cruttenden (1746) and they had five sons and four daughters.

In 1756 Pott was thrown from his horse and suffered a compound, long bone fracture. On Nourse's advice, Pott resisted immediate amputation, and the wound healed successfully. He later wrote about it in his work on fractures. While confined to bed he wrote an essay on ruptures (hernias). His publications helped ensure his election to the Royal Society and to the position of senior surgeon at St Bartholomew's, where he succeeded Nourse (1765). Pott, following William Cheselden (1688–1752), was now firmly established as a leading London surgeon. His position at the hospital allowed him access to large audiences for his lectures. He developed an extensive private practice and moved house to Lincoln's Inn Fields. Among his patients and friends were numerous members of the aristocracy and gentry and such celebrated figures as David Garrick (1717–79), Samuel Johnson (1709–84), and Thomas Gainsborough (1727–88). John Hunter (1728–93) was a pupil. Pott resigned from St Bartholomew's aged seventy-three and was made a governor.

Pott contributed to surgery in two important ways. First, he advanced technical skill and knowledge. Second, like Cheselden, he furthered the social status of the surgeon. Classically learned though he was, Pott had little time for veneration of ancient authorities and, calling on Francis Bacon (1561–1626), advanced the view that surgery was to be improved by concern for the patient, hard work, practical training, and detailed observation. He rejected the writing of a single systematic text, an approach much used by earlier authors, in favor of detailed studies of particular operations or diseases. This whole philosophy he put into practice in his daily life, clinical work, and the writing of a string of short, cheap, and highly popular monographs. Besides the work on ruptures, these included treatises on hydrocele, fistula in ano, wounds of the head, cancer of the scrotum, and lachrymal fistula. Pott is remembered in two eponymous conditions. In his work on palsy he described a relation between spinal curvature (now considered tuberculous) and lower limb paralysis: 'Pott's disease'. In his work on fractures he outlined a distinct fracture dislocation of the ankle: 'Pott's fracture'.

Bibliography

Primary: 1790. *The Chirurgical Works* 3 vols. (London); 1765. *Some Few General Remarks on Fractures and Dislocations* (London); 1779. *Remarks on that Kind of Palsy of the Lower Limbs, which is Frequently Found to Accompany a Curvature of the Spine* (London).

Secondary: Ravitch, M. M., 1974. 'Invective in Surgery.' *Bulletin of the New York Academy of Medicine* 50: 797–816; Lloyd, G. M., 1933. 'The Life and Works of Percivall Pott.' *St Bartholomew's Hospital Reports* 66: 291–336; *Oxford DNB*.

Christopher Lawrence

PRAXAGORAS (b. Cos, Greece; fl. *c.* 340–320 BCE), *medicine.*

Son of the physician Nicarchus, from a prominent medical family in Cos, Praxagoras was a very distinguished figure of ancient medicine. As Diocles' pupil and Herophilus's teacher, he created a bridge between the medical and biological research carried in Aristotle's Lyceum and the spectacular developments in human anatomy and physiology initiated by the Alexandrians. Nothing is known about Praxagoras' life, his chronology is disputed, and there is no evidence of contacts with the Lyceum—but affinities are clear.

Praxagoras related the cause of health and disease to the humors, of which he identified eleven: the healthy humor (blood) and ten morbid ones, including the 'vitreous humor' that caused shivering fevers. Blood was a transformation of nutriment under proportional innate heat, and the pathological humors resulted under various degrees of excess or deficiency of heat.

He practiced dissection and recorded his discoveries. His best contributions were to anatomophysiology, notably his positing of two types of vessel: arteries, originating in the heart, and veins, originating in the liver. Each type of vessel was believed to carry its own substance—veins contained blood; arteries, only air (*pneuma*)—a belief accepted for several centuries and probably inspired by dissecting animals after strangulation. Arterial *pneuma* was an agent of motion and, to explain how it reached the extremities, Praxagoras postulated a third system of vessels, the *neura* ('nerves'). These neura represented the collapsed ends of the arteries and ran more narrowly through the body; thus he inferred the existence of the nerves before their anatomical discovery.

It is not clear to what extent these ideas were independent of the medical milieu, particularly of Praxagoras's father, who was reported by Galen to have associated the arteries with *pneuma*. But Praxagoras thought about these things in a way that led to detailed investigations of the arterial pulse—a natural movement that he attributed to *pneuma* in the arteries, not to the heart. Apart from starting to distinguish various types of pulse (an operation continued by his pupil Herophilus), Praxagoras established for the first time the diagnostic value of the pulse, presumably

making correlations (unknown to us) between disease and pneumatic–arterial movement. *Pneuma* had played substantial roles in the philosophical medicine of the Presocratics, Aristotle, and various doctors, but only with Praxagoras did it become a promising medical entity of interest to the clinician.

Together with Aristotle and cardiocentrist doctors such as Philistion and Diocles, Praxagoras held that the heart was the seat of the soul, the brain being only an excrescence of the spinal cord. He believed, with Empedocles and Diocles, that digestion was a kind of putrefaction. Like Democritus, he regarded respiration as a function designed to nourish the *pneuma* rather than cool the innate heat—the dominant Aristotelian view (Philistion, Diocles).

In pathology, Praxagoras was preoccupied with the precise discovery of the affected site. He contended, for example, that pleurisy was located in the extremities of the lung (not in or around the pleura, ribcage membranes, etc.).

Praxagoras belongs in the tradition, opened by Diocles, of doctors who made dietetics equal—if not superior—to the traditional branches of surgery and pharmacy. Yet he also practiced dangerous therapies, using poisonous substances such as hellebore, or lethal abdominal surgery. It is debatable whether or not he made use of venesection.

Bibliography

Primary: 1958. (Steckerl, F., ed. and trans.) *The Fragments of Praxagoras of Cos and His School* (Leiden).

Secondary: Nutton, V., 2004. *Ancient Medicine* (London) pp. 124–127; Staden, Heinrich von, 1989. *Herophilus. The Art of Medicine in Early Alexandria* (Cambridge); Harris, C. R. S., 1973. *The Heart and Vascular System in Ancient Greek Medicine* (Oxford); Solmsen, F., 1961. 'Greek Philosophy and the Discovery of the Nerves.' *Museum Helveticum* 18: 169–197; Baumann, E. D., 1937. 'Praxagoras of Cos.' *Janus* 41: 167–185; *DSB*.

Manuela Tecusan

PREVOST, JEAN-LOUIS (b. Republic of Geneva [now Switzerland], 1 September 1790; d. Geneva, Switzerland, 14 March 1850), *therapeutics, reproductive physiology, embryology, hematology, muscular contraction, pathophysiology, nerve regeneration.*

The son of a rich merchant and his wife, Jeanne-Emilie Moultou, Prevost initially studied theology, but he later decided in favor of medicine, a profession not taught at that time at the Geneva Academy. After two years of studies at the Medical Faculty in Paris and another couple of years in Scotland, he obtained a medical degree in 1818 in Edinburgh. Following further training in Dublin, he returned to Geneva in 1820 with the goal of practicing both medicine and experimental physiology.

Initially he teamed up with Jean-Baptiste Dumas, a twenty-year-old pharmacy apprentice who later became the well-known French chemist. They embarked on a multifaceted experimental program researching blood, muscular contraction, reproduction, and embryonic development, using animals of different vertebrates and judiciously combining the possibilities offered by the scalpel, the test-tube, the microscope, and the electric battery. In 1821 they reported experiments in which they had injected defibrinated blood into previously bled animals, with only short-lasting beneficial effects. Following bilateral nephrectomy, they convincingly showed that urea was a normal constituent of blood plasma, and not a product of the kidney. A first report on spermatozoa in various animal species also appeared in 1821, indicating that Prevost and Dumas had already started their ambitious study on reproductive processes—their most famous contribution—which they presented before the French Academy of Sciences in Paris in 1823. It was awarded the Montyon prize for experimental physiology for the year 1824. The twenty-three-year-old Dumas settled thereafter in Paris, where he found professional and social opportunities far superior to those that Geneva could offer.

In the following years, Prevost, alone or with new co-workers, published a number of articles—on the comparative anatomy of male and female gonads in fish and in various invertebrates; on gastric juice and digestion (with the Geneva pharmacist A. Le Royer); on animal electricity; and on the development of the cardiovascular system (with the German-born pathologist H. Lebert, then chief-physician in a small thermal bath near Geneva). Among these publications, two short articles published in 1826 (on nerve regeneration) and in 1833 (on inflammation) are striking for the elegance of the experimental design and their potential interest for medicine. In the first study, Prevost used kittens to successfully repeat experiments demonstrating the functional recovery of nerves after bilateral vagotomy, a result first realized by Felice Fontana but later questioned on the Continent by, among others, François Magendie. Having split and then examined the newly formed nerve fibers under the microscope, Prevost observed that the regenerated fibers originated exclusively from the proximal nervous stub. He did not comment on that asymmetry, in which we recognize, with hindsight, the notions of Wallerian degeneration and of the polarity of nerve cells. In the second study, Prevost searched for pharmacological methods that might complement bloodletting to fight inflammation. His method was to observe with the microscope the local blood circulation of the interdigital membrane of the frog leg. Vasoconstriction occurred when he applied a solution of aconite, which significantly decreased the blood flow, under normal conditions, as well as when exacerbated by an experimental lesion. In a control experiment, distilled water applied to the second frog leg was shown to have no effect on the inflammatory response.

Erwin Ackerknecht, the historian of medicine, considered Prevost to be outstanding in his medical practice for his 'French diagnosis' coupled to 'British therapy'. The famous French novelist Stendhal often traveled to Geneva to get medical advice from Prevost. In his autobiography, the botanist Augustin-Pyramus de Candolle describes Prevost as 'one of the most skilful physicians and physiologists of Europe, a gentleman, knowledgeable in all subjects and devoted to his patients'. De Candolle had suffered from severe side effects following the intake of sponge and hemlock extract prescribed by another physician as a remedy for goiter. Prevost was one of the first to propose that minute quantities of iodine should be added to food or water to prevent goiter. He introduced platinum hydrochloride as a remedy for epilepsy. With his colleague and friend Louis-André Gosse, Prevost was, in 1820, among the founders of the *Dispensaire*, the first medical clinic on the Continent where, following the British model, poor patients were treated free of charge.

In 1837 Prevost significantly reduced his medical practice and moved into the country house of his ailing father, on the outskirts of Geneva. He continued to treat patients downtown, and was often asked to give second opinions. Eight handwritten laboratory notebooks, with many drawings of the embryological stages of development and of contracting muscular fibers observed under the microscope, testify to his continuing scientific endeavors. After suffering from a chronic disease since the mid-1840s, he passed away on the eve of his sixtieth birthday. Although Prevost's written output clearly decreased following the departure of Dumas from Geneva, he made several new and important contributions to medicine, to pathophysiology, and to general physiology in his later years.

Bibliography

Primary: 1821. (with Dumas, J. B. A.) 'Examen du sang et de son action dans les divers phénomènes de la vie.' *Ann. Chim.* (Paris) 18: 280–297.

Secondary: De Candolle, A. P., 2004. *Mémoires et souvenirs* (Geneva) p. 512; Richet, G., 1999. 'The Contribution of French-speaking Scientists to the Origins of Renal Physiology and Pathophysiology (1790–1910)'. *American Journal of Nephrology* 19: 274–281; De Morsier, G., 1966. 'Jean-Louis Prévost (1790–1850) et la découverte de l'ovule des mammifères.' *Gesnerus* 23: 117–121; Ackerknecht, E. H., 1966. 'La médecine à Genève, surtout dans la première moitié du XIXème siècle' in *Comptes-rendus Congrès international d'histoire de la médecine* (Basel) pp. 420–425; François, A., 1954. *Stendhal à Genève* (Neuchâtel) pp. 107, 131; Buess, H., 1947. 'The Contribution of Geneva Physicians to the Physiology of Development in the 19th Century'. *Bulletin of the History of Medicine* 21: 871–897; *DSB*.

Jean-Jacques Dreifuss

PRICHARD, JAMES COWLES (b. Ross-on-Wye, Herefordshire, England, 11 February 1786; d. London, England, 23 December 1848), *medicine, psychiatry, ethnology.*

Prichard was the eldest child of Thomas Prichard, a dealer in the iron trade, and Mary Lewis. Both belonged to well-established Quaker families, but Thomas's business concerns meant that he spent time in the port of Bristol, which was where James was educated, mostly by private tuition. Prichard began his medical education in Bristol (1802) before moving to study in London at St Thomas's Hospital (1804) and then to Edinburgh University (1805). He did his MD at Edinburgh (1808), on the varieties of mankind, before short stays at both Cambridge and Oxford. He attended the latter in 1810, having converted to the Church of England that year to make his stay possible. He also returned to Bristol in 1810, set up private practice, and then joined St Peter's Hospital (1811) before being elected to Bristol Infirmary (1816). He served as physician there until 1843. In 1811 he married the daughter of a local Unitarian minister, Anna Maria Estlin; they had ten children, two of whom died in infancy.

Prichard combined his medical career with involvement in Bristol's scientific culture, as well as becoming a medical visitor to madhouses in Gloucestershire (1826–28). He published on insanity as a result, but his reputation as a man of learning was based on the work that grew out of his MD dissertation on the history of human varieties. Five versions of the original were completed, all the product of a man of shyness, quietness of speech, and an immense capacity for reading books in many languages, including German. His most central claims emanating from this wealth of material were the unity of mankind, descended from a single parental pair despite differences in color, culture, and religious beliefs, and the claim that as civilization developed, men turned white. Whiteness of skin was an index of civilization and would eventually come to all human groups, especially as missionary Christianity spread worldwide along with European imperial power. But when that power was used cruelly or greedily, leading to extermination or rank exploitation (as in slavery) Prichard's Quaker origins and his moral revulsion made themselves felt. Man's original father, Adam, was white but (after the Fall) 'the primitive stock of men were Negroes'; the journey of civilization was toward the original truth and the original color of Christian man. The learning that Prichard displayed in his ethnological life's work became legendary, incorporating comparative linguistics (to display links, for example, between the Celtic languages, Sanskrit, and Hebrew) and the study of mythologies and their common aspects across cultures (he made a special study of Egyptian mythology to that purpose). Every detail added by Prichard to each version of the story was at the service of a single thesis: the common origin of all humans, whatever their current physical and moral differences. The foundation for this was the book, read in the private library, not the notes made from travel to foreign lands.

Prichard's contribution to the growing literature on mental illness became most famous when—in the 1830s—he blended the ideas of French alienists as well as Quaker authors on the subject to propose the reality of 'moral insanity'. This was an insanity in which the capacity for reasoning was left intact (a very un-Lockean proposal) but in which the fracture, the lesion, instead occurred in the moral faculty of the agent. A cold-blooded murderer might be fully aware of the nature of his act and how it was performed; he had taken leave, nonetheless, of his moral and emotional understanding of its true nature.

Prichard's ethnology was both a learned and a practical project, since how one conducted oneself in public life— through sobriety, pursuit of science, charitable works, careful and responsible marriage—added to the daily accumulations of the civilizing mission, both at home and abroad. Even the Prichard family dog shared in the process, being given the name of the Roman emperor thought least hostile to Christianity. Thus under Pope Gregory I the emperor was resurrected from the dead through divine intercession and baptized into the Christian faith, this legend being followed by Dante in *The Divine Comedy*. The dog was called Trajan.

Bibliography

Primary: 1813. *Researches into the Physical History of Man* (London) [1973, reprint with an introduction by Stocking, G. W. (Chicago)]; 1835. *A Treatise on Insanity and other Disorders Affecting the Mind* (London).

Secondary: Augstein, H. F., 1999. *James Cowles Prichard's Anthropology: The Remaking of the Science of Man in Early Nineteenth Century Britain* (Amsterdam); Stocking, George W., 1987. *Victorian Anthropology* (Chicago); *DSB*; *Oxford DNB*.

Michael Neve

PRINGLE, JOHN (b. Roxburgh, Roxburghshire, Scotland, 10 April 1707; d. London, England, 18 January 1782), *military medicine, naval medicine.*

Pringle was the youngest son of Sir John Pringle, baronet, and his wife, Magdalen. He was tutored at home and, from 1722, attended St Andrews University, where his uncle Francis Pringle was professor of Greek and a practicing physician. In 1727 he entered Edinburgh University for a year. Following this he visited Amsterdam as part of a plan to enter commerce. But he also visited Leiden and, apparently, after attending a lecture by Herman Boerhaave (1668–1738), determined to study medicine. He matriculated (1728) and graduated MD (1730) at Leiden. During his studies he became a close friend of Gerard van Swieten (1700–72). He furthered his medical education in Paris and returned to Edinburgh to practice.

In 1734 he was appointed joint professor of pneumatics (moral philosophy) at the university. He continued, however, to practice medicine. Around this time Pringle became physician to the Earl of Stair, officer commanding the British army in Flanders and a friend of the Pringle family with lands north of Roxburgh. In August 1742, through the offices of the Earl, Pringle was appointed a physician to the army and took charge of the military hospital in Flanders, where he served for much of the war of the Austrian Succession (1740–48). In 1744 the Duke of Cumberland appointed him physician-general to His Majesty's forces in the Low Countries. In that year he was on duty during the French invasion of the Austrian Netherlands. Pringle then accompanied the army to Scotland and resigned his professorship. He was present at the Battle of Culloden (1745). After this he was again abroad until the peace of Aix-la-Chapelle (1748), after which he returned to take up private practice in London.

Here, just over forty, well bred, learned, experienced, and well connected, Pringle garnered all the glittering prizes. Already, in 1745, he had been admitted FRS. In 1749 he became physician in ordinary to the Duke of Cumberland. Oddly he did not become a licentiate of the RCP until 1758. He was made a fellow, *speciali gratiâ*, the same year in which he became physician in ordinary to the queen (1763). The year 1766 saw him a baronet and he was gazetted physician in ordinary to the king in 1774. Foreign honors rained on him. In 1752 Pringle married Charlotte, the second daughter of William Oliver, Bath physician and creator of the Bath Oliver biscuit. The marriage produced no children.

Pringle's medical life is conveniently divided in two. During the first period, he served as a practical and intellectual contributor to military hygiene. During the second, as president of the Royal Society (1772–78), he patronized and orchestrated experimental work touching on diseases of military and naval populations. During the campaigns in the Netherlands, the Earl of Stair's suggestion (readily accepted by the French) that military hospitals were to be recognized as neutral territory must have come from Pringle. His two works on diseases of institutions and military camps of 1750 and 1752, respectively, are widely recognized as landmarks in the history of epidemic febrile disease. His description of jail fever is regarded as an accurate delineation of the natural history of typhus. More generally his publications were at the forefront of those drawing attention to institutional fevers (in hospitals, jails, ships, military camps, etc.) and their roots in poor sanitation and ventilation. Pringle's studies in these areas were also theoretical and experimental. His work is significant in that he stressed the investigation of 'septic' processes both within and outside the body. In doing so he promoted the growth of the study of living pathology, which was part of the move from mechanism to vitalism that characterized eighteenth-century thought.

Central to these new studies of fever and septic processes was gas chemistry. Scurvy at sea was considered by many to be a septic disease, analogous to fevers. Lloyd and Coulter (1961, p. 308) describe Pringle in 1764 as Surgeon-in-Chief of the army, and through his offices 'wort' (an infusion of malt) was recommended by the Admiralty to be used in trials as a cure for scurvy in the naval hospitals at

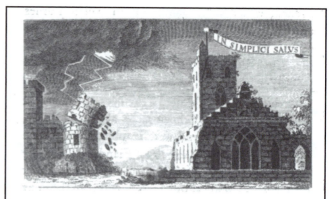

Illustrated page from *Observations on the Diseases of the Army...*, London, 1768. Wellcome Library, London.

Portsmouth and Plymouth. Wort, being acidic, was held to counteract the alkaline basis of septic processes. Wort received a favorable report from James Cook (1728–79) after his first voyage of 1768. Later various preparations of fixed air were used in scurvy trials. (Fixed air, an acidic gas, today's carbon dioxide, had been isolated and described by Joseph Black in 1764.) Central to the gas and scurvy researches of the 1770s was Joseph Priestley (1733–1804), whose work was specifically promoted by Pringle when president of the Royal Society. Priestley's work on the impregnation of water with fixed air for use as a cure of scurvy received the Copley Medal, awarded by Pringle in 1773. In 1776 Cook, whose voyages were strongly backed by Pringle, was awarded the medal, also by Pringle, for a paper on the health of seamen. The Whig and dissenting circle supported by Pringle effectively dissolved with the succession of the Tory, Joseph Banks (1743–1820), to the presidency of the Royal Society in 1778. Nonetheless Pringle's military and naval initiatives were eventually to enter civilian life as constitutive of the public health movement in the nineteenth century.

Bibliography

Primary: 1750. *Observations on the Nature and Cure of Hospital and Jayl-Fevers. In a letter to Doctor Mead* (London); 1752. *Observations on the Diseases of the Army, in Camp and Garrison* (London); 1776. *A Discourse upon some Late Improvements of the Means for Preserving the Health of Mariners* (London).

Secondary: Lloyd, Christopher, and Jack L. S. Coulter, 1961. *Medicine and the Navy. Volume III—1714–1815* (Edinburgh and London); Singer, Dorothea Waley, 1948–50. 'Sir John Pringle and His Circle.' *Annals of Science* 6: 127–180; 229–247; 248–261; [Mac-Michael, W.], 1830. *Lives of British Physicians* (London); *DSB*; *Munk's Roll*; *Oxford DNB*.

Christopher Lawrence

PROUT, WILLIAM (b. Horton, Gloucestershire, England, 15 January 1785; d. London, England, 9 April 1850), *medicine, chemistry, biochemistry.*

Prout was the youngest son of John Prout, a tenant farmer, and Hannah Limbrick. As a child he suffered severe earaches and became deaf in later life. His early education being rudimentary, he was occupied at farming until entering Sherston Academy, Wiltshire (1802), to learn Greek and Latin. After advertising for advice on further education, he joined Reverend Thomas Jones's seminary at Redland, Bristol (1805), which sparked his interest in chemistry, notably Humphry Davy's (1778–1829) electrochemical work. Encouraged by Jones, he studied medicine at Edinburgh University (1808–11), boarding with Alexander Adam, rector of Edinburgh High School. His tutors included Alexander Monro *tertius* and Andrew Duncan. At Edinburgh University he also met John Elliotson (1791–1868), who became a close friend. Prout moved to London (1812), spending a year at Guy's and St Thomas's Hospitals before establishing a practice and marrying Adams' daughter, Agnes (22 September 1814). They had six children.

Prout's chief interests were metabolism and digestion. He differentiated between taste, smell, and flavor (1812), and measured carbon dioxide output (1813), wearing a measurement apparatus for three weeks. His lectures on animal chemistry (1814) attracted attention from Astley Cooper and Alexander Marcet, who sent him a child's abnormal urine specimen from which Prout isolated melanic (homogentistic) acid (1822), excreted in the metabolic disorder alkaptonuria. He was also the first to obtain urea from urine (1814) and after discovering purpuric acid, was elected FRS (1815). He was an early user of iodine (1816) to treat goiter, a remedy adopted by Elliotson at St Thomas's Hospital (1819).

Prout's reputation as a chemist was established with *An Inquiry into the Nature and Treatment of Gravel* (1821), one of the first nineteenth-century medical textbooks to deal with disease from a chemical perspective. The book, translated into French and German, made Prout famous as a urinary specialist. He offered no chemical remedies to dissolve stones, believing that once formed, they could be enlarged by the normal ingredients of urine. In his Gulstonian Lectures delivered to the RCP (1831), he suggested that most bodily changes, normal or pathological, owed much to chemistry. In one important sidestep from organic analysis, he speculated that since the atomic weights of the chemical elements appeared to be whole number multiples of hydrogen (H = 1), elements might be compounds (polymers) of it or some simpler body (1815, 1816). Hydrogen might indeed be the *protyle* (primitive matter) of the ancient Greeks. 'Prout's hypothesis' stimulated chemical analysis and research into the properties of elements, and was later verified by Francis W. Aston's concept of isotopy (1920).

A pale slender figure, usually dressed in black, Prout was described as an accurate and scrupulous experimentalist, rising early to conduct experiments before seeing patients. Meticulous analysis produced the important, if controversial, discovery that gastric juice was muriatic (hydrochloric) acid formed, he suggested, from blood chlorides disunited by electrolysis, the soda residue maintaining the blood's alkalinity (1823). Prout's method for analyzing organic compounds won the Royal Society's Copley Medal with the paper *On the Ultimate Analysis (Composition) of Simple Alimentary Substances* (1827), although his apparatus was soon outmoded by that of Justus Liebig (1831). A vitalist, Prout maintained that blood and tissues were formed by a vital principle from four aliments (foodstuffs) classified as water, saccharinous (carbohydrates), oleaginous (fats), and albuminous (proteins). He expanded on this theory of metabolism in his Bridgewater treatise (1834) in which, in the meteorology section, he coined the word 'convection' to describe the conduction of heat through air or liquids.

Prout's considerable reputation waned during his last fifteen years. Increasing deafness led to his withdrawal from scientific society, and he concentrated on medical practice and revision of his textbooks. With justification, Thomas Wakley criticized him for ignoring or failing to keep up with developments in Continental chemistry so that his achievements became eclipsed by those of Justus Liebig (1803–73) and the German school even though much of his work between 1815 and 1825 foreshadowed theirs.

Bibliography

Primary: 1821. *An Inquiry into the Nature and Treatment of Gravel, Calculus, and other Diseases Connected with a Deranged Operation of the Urinary Organs* (London, 2nd edn., 1825; 3rd edn., 1840; 5th edn., 1848); 1834. *Chemistry, Meteorology, and the Function of Digestion, Considered with Reference to Natural Theology* (London).

Secondary: Brock, W. H., 1985. *From Protyle to Proton: William Prout and the Nature of Matter* (Bristol); Brock, W. H., 1965. 'The Life and Work of William Prout.' *Medical History* 9: 101–126; Kasich, Anthony M., 1946. 'William Prout and the Discovery of Hydrochloric Acid in the Gastric Juice.' *Bulletin of the History of Medicine* 20: 340–358; [Anon.], 1851. 'Some account of the life and scientific writings of William Prout.' *Edinburgh Medical and Surgical Journal* 76: 126–183; *DSB*; *Munk's Roll*; *Oxford DNB*.

Carole Reeves

PUCCINOTTI, FRANCESCO   (b. Urbino, Italy, 8 August 1794; d. Florence, Italy, 8 October 1872), *medicine, psychiatry, hygiene, epidemiology, history, forensic medicine.*

After studying Greek and Latin first at the Seminar and then in the High School of the Italian Kingdom of Urbino, Puccinotti entered the Military School in Pavia (1811) to study natural sciences and philosophy. At the end of the Napoleonic epoch, he moved to the medical school of Rome, receiving his MD in 1816. In 1822 he was appointed to the chair of clinical medicine at Fermo University. He never began teaching because in 1823 he was named first physician of the city of Urbino, but decided to move to Recanati, as a 'medico condotto' [municipal doctor]. Here he had as a patient and lifelong friend the great poet Giacomo Leopardi (1798–1837).

In 1826 he was named to the chair of pathology and forensic medicine at the University of Macerata and became also the director of the local hospital and psychiatric hospice. Because of political riots in which he was implicated, he moved in 1831 to Tuscany, where Leopold II nominated him for the chair of 'medico-civil institutions' at Pisa University (1838). In 1839, at the First Congress of the Italian Scientists in Pisa, he was appointed secretary of the medical section. During these years he collaborated with literary circles and journals such as *Giornale Arcadico* and *Biblioteca Italiana*. In Pisa he created a 'Hippocratic Academy'. Puccinotti's clinical activity was quite limited, but his teaching was much appreciated and his publications were quite influential. In 1855 he became a member of the Academia della Crusca.

In 1860 Puccinotti moved to Florence. The newly created Kingdom of Italy had established an Institute for Advanced Studies here and he occupied the chair of the history of medicine. He was also named 'Senator of the Kingdom', but in 1865 he renounced this position because of his bad health and pessimism.

The first publications by Puccinotti were three discourses read at the Accademia dei Lincei (1820), in which he encouraged establishing a Hippocratic medicine and discussed the nature of the contagion, stating that 'according to the histories and to reason' they are not 'spontaneous', that is

produced by the body itself, but always enter it from outside, even if he confessed 'not to know what contagions are'. In his *Storia delle febbri intermittanti* [History of the Intermittent Fevers] (1824) and in his book on periodical fevers (1826), Puccinotti described malaria epidemics that he had observed as a doctor at the hospital of the Salvatore al Laterano, using the word *malaria* in the modern sense, as a specific disease, without the apostrophe as used before (*mal'aria*, that is bad air).

In 1828 Puccinotti published his book *Inductive Pathology*, in which he suggested a synthesis between two traditional schools, which he called 'dynamism' and 'organicism' (functionalism and solidism).

Because of his publications on nervous diseases (1834) and forensic medicine (1852), Puccinotti was considered for decades to be the founder of modern Italian psychiatry and legal medicine. He analyzed the legal status of 'mania', suggesting that this status cancels the principle of legal responsibility. He attributed the increased number of mental diseases to the changes produced by industrial society and this was part of the rationale for his engagement with social medicine and hygiene. He believed that medicine had a civic responsibility and that the modern state should promote 'social hygiene', produce legislation against epidemic diseases, and create institutions for epidemiological surveys.

Puccinotti promoted experimental physiology, using a wide variety of experimental apparatus, and he published with Pacinotti on the electric currents in living organisms.

In the last part of this life, Puccinotti devoted all his time to the history of medicine. As a devout Christian, he considered the progress of medicine to be a significant demonstration of the divine wisdom.

Bibliography

Primary: 1820. *Dei contagi spontanei e delle potenze e mutazioni morbose credute atte a produrle nei corpi umani* (Rome); 1824. *Storia delle febbri intermittanti perniciose di Roma negli anni 1819–21* (Urbino); 1828. *Patologia induttiva proposta come nuovo organo della scienza clinica* (Naples); 1834. *Lezioni sulle malattie nervose* (Florence); 1836. *Annotazioni cliniche sul cholera-morbus e sulle malattie epidemiche e contagiose in generale: secondo le osservazioni fatte in Firenze e in Livorno nella epidemia del 1835* (Naples); 1850–66. *Storia della medicina* (Livorno); 1852. *Lezioni di medicina legale* (Naples); 1858. *Opere complete edite e inedite* (Naples).

Secondary: Belloni, L., 1974. 'Sull'ippocratismo di S. de Renzi e di F. Puccinotti e sul concorso alla cattedra del testo di Ippocrate e di storia della medicina all'università di Napoli nel 1844.' *Episteme* 8: 2–4, 132–147; Hahn, L., 1889. 'Puccinotti (Francesco)' in Dechambre, A., L. Lereboullet, and L. Hahn. eds., *Dictionnaire Encyclopédique des Sciences Médicales* Deuxième série vol. 27 (Paris) p. 828; Livi, Carlo, 1873. *Della vita e delle opere di Francesco Puccinotti: discorso letto nella pubblica adunanza generale del dì 24 novembre 1872* (Siena and Rome).

Bernardino Fantini

PUIGVERT GORRO, ANTONI (b. Santa Coloma de Gramenet, Barcelona, Spain, 26 April 1905; d. Barcelona, 18 May 1990), *urology.*

Puigvert, the son of a medical doctor, attended Barcelona Medical Faculty from 1923 to 1928), where he was a boarder with Manuel Seres (1898–1928), professor of urology. A misunderstanding with the new professor led him to start an early private medical practice. In 1932, with the support of a grateful patient, he went to Inselspital in Bern and Hôpital Lariboisière in Paris to improve his education. Hans Wildbolz, Felix Legueu, and Georges Marion taught him.

After returning to Barcelona, Puigvert won a post as assistant (1933) in the urology department of *Santa Creu i Sant Pau* Hospital, where he developed a productive career and was appointed physician-in-chief in 1951.

During that period, Puigvert showed bold ability in his reception and application of new technical procedures, which led to several publications, among them *Tuberculosi renal* (1936), *Endoscopia urinaria* (1939), and *La tuberculosis genitourinaria* (1941). Shortly after the development of urography, he published two works on the subject with original illustrations: *Atlas de urografía* (1933) and *Tratado de urografía clínica* (1944). With L. Martínez-Piñeiro and E. Pérez Castro, he participated in strengthening urology as a medical specialty in Spain by creating a medical journal, *Archivos Españoles de Urología* (1944). Beginning in 1944 he set up daily clinical and monthly bibliographical sessions in the hospital urology department to achieve rationality and new standards of quality assistance. Another step toward that objective was the organization in 1946 of yearly schools on urology, which are still held.

Puigvert launched an ambitious program aimed at creating an integral vision of genitourinary diseases. That effort eventually led to great institutional changes such as creation of the Puigvert Foundation (1961), later established on the premises of *Santa Creu i Sant Pau* Hospital (1966), where his private and public practices met.

His private clinic, established in 1928, turned into a well-equipped Urological Institute in 1943. After taking over direction of the hospital urology department (1951), he entered into negotiations with the hospital administration to incorporate his private institute in 1953. He contributed his own resources to establish a powerful Urological Institute in the hospital. Immediately he enlarged the departmental premises with new laboratories, uroendoscopy and urography sections, and new nephrology (1954) and andrology (1955) divisions, which resulted in the establishment of potent teamwork. Also interested in the training of experts in such areas, Puigvert pioneered a three-year syllabus in urology (1952) by admitting two resident doctors to his institute. New training programs were outlined in the recently instituted specialties of nephrology (1965) and andrology (1968).

Puigvert also excelled in the introduction of instrumental procedures in surgical urology, such as a practical adaptation in perineal prostatectomy through a swinging Benique's sound or a pyelography–urography syringe known as Puigvert's tutor sound. In connection with his work on tuberculosis, Puigvert gave his name to the surgical suture of the urethra and bladder used in treating the infection of the urinary tract by tuberculosis, and he also described megacalyosis, a nonobstructive condition of the kidney characterized by an increase in the number and size of renal calyces (1963).

In gratitude for his work in urology, the Spanish Ministry of Education designated Puigvert an extraordinary professor of the new medical school of the Barcelona Autonomous University (1971). During the following two decades, the Puigvert Foundation achieved a dynamic level of activity in the areas of assistance, training, and research, becoming quite influential in the Spanish and Latin American urological world. Puigvert also earned worldwide personal recognition, thanks to his significant work in urology. He was awarded a number of international prizes and received appointments as an honorary professor at several universities.

Bibliography

Primary: 1971. *Tratado de operatoria urológica* (Barcelona); 1976. *Del saber y del hacer urológico* (Barcelona); 1981. *Mi vida . . . y otras más* (Barcelona).

Secondary: Baños, Josep Eladi, and Elena Guardiola, 2002. 'Eponímia mèdica catalan. Els epònims de Puigvert.' *Annals de Medicina* 85: 173–175; Granjel, Luis S., 1986. *Retablo histórico de la urología en España* (Salamanca).

Alfons Zarzoso

PUTNAM, JAMES JACKSON (b. Boston, Massachusetts, USA, 3 October 1846; d. Boston, 4 November 1918), *neurology, psychoanalysis.*

Putnam came from one of Boston's most famous medical families. He graduated from Harvard College in 1866 and received the MD from Harvard Medical School in 1870, where he studied under Brown-Séquard, Jeffries Wyman, and Oliver Wendell Holmes. He took up the study of diseases of the nervous system and formed lifelong friendships with William James, Henry Pickering Bowditch, and Edward Emerson. In 1870 he went to Europe to study electrotherapeutics and neurology. Among others, he studied with Theodor Meynert, Hughlings Jackson, and J.-M. Charcot. On his return to Boston in 1872, he was appointed lecturer on the application of electricity in nervous diseases at Harvard Medical School and in 1875 opened the out-patient clinic for diseases of the nervous system at the Massachusetts General Hospital, where he worked as 'Chief Electrician'. At Harvard Medical School, together with William James and Henry Bowditch, Putnam conducted experiments on the localization of brain functions, the earliest known contributions to brain neuropathology in the United States, according to Walter Cannon.

In 1874 he became a founder of the American Neurological Association. In 1893 he was appointed professor in diseases of the nervous system at Harvard.

In the mid 1880s, largely under the influence of William James, Putnam began experimenting with hypnosis and psychotherapy. Following Meynert, he was initially a staunch materialist critical of the efflorescence of 'functional' neuroses, but he became increasingly convinced, through the debates on railway spine injury, that symptoms that he once considered to be physiological were caused by a 'buried idea'. From 1890 onward, he was a significant member of the 'Boston School of Psychotherapy', a loose-knit network of psychologists, philosophers, neurologists, and psychiatrists, including William James, Josiah Royce, Hugo Münsterberg, Morton Prince, and Edward Cowles, which played a central role in establishing psychotherapy in the United States. The Boston School had close links with the French, English, and Swiss developments in the fields of psychical research, abnormal psychology, and psychotherapy, and the works of Pierre Janet in particular were seminal. In his psychotherapy, Putnam conceived of health as a moving equilibrium of consciousness and the subconscious and of mental and bodily processes. He held that in neurosis, the sense of character and the capacity to act efficiently were lost. Thus the task was one of healing dissociations. Patients were encouraged to reconceptualize themselves and change their character.

In line with the eclectic development of psychotherapy at the turn of the century, Putnam took up Breuer and Freud's work. In 1906 he published a paper detailing his use of what he called 'psychoanalysis' at the Massachusetts General Hospital, dissenting from the specifics of Freud's theories. His early articles convey how loose this term was at this time, for he included the use of hypnosis and automatic writing under the rubric. In 1906, together with Elwood Worcester and others, Putnam launched the Emmanuel Movement, a collaboration of physicians and clergymen that helped to establish psychotherapy in the United States. However, he soon became critical of this movement.

In 1909 he had a personal encounter with Freud during Freud's lectures at Clark University, which proved to be a significant turning point in his allegiance to the psychoanalytic cause, to which he underwent something akin to a conversion experience. Putnam, Freud, Jung, and Ferenczi spent a week together at Putnam's camp in the Adirondacks. In 1911 the American Psychoanalytic Association was founded, with Putnam as the president. In retrospect, Freud claimed that Putnam did more than anyone else to further the cause of psychoanalysis in America, as much because of the respect in which he was held as to his actual work.

During this period, Putnam set about reformulating psychoanalysis. He critiqued Freud's positivism, arguing that this had deleterious consequences in practice: repression, in his view, was always in the service of some 'good', and thus without an inquiry into values, psychoanalysis would be of no avail. He presented a positive melioristic reading of the contents of the unconscious, drawing on Bergson, Hegel, James, and New England Transcendentalism. In 1915 he presented this synthesis in his work *Human Motives*, which began and ended with quotes from Ralph Waldo Emerson. In this work, he argued that the two main sources of human motives were to be found in one's rational aspirations and emotional repressions, and he attempted to show how these could be reconciled. In so doing, Putnam synthesized a rationalized religion as representing man's ideals with Freud's metaphysics of instinct. Thus Putnam's work demonstrates the manner in which the spread of psychoanalysis in the United States came through its Americanization, which emphasized the pragmatic application of indigenous developments in the psychological and psychotherapeutic field.

Bibliography

Primary: 1915. *Human Motives* (Boston); 1921. *Addresses on Psycho-Analysis* (London); 1971. (Hale, Nathan J., Jr., ed.) *James Jackson Putnam and Psychoanalysis: Letters between Putnam and Sigmund Freud, Ernest Jones, William James, Sándor Ferenczi and Morton Prince, 1877–1917* (Cambridge, MA).

Secondary: Taylor, Eugene I., 1988. 'On the First Use of 'Psychoanalysis' at the Massachusetts General Hospital, 1903–1905.' *Journal of the History of Medicine and Allied Sciences* 43(4): 447–471; Taylor, Eugene I., 1985. 'James Jackson Putnam's Fateful Meeting with Freud: The 1909 Clark University Conference.' *Voices: The Art and Science of Psychotherapy* 21(1): 78–89; *DAMB*.

Sonu Shamdasani

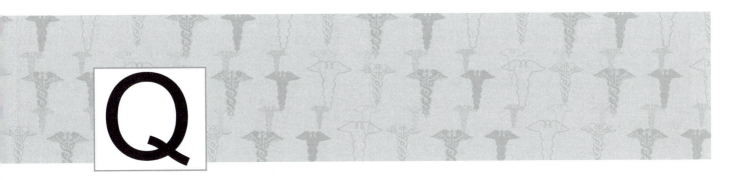

Q

QIAN, YI 錢乙 **(aka QIAN, ZHONGYANG** 錢仲陽**)**
(b. Dongping, Yun prefecture, Shangdong Province, China, 1032;
d. Dongping, China, 1113), *Chinese medicine, pediatrics.*

Qian Yi was a Song dynasty (960-1276) physician. He is
considered China's first pediatrician. Qian's father practiced
acupuncture, although he never received formal training.
When Qian was three years old, his father became a monk.
Shortly thereafter, Qian's mother died and he went to his
aunt's home in Shandong. His uncle had a thriving medical
practice, and Qian spent most of his day learning about
medical treatment. Qian read all the medical classics he
could obtain, including the *Yellow Emperor's Inner Canon*,
the *Canon of Difficulties*, and materia medica collections.
When Qian was ten, his uncle allowed him to see patients in
his clinic. Qian soon established a reputation as a successful
doctor, especially in treating children.

Qian's reputation began during Yuanfeng's reign (1078–
85), when the emperor's cousin became sick. Since all the
court physicians were baffled, Qian was called in to diagnose
and treat her. Following his successful treatment, he was
appointed to the Han Lin Academy. Two years later, the
emperor's son became sick. Once again Qian cured the
child. Subsequently, the emperor appointed him an Imperial
Physician and many members of the imperial family and
high officials sought him for the treatment of their children.
After serving the emperor for a few years, Qian retired from
his post.

Qian's most important book, and the only one that has
survived to the present, was *Direct Instructions for Treating
Pediatric Manifestation Types and Medicines*. In this book,
Qian clarified the special characteristics of pediatrics and
differentiated them from existing medical theories and techniques appropriate for adults. He was the first to describe in
detail how a child's body differed from an adult's. Using the
Yellow Emperor's Inner Canon and the Canon of Problems as
his starting point, he claimed that when a child is born,
the internal organs are not fully formed or, using Chinese
terminology, have not yet 'solidified', thus rendering the
body more susceptible to outside pathogens. Consequently, children's pathogenesis, diagnosis, and treatment
were inherently different. A doctor could not apply the
same techniques he used for adults.

Traditional Chinese diagnosis relied on four methods—
visual inspection, interrogation, auditory and olfactory
examination, and palpation of the pulse. Qian claimed
that, when diagnosing a child, the pulse was not as distinct
as an adult's, the doctor's questioning of a child was nearly
useless, and the visual inspection was often misleading due
to the child's agitation when visiting a physician. Accordingly, he established guiding principles for diagnosing children based on a simple set of observable symptoms, as well
as those reported by the parent. He correlated the internal
organs with hues of sections of the face as a means of dif-
ferentiating normal and pathological signs. He also used

facial complexion to draw on the functionality of the internal organs, whether they were in excess or deficiency, hot or cold. He linked these symptoms with guidelines framed by the correspondences of Yin and Yang, as well as the Five Agents, to construct patterns of pathology associated with the five *zang* 藏 [visceral organs and their system of functions]. By doing this he reshaped clinical diagnosis, adapting it to fit the treatment of children.

From the therapeutic perspective, Qian claimed that common drug formulas would have adverse effects on children. Formulas for children, according to him, should be milder and support the *qi*. Qian devised medicinal formulas and prescriptions specifically designed to treat children's diseases.

Finally, Qian contributed in other fields of medicine. He was among the first physicians to compile a work discussing 'cold damage' disorders during the Northern Song dynasty (960–1127). Although this book did not survive, we do know that it focused on the treatment of febrile diseases in children and newborns.

Bibliography

Primary: 1119. *Xiaoer yao zheng zhi jue* 小兒藥證直訣 [Direct Instructions for Treating Pediatric Manifestation Types and Medicines]; 1032-1113 (lost). *Shanghan lun zhi wei* 傷寒論指微 [Pointing out Subtleties in the Treatise of Cold Damage Disorders].

Secondary: Goldschmidt, Asaf (forthcoming) *The Evolution of Chinese Medicine: Northern Song Dynasty, 960–1127* (London).

Asaf Goldschmidt

QUERVAIN, JOHANN FRIEDRICH DE (b. Sion, Switzerland, 4 May 1868; d. Bern, Switzerland, 24 January 1940), *surgery, clinical statistics, internationalism.*

The first of ten children of a German-speaking Swiss clergyman's family, de Quervain studied medicine in Bern (1887–92). He was a student assistant with the Pathology and Physiology Institutes, having understood the importance of these two disciplines for the development of surgery, his preferred field. After graduation and a study trip through Germany, he worked for two years with Theodor Kocher in Bern. In 1894 de Quervain assumed his first independent post as chief surgeon at the City Hospital of La Chaux-de-Fonds near the French border, where he married his francophone wife.

The combination of the strictly methodical approach to clinical problems as taught by Kocher, and the more 'intuitive' one of the French school that he now experienced, was the secret behind the international success of his *Treatise of Surgical Diagnosis*, published in six languages and ten German editions (from 1907). He also wrote on stenosing tendosynovitis of the thumb muscles, still known by surgeons as de Quervain's disease (1895), and sub-acute inflammation of the thyroid (giant-cell thyroiditis), referred to as de Quervain's disease in internal medicine (1902).

In 1910 de Quervain was appointed to the chair of surgery in Basel. Having declined an offer to the University of Geneva, he ultimately succeeded Kocher in Bern (1918–38). During those years he wrote standard monographs on goiter and cretinism. He was among the first to systematically compare radiological and anatomo-pathological diagnoses of gastrointestinal diseases. Furthermore, de Quervain was scientifically responsible for the state-supported, eminently successful introduction of iodized salt in the prophylaxis of endemic goiter in Switzerland (from the 1920s), not to mention his distinguished work as a medical historian.

A notable accomplishment was his methodical approach to the evaluation of surgical interventions. Atypically for his time, when surgical statistics usually showed merely operation results, de Quervain assessed, retrospectively, the outcomes of patients with acute appendicitis from the surgery units against those from the medical departments of the same Swiss hospitals. Using the timing of operation after onset of symptoms rather than clinical-pathological criteria as variables, he showed the superiority of prompt operation in terms of lethality and costs (1913). This settled a decade-long controversy. In a sophisticated retrospective approach running for ten years, he then attempted the same for breast cancer. This comparative study was the first of its kind in the surgical literature. The analyses, in collaboration with a professional statistician, related relative survival times of both groups to life expectancy in healthy women at the time of diagnosis. The results relativized the value of radical surgery (1930).

De Quervain's general education was by no means limited to medicine. He regarded science as an international—indeed, supranational—venture. The impact of his personality can be seen in the role he played in restoring the international scientific community after World War I. He initiated international student exchanges within Europe and, after a visit there in 1921, with the United States. Completely at home in both the German and French cultures, and publishing regularly in English as well, he made the first attempt to reunite the *Société Internationale de Chirurgie*, which had disbanded according to nationalistic political camps in 1918. His painstaking efforts over more than twelve years were crowned by the first truly international postwar congress of the *Société*, held in Madrid in 1932, with himself in the chair.

Bibliography

Primary: 1895. 'Ueber eine Form von chronischer Tendovaginitis.' *Correspondenzblatt. Schweizer Aerzte* 25: 389–394; 1902. 'Ueber acute, nicht eiterige Thyreoiditis.' *Verhandlungen Deutsche Gesellschaft für Chirurgie* 31: II, 118–126; 1907. *Spezielle Chirurgische Diagnostik* (Leipzig) (English edns., 1913, 1917, 1921, 1926); 1930. *Gesamtergebnisse der Schweizerischen Brustkrebsstatistik* (Bern).

Secondary: Boyes, Joseph, 1976. *On the Shoulders of Giants. Notable Names in Hand Surgery* (Philadelphia) pp. 158–161; Tröhler, Ulrich, 1973. *Der Schweizer Chirurg J. F. de Quervain (1868–1940). Wegbereiter neuer internationaler Beziehungen in der Wissenschaft der Zwischenkriegszeit* (Aarau); Wangensteen, Owen, 1969. 'The Berne Surgical Clinic Revisited in Memory.' *American Journal of Surgery* 117: 388–396.

Ulrich Tröhler

QUESNAY, FRANÇOIS (b. Méré, France, 4 June 1694; d. Grand-Commun, France, 16 December 1774), *surgery, medicine, medical polemics.*

Quesnay was born to a peasant family in Seine-et-Oise, the eighth of thirteen children. Illiterate until age eleven, he was inspired by medical and agrarian writers such as Charles Estienne and Jean Liébault, and decided to follow a career in surgery. In 1711 he moved to Paris to apprentice under Pierre de Rochefort, and he took surgical courses at St-Côme, the Faculté de Médecine, and the Hôtel Dieu. In 1718 he received his *lettres de maîtrise* and began to practice in Mantes, a town outside of Paris. He had just married Jeanne-Catherine Dauphin; two of their children survived infancy.

In Mantes, Quesnay was renowned for his obstetrical talents, and he became first surgeon at the local Hôtel Dieu. In 1723 Quesnay began to collaborate with René Croissant de Garengeot, who was impressed by his skills and introduced him to François Gigot de Lapeyronie, the first surgeon to Louis XV, and the most important advocate for surgical reform. Quesnay picked up the reform cause and endeared himself to Lapeyronie by attacking physician J.-B. Silva's ideas about phlebotomy. After his wife died, Quesnay entered the personal service of the duc de Villeroy, and returned to Paris in 1734.

In Paris, Quesnay launched a meteoric career. In 1736 he published important studies on physiology and venesection, in which he formulated iatromechanistic theories of health and sickness. Under Lapeyronie's patronage, he became a master at St-Côme in 1737, and secretary of the Académie Royale de Chirurgie in 1740 (a post he held for about a decade). He also edited the first volume of the Académie de Chirurgie's *Mémoires.* At the same time, Quesnay engaged in a pamphlet war between surgeons and physicians over a royal decree which mandated that surgical candidates must take an arts degree from a French university. He argued that the country surgeon in fact functioned as a general practitioner for ordinary folk. In 1744 Quesnay himself received a medical degree at Pont-à-Mousson.

During the 1740s Quesnay became a protégé of the Marquise de Pompadour, Louis XV's powerful mistress. In 1749 he moved to Versailles and began treating the royal family, saving the dauphin from smallpox. Although Quesnay never became médecin du roi, the king gave him noble status and appointed him to the Académie des Sciences. In the 1750s Quesnay published several medical works on gangrene, fevers, and suppuration, but he practiced only for the royal family.

During the 1750s, Quesnay redefined himself as a major Enlightenment thinker after he was commissioned to write articles on rural economy for Denis Diderot's *Encyclopédie.* In 1757 he met with Victor de Mirabeau, the best-selling author of *L'Ami des hommes,* and together they launched the economic school of 'physiocracy' (a neologism meaning 'the rule of nature'). In his writings, Quesnay claimed to discover the natural mechanism that shaped economic and social laws, identifying the 'net product' (the disposable surplus over cost) that caused the economy to grow or decline. Unlike A.-M. de Turgot and Adam Smith, Quesnay declared that agriculture alone determined this net product, and the only productive work was farming (rather than manufacturing). Above all, he believed in private property and free markets, and he wanted an enlightened monarch to deregulate the grain trade. Physiocracy enjoyed its greatest popularity during the 1760s, acquiring its own journal, the *Éphémérides*; but it was eclipsed by competing economic schools. In the 1770s Quesnay turned to geometry. After Louis XVI failed to appoint him as médecin du roi, Quesnay retired to Grand-Commun, where he died in 1774.

Although Quesnay started from a humble background, his acumen and talent allowed him to acquire bourgeois and aristocratic patrons, including members of the royal household. He played a key role as spokesman on behalf of the surgeons' professional aspirations and reforms, and he personified the ideal of an enlightened medical practitioner. Most famously, he founded the first modern school of economics, and promoted socioeconomic reform in France.

Bibliography

Primary: 1744. (with Louis, A., et al.) *Recherches critiques et historiques sur l'origine, et les divers états et sur les progrès de la chirurgie en France* 2 vols. (Paris); 1747. *Essai physique sur l'œconomie animale,* 2nd edn., 3 vols. (Paris); 1748. *Examen impartial des contestations des médecins et des chirurgiens* (n.p.); 1768–69. *Physiocratie* 2 vols. (Paris).

Secondary: Spary, E. C., 2003. 'The "spirit of system" in the fortunes of physiocracy' in Schabas, Margaret, and Neil De Marchi, eds., *Oeconomies in the Age of Newton* (Durham, NC); Gelfand, Toby, 1980. *Professionalizing Modern Medicine: Paris Surgeons and Medical Science and Institutions in the 18th Century* (Westport, CT); Hecht, Jacqueline, 1958. 'La vie de François Quesnay' in Sauvy, Alfred, ed., *François Quesnay et la physiocratie* 2 vols. (Paris) 1: 213–214; Schelle, Gustave, 1907. *Le docteur Quesnay* (Paris); Louis, Antoine, 1859. 'Eloge de Quesnay (1775)' in Dubois, E.-F., d'Amiens, ed., *Eloges lus dans les séances publiques de l'Académie Royale de Chirurgie* (Paris).

Sean Quinlan

QUETELET, LAMBERT ADOLPHE JACQUES (b. Ghent, Belgium, 22 February 1796; d. Brussels, Belgium, 17 February 1874), *social statistics.*

Quetelet was the son of François A. J. H. Quetelet and Anne F. Vandervelde. His wife, whom he married in 1825, was a daughter of the French physician Curtet. Initially, Quetelet was a traditional mathematician who in 1819 was the first to receive a doctorate at the newly established University of Ghent. In 1820 he was appointed professor of mathematics at the Athenaeum in Brussels. His interests ranged much wider than his chosen field. He wrote plays, composed an opera, and published a history of mathematics and the natural sciences in Belgium.

As a result of his growing interest in astronomy and meteorology, he proposed the foundation of an observatory in Brussels. In 1823 he went to Paris to gain experience in practical astronomy. Through his contacts with famous French mathematicians such as Pierre Simon de Laplace and Jean Baptiste Joseph Fourier, he became acquainted with probability theory. This influence proved to be decisive for Quetelet's whole life. Following their example, Quetelet tried to relate population figures to probabilities. He developed the idea of applying the 'error curve', or bell curve—the probability distribution of measurement errors, which was well-known in astronomy—to a variety of biological data. As a result, he arrived at the conclusion that this distribution—to become known as the normal distribution—could be applied very broadly.

To Quetelet, the 'average man'—the man who had the mean value for every quality—was the characteristic, even ideal person. He was the center of gravity of society. Quetelet advocated a new science of society, a kind of quantitative sociology, which he called social physics (*physique sociale*), in which this average man would be the focus of study. In 1835 he published *Sur l'homme et le développement de ses facultés. Essai de physique sociale,* through which he became internationally famous. An extended edition appeared in 1869.

He also studied the moral qualities of men. Crime figures, such as the number of murders, but also the number of suicides, could be used to determine the moral quality of a country, because they turned out to be stable. Quetelet's idea was that each nation could be characterized by the tendency to crime (*penchant au crime*), and therefore the moral quality of different nations could be compared.

Quetelet was involved in the founding of the English Royal Statistical Society, and took the initiative of organizing international statistical congresses, the first of which was held in 1853 in Brussels. He was very influential in the sanitary movement; Florence Nightingale, who used statistical arguments to convince politicians to improve the medical and hygienic circumstances of soldiers, was among his many admirers.

In medicine, the importance now attributed to the so-called 'normal values' of substances in the human body, especially in blood, reflects Quetelet's perception of the importance of the mean. Quetelet demonstrated that body weight divided by the square of body length is relatively constant. This Quetelet Index (QI), or Body Mass Index (BMI), is now used as an indicator of obesity.

Bibliography

Primary: 1829. *Recherches statistiques sur le royaume des Pays-Bas* (Brussels); 1835. *Sur l'homme et le développement de ses facultés. Essai de physique sociale* 2 vols. (Paris) [English edn., 1842 *A Treatise on Man and the Development of His Faculties* (Edinburgh)]; 1869. *Physique sociale ou Essai sur le dévelopment des facultés de l'homme* (Brussels) [reprint, 1997, Vilquin, Éric, and Jean-Paul Sanderson, eds. (Brussels)].

Secondary: Stigler, Stephen M., 1999. *Statistics on the Table: The History of Statistical Concepts and Methods* (Cambridge, MA) esp. pp. 51–65; Lottin, Joseph, 1912. *Quetelet, statisticien et sociologue* (Louvain) [reprint 1969, New York]; Hankins, Frank H., 1908. *Quetelet as a Statistician* (New York); *DSB.*

Ida H. Stamhuis

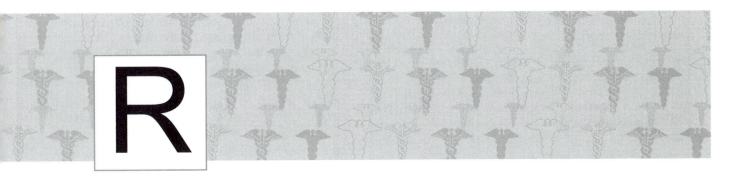

R

RABINOWITSCH-KEMPNER, LYDIA (b. Kowno, Lithuania, 22 August 1871; d. Berlin, Germany, 3 August 1935), *bacteriology.*

Rabinowitsch was the youngest of nine children of a Jewish brewery owner in Lithuania, which was a part of Russia at the time of her birth. As a girl she had two experiences of lasting biographical importance. Frequent poverty and starvation in the rural area around Kowno taught her that health problems, tuberculosis (TB) in particular, could only be fully understood and combated through the social and economic backgrounds of those who suffered from such diseases. In 1881 she experienced the pogroms that were triggered by Tsar Alexander's assassination. For her, the year 1933 was a recurrence of such events.

After her father's death in 1883, Rabinowitsch's mother supported her school and university education. From 1889 on, she studied a variety of subjects in Zurich and Bern, and in 1894 received a doctoral degree for a microbiological study on *gastromycetes.* Immediately thereafter she became an (unpaid) employee in Robert Koch's Institut für Infektionskrankheiten in Berlin, where she was to spend most of her time till 1903. Here Rabinowitsch made contributions in a variety of fields, but finally concentrated on TB and, in particular, on issues related to its transmission from animals to humans. This made her an important collaborator of Koch. During the 1890s she had two one-year stays at the Women's Medical College in Pennsylvania, where she was the head of the bacte-

riological laboratory and was offered a professorship in 1898. That same year, however, Rabinowitsch married colleague Walter Kempner, turned down the offer, and settled in Berlin. Her career in Koch's institute was terminated in 1903 mainly for two reasons: when Koch renounced his earlier views on the identity of bovine and human TB in 1902, Rabinowitsch, the expert on the transmission of the disease from one to the other, found herself in dissent. Although this seems to have left the personal relations intact, there seem to have been intrigues by others. In 1903, while Koch was absent in Africa, a group of institute members succeeded in having her expelled. Koch, after his return, was either unwilling or unable to reverse this step. Rabinowitsch continued her work in Johannes Orth's institute for pathology at Berlin University. Orth, a pupil of Rudolf Virchow, was one of Koch's most prominent critics in the debates on tuberculosis.

In the twentieth century, Rabinowitsch made herself a name as an expert on TB and social hygiene in general. She became a member of important scientific and medical societies, and from 1914 to 1934 was editor of the prestigious *Zeitschrift für Tuberkulose.* From about 1900 on, she fought an endless battle for the bacteriological examination of milk and butter. After her husband's death in 1920, Rabinowitsch finally took a paid position as the director of a bacteriological laboratory in a municipal hospital in Berlin. In these years she continued her intense scientific and political activities. She promoted university education for women, emphasized the role that well-informed mothers played in the successful combating of TB, and was a strong supporter of Calmette's BCG inoculation. Following the National Socialists' takeover of power in 1933, she was removed from office in 1934. Her son, Robert Kempner, who was a stout republican lawyer, was arrested in 1935. He emigrated after his release, and after the war returned as one of the prosecutors in the Nuremberg trials. Rabinowitsch, who suffered from cancer, died in the summer of 1935.

Bibliography

Primary: 1894. *Beitrag zur Entwicklungsgeschichte der Fruchtkörper einiger Gastromyzeten* (Bern); 1900. 'Über die Gefahr der Übertragung der Tuberkulose durch Milch und Milchprodukte.' *Deutsche Medizinische Wochenschrift* 26: 416–419.

Secondary: 2003. Dokumentation: Ärztinnen im Kaiserreich, Freie Universität Berlin, Institut für Geschichte der Medizin, http://userpage.fu-berlin.de/~elehmus/; Bleker, Johanna, and Sabine Schleiermacher, 2000. *Ärztinnen aus dem Kaiserreich. Lebensläufe einer Generation* (Weinheim); Graffmann-Weschke, Katharina, 1999. *Lydia Rabinowitsch-Kempner (1871–1935). Leben und Werk einer der führenden Persönlichkeiten der Tuberkuloseforschung am Anfang des 20. Jahrhunderts* (Herdecke).

Christoph Gradmann

RAJCHMAN, LUDWIK WITOLD (b. Warsaw, Poland, 1 November 1881; d. Chenu, France, 31 August 1965), *public health.*

Rajchman was undoubtedly one of the most important figures of international public health in the first half of the twentieth century, and he also played a crucial part in Polish reconstruction after both world wars. Besides his role as an advocate of UNICEF, he can be considered the spiritual father of the World Health Organization (WHO). Born into a prominent assimilated Jewish family, Rajchman was the son of Aleksander, founder of the Warsaw Philharmonic, and Melania Hirszfeld, a well-known feminist. He himself was involved in Polish national and social causes from an early age. He completed his medical degree in Cracow (1905), specializing in bacteriology and working with Odon Bujwid.

In 1906 Rajchman returned to Warsaw to engage in hospital practice but was arrested by the Russians for socialist activities and exiled to Kazan, from where he escaped to Paris. He pursued his bacteriological studies at the Pasteur Institute (1907–09), working with Elie Mechnikov, Constantin Levaditi, and Antoine Borrel. After a short return to Cracow (1909–10), where he lectured in microbiology and worked in Jan Nowak's laboratory, Rajchman moved to London (1910–18), lecturing first at the Royal Institute of Public Health, then at Kings College (working with William Bulloch). With the outbreak of World War I, he devoted himself to epidemio-logical research at the Medical Research Committee (later Council).

Just before the armistice, Rajchman went back to Poland and established the National Institute of Hygiene [Panstwowy Zaklad Higieny] in 1918, and subsequently a School of Hygiene in 1923. The National Institute of Hygiene attracted prominent Polish microbiologists such as Ludwik Hirszfeld (Rajchman's first cousin) and Casimir Funk. In 1921 Rajchman was named first director of the League of Nations Health Organization. Far from limiting its scope to the control of infectious diseases, Rajchman and his team brought issues of preventive medicine, chronic illness, biological standardization, and health insurance to the forefront of international health.

As a prominent anti-appeaser, Rajchman was dismissed from the League in December 1938 and set out to help nationalist China (where he had been involved in public health projects) reinforce her air force. In September 1939 Rajchman was named commissar for humanitarian affairs by the Polish government in exile and traveled to the United States, where he remained for the next ten years (1940–50). Once the United States entered the war and help for Polish civilians became impossible, Rajchman worked once again with the Chinese, before being called upon to act as consultant in public health for the United Nations Relief and Rehabilitation Administration (UNRRA). He was subsequently named Polish delegate to UNRRA (1944) and participated in the Potsdam conference.

When the United States announced its withdrawal from UNRRA (July 1946), Rajchman proposed the creation of a United Nations International Children's Emergency Fund to provide aid for European and Chinese war-ravaged children. UNICEF was officially established on 11 December 1946, with the political support of Herbert Hoover. Within UNICEF Rajchman launched four major programs: BCG vaccination, production and distribution of powdered milk, access to antibiotics, and DDT (to prevent typhus, one of the major scourges of the previous world war).

The Cold War made Rajchman's position uncomfortable as a Polish national living in the United States and chairman of a prominent UN organization. He was obliged to leave the United States in the wake of McCarthyism, at the same time that Stalinist Poland withdrew his diplomatic passport. He settled in France (1950) and established, with Robert Debré, the International Children's Center in Paris. After 1956 Rajchman retrieved his Polish passport and visited his homeland for the last time in 1963 to mark the forty-fifth anniversary of the National Institute of Hygiene.

Rajchman believed firmly that health was a universal value that must be placed above national interests. He also continuously stressed the responsibility of states for the well-being of their citizens. For him, securing the basic conditions for health and international collaboration were ultimately the surest guarantee for peace.

Bibliography

Primary: 1943. 'A United Nations Health Service: Why Not?' *Free World*, September.

Secondary: Balinska, M. A., 2000. 'A Biographical Sketch of a Polish Jew.' *Polin* 13: 373–382; Balinska, M. A., 1998. *For the Good of Humanity: Ludwik Rajchman, Medical Statesman* (Budapest) [originally published 1995 as *Une vie pour l'humanitaire: Ludwik Rajchman* (Paris)]; Debré, R., 1965. 'Ludwik Rajchman.' *Médecine et enfance*, Sept.–Dec.

Marta Aleksandra Balinska

RAKHMABAI (aka RUKHMABAI) (b. Bombay [now Mumbai], India, 22 November 1864; d. Bombay, 25 December 1955), *medicine.*

Rakhmabai (who used only this name) was the only child of Jayantibai and Janardan Pandurang Save, a civil contractor. Widowed after three years of marriage, Jayantibai married Sakharam Arjun, Assistant Surgeon at the J. J. Hospital, Bombay, in 1870. Arjun was one of the leading surgeons of Bombay, well-known for his eclectic research interests and reformist views. They had three sons and a daughter. Rakhmabai remained under the guardianship of her stepfather from the age of six until his death when she was nineteen.

In 1875 Rakhmabai was married off to a distant relative, Dadajee Bhikaji, at the age of eleven, though she remained in her stepfather's household. In 1883, when Dadajee requested her to return to her marital household, she refused. A court case followed: Dadajee demanded 'restitution of conjugal rights', but Rakhmabai was adamant. Public support for Rakhmabai was elicited in England and India, and a Rakhmabai Protection Committee formed to defend her case at the Privy Council in London. In 1887 Dadajee agreed to an out-of-court settlement and gave up his claims to Rakhmabai.

Free to pursue her long-cherished desire for a medical education, the twenty-two-year-old Rakhmabai went to London on a scholarship, the first Indian woman to do so. Edith Pechey Phipson, Chief Medical Officer at Cama Women's Hospital, Bombay, was her greatest supporter, even arranging for her stay in London at the McLaren household, Rakhmabai's guardians throughout her stay in England. In London, Rakhmabai developed a long and enduring friendship with Alice (first wife of Bertrand Russell).

She completed the mandatory one-year course in arts from Bradford College, Cambridge, and became proficient in English. In October 1890 Rakhmabai entered The London School of Medicine for Women and passed her first two examinations in medicine in 1891and 1892. Her clinical training was at the Royal Free Hospital, London. She also undertook a special study of midwifery and gynecology for two months at the Rotanda Hospital, Dublin, and passed the Operative Midwifery Examination of the London School of Medicine. Success at the LRCP, LRCS (Edinburgh), and LFPS (Glasgow) examinations in 1894 meant Rakhmabai's name (spelled Rukhmabai) was formally included in the British Medical Register. She gained an MD from Brussels the same year.

Upon her return to India, Rakhmabai started her practice as a house surgeon at the Cama Hospital on 16 February 1895. Her life remained constantly in the glare of the media, curiosity having been created by her dramatic court case, which followed her to England and back again. By December 1895 Rakhmabai had moved to the Morarbhai Vajrabhushandas Malawi Hospital, Surat (now known as the Rakhmabai Hospital). Rakhmabai worked toward popularizing the idea of delivery at maternity hospitals within conservative Gujarati society. She carried out a successful delivery of a pregnant sheep at the hospital and arranged for press coverage, thereby ensuring an emphatic victory for the cause of maternity hospitals. Upon the outbreak of an influenza epidemic in Surat, Rakhmabai offered her services free of charge and in 1918 was presented with the Kaiser-I-Hind medal. In the same year, she opened a branch of the Red Cross and started a training course for nurses. Her successful medical practice and devotion made many people affectionately refer to her as 'bai' ('sister' in Gujarati).

In 1918 she accepted the post of chief doctor for the provinces of Kutch and Saurashtra at the Rasulkalji Janaana Hospital, Rajkot. Her reputation for healing and helping made women in an advanced stage of pregnancy from all over Saurashtra come to Rajkot.

At a time when hospital visits for women were particularly tabooed, Rakhmabai's decision to study medicine and serve her countrywomen stands as a shining example of one of the most remarkable medical women of India.

Bibliography

Secondary: Varde, Mohini, 2000. *Dr Rakhmabai. An Odyssey* (New Delhi).

Namrata R. Ganneri

RAMALINGASWAMI, VULMIRI (b. Srikakulam, Andhra Pradesh, India, 8 August 1921; d. Delhi, India, 28 May 2001), *pathology.*

Ramalingaswami came from a family of educators. He went to school in Bobbili, a small town in southern India. He attended A. V. N. College and, later, Andhra Medical College in Visakapatnam, where he took his MBBS degree in 1944. He took his MD from Andhra University in 1946.

Ramalingaswami began his research career at the Nutrition Research Laboratory in Coonoor in southern India, with his pioneering study of the role of essential fatty acids on phrynoderma, a clinical dermatological problem of nutritional origin. He was deputed by his institution to go to Oxford for specialized training in nutritional pathology under the supervision of Hugh Sinclair. He was awarded a

DPhil in 1951. While in England he came into contact with Sir Robert McCarrison, whose work on Himalayan goiter was to remain a lifetime inspiration. Ramalingaswami returned to Coonoor and set up a collaborative study that developed a model of nutritional anemia in primates. The pathology of malnutrition remained one of Ramalingaswami's most important areas of research.

Impressed by Ramalingaswami's potential, C. G. Pandit, at that time Secretary of the Indian Council of Medical Research (ICMR), offered him the position of senior research officer at the ICMR in Delhi. There he continued with clinical research, working on the epidemiology and pathology of the hepatitis epidemic in Delhi (1954). Ramalingaswami played an active role in drawing up the Health Plans for India from 1955 onward.

Ramalingaswami's vision was responsible for the creation of a statistical unit within the ICMR and the Indian Registry of Pathology. In 1957 Ramalingaswami was appointed research professor in pathology in the newly founded All India Institute of Medical Sciences (AIIMS). At AIIMS his study of a new clinical entity, non-cirrhotic portal fibrosis, also known as Indian childhood cirrhosis, contributed to a complex understanding of this fatal form of liver disease. During this period, his earlier interest in iodine metabolism returned. His study of Himalayan goiter, cretinism, and mental retardation paved the way for the National Goitre Control Programme through the iodization of common salt. He also worked on the pathological and physiological dimensions of protein energy malnutrition, which directed the measures adopted by the government of India to rehabilitate and provide nutritional protection to victims of the Bihar famine in 1967 and to the millions of refugees from Bangladesh in 1970–71.

Ramalingaswami soon took on the responsibility of professor and head of pathology and introduced procedural changes that made optimal use of clinical and medicolegal autopsies. As a medical educator, he facilitated scientific interaction by inviting scientists from the West to spend time at AIIMS. In 1969 he became the director of AIIMS. He served as the director-general of ICMR from 1979 to 1986.

Ramalingaswami was awarded a DSc by Oxford University in 1967 and the Lion Bernard Foundation award in 1976 by the WHO, an organization he served in several capacities throughout his life. He was a Fogarty Fellow in the late 1980s and, after that, special professor of toxicology at Harvard. He was elected FRS in 1986.

Throughout his life Ramalingaswami continued to synthesize laboratory, clinical, and community-based research. He also initiated research on HIV in India. His involvement in national policy gave direction to medical research at a time when large-scale health programs were not common in India.

Bibliography

Primary: 1967. 'Cell Regeneration in Protein Deficiency.' *Nature* 216(114): 499–500; 1969. 'Interface of Protein Nutrition and Medicine in the Tropics.' *Lancet* ii: 733–736; 1972. (with Nayak, N. C., S. Visalakshi, M. Singh, V. Chawla, and R. K. Chandra) 'Indian Childhood Cirrhosis—A Re-evaluation of Its Pathomorphologic Features and Their Significance in the Light of Clinical Data and Natural History of the Disease.' *The Indian Journal of Medical Research* 60(2): 246–259.

Secondary: Sriramachari, S., 2001. 'Professor V. Ramalingaswami (1921–2001).' *Indian Journal of Medical Research* 113: iii–vii; Anand Kumar, T. C., 2001. 'V. Ramalingaswami: An Obituary.' *Current Science* 80(12): 1599.

Indira Chowdhury

RAMAZZINI, BERNARDINO (b. Carpi, Italy, 4 October 1633; d. Padua, Italy, 5 November 1714), *medicine, epidemiology, occupational medicine.*

Ramazzini was the second of five brothers. His first biographer was the son of one of these brothers, Bartolomeo Ramazzini, a doctor whose second wife was the sister of the famous historian and man of letters Ludovico Antonio Muratori (1672–1750). Bernardino started his studies under the Jesuits in his hometown and then moved to Parma, where in 1659 he received degrees in philosophy and medicine.

He studied medicine in Rome under Antonio Maria de' Rossi (1588–1671) and then took a practice in the Duchy of Castro near Viterbo until April 1663. Then, after coming down with malaria, which was common in that region, he went back to Carpi, where he married in 1665. Ramazzini and his wife had four children, but two of them, both sons, died young, and his older daughter never had children. Thus, his younger daughter Gismonda was the only one who had offspring. Three of her sons lived with their grandfather in Padua, assisting him in the last years of his life as readers and amanuenses.

In Carpi, Ramazzini combined private practice with an active cultural life as a member of the local Accademia degli Apparenti.

Modena

In 1676 Ramazzini and his family moved to Modena, where he gained a solid reputation at the court of Duca Francesco II d'Este (1660–94) as a physician and a scholar. He was given the professorship in medicine at the newly refounded University of Modena. There he met Francesco Torti (1658–1741), who taught in Modena (from 1685) with a particular focus on physiology and hygiene. In 1690 Ramazzini, who had already stopped working on his comments on the Hippocratic texts, turned his attention to work-related diseases. In 1691 Ramazzini and Torti were named 'court doctors'.

In the short, intense period between 1690 and 1700, Ramazzini published literary texts, accusatory essays against other doctors, and many scientific studies on clinical and epidemiological subjects. Some of these essays would later be reprinted with the recommendation of Gottfried Wilhelm Leibniz (1646–1716) by the Caesareo-Leopoldina Academia Naturae Curiosorum. This institution soon took Ramazzini, with the name of Ippocrate III, into its ranks. Some of Ramazzini's studies—for example *De costitutione Anni M.DC.LXXXX ac de rurali epidemia, quae mutinensi agri epidemica . . .*, *De costitutione Anni M.DC.LXXXXI apud mutinenses dissertatio*, and *De costitutione Annorum M.DC.XCII, XCIII, et XCIV in mutinensis civitate et illius ditione dissertatio*, which was written in 1695—studied the relationship between man and his surroundings, considering the influence that factors such as temperature, barometric pressure, humidity, and winds had on man's health.

Some of his other essays discussed physics and geophysics: the *De fontium mutinensium admiranda scaturigine Tractatus physico-hydrostaticus* (1691), the *Ephemerides barometricae mutinesis* (1695), and the *Francisci Ariosti de Oleo Montis Zibinii, seu Petroleo agri mutinensis libellus* (1698). Other works of the same period treated the relationship between society and work and how they both influenced workers' health.

Workers' Disease

The *De morbis artificum diatriba* [*Diseases of Workers*] (1700) took at least ten years to write. This publication dealt with a subject related to Ramazzini's medical practice and to teaching. One can easily recognize that this work grew from his observations, as a district doctor, on the diseases of the poor and of craftsmen and from the contact he had with workers while doing geophysical field research. For example, one day he observed a workman hurrying to empty a septic tank as rapidly as possible and asked him questions, which the worker answered quite candidly. The worker explained that he worked at such speed in order to diminish the length of exposure to the exhalations of the septic tank, since they caused him such serious ocular irritations that, when he came home, he had to stay in the dark for twenty-four hours and needed to wash his eyes with warm water continuously. He also told Ramazzini that he expected sooner or later to go blind or semi-blind, like many of the people who plied his trade.

Ramazzini divided the risk factors for workers into two main classes: the first one for the noxious effects of the substances handled and of the byproducts of the work process; and the second one for the repetitious movements and the unhealthy stances required by the job. For each of more than fifty types of jobs under consideration, the author set up norms for analyzing the risks. They included a description of the technology and the raw materials used; examination, using strict clinical criteria, of the people currently at work and of ones that had done the same job in the past; surveys of the existing literature; discussion of the therapy, about the individual protective measures and about

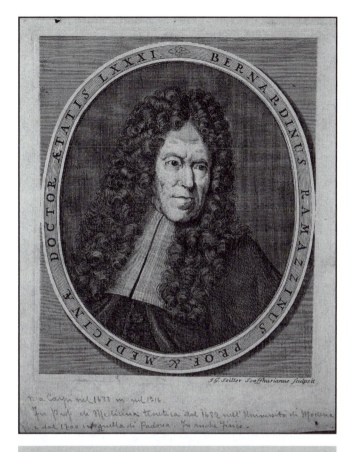

Bernadino Ramazzini. Line engraving by J. G. Seiller, 1716. Iconographic Collection, Wellcome Library, London.

reclaiming land; and proposals for norms of good practice, personal, and social behavior both for individuals and for government, which would substitute traditional codes of behavior that were being abandoned.

Each one of these chapters was written in easily understood, but somewhat affected, Latin. Ramazzini often used citations drawn from every field of knowledge, adding sarcastic and humorous notes. He defined, in essence, the standards for describing poisoning due to exposure to various types of metal and, particularly, for mercury and lead contamination observed in metal miners, gilders, potters, ceramists, tinsmiths, and glassmakers. The symptoms of saturnism (chronic lead poisoning) are described in the biography of the Italian painter Antonio Allegri, known as Correggio (1489/1494–1534), who suffered from pallor and depression. Other workers suffered from exposure to high concentrations of mineral or vegetable dust; this was true for plasterers and lime workers, tobacco workers, bakers and millers, stone cutters, as well as workers who handled flax, hemp, and silk. In order to limit the effects of such exposure (including the asthma due to breathing dust from organic sources, which he described in great depth), the author suggested that such work should be done in large, open spaces, that workers should turn their backs to the wind, wash out their mouths frequently with water and vinegar, and leave their jobs as soon as they came down with pulmonary disease. A whole chapter of his study dealt with corpse bearers, since Ramazzini felt that 'We must safeguard the health of corpse bearers, whose services are so necessary, and because it is only fair, seeing that they bury not only the dead but the doctor's mistakes as well, that the art of medicine should do them a good turn and repay them for saving the reputation of our profession.' (Ramazzini, 1964, p. 157). Workers who stand; sedentary workers who make minute objects, such as goldsmiths and carvers; lackeys; shoemakers; tailors; potters and weavers; porters; athletes; voice trainers; and singers were studied with precise reference to muscular and skeletal ailments. Ramazzini noted, 'It is an ironic sight to see those guilds of cobblers and tailors on their own special feast days when they march in procession two by two through the city or when they escort a member of their guild who has died to the tomb. Indeed; it makes one laugh to see that troop of stooping, round shouldered, limping men swaying from side to side; they look as though they had all been carefully selected for an exhibition on these infirmities' (Ramazzini, 1964, p. 283).

Ramazzini lived to see a new edition of the *De morbis artificum diatriba*, a 'Supplement' published in 1713 that added thirteen new chapters, including ones concerning printers, weavers, carpenters, razor sharpeners, brickmakers, sailors and rowers, hunters, soapmakers, and nuns. Ramazzini noticed a high incidence of breast cancer in nuns and, in general, in women who were virgins, which would be confirmed in later epidemiological studies.

Few medical studies can match *De morbis artificum diatriba*'s editorial success story. This publication has been republished, imitated, and translated into a great number of languages many times. It was one of the most frequently cited texts in the past and is still consulted today.

Padua

In 1700 Ramazzini was given a position at the University of Padua. Although his publications brought him little income, in this period Ramazzini reached a certain level of economic security thanks to his work as a doctor and to teaching. He invested money in agricultural property near Modena. He also received many academic honors: in 1704 he became a member of the society of the Arcadi with the academic name of 'Licoro Langiano'; in 1707 he was admitted to the Societas regia scientiarum in Berlin on the recommendation of its president, Leibniz; in 1708 he was elected to the Collegio dei filosofi e dei medici; and for three years, from 1708 to 1711, he was president of the Collegio degli artisti.

During his Paduan period, Ramazzini also produced a great number of important scientific studies, including the fifteen inaugural *Orationes*, academic essays mostly of a philosophical nature. In the *Oratio saecularis*, written on 12 December 1700, he discussed the progress of medicine during the seventeenth century and emphasized the important developments of his time. In the 1711 *Oratio*, he dealt with public health issues concerning bovine epizooty, which was rife in the countryside around Padua that year. He recognized the sick animals as the prime causes of this infection, confuting the hypotheses that linked the disease to the nature of the pastures and the air or to the influence of stars. He suggested that the corpses of animals should be buried. In this essay appeared the much cited sentence '. . . longe praestantius est praeservare, quam curare, sicuti satius est tempestatem praevidere, ac illam effuggere, quam ab ipsa evadere' [It's better preventing than curing, as it's better previewing a storm than escaping when it's already begun] (Ramazzini, 1742, p. 103). In his last *Oratio*, written in 1714, the year of his death, Ramazzini insisted that doctors must widen their cultural horizons by travel and contact with other scholars

De principum valetudinem tuenda commentatio (1710) is a sort of second monographic supplement to *De morbis artificum diatriba*. However, it is more of a dissertation on the health of men of letters than a study comparable to the ones he wrote about the health of workers involved in manual labor. It presents far more research done using a clearer physiopathological approach and more in-depth descriptions of the complexity and specificity of the risk factors.

During the last year of his life, Ramazzini published *Dissertatio de abusu chinae chinae*, a work of medical criticism, and *Annotationes in librum Ludovici Cornelii de vitae sobriae commodes* (1714). In the latter, he wrote medical annotations for each paragraph of the famous pamphlet, correcting its inaccuracies and overstatements, as an attempt to turn it into a true treatise of personal hygiene.

In 1705 Ramazzini experienced the first symptoms of an eye ailment that would gradually lead to blindness. He also had cerebral vascular problems, which caused, during the last years of his life, several attacks witnessed by Giovanni Battista Morgagni, his personal doctor and university colleague. Morgagni also diagnosed the cerebral hemorrhage that invaded Ramazzini's ventricles one day while he was going to teach a class at the University and killed him twelve hours later.

Bibliography

Primary: 1742. *Opera Omnia* (London); 1700. *De morbis artificum diatriba* (Modena); 1713. *De morbis artificum diatriba nunc accedit supplementum eiusdem argumenti, ac dissertatio de sacrarum virginum valetudine tuenda* (Padua); 1713. *De principum valetudine tuenda commentatio* (Padua); 1964. *Diseases of Workers* (translated from the Latin text, *De morbis artificum*, of 1713 by Wright, Wilmer Cave) (New York).

Secondary: Carnevale, Francesco, and Alberto Baldasseroni, 2000. 'The *De Morbis Artificum Diatriba* Editions since 1700 and Their Heritage.' *Epidemiologia e Prevenzione* 6: 270–275; Franco, Giuliano, 2000. 'Ramazzini's "De Morbis Artificum Diatriba" and Society, Culture, and the Human Condition in the Seventeenth

Century.' *International Journal of Occupational and Environmental Health* 6: 80–85; Zocchetti, Carlo, 2000. 'Bernardino Ramazzini (1633–1714) Epidemiologo ante litteram.' *Epidemiologia e Prevenzione* 6: 276–281; Di Pietro, Pericle, 1999. 'Bernardino Ramazzini, Biography and bibliography.' *European Journal of Oncology* 4: 253–317; Felton, Jean S., 1997. 'The Heritage of Bernardino Ramazzini.' *Occupational Medicine* 47: 167–179; Maggiora Vergano, Arnaldo, 1933. 'Nel III centenario della nascita di Bernardino Ramazzini.' *Rassegna di Medicina Applicata al Lavoro Industriale* 4: 449–496.

Franco Carnevale

RAMÓN Y CAJAL, SANTIAGO   (b. Petilla de Aragón, Navarra, Spain, 1 May 1852; d. Madrid, Spain, 17 October 1934), *histology, neurology.*

The son of a rural surgeon, Cajal attended secondary school at Jaca and Huesca, and pursued medical studies at the University of Zaragoza, where he graduated in 1873. After graduation he obtained a post as physician in the army, took part in the campaigns in Catalonia, and went to Cuba where a colonial war was taking place. He came back to Spain in 1875, affected by malaria. His father persuaded him to return to the University of Madrid to pass the doctorate courses. Under Areliano Maestre de San Juan and Leopoldo López García, he was introduced to histology, a discipline that attracted him more than any other. Convinced that he desired an academic career, he failed in his first attempt to obtain a chair in 1880, but three years later was appointed to the chair of anatomy in Valencia. During the following four years he focused on neurohistological research, and started the publication of a handbook of histology in 1884. In 1887 he visited some micrography laboratories in Madrid, and learned from Luis Simarro the chrome-silver impregnation method introduced by Camillo Golgi.

In 1887 the medical syllabus changed at the Spanish universities, and histology was moved from the doctorate to the graduate level. New chairs were promoted, and Cajal moved first to Barcelona (1887) and then to Madrid (1892), where he occupied the chair in histology until his retirement. In 1901 Cajal was appointed director of the Laboratorio de Investigaciones Biológicas [Laboratory of Biological Research], later called Instituto Cajal to acknowledge the international dimension of his work, crowned in 1906 by the Nobel Prize he shared with Golgi.

From Reticularism to the Neuron Theory

It is accepted that Otto F. K. Deiters defined the basic constitution of the nervous cell as consisting of a body (or soma) containing the nucleus, and the protoplasmic expansions—dendrites and axons, in the terminology of Wilhelm His. Although the first experiments of Albrecht von Kölliker during the 1840s focused on the independence of nerve cells and suggested an anatomical autonomy, the prevailing image of the nervous structure since the beginning of the 1870s was the reticular theory postulated by Joseph von Gerlach. Using observations based on a chloride of gold staining material, Gerlach observed a continuity among the terminal fibers of dendrites and those of the neighbor cells, and interpreted the gray substance of the nervous centers as a complex network consisting of joined dendrites and the last branches of neurites.

Some years later, Gerlach's theory was modified by the Italian Camillo Golgi. He applied a new, original tincture technique, the so-called 'black reaction', a chrome-silver impregnation, to his investigations of the structure of the gray brain substance, cerebellum, olfactory lobes, and others, from 1873. A decade later he proposed the hypothesis of a slight network spread through the gray substance in the nervous centers. Instead of a continuity of dendrites, as stated by Gerlach, Golgi observed that they were free, but a union at the level of the neurites seemed to exist.

Although reticularism was the prevailing theory at the moment, it was not an unquestioned doctrine. A certain number of outstanding neurohistologists proposed a set of coherent proofs against the reticular model advocated by Gerlach and Golgi. In 1886 Wilhelm His gave the histogenetic basis for the independence of the nervous cell and, one year later, August Forel contradicted Golgi's results, inasmuch as his experiences showed a completely free termination also in the case of neurites.

This was the time and the scientific context in which Cajal began his most significant research. Recently appointed professor at the University of Barcelona (1887), Cajal modified Golgi's tincture method—the silver staining technique—in the sense of a 'double impregnation', which allowed him to obtain clear and persistent images of the nervous structures. A second point was the decisive factor: he adopted an 'ontogenetic method and perspective'; i.e., he applied the new techniques to embryos—mainly bird and mammalian—not to adults, since he thought that the fundamental histological plan of composition of the gray substance is better drawn and easier to investigate during the stages of development of the embryo. At this time Cajal was a fervent follower of Darwinian ideas on evolution. As a member of the scientific community, he took part in some of the controversies, but he always preserved a microscopic and histological approach to the constitution of the brain substance, and never took part in scientific debates around other questions such as the structures of the brain, or the problem of brain localizations.

The Dynamic Polarization of Neuron Cells and the Histology of the Nervous Centers

During his period in Barcelona (1888–92) Cajal was especially active, publishing almost fifty papers and founding a journal, the *Revista Trimestral de Histología Normal y Patológica* [Quarterly Journal of Normal and Pathological Histology], with the principal aim of publishing the results of his observations about the structural organization of the nerve tissues. The first contributions focused on the cerebellum molecular coat, where he could never observe the reticular frame described by Gerlach and Golgi. His observations brought him to a firm conviction about the absolute independence of each nerve cell as a physiological unit.

Aware that this argument contradicted the reticularist perspective, Cajal brought forward new features, exploring other cerebellum regions and parts of the retina. He proposed finally as a hypothesis the possibility that the transmission of the nerve actions could be not by continuity of the dendrites' and neurites' terminal branches, but by contact or contiguity—i.e., by means of a sort of inductive phenomenon able to transfer the nerve impulse through the surrounding substance from cell to cell. Following an imaginative plan of research, he began his investigation of the cerebellum and retina. This new plan had advantages that helped to explain certain problems of form and relation among ganglion corpuscles. Cajal proceeded with investigating the nerve structures in the brain centers and the spinal cord.

In 1888 some of Cajal's papers relating to the nerve centers of birds showed that there was no strong evidence for a nerve net in the central nervous system. The same idea was verified when investigating the structure of the cerebellum. He stated, 'We have made careful investigations of the course and connections of the nerve fibers in the cerebral and cerebellar convolutions of man, dog, etc. and have never seen an anastomosis between ramifications of two different protoplasmic expansions' (Cajal, 1888, p. 450).

In 1889 Cajal was awarded membership in the German Society of Anatomy, and in the same year he took part for the first time in an international congress in Berlin. Cajal showed his neurohistological preparations and received the indifference and incredulity of the majority of the participants. Nevertheless, he managed to attract the attention of Albrecht von Kölliker and convinced him of the importance of his discoveries and the possibilities of the new tincture methods. A few months later, Kölliker could confirm Cajal's contributions. One of the German professors present at his demonstration was Wilhelm Gottfried von Waldeyer, head of the Berlin Anatomical Institute, who helped Cajal two years later in the publication of a series of brief articles in the *Deutsche medizinische Wochenschrift*. In this publication Cajal summarized the evidence of the neuronist point of view. These facts were decisive for the international diffusion of his work, and the acceptance of his new conception of the structure of the nervous tissue stimulated his enthusiastic devotion to research.

Further contributions based on embryological research led Cajal to conclude that 'the neuroblast, primitive nerve cell, generates the nerves through the emission of a bud or appendix, the *axon*, which grows through the other tissues until the terminal structures, where it finishes in independent ramifications' (Cajal, 1923, p. 223). Following his

observations of the retina, cerebellum, spinal cord, and olfactory bulb, Cajal attributed to the dendrites and the neuron body the role of receptor and conductor, inasmuch as those elements are concerned with the terminal branches of other neurons' axons. He summarized his points of view in 1891 in a general explanation, reviewed in 1897 as the 'law of the dynamic polarization of neurons', stating that 'The transmission of the nerve movement always takes place starting from the protoplasmic branches and the cell soma into the axis cylinder or functional expansion. Each neuron cell owns, then, an apparatus of reception, the soma or cell body, and the protoplasmic extensions, an apparatus for emission, the axis cylinder, and an apparatus of distribution, the terminal branching' (Cajal, 1894, p. 85).

Despite the enormous amount of research work undertaken by Cajal at the end of the 1880s and the beginning of the 1890s, he found time to write a handbook, *Manual de Anatomía Patológica* [Handbook of Pathology], intended for his medical students. His research focused on the structure of the mammalian brain cortex; he was attracted not only by its incredible complexity, but also by the perfect architectural plan and disposition of the nerve elements and their functionality. During this time Cajal observed a 'growth cone' in the spinal cord of chicken embryos after the third day of incubation, which confirmed His's neurogenetic conception.

Once he moved to Madrid in 1892, Cajal offered his first general views of the structure and functioning of the nervous system. In March 1892 he returned to Barcelona, and at the Acadèmia de Ciències Mèdiques de Catalunya [Medical Sciences Academy of Catalonia] gave a series of lectures which summarized his contributions to the understanding of the nervous system, later published in a medical journal under the title *Nuevo concepto de la histología de los centros nerviosos* [New concept of the histology of the nerve centers]. These lectures achieved great success and were translated into French and German. Taking the same perspective, he wrote several theoretical papers and *Consideraciones generales sobre la morfología de la célula nerviosa* [General considerations on the morphology of the nerve cell], submitted to the International Congress of Medicine held in Rome in 1894. In these papers he tried to furnish new evidence supporting Haeckel's fundamental biogenetics law, which related ontogeny to phylogenetic evolution of each particular species. He stated a law of morphological process, relating the functional adaptation of neuron cells to the settlement of new adaptive interneuronal connections, so that the most perfect functioning is seen as depending not on the quantity of cells, but on their functional ability to develop an upper associative capacity (1894).

The international reception of his work increased, and in 1894 Cajal was invited by Sir Charles S. Sherrington to read the Croonian Lecture at the Royal Society in London. He summarized his work and his ideas in French in a lecture entitled *La fine structure des centres nerveux* [The fine structure of the nervous centers]. This has been considered as a landmark paper in the history of neurosciences. Cajal stated that the connections established between fibers and the nerve cells take place by means of contact, i.e., with the help of genuine articulations. He offered as a general conclusion that 'the cells are polarized, that is to say, the nerve current always enters by way of the protoplasmic apparatus of the cellular body, and leaves it by the axis cylinder which transmits it to a new protoplasmic apparatus' (Cajal, 1894, p. 465).

Some years later Sherrington recognized the several aspects of Cajal's contributions: 'It is much to say of him that he is the greatest anatomist of the nervous system ever known. . . . He solved at a stroke the great question of the direction of the nerve current in its travel through brain and spinal cord. . . . The nerve circuits are valves, he said, and he was able to point out where the valves lie, namely where one nerve cell meets the next one' (cited in Smith, 1997, pp. 49–51).

The Texture of the Nervous System

In 1897 Cajal entered a new stage distinguished by his intellectual maturity, centering around an ambitious project consisting of a general exposition of all the neurological knowledge obtained supporting the independence of neuron cells. From this perspective he conceived his *Textura del sistema nervioso del hombre y los vertebrados* [Texture of the nervous system in man and vertebrates], published successively as a collection of booklets, a common literary genre in those days. According to Cajal's own testimony, this was to be considered his *opera magna,* or at least the most ambitious one, in which he proposed a global synthesis of the up-to-date knowledge in comparative neurohistology. In the *Textura* he made a thorough review of the research on the central and peripheral nervous system, summarizing in each chapter the prevailing theories and offering the results of his own work in the systematic application of Golgi's staining method. The perspective Cajal gave in his work is that of a follower of evolutionary morphology, inasmuch as he stated that the nervous system represents the last step in the evolution of living matter and, as a consequence, it is the most complex machine and the site of the most noble activities in nature. Cajal's *Textura* also demonstrated the intellectual influence of Herbert Spencer, an author he widely cited and commented upon, especially in the report presented by him to obtain the chair in Valencia (1884). Globally speaking, the *Textura* can be seen as the most significant Spanish-language contribution to contemporary science.

After publication of the *Textura* in 1904, Cajal was able to contribute to the comprehension of the nervous system in three basic aspects: (a) he collected a lot of evidence supporting the individuality of the neuron cells; (b) he described its phylogenetic evolution; and (c) he put forward an explanation of the structural functioning of the nervous system as a whole.

At the beginning of the twentieth century, new staining methods allowed neurohistologists to investigate in greater detail the internal structure of the nerve cell. The new features and the fibrous morphology of the nerve cells gave new arguments to the reticular theory which reappeared strongly, mainly supported by the contributions of Albrecht Bethe (1872–1954) in his investigations on neurofibrils in vertebrates. The main point of discussion was whether or not the protoplasmic fibrils, the so-called neurofibrils, were independent as elemental units composing the structure of the nervous system and conducting nerve impulses without intervention of the neuroplasma. Another important point was to determine the role of neurofibrils as a universal component of the neuron cells.

These new points of controversy stimulated Cajal to essay new methods of research. After many unsuccessful attempts, in 1903 he obtained a fruitful and encouraging method based on Simarro's staining technique, the so-called reduced silver nitrate method, the only one at the time that allowed him to color the neurofibrils clearly and permanently, showing two organizations: a compact network surrounding the neuron nucleus, and another soft one around the surface of the protoplasma following the dendrites and neurite fibrils. The new technique showed the nerve fibers as free tree-shaped endings stretching into the nerve centers, and their presence in even the smallest cells, like the cerebellum particles. It confirmed the existence of a neurofibrilar network in ganglion corpuscles of invertebrates and, at the same time, refuted the reality of interstitial networks.

The application of the reduced silver nitrate method characterizes a new period in Cajal's scientific research. One of the most relevant discoveries, achieved in collaboration with his pupils Tello and García Izcara, was the morphological variability of the neurofibrils under the effect of temperature and rabies virus, as evidence of the sharp sensibility felt when stimulated by physiological and pathological agents. Moreover, he analyzed motor and sensitive structures in bird embryos (something researched before only in mammals) and the optical reflex descending track of the quadrigeminal tuberculum in mammals; and he described, for the first time, the structure of the human sympathetic ganglia. Globally considered, the results obtained with this method allowed him to elucidate the controversy about the independence of neurofibrils, furnishing new evidence against the arguments of the new reticularists headed by Bethe, István Apáthy, and Max Bielschowsky. Cajal's work demonstrated that the faculty of conducting impulses is located in the neuroplasma, and not in the neurofibrils.

Regeneration and Degeneration of Nerves

Between 1905 and 1907, Cajal focused his investigations on the regeneration and degeneration of nerves, and on the neurogenetic process developed in embryos. Although after the work of Bethe it was widely accepted that the regenerative faculty of the nervous fibers, previously divided, could restore their functionality, Cajal showed the unfailing degeneration of the divided nerve. He saw how its regeneration was always due to new fibers originating from the axons of the central segment (body). Concerning neurogenesis, the new experiments verified his old discoveries since neuroblasts appeared to be free corpuscles endowed with a fundamental extension (axis cylinder), possessing a growth cone, which moves itself between the cell interstices.

After 1907 Cajal developed experiments comparing the structure of the brain and that of the medulla oblongata using the same staining procedure followed in his experiments on the regenerative and degenerative processes. He also analyzed the structure of the neuron nucleus. The results of these wide research activities laid the principal foundations of the final triumph of neuronism over newer versions of reticularism.

During the first years of the twentieth century, Cajal received the highest awards to which a scientist could aspire. In 1905 he received the Helmholtz Medal conferred by the Imperial Academy of Sciences in Berlin; a year later he was awarded from the Karolinska Institutet in Stockholm the Nobel Prize in Medicine or Physiology, shared with Camillo Golgi. The Nobel lectures given by both scientists offered general overviews on the structure and connections of neuron cells and neuron theory. In March 1906, he was received as a member of the Royal Academy of Medicine in Madrid. In the ceremony of reception he lectured on the *Mecanismo de regeneración de los nervios* [Mechanism of nerve regeneration].

This was his main topic of research during the following years, particularly focused on the compensatory functional adaptation of neuron cells after being damaged. The development of many experiments furnished a great deal of material for his monograph of 1913–14 on the degeneration and regeneration process in the nervous system. At the same time, Cajal continued his investigations on subtle anatomy of the nerve centers developed in different species of animals. Furthermore, he discovered the interstitial ganglion in the posterior longitudinal fascicle, investigated the reticular substance in the medulla oblongata, and devised a new method to observe Golgi's apparatus by means of uranus nitrate, the so-called formol uranus technique (Cajal, 1912). But this was not the only technical novelty introduced by Cajal at the end of his career as a researcher. He also invented the sublimated gold technique (Cajal, 1913), an excellent novelty for the study of the neuroglia, the tissue constituting the material support in the nerve centers, extremely difficult to observe through traditional methods of staining.

In 1915, with the collaboration of his pupil Domingo Sánchez, Cajal developed a series of experiments on the eye and retina of several types of insects. The Darwinian evolu-

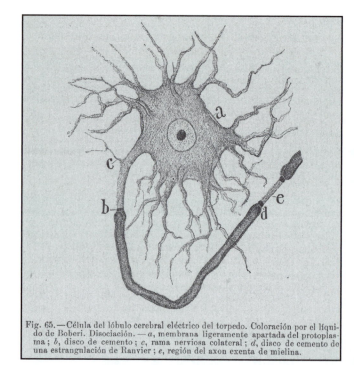

Fig. 65.—Célula del lóbulo cerebral eléctrico del torpedo. Coloración por el líquido de Boveri. Disociación. — *a*, membrana ligeramente apartada del protoplasma; *b*, disco de cemento; *c*, rama nerviosa colateral; *d*, disco de cemento de una estrangulación de Ranvier; *e*, región del axon exenta de mielina.

Cell of the electrical cerebral lobe of the torpedo fish. Halftone reproduction from *Textura del sistema nervioso del hombre y de los vertebrados . . .*, 1904. Wellcome Library, London.

tionary paradigm experienced a crisis in that period, and Cajal admitted some years later in his memoirs how the marvelous organization of the retina and the optical apparatus of the eye that he saw in the insects raised in his mind serious doubts about the mechanism of natural selection as a general law in nature.

Cajal devoted the last three years of his life to a detailed review of all the features supporting the individuality of the neuron cells, always worried by the persistence of reticularism in certain scientific groups. The main fruit of this thorough task was the publication of an extensive work. It was initially written to be included in a handbook of neurology edited by O. Bumke and O. Förster, but Cajal published it first in Spanish (1933) as *¿Neuronismo o reticularismo? Las pruebas objetivas de la unidad anatómica de las células nerviosas* [Neuronism or reticularism? Objective proofs of the anatomical unity of the nervous cells]. It finally appeared in German in 1935, one year after Cajal's death, as *Die Neuronlehre*. It is to be considered his true scientific testament.

During the last period of his life, Cajal devoted his social and political influence to support the public policies developed by the Spanish government for the promotion and institutionalization of science. From the founding in 1907 of the *Junta para Ampliación de Estudios e Investigaciones Científicas (JAE)* [Board for Advanced Studies and Scientific Research] until his death in 1935, Cajal was its president. The fruitful policy followed by the JAE contributed decisively to what has been considered the silver age of Spanish science.

Bibliography

Primary: 1888. 'Estructura de los centros nerviosos de las aves.' *Revista trimestral de Histología normal y patológica* 1: 305–315; 1888. 'Estructura del cerebelo.' *Gaceta Médica Catalana* 11: 449–457; 1890. 'Sobre la aparición de las expansiones celulares de la médula embrionaria.' *Gaceta Sanitaria de Barcelona* 2: 413–418; 1890–92. *Manual de Anatomía Patológica general, seguido de un resumen de Microscopia aplicado a la Histología y Bacteriología Patológica* (Barcelona); 1892. 'Nuevo concepto de la histología de los centros nerviosos.' *Revista de Ciencias Médicas de Barcelona* 18: 336–376, 457–476, 505–520; 529–540; 1894. 'La fine structure des centres nerveux.' *Proceedings of the Royal Society of London* 55: 444–468; 1897. 'Leyes de la morfología y dinamismo de las células nerviosas.' *Revista Trimestral Micrográfica* 2: 1–12; 1897–1904. *Textura del sistema nervioso del hombre y los vertebrados* (Madrid); 1903. 'Un sencillo método de coloración del retículo protoplásmico y sus efectos en los diversos centros nerviosos de vertebrados e invertebrados.' *Trabajos del Laboratorio de Investigaciones Biológicas* 2: 219–221; 1906. 'Estructure et connexions des neurones.' in *Les Prix Nobel en 1906* (Stockholm) pp. 1–27; 1912. 'Fórmula de fijación para la demostración fácil del aparato reticular de Golgi.' *Boletín de la Sociedad Española de Biología* 1: 263–269; 1913. 'Sobre un nuevo proceder de impregnación de la neuroglía y sus resultados en los centros nerviosos del hombre y los animales.' *Trabajos del Laboratorio de Investigaciones Biológicas* 11: 219–237; 1914. 'Comunicación acerca de la significación fisiológica de las expansiones protoplásmicas y nerviosas de la sustancia gris.' *Primer Congreso Médico–Farmacéutico Regional* (Valencia), pp. 70–85; 1915. (with Sánchez, D.) 'Contribución al conocimiento de los centros nerviosos de los insectos.' *Trabajos del Laboratorio de Investigaciones Biológicas* 13: 1–167; 1923. *Recuerdos de mi vida: historia de mi labor científica* (Madrid) [English trans., 1989, *Recollections of My Life* (Cambridge, MA)]; 1935. 'Die Neuronlehre' in Bumke, O., and O. Förster, eds., *Handbuch der Neurologie* (Berlin) pp. 887–994.

Secondary: Barona, Josep Lluís, 2001. 'Ramón y Cajal, Santiago, 1852–1934. Spanish Neurohistologist' in Hessenbruch, Arne, ed., *Reader's Guide to the History of Science* (London) p. 630; Barona, Josep Lluís, 1999. 'Images of the Nervous System in Cajal's Scientific Thought.' *Physis* 36: 473–485; Calvo Roy, Antonio, 1999. *Cajal. Triunfar a toda costa* (Madrid); Smith, C. U. M., 1997. 'Centenary of the Synapse.' *Endeavour* 21(2): 49–51; Lewy, Enriqueta, 1987. *Santiago Ramón y Cajal. El hombre, el sabio y el pensador* (Madrid); López Piñero, José María, 1985. *Ramón y Cajal* (Barcelona); Durán Muñoz, García, and Francisco Alonso Burón, 1983. *Cajal. Vida y obra* (Barcelona); Castro, Fernando de, 1981. *Cajal y la escuela neurológica española* (Madrid); Albarracín, Agustín, 1978. *Santiago Ramón y Cajal, o la pasión de España* (Barcelona); Ferrer, Diego, 1965. *Santiago Ramón y Cajal y las células nerviosas* (Madrid); Jiménez de Asúa, Francisco, 1941. *El pensamiento vivo de Cajal* (Buenos Aires); Tello, Jorge Francisco, 1935. *Cajal y su labor histológica* (Madrid); Sherrington, C. S., 1935. 'Santiago Ramón y Cajal.' *Obituary Notices of Fellows of the Royal Society of London* 1(4): 425–441; *DSB.*

Josep Lluís Barona

RASORI, GIOVANNI   (b. Parma, Italy, 20 August 1766; d. Milan, Italy, 15 April 1837), *medicine.*

Rasori, son of Francesco, a cultivated pharmacist, and Gaetana Vezzani, was born in the duchy of Parma. He soon distinguished himself for his intelligence and, upon his medical degree (1785), was sent by the government to improve his medical skills abroad. He spent three years with Michelangelo Giannetti in Florence (1788–91), and two years with Antonio Scarpa, Alessandro Volta, Lazzaro Spallanzani, and Johann Peter Frank at Pavia (1792–93). He also met Pietro Moscati, who had just translated the *Elementa* of John Brown. In these years of revolutionary heat throughout Europe, Rasori found in Brown's new system the medical counterpart that offered a simple, global, and new vision of health and illness, easily learned and applied, suited to breaking definitively with the traditional medical and political systems. After honing his surgical skills in London, Oxford, and Cambridge and visiting John Brown in Edinburgh and Samuel Thomas von Soemmering in Frankfurt, Rasori did not return to Parma. He preferred to participate in the Jacobin circles in Milan, working as a journalist and editor.

In 1796 Napoleon conquered northern Italy, and Rasori became professor of pathology, rector of the University of Pavia, and director of the Collegio Ghislieri. He applied his 'scientific Jacobinism', attracting numerous students and translating Brown's *Compendium of the New Doctrine*. He became the main popularizer of 'Brownism' in Italy and introduced a new aspect: the 'counter-stimuli'. Life was not considered to be a forced state, provoked by external stimuli; rather, it was a spontaneous and active phenomenon that could alter into a hypoactive or hyperactive state during illness. Rasori's medical therapy aimed at restoring the natural equilibrium by increasing or reducing the vital stimuli. Frequent 'counter-stimuli' prescribed were emetics, laxatives, and bloodletting. 'Rasorism' required little anatomical knowledge but involved pharmacological experimentation on animals, and it divided Italian physicians into enthusiastic adherents and harsh opponents.

With his polemics against traditional academic medicine, Rasori soon got into trouble with his colleagues, who succeeded in removing him after a few months. Rasori became 'general secretary of the minister of the interior', Antonio Tadini, at Milan but returned to Pavia in 1798 as professor of clinical medicine. Again his opponents, above all the anatomist Antonio Scarpa, succeeded in removing him. Rasori then enrolled as head physician in the French army. During the siege of Genoa (1799), an epidemic of petechial fever broke out, and Rasori had the opportunity to 'experiment' with his medical system. His results were very positive, procuring him praise and scientific authority.

As general inspector of public health at Milan, he obtained further success fighting against epizootics. Together with Agostino Bassi, he was convinced that they were a parasitic contagion, and he put into practice some successful countermeasures.

Upon his coronation, Napoleon reorganized the institutions under his domain. Rasori was appointed director of the two new clinical institutes of the Ospedale Maggiore and of the military hospital Sant'Ambrogio at Milan (1806). Once more Rasori's enemies plotted against him. There were frequent reports about shortcomings of institutional duties, 'scientific' attacks against his system, and personal intrigues ridiculing him as a charlatan. After the Restoration of 1814, Rasori lacked institutional support and lost all his positions. He participated in a conspiracy against the Austrian authorities and was imprisoned. After his liberation (1818), he was a poor man, unable to find any scientific or medical position, surviving thanks to the proceeds from the sale of his books and with the help of former students and friends, among them poets such as Stendahl, Silvio Pellico, and Ugo Foscolo. In 1837 he died during an epidemic of influenza.

Bibliography

Primary: 1837. *Opere complete* (Florence); 1792. *Compendio della nuova dottrina medica di G. Brown* (Pavia); 1800. *Storia della febbre petecchiale di Genova negli anni 1799 e 1800* (Milan).

Secondary: Cosmacini, Giorgio, 2002. *Il medico giacobino: la vita e i tempi di Giovanni Rasori* (Rome); Ongaro, Giuseppe, 1994. 'Rasori, Borda e le dottrine dello stimolo e del controstimolo.' *Medicina nei secoli* 6: 495–514.

Ariane Dröscher

RAWSON, GUILLERMO (b. San Juan, Argentina, 25 July 1821; d. Paris, France, 20 February 1890), *public health.*

Son of Amán Rawson, an American surgeon, and Justina Rojo Frías, a member of a prominent family in San Juan, he started school in his home province. In 1839 he moved to Buenos Aires, where he finished high school at Colegio de los Jesuitas and then studied medicine. He earned a doctorate with a thesis on pathological heredity (1845) that, influenced by phrenologist Franz Joseph Gall, claimed a relationship between specific brain locations and the inclination to some illnesses. For Rawson, however, this biological inclination could be buffered by a hygienic environment.

In 1844 Rawson returned to San Juan, where he combined professional practice with political activities. In 1853 he was persecuted and imprisoned by the local authorities because of his opposition to the governor. A year later, he was elected senator in the national parliament as a representative of the Liberal Party. Thanks to his speeches and activities in Congress, he was appointed Minister of the Interior by president Bartolomé Mitre (1862–68), an administration crucial to Argentina's progress and social

reform. During his term in office, Rawson promoted the relocation of Welsh immigrants in the south of Argentina, advocated the metric system, and paved the way for the first census (1869). Quantifying the population and learning about its geographical distribution, among other features, was considered crucial for the designing and implementing of public policy.

Following the creation of the new School of Medical Sciences of the University of Buenos Aires in 1873, Rawson was appointed full professor of the first chair of hygiene in Argentina. This was a milestone which fostered the training of a new generation of doctors, who promoted sanitary activities aimed at improving living conditions in the cities.

In his lectures, Rawson underscored the futility of quarantines to control epidemic outbreaks. Rawson's ideas were part of the context of free trade health policies that postulated that restrictive measures paralyzed commerce, limited people's mobility, and were irrelevant to a population's health. His main preventive measure was housing improvements for the lower classes. According to Rawson, the responsibility for such projects lay both with governmental authorities and individuals who had to work jointly in philanthropic or business partnerships.

In 1876 Rawson attended the International Medical Congress in Philadelphia, where he delivered a paper on vital statistics in Buenos Aires, the first study of its kind in Argentina. This work combined demographic data and public hygiene-related concepts to reinforce Rawson's idea that good and safe housing, plus the building of a sanitary infrastructure such as sewers and drains, would have a positive impact on the reduction of mortality rates. After the meeting Rawson visited medical establishments in France and Italy, and returned to Argentina in 1880. Upon his return he created the Argentine Red Cross, an important achievement of his career.

In 1881 Rawson settled in Paris, where he shared with Alfonso Bertillón his concern about higher male mortality as opposed to female, especially during early childhood. According to Rawson, the explanation for this difference resided in the fact that women had richer brain and marrow centers. However, he also pointed out that this supposedly higher resistance decreased when sexual activity began.

Rawson officially retired in 1883 from any university activity in Argentina, and allocated part of his pension to fund an award for the best work in public hygiene. The first physician who received such award was Emilio Coni.

Bibliography

Primary: 1876. *Estadística vital de Buenos Aires* (Buenos Aires); 1883. *Estudio sobre las casas de Inquilinato en Buenos Aires* (Buenos Aires).

Secondary: Armus, Diego, 2000. 'El descubrimiento de la enfermedad como problema social' in Lobato, Mirtaed., ed., *El progreso, la modernización y sus límites (1880–1916)* (Buenos Aires) pp. 507–

552; González, Leandri, 1999. *Curar, persuadir y gobernar. La construcción histórica de la profesión médica en Buenos Aires, 1852–1886* (Madrid).

Karina Ramacciotti

RAY, ISAAC (b. Beverly, Massachusetts, USA, 16 January 1807; d. Philadelphia, Pennsylvania, USA, 31 March 1881), *psychiatry.*

Ray, son of Captain Isaac Rea and his second wife, Lydia Symonds, was educated at Phillips Academy in Andover, Massachusetts. Subsequently, he attended, but did not graduate from, Bowdoin College in Maine, where his classmates included Luther Bell, the poet Henry Wadsworth Longfellow, and Franklin Pierce, later fourteenth president of the United States.

Ray began his medical training as an apprentice to Samuel Hart in his birthplace, Beverly, Massachusetts. Enrolling at Harvard Medical School, he continued his apprenticeship under George Cheyne Shattuck before transferring to the Medical School of Maine, located at Bowdoin College, and receiving his medical degree in 1827, at the age of twenty.

Ray first attempted to build a general medical practice in Portland, Maine, with little success. He moved to Eastport, Maine, in 1829 and, the following year, married Abigail May Forthingham. In 1838 he published *A Treatise on the Medical Jurisprudence of Insanity*, a textbook that appeared in British editions the following year from publishers in Edinburgh and London and in four subsequent American editions (1844, 1853, 1860, and 1871), quickly establishing him as the leading New World authority on the subject. In 1841 his interest in insanity secured him the post of superintendent at the Maine Insane Asylum, in Augusta, after a scandal forced the resignation of its first superintendent, Cyrus Knapp. He remained in that post for four years, adopting the moral treatment approach then widely in vogue in both European and American asylums. In 1844, with a dozen others, including his former college classmate Luther Bell, he helped launch a national organization for the nascent psychiatric profession, the Association of Medical Superintendents of American Institutions for the Insane (AMSAII), the ancestor of the American Psychiatric Association.

In 1845 Ray resigned his position at Augusta on being offered the superintendency of a new private institution, the Butler Asylum in Providence, Rhode Island. That asylum did not receive its first patient until 1847, and Ray spent some of the intervening months traveling in Europe, inspecting a variety of asylums and preparing for his new post. For almost two decades, until 1866, Ray served as Butler's superintendent, becoming one of the most prominent mental specialists of his generation and occupying the presidency of the AMSAII from 1855 to 1859. He published extensively on psychiatric subjects and continued to display a particular interest in the intersection of mental illness and the law. His work there encompassed both a set of reflections on the law regarding the involuntary hospitalization of the mentally ill and further discussions of the intersection between crime and insanity. His extensive correspondence on the latter issue with Charles Doe, an associate justice of the New Hampshire Supreme Court, eventually led to the formulation of the extremely influential 'New Hampshire doctrine', the notion that any act that was the product of insanity could not constitute a crime or form the basis of a valid contract or will.

In 1859 Ray's son Benjamin, who had trained at Harvard Medical School, became an assistant physician at Butler. When the senior Ray retired, however, both men relocated to Philadelphia, and the younger Ray abandoned the field in favor of general practice. Even in retirement, Ray continued to involve himself with the treatment of the mentally ill, serving as one of the committee supervising the insane department of the Philadelphia Almshouse, until his complaints about the ill-treatment of patients led to the discontinuance of his appointment. The death of his son from a stroke in 1879 effectively brought Ray's career to an end. He became withdrawn and depressed and died in his sleep.

Bibliography

Primary: 1838. *A Treatise on the Medical Jurisprudence of Insanity* (Boston); 1863. *Mental Hygiene* (Boston); 1871. *Insanity and Its Treatment* (Philadelphia); 1873. *Contributions to Medical Pathology* (Boston).

Secondary: McGovern, Constance, 1985. *Masters of Madness: Social Origins of the American Psychiatric Profession* (Hanover, NH); *DAMB.*

Andrew Scull

RAYER, PIERRE-FRANÇOIS-OLIVE (b. Saint-Sylvain near Caen, Calvados, France, 8 March 1793; d. Paris, France, 10 September 1867), *dermatology, nephrology, comparative medicine.*

Rayer was the son of a merchant, Olive-Jean-François Rayer, and Marie-Jeanne Guerard. He studied under a private tutor at Caen, possibly also attending a local school, Saint-Sylvain. He then entered the École de médecine at Caen, but shortly after went to the École de médecine in Paris in 1810. He was named an interne in 1813, winning prizes at the École pratique and as an interne. He became a doctor in 1818, writing a thesis on anatomical pathology.

Rayer married Françoise de LaCoste in 1822 and, four years later, published a well-received book on skin diseases. He also made a number of studies of epidemic diseases such as cholera. Although he had become known as an excellent physician, he was prevented from competing for a teaching position as agrégé on the grounds that he had married a Protestant. He became a hospital physician at Saint-Antoine Hospital in 1827, and subsequently chief of service at La Charité in 1832. He had an active private practice as a physician to wealthy financiers, and later to the household of Napoleon III. In 1837 he expanded his work on contagious diseases by demonstrating the transmissibility of glanders between horse and human.

Noted for his interest in scientific medicine, Rayer taught many young physicians who later became famous, including Casimir Davaine, Claude Bernard, Edouard Brown-Séquard, Jean-Martin Charcot, and Charles Robin. Rayer also taught Emile Littré medicine, remained his friend throughout his life, and introduced Robin to both Littré and scientific positivism. When Robin founded the Société de Biologie in 1848 under the banner of scientific positivism in order to promote laboratory medicine, Rayer was named perpetual president. He remained one of the most active members until his death, presenting before the Société his experimental studies on the transmission of anthrax in sheep. He was made a commander of the Legion of Honor in 1854. In 1862 Napoleon III, without consulting the Faculté de Médecine, named Rayer dean of the Faculty as well as to a new chair of comparative medicine. Faculty and student protest against this political imposition led to Rayer's resignation two years later. In his introductory lecture he had outlined a course of medical investigation to study morbid processes in the entire animal and plant kingdoms.

Rayer wrote significant works on skin diseases, and he was the first to distinguish between acute and chronic eczema. He identified pituitary obesity, but he is best known for his contributions on diseases of the kidney. In his study of renal disease, he incorporated extensive investigations on the chemistry and microscopical analysis of urine, classified different forms of albuminuric nephritis, demonstrated the existence of albuminuria in diabetes mellitus, and described renal vein thrombosis. In his final contributions before the Société de Biologie, he emphasized his investigations on comparative pathology.

Bibliography

Primary: 1826–27. *Traité théoretique et pratique des maladies de la peau* 2 vols. with atlas (Paris) [English trans. 1835]; 1837. 'De la morve et du farcin chez l'homme.' *Mém. Acad. Roy Méd.* 6: 625–873; 1837–41. *Traité des maladies des reins et des alterations de la sécrétion urinaire* 3 vols. with atlas (Paris) [2005. part English trans. as *The History of Albuminous Nephritis (1840)*, French trans. Berry, Diana, and Stewart Cameron, Latin trans. Booker, Michael, intro. and commentary, Mackenzie, Campbell, *Medical History Supplement* 24 (London)].

Secondary: Théodoridès, Jean, 1997. *Pierre Rayer (1793–1867): un demi-siècle de médecine française* (Paris); Richet, G., et al., 1991. 'Pierre Rayer.' *Histoire des Sciences Médicales* 25(4): 261–302 (entire issue devoted to Rayer with articles by G. Richet, P. Fleury, J. Poirer, J. Théodoridès, G. Tillès, D. Wallach); Ackerknecht, Erwin H., 1967. *Medicine at the Paris Hospital 1794–1848* (Baltimore).

Joy Harvey

RAZETTI, LUIS (b. Caracas, Venezuela, 19 September 1862; d. Caracas, 15 May 1932), *surgery, obstetrics, ethics, Darwinism.*

Razetti was born to the Genovese businessman Luigi Razetti and a Venezuelan lady. He graduated in 1884 from the Central University of Venezuela as a medical surgeon, becoming a general practitioner in the provinces for a time. He later returned to Caracas and in 1890 moved to Paris, where he took courses (1890–93) to specialize in surgery and obstetrics. Upon his return to Caracas, and jointly with other Venezuelan colleagues who had also studied in Paris, he led a series of initiatives to renovate Venezuelan medicine. He founded the Society of Physicians and Surgeons of Caracas (1893) that undertook the publishing of the *Medical Gazette of Caracas* (1893), still extant; he collaborated with Santos Aníbal Domínici in founding the Pasteur Institute (1895); and in 1904 he induced Congress to approve the charter for the creation of the National Medical Academy. Additionally, he promoted medical training based on clinical practice (1895); the systemization of medical student practices in Caracas through the Hospital Competition for Interns and Externs (1895); and the reform of the chairs of anatomy and operating medicine (1895–96).

Razetti jointly held the chairs of external pathology, operating medicine, obstetrics, descriptive anatomy, and clinical surgery. As professor of obstetrics, he taught the principles of Pinard's French school relating to the treatment of uterine hemorrhages at childbirth, also getting involved with puerperal eclampsia and miscarriage. He was an outstanding teacher of surgery, establishing his own school as exemplified by his textbook, *Lecciones y Notas de Cirugía Clínica* (1917). Among many other surgical innovations, he performed the first total retrogressive ascending laryngectomy in the country (1914). As professor of anatomy, in 1911 he founded the Anatomical Institute, where it was compulsory for medical students to carry out practical dissections.

Razetti additionally engaged in various public health activities, such as campaigns to combat alcoholism, venereal diseases, tuberculosis, and cancer; and to promote maternal and child hygiene, and eugenics and birth control. The latter two campaigns brought about several polemics, especially with the Catholic Church.

Razetti was a keen polemicist; for instance, following his lead, the National Medical Academy based its doctrine of biology on Darwin's evolutionary theory. Razetti let his position be known with the book *La Doctrina de la Descendencia* (1906). Also through the Academy he promoted the approval (1918) of the *Medical Ethics Code*, which established guidelines regarding patient care, professional dignity, medical meetings and consulting, specialists, medical secrecy, and professional fees, among others. This Code became an inspiration to others in Latin America, although in Venezuela it was not applied because of federal court annulment.

Razetti promoted science-based medicine and fought against quacks and medical malpractice; for him, the aim of medicine was to do good, hence his interest in developing medical ethics.

Bibliography

Primary: 1979. *Obras Completas* 9 vols. (Caracas).

Secondary: Glick, Thomas F., 1984. 'Perspectivas sobre la recepción del darwinismo en el mundo hispano' in Sociedad Española de Historia de las Ciencias, *Actas, II Congreso de la Sociedad Española de Historia de las Ciencias* 3 vols. (Zaragoza) vol. 1, pp. 49–64; Archila, Ricardo, 1982. 'Luis Razetti' in Fundación, Eugenio Mendoza, ed., *Venezolanos del siglo XX* 3 vols. (Caracas) vol. 1, pp. 40–60; Archila, Ricardo, 1963. *Luis Razetti o biografía de la superación* (Caracas).

Yajaira Freites
English translation by Claudio Mendoza

AL-RĀZĪ, ABŪ BAKR MUḤAMMAD B. ZAKĀRIYYA' (aka RHAZES) (b. Rayy, Iran, c. 865, d. Rayy, 925 or 932), *medicine, philosophy, alchemy, music.*

Muḥammad ibn Zakāriyya' al-Rāzī, known in medieval Europe as Rhazes, was born in the Persian city of Rayy, near present-day Tehran. Few facts of his life are known, since most recorded information consists of contradictory, anachronistic, or even malicious anecdotal details. Although the literary topos concerning his interest in medicine after his thirties or forties has been accepted until recently, he did study medicine in his youth. Al-Rāzī was a court physician and a prolific medical writer, but more importantly he was also a practitioner, a true clinician, and a medical teacher. He directed his town hospital in Rayy and, later on, was appointed to head the hospital at Baghdad. Probably as a consequence of excessive work, his right hand became paralyzed near the end of his life, and he became blind from cataracts. Although it might well be an anecdote playing on the reversal of the roles of doctor and patient, al-Rāzī, at the suggestion of having his cataracts couched, is said to have kindly refused because it was not worth undergoing such pain and discomfort at the end of his life. Sources disagree regarding the date of his death, but he died in his hometown Rayy, in which he seems to have spent most of his life.

Al-Rāzī was one of the most influential medieval Islamic physicians, and he is also considered the most freethinking of the major philosophers of Islam. Additionally, this multifaceted scholar was well versed in music and alchemy, and he also wrote a number of treatises on logic, cosmology, mathematics, and theology. He refused to accept the principle of absolute authority, and he distrusted established spiritual or intellectual verities. In contrast, he strongly believed in reason, experience, and the continuing progress of the sciences. Hence, his philosophical ideas—mainly anti-Aristotelian and anti-prophetic—met with hostility

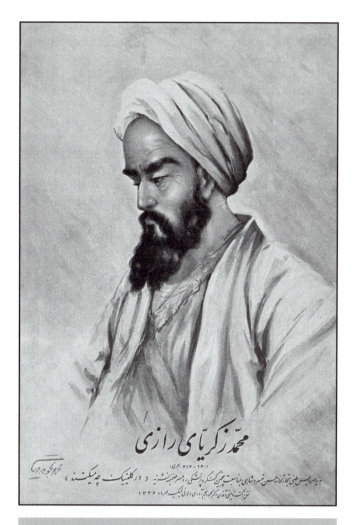

Al-Rāzī. Color process print, Wellcome Library, London.

from religious authorities and contemporary scholars, as well as from their medieval successors. As a consequence, few of his nonmedical works were copied and are known to us only through quotations by later authors and his critics, for the most part members of the Isma'ili sect, who against al-Rāzī's equalitarian views, defended a strict hierarchical principle. Only two treatises on ethics have been preserved: *Kitāb ṭibb al-ruḥānī* [The Book of Spiritual Physick], which embodies al-Rāzī's largely Epicurean ethical system, and *Sirat al-falsafiyya* [The Philosophical Way of Life], in which he claims that his has been a life of moderation, excessive only in his devotion to learning. His treatise *K. al-Shukūk ʿalā Jālīnūs* [Doubts concerning Galen], deals with philosophical as well as with medical issues and clearly reflects his critical attitude toward dogmatism and authority. Likewise, al-Rāzī's alchemy dismisses the idea of potions with an appeal to magic when the latter means reliance on symbols as causes. For him, the theory and practice of alchemy were part of philosophy, and he brought a new, more empirical and naturalistic approach to the discipline than that of the Greeks and Jabir ibn Hayyan.

As a physician, al-Rāzī stands out as the sole medical theoretician of medieval Islam whose actual medical practice is profusely attested. His tireless medical activity resulted in the K. al-Tajārib, or Casebook, which contains nearly 900 cases treated or supervised by him. After his death, one of his students compiled the information, and it seems to have circulated later as a textbook. Throughout his life he also extracted and recorded useful passages regarding pathology and therapy from earlier Greco-Roman, Indian, Syriac, and Islamic sources, to which he added his own opinions and experiences, often in the form of case histories. Although the material was intended for his private use, it was arranged for publication after his death, resulting in a huge compilation known as Kitāb al-Ḥāwī [The Comprehensive Book on Medicine]. Several unfinished works can be discerned in this collection of medical study; files are arranged by subject, such as a group of thirty-three clinical observations in the volume devoted to fevers, to be read alongside the case histories found in the Hippocratic book Epidemics. Because of its voluminous size, complete copies of the K. al-Ḥāwī were rare, but it proved to be very influential, particularly in the Western tradition. Translated as Continens by the Jewish physician Farāj ibn Sālim (Farragut) in 1279 for King Charles of Anjou, it was first printed at Brescia in 1486. Another work containing a number of case histories—this time concerning rulers and distinguished men—is a short treatise entitled Sirr ṣināʿat aṭ-ṭibb [The Secret of the Medical Art]. Al-Rāzī disagreed with the section in the Hippocratic Oath relating to the rule of hiding medical knowledge or making it obscure in order to prevent its vulgarization among the ignorant, and his aim in this work is to present medical knowledge in an easy, concise, and accessible way. Al-Rāzī dedicated some of his most famous writings to the princes and governors whom he attended, such as his K. Ṭibb al-mulūkī [Medicine for the Princes], addressed to the governor of Rayy, ʿAli ibn Wahsudhan (g. 920), and the K. manāfiʿ al-aghdhiya wa-dafʿ madarri-ha [On the Usefulness of Foodstuffs and Its Harmfulness], dedicated to the local ruler Abu l-ʿAbbās Ahmad ibn ʿAlī. One of his most successful works was his Kitāb al-Manṣurī [Book for al-Mansur], dedicated to the Samanid ruler—and also governor of Rayy between 903 and 914—Abu Ṣalih al-Manṣūr ibn Isḥāq. Comprising theory as well as practice, it is divided into ten chapters: I. Anatomy; II. Humoral physiology and physiognomy; III. Materia medica; IV. Hygiene and preservation of health; V. Cosmetics; VI. Regimen for travelers; VII. Surgery; VIII. Poisons; IX. Diseases and their treatment; and X. Fevers. Translated by Gerard of Cremona (d. 1187), this short but condensed medical compendium exerted a considerable influence in the Latin tradition under the title Liber ad Almansorem. The ninth chapter, devoted to therapy for diseases of specific parts of the body from head to toe, was printed separately and gained wide circulation, becoming the subject of several commentaries by university scholars as well as by the Renaissance anatomist Andreas Vesalius.

Other general manuals composed by al-Rāzī and translated into Latin by Gerard of Cremona are the K. al-Madkhal ilā ṣināʿat aṭ-ṭibb (also known as Isagoge, Introduction to the Art of Medicine), the K. Taqsīm al-ʿilal [Book of Classification and Tabulation of Diseases], and the K. al-Aqrabādhin, or Antidotarium. Al-Rāzī's literary production of nearly 200 titles on different topics also includes treatises on minor topics, such as the K. al-Murshid or al-Fuṣūl [Aphorisms], the Kitāb al-Ḥaṣā fī l-kulā wa l-mathāna [Stones in the Kidney and the Bladder], and the famous Fi l-judarī wa-l-ḥaṣba [On Smallpox and Measles], a medical issue about which Greco-Roman and Byzantine literature are silent. This treatise was not the earliest Islamic monograph on the subject (the first one was written by Thābit b. Qurra, d. 901). However, in addition to the Medieval Latin translation by Gerard of Cremona, al-Rāzī's clinical and therapeutic observations still deserved an edition and new translation in 1766 by the London apothecary John Channing (d. 1775), and they were edited again and translated into English in 1847 by W. A. Greenhill. Minor works focus on colic, on the ingestion of fruit before food, on the allergy caused by roses in spring (dedicated to his teacher of philosophy Abū Zayd Ahmad ibn Sahl al-Balkhī, d. 934), on the excellence of bloodletting among all methods of bodily evacuation (dedicated to the emir Ahmad ibn Ismaʿīl ibn Ahmad, g. 907–13), on the examination of physicians, on intercourse, or on passive anal eroticism (ubna, or 'the hidden illness') and its cure, thus defining this type of homosexuality as a medical condition. Concerned for the health of ordinary people, he also wrote a treatise intended for those without a physician to attend them, as well as another entitled Cure in One Hour. Likewise, aware of the psychological factors in medicine and their impact on therapy, he devoted several writings to discussing why an intelligent physician cannot heal all diseases, people's preference for quacks over competent doctors, and why ignorant physicians, common folk, and women in the cities are more successful than scientists in treating certain diseases, among other subjects. He also produced a work, still unpublished, on khawaṣ, or occult properties of things, a topic that is not at odds with his rationalism since he firmly believed that Nature conveys secrets or phenomena that man cannot understand and explain.

Throughout his works, al-Rāzī often referred to his Kitāb al-Jāmiʿ (also to be translated as The Comprehensive Book on Medicine) as a published work, although no copy is as yet known to exist and some scholars identify it with the Kitab al-Ḥāwī. Like Galen, he wrote an autobiography and believed that the best physician must also be a philosopher, but otherwise al-Rāzī rejected a number of Galenic theories and observations, and even claimed that in some aspects his experience was much more abundant than that of his predecessor.

Bibliography

Primary: Greenhill, W. A., trans., 1847. *A Treatise on the Smallpox and Measles* (London); Koning, P., de, ed. and trans., 1896. *Traité sur le calcul dans les reins et dans la vessie* (Leiden) [Reprint 1996 (Frankfurt)]; Guigues, P., 1903. 'La guérison en une heure de Razès.' *Janus* 8: 363–370, 411–418; Meyerhof, M., 1935. 'Thirty-Three Clinical Observations by Rhazes.' *Isis* 23: 321–356 [Reprinted 1984 in Johnston, P., ed., *Studies in Medieval Arabic Medicine*, (London)]; Iskandar, A. Z., 1960. *Kitāb Miḥnat aṭ-ṭabīb* [On examining physicians]. *al-Machriq* 54: 471–522; Iskandar, A. Z., 1961. 'Rhazes' *K. al-Murshid aw al-fusul* (The Guide or Aphorisms) with texts selected from his medical writings.' *Revue de l'Institute des Manuscrits Arabes*, 7, fasc. 2; 1965–68. *K. al-Ḥāwī fi l-tibb* 23 vols. (Hyderabad); Hau, Friedrun R., 1975. 'Rāzīs Gutachten über Rosenschnupfen.' *Medizin-historisches Journal* 10: 94–102; Vázquez de Benito, C., ed., 1979. *K. al-Madjal ilà sinaʿat al-tibb. Introducción al arte de la medicina o 'Isagoge'* (Salamanca); Brabant, R. Kuhne, 1982, 1984, 1985. 'El *Sirr sinaʿat al-tibb* de Abu Bakr Muḥammad b. Zakāriyya' al-Rāzīs.' *Al-Qantara* 3: 347–414, 5: 235–292, 6: 369–395; Hammami, S. M., ed. and French trans., 1983. *K. al-Qūlanj* (Aleppo); 'Aytanī, A., ed., 1985. *K. Manāfiʿ al-aghdiya wa-dafʿ madarri-ha* (Beirut); Hammami, S. M., ed. and French trans., 1992. *K. Al-Taqsīm wa-al-tashjīr: Taqāsīm al-ʿilal* (Aleppo); Mohaghegh, M., ed., 1993. *K. al-Shukūk ʿalá Jālīnūs* (Tehran).

Secondary: Goodman, L. E., 2003. [*s.v.* al-Rāzīs], [in *Encyclopaedia of Islam*, CDRom Edition (Leiden)] *The Encyclopaedia of Islam* (New edn., 11 vols., Leiden 1960–2002), VIII, pp. 474–477; Álvarez Millán, C., 2000. 'Practice *versus* Theory: Tenth-Century Case Histories from the Islamic Middle East' in Savage-Smith, E., and P. Horden, eds., *The Year 1000: Medical Practice at the End of the First Millennium*, Special volume of *Social History of Medicine*, 13: 293–306; Álvarez Millán, C., 1999. 'Graeco-Roman Case Histories and their Influence on Medieval Islamic Clinical Accounts.' *Social History of Medicine* 12: 19–43; Richter-Bernburg, L., 1994. 'Abu Bakr Muhammad al-Rāzīs's Medical Works.' *Medicina nei secoli* 6: 377–392; Brabant, R. Kuhne, 1993. 'Al-Rāzīs on When and How to Eat Fruit', in De Jong, F., ed., *Miscellanea Arabica et Islamica (Dissertationes in Academia Ultrajectina prolatae anno MCMXC)* (Leuven) pp. 164–174 (Orientalia Lovaniensia Analecta, 52) [Reprinted 2002 in Waines, D., ed., *Patterns of Everyday Life* (Aldershot) pp. 317–327 (The Formation of the Classical Islamic World, 10)]; Iskandar, A. Z., 1990. 'Al-Rāzīs' in Young, M. J. L., J. D. Latham, and R. B. Serjeant, eds., *Religion, Learning and Science in the ʿAbbasid Period* (Cambridge) pp. 370–377; Rosenthal, F., 1978. 'Al-Rāzīs on the Hidden Illness.' *Bulletin for the History of Medicine* 52: 45–60 [Reprinted 1990 in *Science and Medicine in Islam. A Collection of Essays* (Aldershot)]; Ullmann, Manfred, 1970. *Die Medizin im Islam* (Leiden and Cologne) pp. 128–136; Sezgin, Fuat, 1967–1984. *Geschichte des arabischen Schrifttums* 9 vols. (Leiden) III, pp. 274–294; Temkin, O., 1942. 'A Medieval Translation of Rhazes' Clinical Observations.' *Bulletin for the History of Medicine* 12: 102–107; DSB.

Cristina Álvarez Millán

READ, GRANTLY DICK   (b. Beccles, Suffolk, England, 26 January 1890; d. Wroxham, Norfolk, England, 11 June 1959), *obstetrics.*

Read, the son of Robert Read, a miller, and Frances Sayer, attended Bishop's Stortford College and St John's College, Cambridge. After obtaining a third class degree, he entered the London Hospital as a clinical student in 1911. There he studied under the neurologist Henry Head (1861–1940) and the obstetrician Eardley Holland (1879–1967). Their theories on the pain of childbirth and his experiences as a student obstetrician in the East End of London convinced Read that childbirth was not an inherently painful process.

After qualifying in 1914, Read volunteered for the RAMC and was injured in the Gallipoli campaign of 1915. At the end of the war, he returned to Cambridge and received his MD in 1920. In 1921 he set up a private practice in Woking and married Dorothea Cannon. Read used his experiences as a general practitioner to develop the notion of a 'fear-tension-pain' cycle. Obstetricians portrayed childbirth as a painful event; fear of this pain led women to become physically and emotionally tense; tension led to pain; and pain in turn led to more fear. If women were taught to understand the processes of childbirth and to look forward to it, rather than to fear it, this vicious circle would be broken. By teaching methods of relaxation that could be used during labor, obstetricians could eliminate the tension that led to pain.

Read published his ideas in *Natural Childbirth* (1933), a book whose title became the name of his method. The book was a small success, but, more importantly, it prompted women from across the world to write to Read with their experiences of childbirth and their comments on his theories. This cascade of correspondence continued until Read's death and formed a major influence on his thought. Read incorporated their testimony into his most popular book, *Revelation of Childbirth* (1942). He became increasingly interested in becoming a full-time obstetrician but refused to take the membership examination for the Royal College of Obstetricians and Gynaecologists, claiming that the College perpetuated the myth of painful childbirth. Public interest in natural childbirth prompted the College to offer Read a small clinic in which he could put his methods into practice, but he refused, dismissing the offer as an insult.

Feeling that his work was unappreciated in England, Read moved to South Africa in 1948 and began to practice at a small maternity hospital. He divorced Dorothea Cannon in 1952 and immediately married Jessica Bennett. Two years later he embarked on a tour of Africa, seeking to record tribal birth customs. In his later writings, he used his observations from this tour to support his critique of Western obstetric practice. He returned to England in the winter of 1954 and almost immediately set off on a worldwide lecture tour. In 1956 he was granted a papal audience and was presented with a medal for his work. In the same year he issued a record of women experiencing natural childbirth, and the year after a series of films he had made, showing African women giving birth in a 'natural' way, were broadcast on BBC television.

Read's influence is difficult to judge. His writings gave women the opportunity to express their feelings about childbirth and to question the medicalization of what, to many, seemed a natural process. However, his refusal to engage with orthodox obstetric opinions and his overwhelming concern for public rather than professional approval limited the incorporation of his theories into obstetric practice.

Bibliography

Primary: 1933. *Natural Childbirth* (London); 1942. *Revelation of Childbirth* (London).

Secondary: Thomas, Mary, ed., 1997. *Post-War Mothers: Childbirth Letters to Grantly Dick-Read* (London); Thomas, Anthony N., 1957. *Doctor Courageous: The Story of Dr Grantly Dick Read* (London); *Oxford DNB*.

Richard Barnett

REDI, FRANCESCO (b. Arezzo, Italy, 18 February 1626; d. Pisa, Italy, 1 March 1697), *medicine, natural history, parasitology, poetry.*

The eldest son of Gregorio Redi, physician of the Medici Court, and Cecilia de' Ghinci, Redi moved with his family at the age of thirteen (1639), first to Prato and then in 1642 to Florence, where he lived for the rest of his life, with frequent journeys to his native Arezzo and to Prato, Pisa, and Livorno. In 1643 Redi moved to Pisa University, where in 1647 he obtained his doctoral degree in philosophy and medicine. Immediately after, he joined his family in Florence, and the following year he passed the habilitation examinations to practice medicine. After traveling to Rome, Naples, Bologna, Padua, and Venice, he began to practice medicine. In 1648 he entered the Medici Court, as a physician and supervisor of the grand-ducal pharmacy, and in 1666 he became first physician of Ferdinando II, an appointment confirmed by the successor, Cosimo III.

In 1655 Redi was named to the Accademia della Crusca, a literary society founded in Florence in 1582 to unify literary Italian and to produce a dictionary. He participated in the activities of the small but influential Accademia del Cimento, which, between 1657 and 1667, fostered Galilean science and the experimental method.

Redi's first scientific essay, 'Observations on Vipers' (1647), took advantage of the availability in the grand-ducal pharmacy of snakes, used to prepare the traditional remedy theriac. Through careful observations on living specimens and repeated experiments with injections of poison in the body of animals, Redi was able to show that the poison was produced by two special organs of the head

and stored in cavities of the teeth. Following Harvey's idea on the circulation of the blood, Redi showed that the venom acted only when it entered the blood circulation and was harmless if ingested. He suggested stopping the circulation of the blood near the wound with a tourniquet as a remedy.

Redi's most influential book was his *Experiments on the Generation of Insects* (1668), in which he disproved the classical idea of 'spontaneous generation' in a variety of small animals (frogs, flies, bees). Using a precise experimental method, Redi prepared eight jars and put meat in each. Then he sealed half of them to avoid contact between meat and flying insects. Maggots appeared on meat in the open jars, but not in the sealed ones. Maggots also hatched to produce new insects of the same species that the experimenter had seen depositing eggs.

This experiment, however, was not considered conclusive. Redi's results attacked the influential ideas on generation of the Jesuit Athanasius Kircher (1601/2–80), and another Jesuit, Filippo Buonanni, suggested that the sealing of the jars in Redi's experiments had impeded the circulation of the air, necessary for life. Redi conducted a new series of experiments, leaving open half of the recipients and covering the other half only with gauze that did not prevent contact with the air. The results of these control experiments confirmed that maggots were not produced by a mysterious principle, but exclusively from the eggs deposited on meat by insects.

Over the same period, Redi performed many experiments on what he considered another kind of generation. He observed 'more than twenty thousands oak galls', finding in them maggots that he considered to be produced by a 'zoogenic' power, as was also the case of worms in cherries. His general idea was that life itself is the 'immediate cause' of the generation. The manuscript summarizing these researches ('History of fruits and worms produced by oaks and other trees') was never published, and the explanation of the presence of maggots in galls was later found by Marcello Malpighi (1628–94) and Antonio Vallisneri (1661–1730).

The Danish anatomist Nicolas Steno arrived in Florence in 1666, and Redi established a very firm and friendly collaboration with him, which produced many public anatomy demonstrations on numerous species of living organisms, especially at the court, and experiments in botany, zoology, and geology.

Applying his simple and rational experimental method, Redi refuted another observation made by the Jesuits, according to which a stone found in the heads of cobras had unusual medical powers, curing many diseases, when attached to a wound, by sucking out the poison causing the disease. Redi repeatedly failed to confirm the results described by the Jesuits experimentally, and therefore he denied the supposed therapeutic value of the stones. These experiments were summarized in a book published in

1671, which remains a beautiful illustration of the experimental method of the seventeenth century.

In this same book Redi also summarized his experiments on digestion in birds, coming to the conclusion that this process was not produced by mechanical causes, as suggested by the presence of small stones in the intestines of birds, but was a fermentation produced by a special liquid ('mestruo'), with the stones playing the same function as teeth in other animals.

In 1684 Redi published another book, which reported his several hundred observations on various parasites, worms, and insects living in a hundred different species of animals. In this book, which is incomplete but is still considered as the first treatise in parasitology, Redi suggested that these parasites are always generated from eggs deposited in the organism and fertilized through sexual intercourse.

In 1680, at the occasion of a visit to Livorno with the Court, Redi met the pharmacist Diacinto Cestoni. That was the beginning of a long friendship and a productive scientific collaboration. Redi played an important role in the discovery by Giovan Cosimo Bonomo, in collaboration with Cestoni, of the etiology of scabies. These observers followed Redi's instructions and theory and demonstrated, observing the mite laying eggs, that the parasite reproduces through the union of a male and a female. These observations were published as a letter to Redi, which was included in the nineteenth-century edition of Redi's works.

In his scientific writing, Redi always used Italian, as he did in his medical consultations, which have a substantial literary value. Redi was also a poet, his chief poetical work being the ode *Bacchus in Tuscany* (1685).

Bibliography

Primary: 1712. *Opere* (Venice); 1858. *Opuscoli di storia naturale* (Florence); 1664. *Osservazioni intorno alle vipere, fatte da Francesco Redi e da lui scritte in una lettera a Lorenzo Malagotti* (Florence) [English edn., 1988]; 1668. *Esperienze intorno alla generazione degli insetti scritte in una lettera a Carlo Dati* (Florence) [English edn., 1909]; 1671. *Esperienze intorno a diverse cose naturali, e particolarmente a quelle che ci son portate dall'Indie, scritte in una lettera al reverendissimo padre Atanasio Chircher della compagnia di Gesù* (Florence); 1684. *Osservazioni intorno agli animali viventi che si trovano negli animali viventi* (Florence).

Secondary: Bernardi, W., 2004. 'Tra 'città' e 'corte'. Promozione sociale e vocazione scientifica nella Toscana del Seicento: Francesco e Gregorio Redi.' *Medicina & Storia* 8: 3–48; Straker, Stephen, 2000. 'Redi, Francesco' in Applebaum, Wilbur, ed., *Encyclopedia of the Scientific Revolution from Copernicus to Newton* (New York and London) pp. 554–556; Bernardi, W., and L. Guerrini, eds., 1999. *Francesco Redi. Un protagonista della scienza moderna. Documenti, esperimenti, immagini* (Florence); Findlen, P., 1993. 'Controlling the Experiment: Rhetoric, Court Patronage, and the Experimental Method of Francesco Redi (1626–97).' *History of Science* 31: 35–64; Belloni, L., 1958. 'Francesco Redi, biologo' in *Celebrazione dell'Accademia del Cimento nel tricentenario della fondazione. Domus Galilaeana, 19 giugno 1957* (Pisa) pp. 53–70; Viviani, U., 1924–31. *Vita, opere, iconografia, bibliografia, vocabolario inedito delle voci aretine e libro inedito de' Ricordi di Francesco Redi* 3 vols. (Arezzo); *DSB.*

Bernardino Fantini

REED, WALTER (b. Gloucester County, Virginia, USA, 13 September 1851; d. Washington, D.C., USA, 23 November 1902), *bacteriology, epidemiology.*

Reed was the last of five children born to Lemuel Sutton, a Methodist minister, and Pharaba White, daughter of a North Carolina planter. Although he was born in Gloucester County, Virginia, Reed and his family moved soon and frequently, following Lemuel's changing ministerial assignments through several small towns in Virginia and North Carolina. Shortly after the Civil War ended, the Reeds were sent to Charlottesville, Virginia. Mrs Reed died shortly thereafter. In 1867 he enrolled at the still new University of Virginia. His intellectual inclinations drew him to classical languages and philosophy, but his more pragmatic nature soon led him to medicine. Despite remarriage to a financially secure widow, Reed's father could not support the university education of all of his sons. Reed thus struck a deal with the university's medical faculty: if he passed the requisite examinations, the university would grant him the MD. Nine months later (1869), he successfully completed his exams, and Virginia accordingly conferred a medical degree on the seventeen-year-old. Lacking experience with patients, however, Reed went to New York City that autumn, spending the academic year at Bellevue Hospital. He worked briefly at King's County Hospital before accepting a residency at Brooklyn City Hospital (1871–72). At twenty-two, Reed was appointed an inspector on the Brooklyn Board of Health and set about establishing a medical practice in Brooklyn.

During a visit to his family, then living in North Carolina, he developed a romantic attachment to Emily (Emilie) Lawrence, who, like his own mother, was the daughter of a planter. Looking to support his new fiancée, Reed abandoned the challenging task of building up a profitable private medical practice (having few social contacts) and turned instead to the U.S. Army. Passing the army's extensive examinations for prospective medical officers, he was commissioned first lieutenant and received his first military assignment (1875). In 1876 he was stationed on the American West frontier, in Arizona, where his new wife Emilie eventually joined him. Son Walter Lawrence was born in 1877, and daughter Emily ('Blossom') Lawrence in 1883. Between the birth of their first and their second child, the Reeds returned briefly to the East Coast. Reed, now an army captain, was stationed at Fort McHenry (1881). He took full advantage of his Baltimore location, studying physiology at the Johns Hopkins University. The next year, Reed was again sent west, eventually returning to Baltimore in 1890. Medicine had been changing rapidly in his absence from the centers of American medical education, and he was eager to learn the new bacteriology. The army granted him special leave to follow a course in bacteriology and pathology under William Welch at Johns Hopkins Hospital; he was then sent to Minnesota (1891).

Reed made what would be a permanent move to Washington, D.C., in 1893, when he was assigned to the office of the new Surgeon General, George Miller Sternberg. Appointed curator of the Army Medical Museum and professor of 'clinical and sanitary microscopy' at Sternberg's newly created U.S. Army Medical School, Reed was soon promoted to full surgeon and major. Subsequently, he was given the task of investigating a number of diseases, including malaria, diphtheria, and smallpox; in the process, he developed his epidemiological abilities. By 1898, when the Spanish-American War brought typhoid to the fore, Reed was well prepared to head up the army's typhoid commission. With Victor C. Vaughan and Edward O. Shakespeare, Reed inspected a series of army camps in the United States where typhoid was rampant. The commission soon discovered that medicine's recent advances, both in the laboratory and in the field, had yet to find a place in military routine. It was known that typhoid was spread by fecal-oral transmission and so could be avoided through proper sanitation; the Army was not taking proper steps to separate living quarters and toilets. The Commission further demonstrated the role that flies played in moving improperly treated waste matter to the mess tents. Moreover, although typhoid could be diagnosed with Fernand Widal's serological test, the camps lacked laboratories, and line officers tended to deny that their soldiers were suffering from the deadly but largely preventable disease. Surgeons were often too young or too inexperienced to oppose the line officers and lacked the military authority to do so, even when they did understand typhoid transmission. Reed was called away before the commission processed its data and wrote its preliminary report. He did, however, collaborate substantially on the report abstract (1900). The full report appeared only after both Reed and Shakespeare had died (1904).

Even after the Spanish-American War had ended, Reed continued to deal with its consequences. The victorious Americans had kept troops in Cuba, and those troops were now fighting another deadly foe: yellow fever. The United States was, unfortunately, familiar with the disease, its residents having survived a number of devastating epidemics over the years. Familiarity, however, had not brought with it an understanding of the disease, far less the power to control it. Yellow fever was not transmitted by direct contact, like smallpox, but seemed still to be infectious, and, geographically, it appeared to move erratically. Efforts to inoculate humans and animals directly with infected blood

had proven futile, and the disease required some time to develop its characteristic symptoms in an exposed individual. What causal agent and means of distribution might explain these patterns? What laboratory could test possible explanations? Italy's Giuseppe Sanarelli had identified what he believed to be the causal microbe of the disease (*Bacillus icteroides*; 1897), but many, including Surgeon General Sternberg, were unconvinced. Some thought Sanarelli had the wrong organism; others continued to believe that the disease was not caused by any living organism, but by 'fomites'—minute particles that emanated from waste materials, could be carried on clothing and other effects, and seemed to account for the disease's strange dispersion patterns. By the time Reed came to the subject (1899), it was becoming clear that the agent of yellow fever belonged to the recently recognized group of disease-causing organisms that were so small they passed through ceramic filters. (Many of these so-called filterable viruses, including the agent of yellow fever, were eventually called 'viruses'.) In June 1900 Reed, as head of the Army's Yellow Fever Commission, sailed to Cuba with longtime assistant James Carroll. They arrived to find the two other members of their commission, Jesse W. Lazear and Aristides Agramonte, already in Havana.

Although the commission was principally interested in determining the causal organism of yellow fever, its members soon turned to the problem of its epidemiology. They had at hand a local expert on the disease with an intriguing theory: Carlos J. Finlay, president of Cuba's Board of Health, had suggested some twenty years earlier that the *mosquito* transmitted yellow fever between humans. He had even determined the mosquito species most likely to act as the disease's vector (now called *Aedes aegypti*). In the intervening years, a number of other diseases, including Texas cattle fever, plague, and malaria had been linked to insect vectors. (Indeed, Patrick Manson had demonstrated the mosquito transmission of filariasis before Finlay suggested it for yellow fever.) Still, Finlay had not successfully demonstrated his theory. British malariologist Ronald Ross, however, had recently shown (1898) that mosquitoes not only spread malaria, but also served as the intermediary host of the disease: malaria parasites developed in the mosquitoes before migrating to the insects' salivary glands, from which they were inoculated into humans. The Army commission consulted with Finlay and soon began experimenting with mosquitoes. Mosquito transmission, however, could only be demonstrated on *human* subjects, which required special permission that the commission was soon granted. In uncontrolled circumstances, two of the commission members received bites that resulted in yellow fever. Carroll was bitten in late August and developed a serious, but ultimately nonfatal, case of the disease. Just as he was recovering, however, Lazear, previously bitten by a mosquito in a hospital ward, fell ill. He died on 25 September. Reed, deeply saddened by his colleague's death, now had evidence of yellow fever's transmission by mosquitoes but still lacked demonstrative proof.

That October, Reed, back in the United States, presented his preliminary findings to a meeting of the U.S. Public Health Service and convinced the military to support a controlled trial to substantiate the mosquito hypothesis. He returned to Cuba with approval and funding to construct an experimental sanitary station. The chosen location was a field about a mile outside Quemados, Cuba, which would be named 'Camp Lazear'. Reed oversaw the construction of special buildings and designed a special contract—Bean (1977, p. 75), called it a 'covenant'—to be signed by (non-immune) volunteers, informing them about the experiment and its risks. By November the buildings were ready. The first building tested the 'fomite' theory. Volunteers slept in one building, surrounded by the soiled clothing and bedding of yellow fever patients. The space was dark; it was filthy and poorly ventilated; but it was free of mosquitoes. None of these volunteers contracted the disease, even after spending a considerable number of nights in the unpleasant surroundings. A second building was clean, light, and well ventilated; yet, on one side of a floor-to-ceiling screen, it contained mosquitoes that had fed on yellow fever patients during the time those patients were suspected to be infectious. Nonimmunes were brought into this building, with those on the mosquito side being exposed only for short periods of time. The volunteers were carefully quarantined after leaving the controlled space. Still, only those exposed on the mosquito side, and bitten, contracted yellow fever. The commission published its findings. Moreover, it confirmed the timing of disease transmission through direct transfer of infected blood and, particularly through Carroll's efforts, verified that the causal agent of yellow fever was a filterable virus.

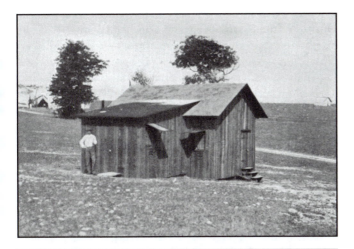

'Yellow fever hut' at Camp Lazear. Halftone reproduction from Howard A. Kelly, *Walter Reed and Yellow Fever*, New York, 1906. Wellcome Library, London.

Reed left Cuba in February 1901, returning to Washington and to teaching. His yellow fever work was the subject both of acclaim and of criticism. The acclaim apparently did not make the charges—that he had recklessly endangered human life, had stolen Finlay's ideas, or was otherwise wrong—any easier to endure. Reed appeared increasingly exhausted. In the autumn of 1902, his health began to fail. By mid-November, his condition reached a crisis. Finally, suspecting appendicitis, he consulted a doctor. Suddenly quite improved, however, Reed decided to delay surgery, but then he quickly declined again. By the time of his surgery, Reed's condition was quite poor. He died six days after the operation, on 23 November 1902, and was buried in Arlington National Cemetery. The Walter Reed Army Hospital opened in 1909. His wife Emilie was alive to see the creation of the Walter Reed Army Medical Center in 1923. She survived until 1950.

Bibliography

Primary: 1900. (with Vaughan, Victor C., and Edward O. Shakespeare) *Abstract of Report on the Origin and Spread of Typhoid Fever in U. S. Military Camps during the Spanish War of 1898* (Washington, DC); 1900. (with Carroll, James, Aristides Agramonte, and Jesse W. Lazear) 'The Etiology of Yellow Fever.' *Philadelphia Medical Journal* 148: 790–796; 1901. (with Carroll, James, and Aristides Agramonte) 'The Etiology of Yellow Fever: An Additional Note.' *JAMA* 36: 431–440; 1901. 'The Propagation of Yellow Fever; Observations Based on Recent Researches.' *Medical Record* 60: 201–209; Hench, Philip S., 'Walter Reed Yellow Fever Collection, University of Virginia': http://yellowfever.lib.virginia.edu/reed/ [archival materials available online].

Secondary: Pierce, John R., and James V. Writer, 2005. *Yellow Jack: How Yellow Fever Ravaged America and Walter Reed Discovered its Deadly Secrets* (Hoboken, NJ); Delaporte, François, 1991. *The History of Yellow Fever: An Essay on the Birth of Tropical Medicine*, trans. Goldhammer, Arthur (Cambridge, MA); Bean, William B., 1982. *Walter Reed: A Biography* (Charlottesville, VA); Bean, William B., 1977. 'Walter Reed and the Ordeal of Human Experiments.' *Bulletin of the History of Medicine* 51: 75–92; Kelly, H. A., 1906. *Walter Reed and Yellow Fever* (New York); DSB; DAMB.

Kim Pelis

REFSUM, SIGVALD BERNHARD   (b. Gransherad, Norway, 8 May 1907; d. Oslo, Norway, 8 July 1991), *neurology.*

Refsum was born in a rural area in Telemark county in southern Norway, where his father was a church minister. He was the youngest of five brothers. Originally he wanted to study theology, and in 1925 he passed secondary school in Oslo with both Latin and Greek in his range of subjects. He then became interested in medicine, and graduated as a medical doctor from the University of Oslo in 1932, planning to specialize in psychiatry. Before doing that, he wanted to gather as much knowledge as possible about the functions of the brain and nervous system. In the years

1936–47, he held several appointments as junior and senior physician at the department of neurology, Rikshospitalet, Oslo. He then spent several years in academic centers in the United States, before being appointed as professor of neurology at the University of Bergen, Norway, in 1952. Two years later, Refsum was called to the chair as professor of neurology at the University of Oslo and head of department of neurology at Rikshospitalet. He remained in this combined position until he retired in 1978.

From 1937 to 1943, while at Rikshospitalet, Refsum was able to single out five patients with certain symptoms in common, and with a disease picture which did not fit with any others in the cobweb of different neurodegenerative disorders. He concluded from his thorough clinical studies that the patients suffered from a previously undescribed inherited neurological disorder. Four features were characteristic: pigmentary retinal degeneration (retinitis pigmentosa); chronic polyneuropathy; ataxia and other cerebellar signs; and increased cerebrospinal fluid protein with normal cell count. Later on, Refsum and others found that many patients also had pupillary abnormalities, lens opacities, anosmia, skeletal malformations, and skin changes which sometimes resembled ichthyosis. First he named the disorder 'heredoataxia hemeralopica polyneuritiformis'; later he changed the name to 'heredopathia atactica polyneuritiformis'. This name, however, proved to be too difficult for most users, and the disorder is usually called Refsum's disease. The disease is rare; only about 120 cases have been reported in the literature.

In his comprehensive monograph of 1946 Refsum wrote, 'It is perhaps permissible to say that the patients suffering from our syndrome are particularly subject to the influence of extraneous factors of various kinds.' Later research confirmed this assumption. In 1963 two German scientists, Klenk and Kahlke, found large amounts of a peculiar branched-chain fatty acid, phytanic acid (3,7,11,15-tetramethylhexadecanoic acid) in the body lipids of a young girl who had died from Refsum's disease. Accumulation of phytanic acid was then found in all the known patients. The phytanic acid is of exogenous origin; large amounts are found in marine oils and plant fats. Refsum's disease patients have a biochemical defect in the degradation mechanism for phytanic acid, in the first step of the so-called a-oxidation pathway. The fact that phytanic acid was of exogenous origin opened the possibility of a dietary treatment—choosing foods with a low phytanic acid content. This treatment has been successful in many patients. For the rest of his life, Refsum retained an active interest in the disease, and contributed from the clinical side to its clarification.

Refsum was an international figure in neurology for the last half of the twentieth century. He published more than 120 articles, along with several chapters and monographs, mainly in the field of inherited neurological disease. He served on numerous national and international neurologi-

cal bodies, and was the president of the World Congress of Neurologists in 1977 and 1981. Refsum received many academic and civil honors and awards, many honorary doctorates, memberships, and fellowships. During his retirement, he continued his enduring work as a medical consultant to the Norwegian Organization for Disabled War Veterans.

Bibliography

Primary: 1946. *Heredopathia Atactica Polyneuritiformis. A Familial Syndrome Not Hitherto Described* (Oslo); 1975. 'Heredopathia Atactica Polyneuritiformis. Phytanic Acid Storage Disease (Refsum's disease)' in Vinken, P. J., and G. W. Bruyn, eds., *Handbook of Clinical Neurology*, XXI (Amsterdam) pp. 181–229.

Secondary: Wanders, Ronald J. A., Cornelis Jakobs, and Ola H. Skjeldal, 2001. 'Refsum Disease' in Scriver, C. R., A. L. Beaudet, W. S. Sly, and D. Valle, eds., *The Metabolic & Molecular Bases of Inherited Disease* (New York) pp. 3303–3321.

Oddvar Stokke

REICH, WILHELM (b. Bukovina, Galicia, Austro-Hungarian Empire [now Ukraine], 24 March 1897; d. Lewisburg, Pennsylvania, USA, 3 November 1957), *psychoanalysis, biology, sex therapy.*

Reich grew up on a farm in Bukovina. He was educated at home in German until he was thirteen, but then his education was disrupted after the suicide of his mother in 1910 and, four years later, the death of his father. He entered the German high school, although he also took responsibility for running the family farm—a situation that soon changed when the Russian Army invaded Bukovina. Reich fled his home and joined the Austrian Army, reaching the rank of lieutenant. After the war Reich entered the Medical School of the University of Vienna, graduating in 1922. He took postgraduate studies in Wagner-Jauregg's Neurological and Psychiatric University Clinic until 1924; he also worked in the psychiatric wards with Paul Schindler. More significantly, Reich became a member of the Vienna Psychoanalytic Association in 1920. He began his private psychoanalytic and psychiatric practice in 1922 and gained various university posts, including vice-directorship of the Polyclinic (1928–30) and directorship of the Seminar for Psychoanalytic Therapy (1924–30).

Reich's clinical work at this time was centered around social causation of neuroses; he also developed an interest in biopsychiatric theories that ultimately led to clashes with Sigmund Freud. These struggles grew out of Reich's development of Freud's libido theory, in which neuroses were caused by the conflict between a natural sexual instinct and the social denial of these instincts. Freud's early works relied upon a biological model of sexual energy building up and being channeled, although later work by Freud and other analysts diluted the libido concept. Reich, on the other hand, insisted that the libido energy was not simply a theoretical development and drew upon his clinical studies to show that sexually satisfied patients overcame their neurotic symptoms caused by frustration. Reich's notion of energy discharge through orgasm as a means to alleviating neurosis led to his belief that libido was a real and quantifiable energy. Failure to release this energy created physical and psychological problems. The energy discharge concept also led Reich to develop methods through which individuals could best achieve their 'orgastic potential': the capacity for total discharge of tumescent excitation.

According to Reich's theories, individuals failed to reach their orgastic potential because of cultural barriers to sexual pleasure. Through the opening of sex clinics, Reich aimed to change the way people thought about sex. The desire to overcome misery also led to Reich's involvement with the Socialist and Communist parties in Vienna and Berlin. Apart from keeping the population happy through better orgasms, Reich also dealt with the concomitant problems of sex education, contraception, and divorce. Unlike many Berlin psychoanalysts, Reich was also critical of rising National Socialism. In 1934 he was forced to flee the Nazis and was expelled from the Psychoanalytic Association. His ensuing travels took him to Sweden, Norway, and finally to America in 1939, where he taught at the New School for Social Research in New York.

Reich's commitment to a universal biological energy force, which he called 'Orgone energy', was not tied solely to the orgasm. He thought it caused the emotions, as well as being linked to other phenomena such as cancer. Because Orgone energy was a part of the natural world, Reich also linked it to the weather—which led to a series of experiments with rainmaking that did not impress the wider scientific community. One of the points of conflict that ended Reich's career was his work on cancer treatments. Just as neuroses were caused by the ineffective release of Orgone energy, so, too, the energy could have a detrimental physical effect. He thought cancer tumors to be local manifestations of the deeper systemic disorder. In order to treat this problem, Reich devised a method by which a cancer patient sat in a large box that had been adapted to draw out Orgone energy. Such techniques were thought to show a decrease in tumor size, as well providing pain relief and effecting weight gain. Nevertheless, patients died. The Food and Drug Administration (FDA) was not impressed with Reich's oncologic efforts. From 1947 to the end of his life, the FDA closed Reich's research institute, destroyed Orgone accumulators, and burned numerous of his publications. After his appeals against further charges of involvement in unregistered cancer treatments failed, Reich was incarcerated in the federal penitentiary in Lewisburg, Pennsylvania, where he died of heart failure after eight months of imprisonment.

Bibliography

Primary: 1927. *Die Funktion des Orgasmus: zur Psychopathologie und zur Soziologie des Geschlechtslebens* (Leipzig) [English edn., 1948, *Discovery of the Orgone, I: Function of the Orgasm*, 2nd edn. (New York)]; 1933. *Massenpsychologie des Faschismus* (Vienna) [English edn., 1946]; 1945. *The Sexual Revolution* (New York); 1948. *Discovery of the Orgone, II: The Cancer Biopathy* (New York).

Secondary: Corrington, Robert S., 2003. *Wilhelm Reich: Psychoanalyst and Radical Naturalist* (New York); Robinson, Paul A., 1969. *The Freudian Left* (New York); *DAMB*.

Ivan Crozier

REIL, JOHANN CHRISTIAN (b. Rhaude, Germany, 20 February 1759; d. Halle, Germany, 22 November 1813), *medicine, anatomy, physiology, psychiatry.*

Reil, son of a Lutheran pastor, received his first education in a small town on the North Sea. He studied medicine at the Universities of Göttingen and Halle. One of his teachers was the anatomist and surgeon, Phillip Friedrich Theodor Meckel (1756–1803). Reil graduated with a dissertation on biliary diseases (1782). Five years later he became extraordinary professor, and one year after that (1788), was appointed clinical professor and director of the Clinical Institute in Halle. During the Napoleonic occupation of Germany (1806–13), Reil spent much time with care of the wounded, and was also involved in reorganizing Halle's Medical School. The famous poet Johann Wolfgang von Goethe visited Reil in Halle for scientific discussions, and also consulted him as a physician. Reil was a stimulating teacher who attempted to close the gap between physicians and surgeons in Germany by proposing better educational standards for the latter. He was particularly interested in training paramedical personnel who could meet the medical needs of the rural population. Reil's reputation grew enormously, and he attracted many students to Halle. In 1810 Wilhelm von Humboldt invited him to participate in the organization of the medical school at the newly founded University of Berlin. After Reil's death some of his ideas for the university's medical clinic were adopted by the clinician Christoph Wilhelm Hufeland (1762–1836). In the battle of Leipzig (1813) Reil risked his own life in the evacuation of victims. He was infected with typhus and died in his sister's house in Halle.

Reil was one of the leading representatives of romantic medicine, which was based on the ideas of natural philosophy presented by Friedrich Wilhelm Joseph Schelling (1775–1854) in his *System der Naturphilosophie*. In connection with the natural philosophical approach of the time to life sciences, physiological explanation and experiment were extensively pursued. In this respect, medicine found itself in the center of the search for leading forces such as irritability, sensibility, and Blumenbach's nisus formativus, forces that were thought to generate and organize organic life. Reil founded the first journal (1796) dealing with physiological problems in Germany. The *Archiv für die Physiologie* published articles on physics, chemistry, histology, biology, and comparative anatomy, as well. Reil's journal was continued by Johann Friedrich

Meckel, the younger (1781–1833), and later by Johannes Müller (1801–58). The initial article of *Reil's Archive* was an extended contribution by the editor on his concept of the vital force of the organism, 'Über die Lebenskraft' [On vital force]. In this work he advocated the concept of vitalism. Like Francis Glisson (1597–1677) and John Hunter (1728–93), Reil recognized irritability as a specific tissue property. He advanced the doctrine of the life force as a chemical expression of physiological function. Reil's explanation that the vital force was located in the chemical transformation of organic matter gained great attention within the medical sciences of his time. Reil argued that, instead of dealing with mechanical principles, medicine had to be guided by certain fundamental ideas, and by this observation could reach a higher level from which all objects could be seen in their natural relationships.

As a versatile physician and physiologist, he was an advocate of humane and ethical treatment for the dying. In *Rhapsodieen über die Anwendung der psychischen Curmethode auf Geisteszerrüttungen* (1803), he pleaded for an understanding and the acceptable care of the mentally ill. Reil's *Entwurf einer allgemeinen Therapie* and *Entwurf einer allgemeinen Pathologie* were published after his sudden death in 1813.

Bibliography

Primary: 1796. 'Von der Lebenskraft.' *Archiv für die Physiologie* 1: 8–162; 1799–1816. *Ueber die Erkenntniss und Chur der Fieber* 5 vol. (Halle); 1803. *Rhapsodieen über die Anwendung der psychischen Curmethode auf Geisteszerrüttungen* (Halle).

Secondary: Broman, Thomas H., 1996. *The Transformation of German Academic Medicine, 1750–1820* (Cambridge); Lohff, Brigitte, 1990. *Die Suche nach der Wissenschaftlichkeit der Physiologie in der Zeit der Romantik* (*Medizin in Geschichte und Kultur*, Vol. 17) (Stuttgart); *DSB*.

Brigitte Lohff

REIMANN, CHRISTIANE ELISABETH (b. Copenhagen, Denmark, 6 May 1888; d. Syracuse, Sicily, 12 April 1979), *nursing.*

Reimann was an only child of stockbroker Carl Christian Reimann and Margit Meisterlin. After primary school (1904) she went abroad for a period, but otherwise remained at home. At the age of twenty-five she decided to become a nurse. Her family opposed this, arguing that 'a nurse is not a lady'; but she pursued her ambition and trained as a nurse from 1913 to 1916 at Bispebjerg Hospital in Copenhagen. The matron of the hospital persuaded her to enroll at Teachers College, Columbia University, New York, and she graduated BS in 1921 and MA in 1925. In 1922 she was elected secretary for the International Council of Nurses (ICN).

The ICN was founded in 1899 by the British suffragist and nurse Ethel Gordon Fenwick, who stated, 'The nursing profession above all things requires organization; nurses, above all other things, require to be united' (Brush et al., 1999, p.1). The vision was that the ICN should be a union of national nursing organizations, led by and representing nurses only, independent of governmental control. Reimann was elected honorary secretary, an unpaid position, at the 1922 ICN meeting at which Henny Tscherning of Denmark passed on her presidency to Sophie Mannerheim from Finland. In 1925 Reimann was reelected—with salary—and given the title of executive secretary. She was located in Geneva, where the ICN established headquarters that same year.

Full of enthusiasm, Reimann started reconstructing the ICN, which had almost ceased functioning during World War I. The coffers were nearly empty, and Reimann contributed generously from her large personal fortune. Part of her time was spent following up on ICN meetings, but her overriding objective was 'to make ICN a recognized international organization, an international spokesman for nurses, an international center for nursing and health care' (Kruse, 1979, p. 22). She pursued this objective by establishing an advisory service in nursing matters for governments and health authorities, and partnerships with international organizations that employed nurses or dealt with questions relating to health. Another objective was to keep in touch with ICN member organizations, and generally inspire nurses throughout the world to form organizations. To that end Reimann traveled extensively at her own expense, visiting twenty European nurses' organizations between 1925 and 1927. Her policy and efforts succeeded in raising the number of member organizations from fourteen to twenty-nine during her twelve years as executive secretary.

In 1922 Reimann took the initiative of publishing, at her own expense, the ICN's first official periodical, *The Bulletin*. The name was changed in 1926 to *The ICN*, and again in 1930 to *International Nursing Review*. Reimann served as editor of the journal and wrote most of the articles herself. She furthermore founded and financed an extensive specialized library in Geneva.

In 1934 Reimann resigned from the ICN due to bad health. Allegedly, her decision was also because of disagreements with board members who felt uncomfortable about Reimann's position of power resulting from her financial support. Another reason was that, in the same year, Reimann married Wilhelm F. C. Alter. The marriage, however, remains a mystery, as there is no evidence of it other than its announcement.

Reimann settled in Sicily, where she bought a property close to Syracuse. In 1967 she offered her property to ICN as a resort for nurses, but ICN declined it as too expensive to maintain. Reimann kept to another decision, namely to fund a prestigious international award in nursing to be considered 'the Nobel Prize for nursing', but named the Christiane Reimann Prize. The first awarded, in 1985, was to Virginia Henderson from the United States.

Reimann played a crucial role in building up the ICN after World War I. Her professional skills and great capacity for work, as well as her intelligence and generosity, made her a devoted pioneer in the international nursing community. In 2002, Reimann was inducted into the Nursing Hall of Fame of Teachers College, Columbia University, New York.

Bibliography

Secondary: Malchau, Susanne, 2001. *Christiane Reimann 1888–1979* (Copenhagen); Brush, Barbara L., et al., 1999. *Nurses of All Nations* (Philadelphia); Kruse, Margrethe, 1979. 'In memoriam.' *Tidsskrift for Sygeplejersker* 18: 22–23.

Susanne Malchau

RENAUDOT, THEOPHRASTE (b. Loudun, France, 1586; d. Paris, France, 25 October 1653), *journalism, philanthropy, chemistry.*

Renaudot was born to bourgeois Protestant parents who were affluent enough to provide a good education. At about age thirteen, Renaudot went to the University of Poitiers. After a conventional classical education, he studied medicine at the University of Montpellier, which welcomed Protestants and offered a more innovative curriculum than the text-based education of the Faculty of Medicine of Paris. After receiving his medical degree on 16 January 1606, Renaudot traveled and then studied surgery at the College of Saint-Côme. The surgeons relied on experience rather than on Aristotelian or Galenic theory as a foundation of medical practice. In later polemics, the Faculty of Medicine indicted Renaudot for his surgical study.

Renaudot returned to Loudun in 1609 to set up a medical practice and begin a family. He married Marthe Dumoustier, daughter of a prominent Protestant family; they had three sons and two daughters. His first medical work favorably discussed polychréton, another name for antimony, which identified him as a proponent of chemical medicine and further distanced him from the medical establishment. He pursued interests in botany and anatomy, and proposed remedies for poverty in Loudun, defining the crucial interests of his subsequent public career in practicing avant-garde medicine, disseminating new knowledge, and implementing relief to the poor. Renaudot wrote a treatise on the poor, which brought him to the attention of Richelieu, then bishop of nearby Luçon. After the death of his first wife in 1624, Renaudot converted to Catholicism (1626), greatly improving his chances for success in Paris, to which he moved the same year.

In the 1630s, with the support of Richelieu, then Louis XIII's prime minister, Renaudot launched many institutions designed to serve the poor. He founded the Bureau d'adresse, designed to offer practical solutions to urban problems and to provide poor relief. Offering information about employment opportunities, real estate, missing persons, etc., the Bureau brought those with services to offer into contact with those who needed them. At the Bureau, Renaudot also operated chemical furnaces to produce medications, offered free medical consultations, introduced monts de piété (pawnshops offering low-interest loans to the poor), and sponsored public conferences on contemporary topics, many of them medical.

The Bureau attracted the enthusiasm of reform-minded physicians. Renaudot's medical consultations functioned as teaching clinics, offering the practical medicine the Faculty abhorred. In the early 1640s, Renaudot proposed to send to patients in remote areas a questionnaire to be submitted to physicians at the Bureau for diagnosis. He also planned to build, with the endorsement of Louis XIII and Richelieu, a teaching hospital in Paris.

The Faculty of Medicine saw Renaudot's medical activities as a direct threat to its monopoly over medical practice and education in Paris. It generated pamphlets and lawsuits to discredit Renaudot, but could not prevail as long as Richelieu protected him. (Guy Patin was the chief spokesman for the Faculty.) After the death of Richelieu (1642) and Louis XIII (1643), the Faculty successfully sued Renaudot for illegal medical practice. On 19 December 1643, the court condemned all of Renaudot's activities. Only his publication, the *Gazette de France*, survived the death of his patrons; the crown supported it, the first newspaper in France, for its propaganda value.

Bibliography

Primary: 1634. *Première Centurie des Questions traitées ez Conférences du Bureau d'adresse* (Paris) [Four subsequent volumes of 100 conferences each, 1635–1652 (Paris)]; 1643. *Requeste présentée à la Reyne par Théophraste Renaudot, en faveur des pauvres malades de ce Royaume* (Paris); 1643. *Factum du Procez, d'entre Théophraste Renaudot, demandeur en rapport d'arrest: Et les Médicins de l'eschole de Paris deffendeurs* (Paris).

Secondary: Wellman, Kathleen, 2003. *Making Science Social: The Conferences of Théophraste Renaudot, 1633–1642* (Norman, OK); Mazauric, Simone, 1997. *Savoirs et philosophie à Paris dans la première moitié du XVIIe siècle* (Paris); Solomon, Howard, 1972. *Public Welfare, Science, and Propaganda in Seventeenth-Century France: The Innovations of Théophraste Renaudot* (Princeton).

Kathleen Wellman

REVERDIN, JAQUES-LOUIS (b. Frontenex, near Geneva, Switzerland, 28 August 1842; d. Geneva, 9 January 1929), *surgery.*

Reverdin was born to a family of Huguenot descent, established in Geneva since 1709. His father, Adolphe (1809–1901), worked as an architect, and his mother, Catherine Mayor, was the daughter of a well-established physician, François Mayor (1779–1854), renowned for being the first to hear the heartbeat of a fetus in 1818. Jaques-Louis was the eldest of four brothers. His elementary education was provided by Geneva College, from where he went on to study at the town's Academy, graduating BA in 1860, and then BSc in 1862.

Reverdin then left Geneva for Paris, where part of his family was established. He was twenty years of age and had decided to study medicine. One can only surmise that the regular contacts he had with his great uncle François Mayor influenced his decision. He was admitted as an interne in 1865, having come nineteenth in the prestigious Parisian competition for internship. His clinical work was carried out under Alphonse Guérin, Félix Guyon, and Léon Gosselin, and his special interest was surgery. His years in Paris were important both for learning and for the social contacts he had with fellow students, including a number of fellow countrymen such as Constant Picot, Adolphe D'Espine, Louis Odier, and Jean-Louis Prevost, a group with whom he was to remain in contact during the rest of his professional life.

In 1869, as he was preparing to return to Geneva, Reverdin won the gold medal of the internship competition, and was therefore invited to prolong his internship for an extra two years. He used the extra time to pursue his expertise in surgery. As a student, he observed the natural formation of what he called 'islets of epidermis on wounds', and envisaged performing a skin graft in order to enhance the healing process. This was to be his first major discovery, and his director, Félix Guyon, encouraged him to present it to the Société impériale de chirurgie [Imperial Surgical society], which he did on 9 December 1869. Subsequently, the technique was rapidly adopted in European hospitals.

In 1870 Reverdin published his doctoral dissertation, *Etude sur l'uréthromtomie interne*, which received the civil prize from the Académie de médecine and the bronze prize from the Faculty of Medicine. He remained in Paris during the German siege and the Commune, taking charge, on top of his normal duties, of an ambulance subsidized by the Swiss community. After the Commune, at the end of 1871, Reverdin visited hospitals in Italy, Prussia, Austria, and Great Britain. In the summer of 1872, after having pondered a career in Paris, he decided definitively to return to Geneva. A little more than a year later, on 15 January 1874, he married Marguerite Bron with whom he would have five children—three girls and two boys.

The same year Reverdin was appointed assistant surgeon in the Cantonal hospital, and then surgeon in charge (1878–82). In 1876, the year of the founding of Geneva's medical school, he was promoted professor of external pathology. As this was a part-time activity, Reverdin was also active in private practice. In 1879 he founded with his cousin, Auguste Reverdin (1848–1908), a private surgical clinic, the first institution of its kind in Geneva. He was also active in the professional sphere, and in 1892 was a founding member of the Association des médecins du canton de Genève (AMG).

Reverdin was a good friend of Lucas Championnière, a key figure in the diffusion of Lister's practices in France. Possibly due to Championnière's influence, he was an early supporter of Lister's bandages, and his taking a position at the Cantonal hospital coincided with Louis Odier's decision to introduce Lister's techniques into Geneva's wards. In 1879 Reverdin modified a suture needle, which was later improved by his cousin Auguste and was then known as 'the Reverdin needle'. In 1882 he presented a paper that was the first to call attention to the danger of totally removing goiters, the solution accepted at the time for healing 'endemic goiter conditions' (goîtres endémiques). In a long paper published the following year, he retraced the cases of all known operations in the Geneva area. The conclusion the cousins came to is that the secondary effects of total removal of the goiter were serious enough for them to recommend partial excision wherever possible.

For many years, Reverdin was a respected surgeon, professor, and editor of the *Revue médicale de la Suisse romande*. He retired from practice and teaching in 1910, some ten years before the legal age, impeded by growing deafness. He spent his last active years studying and publishing widely on the anatomy and the physiology of butterflies.

Bibliography

Primary: 1870. 'Greffe épidermique.' *Bull. Soc. imp. Chir. Paris* (1869) 2 sér 10: 511–515; 1882. 'Accidents consécutifs à l'ablation totale du goiter.' *Rev. méd. Suisse rom.* 2: 539; 1883. 'Note sur vingt-deux opérations de goiter.' *Rev. méd. Suisse rom.* 3: 169–198, 233–278, 309–364; 1887. 'Contribution à l'étude du myxoedème consécutif à l'extirpation totale au partielle du corps thyroïde.' *Rev. méd. Suisse rom.* 7: 275–291, 318–330.

Secondary: Saudan, Guy, 1993. 'Jaques-Louis Reverdin (1842–1929) et son cousin Auguste (1848–1908), ou quand la clinique chirurgicale précède la physiologie expérimentale.' *Revue médicale de la Suisse romande* 113: 567–581; Reverdin, Henri, 1971. *Jaques-Louis Reverdin, 1842–1929. Un chirurgien à l'aube d'une ère nouvelle. Publications de la Société suisse d'histoire de la médecine et des sciences naturelles* (no 25) (Aarau).

Philip Rieder

RIBAS, EMÍLIO (b. Pindamonhangaba, Brazil, 11 April 1862; d. São Paulo, Brazil, 19 December 1925), *public health, microbiology.*

Ribas was born in the countryside of the state of São Paulo, then the center of a dynamic coffee economy. In 1887 he graduated from Rio de Janeiro's School of Medicine and returned to his hometown to work as a physician. He also took part in the political effervescence of republican and abolitionist movements of the time. In 1896–97 he directed the sanitary services of Campinas, an important town within the coffee economy, then threatened by yellow fever.

Under the new republican regime, Ribas was appointed in 1898 director of the Sanitary Services of the State of São

Paulo, and initiated an administration characterized by the creation of permanent services against the main diseases, by hygienic education, and by a clear distribution of responsibilities among the state and the municipalities. One year after his appointment bubonic plague struck Santos, the main port for coffee exports. Local merchants and physicians rejected Ribas' diagnosis and provoked a national debate on the origins of the epidemic. Ribas upheld the plague's microbial origin, supported by medical doctors such as Oswaldo Cruz, who formed part of an emergent network linked by the microbiological paradigm. Ribas's success in the control of plague (and in the related debate) facilitated his creation of a permanent São Paulo laboratory for the production of antiplague sera. Eventually, the initiative resulted in the Butantan Institute, which became best known for its work on snake poisons.

An article by Ribas published in January 1901 reinforced the idea that the *Aedes aegypti* mosquito transmitted yellow fever, and praised the work done in Cuba a year before by U.S. medical scientists. In December 1902 he reproduced the Cuban experience in São Paulo. Ribas dismissed critics that discredited him because Havana was an epidemic town, in contrast to São Paulo that was free from endemic yellow fever. Initially, six volunteers, among them Ribas, allowed themselves to be bitten by mosquitoes infected with mild forms of the disease. In a second stage, three volunteers—Italian immigrants who were not immune—were confined in a sealed room for ten days with the clothes and fluids of yellow fever patients. A report of an independent medical committee, issued in May 1903, legitimized the experiment. It concluded that yellow fever's sole means of transmission was the *Aedes*' bite. Ribas's work was immediately associated with the leading role assumed by microbiology in Brazilian medicine at the turn of the twentieth century.

The experience also gained national and international visibility. For Cruz, national director for Brazil's public health, the experience was instrumental for his successful anti-*Aedes* sanitary campaigns in Rio de Janeiro and other cities. The sanitation of São Paulo, Rio, and the main Brazilian ports contributed to an image of security and safety for Brazil during the early twentieth century. This image was crucial to Brazil's commercial interests, as well as to coveted European immigration. In 1909 Ribas was invited by Patrick Mason to a meeting in London to deliver a paper on the yellow fever work he had performed with Cruz.

Between 1913 and 1917 Ribas intensified his interest in leprosy, publishing works against the confinement of the sick in remote leper asylums, on leprosy as a hereditary disease, and on the domiciliary treatment of lepers. Ribas retired in 1917, after nineteen years of leading the modernization of public health in the richest Brazilian state. His research contributed to the validation of microbiology as the basis of sanitary interventions against contagious diseases. His work was also a remarkable example of the articulation of politics, biomedical research, and public health.

Bibliography

Primary: 1901. *O mosquito como agente de propagação da febre amarela* (São Paulo); 1903. 'Profilaxia da febre amarela.' *Revista Médica de São Paulo* 22: 477–485; 1909. 'The extinction of yellow fever in the State of São Paulo (Brazil) and in the city of Rio de Janeiro.' *Revista Médica de São Paulo* 10: 198–205.

Secondary: Almeida, Marta de, 2003. *República dos Invisíveis: Emílio Ribas, Microbiologia e Saúde Pública em São Paulo (1898–1917)* (São Paulo).

Gilberto Hochman and
Marta de Almeida

RICHARD THE ENGLISHMAN (fl. England, early thirteenth century), *medicine.*

Little is known about the life of this early thirteenth-century, prolific author of Latin texts. Plagued by homonyms, this Richard is unlikely to be the theologian of early thirteenth-century Paris. He has been variously linked with Paris, Salerno, and Montpellier; Talbot, in particular, pointedly attaches him to the latter two centers. In addition, it is thought that he was part of the papal court. Paravicini firmly links him with the more historically identifiable Richard of Wendover, canon of St Paul's and doctor to pope Gregory IX. If Richard is he, Wendover is known to have died in London in 1252; his name is first found in a grant in 1233, in a charter of 1237, and variously thereafter. Matthew Paris refers to Wendover's donation of an ivory cross given to him by the pope, who lay on his deathbed. Wendover also was likely an attendant to Bishop Suffield. He held prebends of Rugmere and Neasden, and amassed considerable holdings, distributed at his demise.

The one compelling biographical detail is that his principle text was written for Lancelinus de l'Isle-Adam, the dean of Beauvais (1178–90, not his own homonym from a century earlier). However, this makes problematic the above mid-thirteenth-century associations. Richard was referred to specifically by his near contemporary, Gilbert the Englishman as, 'of all the doctors the most learned and experienced' (Getz, 1998, pp. 39–40).

While his life is enigmatic at best, Richard is known as the author of the *Micrologus*. No complete extant copy survives, although its constituents exist in separate witnesses. The *Micrologus* consisted of *On the Causes, Signs and Cures of Diseases (Practica); Rules on Urines; Anatomy; A Short Treatise on Acute Medicines and Violent Laxatives;* and *On Prognostic Signs of the Sick (On Signs).* The *Practica* employed the head-to-foot organization for disease-based therapies common at the time. *Anatomy* innovated well beyond the Salernitan porcine anatomies in both detail and synthesis. In general, the *Micrologus* made abundant use of Salernitan authors, including Archimateus, Copho, Ferrarius, Petrocellus, and Platearius, as well as of the *Antidoary of Nicholas.*

Karl Sudhoff identified some thirty-eight manuscripts associated broadly with Richard. But given the paucity of details about his life, identification of Richard as the author of other texts is highly uncertain. Those with which his name has been linked include: *The Compendium of Medicine*, *A Treatise on Fevers and Other Diverse Diseases*, *On Pulses*, *On Critical Days*, *On Phlebotomy*, and *On Cosmetics*. Recent scholars have rather definitively disassociated from his name a variety of other texts.

Bibliography

Primary: 1902. *Anatomia Ricardi Anglici (c. 1242–1252): ad fidem codicis ms. n. 1634 in Bibliotheca Palatina Vindobonensi asservati; primum edidit Robertus Toply eques.* (Vienna); Beusing, Hermann H., 1922. *Leben und Werke des Ricardus Anglicus, samt einem erstmaligen Abdruck seiner Schrift "Signa"* (Leipzig); Frers, Erich, 1934. *Die 'Practica' aus dem Micrologus Richards des Engländers* (Leipzig).

Secondary: Paravicini Baglinai, Augustino, 2000. *The Pope's Body* trans. Peterson, David S. (Chicago); Getz, Faye Marie, 1998. *Medicine in the English Middle Ages* (Princeton); Paravicini Bagliani, Augustino, 1991. *Medicina e scienze della natura alla corte dei papi nel duecento* (Spoleto); Baader, Gerhard, 1974. 'Mathematische und alchimistische Traktate, angeblich von Ricardus Anglicus.' *Actes du XIIIe Congrès International d'Histoire des Sciences 1971* 3–4: 185–189; Talbot, Charles H., 1967. *Medicine in Medieval England* (London); Talbot, Charles H,. and E. A. Hammond, 1965. *The Medical Practitioners in Medieval England: A Biographical Register* (London) pp. 270–272, 284–285.

Walton O. Schalick III

RICHARDS, ALFRED NEWTON (b. Stamford, New York, USA, 22 March 1876; d. Bryn Mawr, Pennsylvania, USA, 24 March 1966), *pharmacology, physiology, administration.*

In Richards's laboratory at the University of Pennsylvania, micropuncture of the nephron was born; it provided the first convincing demonstration of how the kidney fundamentally worked. Richards was born in Stanford, New York, studied at Yale College and its Sheffield Scientific School, and received the PhD from the Department of Physiological Chemistry of Columbia University in 1901. Moving to Columbia's College of Physicians and Surgeons, he worked with physiological chemist Christian Herter and pediatrician John Howland on chloroform poisoning, while creating a laboratory course in pharmacology for 'P & S' medical students. Following additional years of teaching and research at Columbia and, from 1908, at Northwestern Medical School in Chicago, Richards came to the University of Pennsylvania in Philadelphia as professor of pharmacology in 1910.

In this period, debate continued on the question of whether the kidney fashioned urine by way of a dominantly 'mechanical' ultrafiltration process or by 'active' tubular secretion, a theory some condemned as 'vitalistic'. Richards was interested in this question as early as 1913–14 when,

with Cecil Drinker, he constructed a pump for the perfusion of isolated organs, including the kidney, which he used to study the diuretic effect of caffeine. In 1919 Richards and recent Pennsylvania medical student Carl Schmidt began observations on the exposed kidney of the frog. Joseph Wearn, a young Harvard medical graduate, replaced Schmidt in 1921, soon after Richards had learned of a technique for puncturing a red cell using an extraordinarily fine glass pipette. Richards thought such a pipette might be used with the frog kidney preparation to place adrenalin on the efferent arteriole and observe its effect. Wearn proposed instead that they puncture the glomerulus, obtain some fluid, and see what it was like. After extensive tinkering, they succeeded. Results supported glomerular ultrafiltration and tubular reabsorption. Subsequently, Richards's team (mainly Phyllis Bott, Jean Oliver, and Arthur Walker) extended the work to the mammalian kidney, providing a firm foundation for understanding nephron function. From 1931 the Commonwealth Fund, based in New York City, supported Richards's laboratory. It expected prompt clinical yield, so Richards established a 'small hospital unit in which renal disease in man can be studied by modern methods of blood and urine analysis and dietary control'.

Richards's reputation for quiet but effective leadership led to his appointment as vice-president for medical affairs at the University of Pennsylvania. In 1941 he was named chairman of the Committee on Medical Research of the Office of Scientific Research and Development, which oversaw war-related investigation, and his laboratory closed. Under his guidance, methods were attained for the mass production of penicillin. Following his wartime work (and retirement from Pennsylvania), Richards—now medical statesman rather than active scientist—served as president of the National Academy of Sciences and a director of the pharmaceutical house Merck and Company. Phyllis Bott moved to Philadelphia's Woman's Medical College, where she alone kept micropuncture alive until it was revived in the 1960s as the pre-eminent tool of renal physiology.

Coworkers have recalled Richards's integrity, self-deprecation, commitment to education, and sense of humor. Not a brilliant theorist, his career illustrates how scientific accomplishment, enabled by a university that needed it and a foundation that was eager to pay for it, might propel a nonphysician into the highest realm of leadership in what came to be known as 'biomedicine'. Richards received numerous awards (including the Flexner Award of the Association of American Medical Colleges) and honorary degrees. In 1908 he married Lillian Woody, with whom he had one son.

Bibliography

Primary: 1924. (with Wearn, Joseph) 'Observations on the Composition of Glomerular Urine with Particular Reference to the Problem of Reabsorption in the Renal Tubules.' *American Journal of Physiology* 71: 209–227; 1929. *Methods and Results of Direct Investi-*

gations of the Function of the Kidney (Baltimore); 1964. 'Production of Penicillin in the United States (1941–1946).' *Nature* 201: 441–445.

Secondary: Peitzman, Steven J., 1991. 'Micropuncture and the Mechanistic Kidney: A New Look at a Classic Experiment.' *Bulletin of the History of Medicine* 65: 366–375; Schmidt, Carl F., 1971. 'Alfred Newton Richards.' *Biographical Memoirs of the National Academy of Sciences* 42: 271–318; *DAMB.*

Stephen J. Peitzman

RICHARDS, DICKINSON WOODRUFF (b. Orange, New Jersey, USA, 30 October 1895; d. Lakeville, Connecticut, USA, 23 February 1973), *cardiology, respiratory physiology.*

The son of the lawyer Dickinson Woodruff Richards and his wife Sally, Richards was a shy and modest child with an aptitude for learning. At Hotchkiss School in Lakeville, Connecticut, he received a classical education in the humanities, Greek, English, and history. He excelled, won numerous prizes, and went to Yale for undergraduate studies, where he communicated in Greek with his roommate and added a solid foundation in mathematics and sciences to his achievements in the humanities. Upon his graduation (1917), he enlisted in the U.S. Army and served in France. After the war, he decided to follow his maternal grandfather and three uncles into the medical profession. He obtained an MA in physiology from Columbia University (1922) and an MD from Columbia University College of Physicians and Surgeons (1923).

Richards's approach to scientific medicine, according to his own account, was shaped above all by two physiologists, Lawrence J. Henderson (1878–1942) and Henry Dale (1875–1968). Henderson, with whom he corresponded frequently during his internship and residency at Presbyterian Hospital in New York, provided him with the theoretical foundations for his work on cardiac and pulmonary physiology. In 1927 Richards went to London for a year, with a research fellowship from Columbia, to train with Dale at the MRC-funded National Institute for Medical Research, where he was impressed by Dale's skills and creativity as an experimenter. When he returned to New York in 1928, Richards joined a group of full-time clinicians and researchers at the newly created Columbia University–Presbyterian Hospital Medical Center as an assistant physician. The year 1932 marked the beginning of Richards's collaboration and lifelong friendship with André Cournand (1895–1988), then chief resident of the Chest Service at Bellevue Hospital, which led to their Nobel Prize in Physiology or Medicine in 1956 (which they shared with the German Werner Forssmann, 1904–79). Their collaboration was dedicated to detailed studies of cardiopulmonary function, starting from L. J. Henderson's hypothesis that lung, heart, and circulation form a single system for the exchange of respiratory gases between the environment and the tissues of an organism.

In 1936 they began experiments with the introduction of a catheter into the right atrium of the heart, first with dogs and later with a chimpanzee. In 1940 they applied this technique to a human patient, and, in subsequent years, they demonstrated that it was also possible to introduce catheters into the right ventricle and the pulmonary artery. During the war, they worked on shock and the effects of severe injuries on the circulation (under the Committee on Medical Research of the Office of Scientific Research and Development, in which Richards later assumed the role of deputy director of physiologic studies). Catheterization provided them with a means of adequately measuring gas concentrations and blood pressures at crucial points of the circulatory system and contributed, in the postwar period, to the treatment of various forms of cardiac and pulmonary disease. Today, catheterization is a routine procedure.

In 1945 Richards was appointed professor of medicine at Columbia University, director of the Columbia University Medical Service at Bellevue Hospital, and in 1947 Lambert Professor, positions he held until his retirement in 1961. Richards was a popular director who left his mark as a campaigner for a reform of the hospital system in New York. From 1934 he also acted as medical advisor to the Merck pharmaceutical company. After his retirement, his interests in the medical humanities intensified. He published on ancient Greek medicine and Hippocrates, as well as on the history of circulatory physiology; he directed a program in the history of biomedical sciences at Columbia; and he took part in seminars on sociomedical issues and ethical problems in medicine.

Bibliography

Primary: 1957. 'Right Heart Catheterization. Its Contributions to Physiology and Medicine.' *Science* 125: 1181–1185.

Secondary: Cournand, André, 1989. 'Dickinson Woodruff Richards.' *Biographical Memoirs of the National Academy of Sciences* 58: 459–487; Cournand, André, 1974. 'Dickinson Woodruff Richards: 1895–1973.' *American Journal of Medicine* 57: 312–328; *DAMB.*

Carsten Timmermann

RICHARDS, LINDA ANN JUDSON (b. Potsdam, New York, USA, 27 July 1841; d. Boston, Massachusetts, USA, 16 April 1930), *nursing.*

Christened Melinda Ann Judson Richards after the missionary Ann Hasselton Judson (1789–1826), Richards grew up to be a devout Christian who aspired to the missionary life. She was the youngest daughter of Sanford and Betsy Sinclair Richards, both of whom were dead of tuberculosis before she was out of her teens. Cared for by her maternal grandfather, she lived in Derby and Lyndon in Vermont and attended the Barton Academy. Some accounts say that she often nursed friends and relatives in the community. For about seven years, she worked at the Union Straw

Works in Foxboro, Massachusetts, and then briefly as an assistant nurse at Boston City Hospital. Then, in 1872, she learned of the formation of the nurses' training school at the New England Hospital for Women and Children in Boston and enrolled in the first class.

After completing the one-year program, Richards first worked as night superintendent at Bellevue Hospital in New York City and then helped develop the Boston Training School for Nurses in Massachusetts. In 1877 she spent eight months in England and Scotland observing the nurses' training systems at St Thomas' Hospital and King's College in London and the Royal Infirmary in Edinburgh. On her return, she developed a successful new training program at Boston City Hospital. Then, in 1879, she became ill and was unable to work for three years. The illness was variously described as pulmonary and nervous troubles. Given her family history, it seems tuberculosis was the likely cause.

When she recovered, she was determined to follow her renewed missionary ideal and left for Kyoto, Japan, in 1885 to establish a training school for nurses. The Boston-based Women's Board of Missions underwrote the expenses of the training school and hospital and found Richards to be an outstanding candidate for the task. The project proved to be full of difficulties, but the school did open in the fall of 1886 with five students and graduated four trained nurses in June 1888. Richards was anxious to fulfill her main goal, which was to convert the Japanese to Christianity, but she was distracted and exhausted by the exigencies of training nurses and caring for patients. She received little help and was not able to bridge the cultural and religious differences she encountered. Once again she became ill and was forced to resign in early 1890.

After a year of recovery, Richards, now back in the United States and sought after due to her excellent reputation as a reforming nurse, embarked on a series of ten short-term positions, which she fulfilled as her health permitted. She worked at founding nurses' training schools and improving programs in Philadelphia and Boston. Disturbed by the appalling conditions she found in the insane asylums of the day, she turned her attention to improving the standards of nursing by developing training schools in several asylums.

In 1911, at age seventy, she wrote her *Reminiscences,* which was privately published. She retired, living with relatives near Lowell, Massachusetts. Her health declined; in 1925 she suffered a cerebral hemorrhage. She died at the New England Hospital in 1930 and was buried in Forest Hills Cemetery in Boston.

Bibliography

Primary: 1894. 'Mission Training Schools and Nursing' in Billings, John S., and Henry M. Hurd, eds. *Hospitals, Dispensaries, and Nursing* (Baltimore) pp. 565–569 [reprint, 1984 (New York)]; 1911. *Reminiscences of Linda Richards* (Boston); 1915. 'Early Days in the First American Training School for Nurses.' *American Journal of Nursing* 16: 174–179.

Secondary: Doona, Mary Ellen, 1996. 'Linda Richards and Nursing in Japan, 1885–1890.' *Nursing History Review* 4: 99–128; Hawkins, Joellen Watson, 1988. 'Richards, Linda Ann Judson' in Kaufman, Martin, ed., *Dictionary of American Nursing Biography* (New York) pp. 301–306; Goostray, Stella, 1971. 'Richards, Linda.' in James, Edward T., ed., *Notable American Women* (Cambridge, MA, and London) pp. 148–150; *DAMB*.

Joan E. Lynaugh

RICHERAND, ANTHELME BALTHASAR [also BALTHAZARD] (b. Bellay, France, 4 February 1779; d. Villecresnes, France, 23 January 1840), *surgery, physiology, medical education.*

Richerand grew up in modest circumstances in the Bugey region of eastern France, at the southern end of the Jura mountains, the son of a royal notary who died when Richerand was three. With the encouragement of a local physician, he went to the French capital at the age of sixteen to study medicine. He enrolled from 1796 to 1798 at the Paris School of Health, one of three new medical schools established by the revolutionary National Convention at the end of 1794. To help make ends meet, he offered private instruction in physiology. He received his doctorate in 1799, with a thesis on fractures of the collarbone and femur.

The young Richerand became the protégé of the physician-philosopher Georges Cabanis (1757–1808) and the lawyer, economist, and gastronomist Anthelme Brillat-Savarin (1755–1826), who came from his hometown of Bellay. Brillat-Savarin later lauded Richerand in his celebrated *Physiology of Taste* (1825). Richerand's patrons introduced him to the world of Parisian literary, intellectual, and scientific elites, particularly the circle known as the Idéologues, followers of the sensationalist philosophy of the Enlightenment thinker Condillac (1714–80), which linked mental functions to sensory experience.

Richerand enjoyed a rapid rise in the surgical profession and medical academia. He was named associate chief of surgery at Saint-Louis Hospital in 1801, the year when the government confirmed the hospital's role as a special institution for skin disease. He subsequently became chief. In 1807 he was appointed to the chair of external pathology, and the directorship of the Institute of Surgical Pathology, of the Faculty of Paris; in 1818 he moved to the chair of surgical operations and apparatus. Richerand was one of the original members of the Royal Academy of Medicine, founded in 1820. His many other honors included membership in the Legion of Honor and, under the Bourbon Restoration, letters of nobility as a chevalier (1815), and then as a baron (1829).

Whether Richerand's accomplishments merited such distinctions was a subject of debate among his contemporaries, some of whom accused him of leaning too heavily on the work of others, including that of François Chaussier and Xavier Bichat. Richerand returned their contempt; he had a notably bitter feud with Guillaume Dupuytren. Whatever his skills as a practitioner and teacher, he was not responsible for any notable innovations or discoveries. He took great pride in his own position at Saint-Louis, and even included a picture of its building in his baronial coat of arms; but he was remembered there mainly for his reorganization of the institution as a military hospital to care for the casualties of the Battle of Paris in 1814.

Richerand owed his celebrity mainly to his many publications. He published a major text on physiology while still in his early twenties; it reached a total of ten editions and was widely translated and reprinted. His caustic book on popular medical errors became a minor classic. Other works included a study of the links between politics and demography. An increasingly strong conservative streak ran through Richerand's writings, even though the reforms of the French Revolution had made his medical career possible. He attacked democracy, which he feared would be encouraged by population growth in Europe, and also Enlightenment ideas on the science of government.

Richerand is remembered primarily as a medical man of letters. His oeuvre provides a distinctive perspective on the French medical world of the first half of the nineteenth century, from someone who stood at its very center.

Bibliography

Primary: 1801–02. *Nouveaux éléments de physiologie* 2 vols. (Paris); 1810. *Des erreurs populaires relatives à la médecine* (Paris); 1825. *Histoire des progrès récents de la chirurgie* (Paris).

Secondary: Moinet, Lyliane, and Joseph Dumazel, 2000. 'Un citoyen illustre de Villecresnes: Anthelme Balthazard Richerand (1779–1840).' *Clio 94* 18: 133–136.

Matthew Ramsey

RICHET, CHARLES   (b. Paris, France, 25 August 1850; d. Paris, 4 December, 1935), *physiology, immunology.*

Richet was the son of a noted surgeon and professor of the Paris Faculty of Medicine. His preference for experimental science resulted in his being named to the chair of physiology at the early age of thirty-seven (he had taken his MD at nineteen). In 1913 he received the Nobel Prize for his discovery of anaphylaxis.

When Richet was still an intern in surgery, his mentor, Aristide Verneuil, treated a patient who had swallowed a caustic, requiring his esophagus to be removed and replaced with a tube to the stomach. The experiments Richet conducted, while observing the action of the stomach directly, led him to conclude that gastric juice was primarily hydrochloric acid, thus confirming the observations of William Beaumont. Richet's credentials as a researcher were further enhanced by his work on animal body temperature (it was Richet who showed that dogs cooled themselves by panting) and, most importantly, by his discovery of anaphylaxis—the increased sensitivity of the body to moderate doses of some poisons.

According to his unpublished memoirs, Richet's discovery of anaphylaxis was prompted by a remark made by Prince Albert of Monaco, who suggested to Richet during a yachting cruise that someone should study the poisonous sting of the Portuguese man-of-war jellyfish. Richet found that exposure produced fatal reactions to even the slightest subsequent injections. Anaphylactic shock, as Richet called it, helped explain the mechanism of poisoning. Additionally, the similarities to infection led him to suggest the creation of poisons within the body as a mechanism for infection.

Richet conducted research with more ambiguous results, such as his attempts to immunize against tuberculosis and cancer using Pasteur's method of injections with serum from those previously immunized. His lack of success led Richet to explore another means of preventing and curing TB based on observations of dogs fed a raw meat diet who were found to be more resistant to tuberculosis. Those in the early stages of the disease showed improvement with a meat juice diet. This approach proved disappointing when applied to humans, however, in part because of the amount of meat required (400 grams per day of raw meat, or forty grams of an extract).

Richet's interests led him to the outer bounds of science and beyond. Most important was his work on psychic phenomena. Despite a warning from his father, he studied hypnotism during medical school and published a work on somnambulism based on experiments he continued while an intern in the 1870s. In 1895 Richet, the Englishman William Crookes, and others founded the Society for Psychical Research, with Richet as the first president. He wrote novels on the subject, two of which were later performed on stage with Sarah Bernhardt in the lead.

Not long after his appointment to the Faculty of Medicine, Richet began his dictionary of physiology which ran to ten volumes by 1922. In addition, at the turn of the century, Richet devised a classification system for all medical literature, and then edited and published his *Bibliographia Medica* when the *Index Catalogue of the American Surgeon-General* (precursor of *Index Medius*) ceased publication due to lack of subscribers. Three years later Richet was forced to drop the project for similar reasons. Beginning in 1881 and continuing for twenty-five years, Richet edited the *Revue scientifique*. In 1889 he bought the highly respected *Revue des deux mondes*.

Richet's curiosity led him to indulge a wide variety of interests. A trip to Egypt, Palestine, and Syria in 1876 spawned a lifelong interest in Egyptology. He joined Frederic Passy's Société des pacifistes in 1884, thus beginning his work on the problem of war that included articles, books, and his presidency of the French Peace League. When Richet received his Nobel Prize for physiology, the

German pacifist Bertha von Suttner wrote him that he should have been awarded the Nobel Peace Prize instead.

Richet met Victor Tatin while both were working in the laboratory of the physiologist Jules Marey; and from the late 1880s to the time of the Wright brothers' flight in 1904, they experimented, along with Louis Breguet, on the construction of a heavier-than-air craft. Richet's writings on the declining French birth rate prompted him to become a cofounder of the French Alliance against Depopulation in 1896. He was also an active member of the French Eugenics Society in the years before and after World War I.

Bibliography

Primary: 1895–1928. *Dictionnaire de physiologie* 10 vols. (Paris); 1911. *L'anaphylaxie* (Paris); 1933. *Souvenirs d'un physiologiste* (Paris).

Secondary: Schneider, William H., 2001. 'Charles Richet and the Social Role of Medical Men.' *Journal of Medical Biography* 9: 213–219; Kroker, Kenton, 1999. 'Immunity and Its Other: The Anaphylactic Selves of Charles Richet.' *Studies in the Philosophy of Biology and the Biomedical Sciences* 30: 273–296; Wolf, Stuart, 1993. *Brain, Mind and Medicine: Charles Richet and the Origins of Physiological Psychology* (New Brunswick, NJ).

William H. Schneider

RICORD, PHILIPPE (b. Baltimore, Maryland, USA, 10 December 1800; d. Paris, France, 22 October 1889), *venereal disease.*

Born in the United States to French immigrant parents, Ricord emigrated to France in 1818. He studied at the Paris Faculté de Médecine (1820–26), interning first with Guillaume Dupuytren and later with Jacques Lisfranc. After receiving his MD, Ricord established a private practice in several small towns in the environs of Paris. He returned to Paris in 1831 after obtaining a position with the Paris hospital administration. Shortly thereafter he was posted to the Hôpital des vénériens (renamed Hôpital du Midi in 1836), where he remained until his retirement in 1860.

Ricord is best known for his demonstration, by means of experimental inoculation, that gonorrhea and syphilis were two distinct diseases. In the early formulations of his 'new doctrine' of venereal disease, Ricord also maintained that, unlike syphilis, gonorrhea was not caused by a specific material agent, and that only the primary symptom of syphilis, the syphilitic chancre, was contagious. He would subsequently revise both positions. He played an important role in popularizing the use of the speculum, and was largely responsible for the widespread acceptance of the division of syphilis into three distinct stages (1838), a theory that was linked to his introduction of potassium iodide as a standard treatment for the advanced stages of syphilis (1839). In addition, Ricord wrote on a wide range of related topics, including gonor-

rheal conjunctivitis (1834), syphilitic sarcocele (1840), the rarity of reinfection (1846), and numerous surgical procedures. In his last important scientific contribution, published in 1858, Ricord lent his prestige to his student Léon Bassereau's recognition of cancroids (Ducrey's bacillus, or soft chancre) as a distinct disease, a position that directly contradicted one of the central tenets of Ricord's own theory.

Although Ricord largely ceased original scientific research in the mid-1840s, he long remained one of France's most prominent doctors. Elected to the Academy of Medicine in 1850, he immediately became embroiled in major controversies concerning the contagiousness of the secondary symptoms of syphilis, as well as Auzias-Turenne's theory of syphilization. These polemics were the motivation behind his most widely read work, *Letters on Syphilis* (1851). Ricord was thrice awarded a Montyon Prize by the Academy of Science (1838, 1841, and 1842). He was twice appointed physician-in-ordinary to the family of Napoleon III, and was one of the Emperor's consulting physicians in 1870. He was named Chevalier of the Legion of Honor in 1838, promoted to Commandant in 1860, and attained the rare honor of Grand Commandant in recognition of his role in organizing an ambulance service during the siege of Paris in 1870–71. At the time of his death, Ricord could claim in excess of 200 decorations from countries the world over.

Known for his sharp wit, generosity, and good humor, Ricord's lectures in the courtyard at the Hôpital du Midi were for many years popular among medical students (who struck a gold medal for him in 1842). Ricord possessed one of the most lasting and lucrative private practices in Paris. In 1845 he purchased the enormous mansion at 6 rue Tourna, where he maintained a famously lavish lifestyle. According to police reports, his burial at Père Lachaise cemetery was attended by 3,000 persons, ample testimony to his enduring reputation as one of the founders of modern syphilology.

Bibliography

Primary: 1838. *Traité pratique des maladies vénériennes* (Paris) [English edn., 1842 (New York)]; 1851. *Lettres sur la syphilis* (Paris) [English edn., 1857 (Philadelphia)]; 1858. (Fournier, Alfred, ed.) *Leçons sur le chancre* (Paris).

Secondary: Dracobly, Alex, 2004. 'Theoretical Change and Therapeutic Innovation in the Treatment of Syphilis in Mid-Nineteenth-Century France.' *Journal of the History of Medicine and the Allied Sciences* 59: 522–554; Dracobly, Alex, 2003. 'Ethics and Experimentation on Human Subjects in Mid-Nineteenth-Century France: The Story of the 1859 Syphilis Experiments.' *Bulletin of the History of Medicine* 77: 332–366; Perett, Diane Beyer, 1977. 'Ethics and Error: The Dispute between Ricord and Auzias-Turenne over Syphilization.' PhD dissertation, Stanford University.

Alex Dracobly

RIVERS, WILLIAM HALSE RIVERS   (b. Chatham, Kent, England, 12 March 1864; d. Cambridge, England, 4 June 1922), *psychology, anthropology.*

Rivers, the eldest child of the curate Henry Frederick Rivers and his wife Elizabeth Hunt, was educated at Tonbridge School in Kent and then at the University of London and St Bartholomew's Hospital. He was awarded MB and MRCS (1886), thereby becoming the youngest medical graduate in the history of St Bartholomew's. He already suffered from poor health and took a post as ship's surgeon on a journey to Japan and North America (1887) to help alleviate this condition.

Rivers worked in Sussex and London in the late 1880s, and in 1891 he became house physician at the National Hospital in Queen Square. As a result, he met eminent neurologists such as John Hughlings Jackson (1835–1911), Henry Head (1861–1940), and Charles Sherrington (1857–1952). He left the National Hospital in 1892 and decided on a career change, focusing on insanity and psychology. In 1897 he was appointed lecturer in psychology at Cambridge, becoming, in 1902, a fellow of St John's and eventually director of the university's new psychology laboratory (1907). Equally important, he went on the Cambridge anthropological expedition to the Torres Strait (1898), where he developed experimental cross-cultural psychology techniques; then he spent time in southern India (1901–02), where he studied the ethnology of the Toda people and finally traveled in 1907–08 to Melanesia and Polynesia, putting his experiences and observations there to supporting a diffusionist model of the movement of cultural practices from place to place.

Alongside this anthropological work ran Rivers's collaborations with the neurologist Henry Head on sensory perception and its recovery after the severing of the cutaneous nerves. After the outbreak of World War I, Rivers joined the Maghull military hospital in Lancashire as a physician and then moved in 1916 to Craiglockhart Hospital for Officers near Edinburgh. There Rivers, an intensely shy man with a bad stammer, became much more publicly confident. He felt free to employ dream analysis—both Freudian and Jungian—with his patients and, given the relative luxury of an officers' hospital far from the front line, gave himself the time to endorse psychological approaches to trauma and to shellshock that were not widely available within the military medicine of the period. He became the champion, in written texts and in practice, of both a psychotherapeutic psychiatry and a rather elitist ideal of socialism, both of these based on the wider foundations of his anthropological and cultural studies. His ambition to become a Labour Member of Parliament for the University of London (he was elected Labour candidate in 1922) was thwarted only by his death that year before the election was called.

In some ways Rivers's interests were so widespread that any judgment as to his legacy is difficult. His diffusionist anthropological model was widely criticized, and the inno-

vations and techniques practiced at Craiglockhart were very much confined to a particular class of military personnel. But innovations in the formation of experimental psychology and social anthropology within the universities, as well as the neurological work with Head, owe a lot to Rivers and his eclecticism. He remained, in ways open to varieties of interpretation, unmarried.

Bibliography

Primary: 1914. *A History of Melanesian Society* 2 vols. (Cambridge); 1926. *Psychology and Ethnology* (London).

Secondary: Stocking, George, 1996. *After Tylor: British Social Anthropology 1888–1951* (London); Barker, Pat, 1992. *Regeneration* (London); *Oxford DNB*.

Michael Neve

RIZAL, JOSÉ PROTACIO ALONSO MERCADO (aka DIMASALANG; LAONG LAAN)   (b. Calamba, Laguna, Philippines, 19 June 1861; d. Manila, Philippines, 30 December 1896), *medicine, ophthalmology, nationalism, literature, art.*

Rizal received his early education from his mother and private tutors. He obtained a bachelor's degree in land surveying from the Ateneo Municipal de Manila (1877). He enrolled in medicine at the Dominican-run Royal and Pontifical University of Santo Tomas, then sailed for Europe in 1882. He obtained his licentiate in medicine in 1884, and a licentiate in philosophy and letters in 1885, from the Universidad Central de Madrid. Although he became a licensed physician, he was unable or unwilling to sit for the exams that would have qualified him for the academic degree, Doctor of Medicine. While in Spain, Rizal became one of the leading figures of the patriotic movement for reform in the colonial Philippines. In 1887 in Berlin, he published his first novel, *Noli me tangere* [Touch me not], which exposed the ignorance, cruelty, and greed of the Spanish colonizers, as well as the apparent weaknesses and follies of his own people.

Rizal returned to the Philippines and practiced medicine in his birthplace, Calamba, but the negative Spanish reaction to his novel persuaded him to return to Europe in 1888. There he researched the precolonial past in the British Library in London, and published in Paris in 1890 an annotated edition of the 1609 *Sucesos de las islas Filipinas* by Antonio de Morga. In 1891 he published his second novel, *El Filibusterismo* [Subversion], and wrote for the fortnightly Filipino newspaper in Spain, *La Solidaridad*. Political differences with other expatriate Filipinos led him to leave Europe, and he settled in Hong Kong, where he established an eye clinic.

In mid-1892 Rizal returned to the Philippines; he was exiled to Dapitan in the southern Philippines, where he established a school for boys and a medical clinic. He engaged in farming, fishing, and other business ventures.

He also did civic work: he established a water supply system, designed the town plaza, installed public lighting, and adorned the town park with a relief map of Mindanao.

Rizal wrote a Tagalog grammar; began, but did not finish, a Spanish-Tagalog dictionary; and explored the caves and correctly identified 'lightning teeth' as precolonial, stone age tools, thus making his amateur digging (which had already yielded Ming ceramics and gold jewelry) the first archaeological excavation by a Filipino. He collected plant, bird, insect, and shell specimens, sending these to scientists in Europe. Some of these specimens are reported to have survived World War II and are sill extant in Dresden; thus, a frog, a winged lizard (*Draco rizali*), and an insect now bear his name in scientific classifications. He wrote a psychological essay, '*La curacion de los hechizados*' [Treatment of the Bewitched], and the sources make reference to another essay not extant on the 'Mai-mali', a nervous disorder also known in Malay as 'sakhit latar'. Rizal competed with the only other doctor in Dapitan, a homeopathic physician. To end his four-year exile, he applied for and received permission to work as a medical doctor in Cuba. The Philippine Revolution against Spain broke out in August 1896 while Rizal was en route to Cuba; he was arrested in Barcelona and returned to Manila, where he was tried for treason and executed by firing squad.

Bibliography

Secondary: Martensen, Robert L., and David S. Jones, 1997. 'When US Medicine Became Imperial.' *Journal of the American Medical Association* 277(24): 1917; Ocampo, Ambeth R., 1990. *Rizal without an Overcoat* (Manila); Palma, Rafael, 1949. *The Pride of the Malay Race: A Biography of José Rizal* (trans. Ozaeta, Roman) (New York).

Ambeth R Ocampo

RIZZOLI, FRANCESCO (b. Milan, Italy, 11 July 1809; d. Bologna, Italy, 24 May 1880), *surgery, orthopedics.*

Rizzoli was the son of Gaetano, a lieutenant in Napoleon's and Murat's army, and Maria Trovamala. When he was five years old, his father was shot by brigands in Calabria. His mother married again, and Francesco was sent, together with his sister Teresa, to live with his paternal uncle Vincenzo in Bologna. Notwithstanding his modest standard of living, Rizzoli succeeded in obtaining degrees in philosophy, medicine (1828), and surgery (1831) at the University of Bologna, which was still under the dominion of the Pontifical State. He then obtained the (very poorly paid) position as assistant to Paolo Baroni, his brother-in-law, professor at the university and director of the Ospedale degli Abbandonati e Ricovero. When Baroni became head physician and archiater of Pope Gregory XVI in Rome, Rizzoli was nominated head surgeon of the hospital and substitute (1836) and then regular professor (1840) of theoretical surgery and obstetrics. In 1855 he became professor of clinical surgery and director of the Ospedale

Azzolini. The following year, he visited the surgical institute of Joseph François Malgaigne in Paris. Upon the unification of the Italian Kingdom, Rizzoli repeatedly lobbied to improve the horrid sanitary and didactical conditions of the hospital. Seeing his requests ignored, he resigned from his chair and as director of the hospital (1864), and dedicated his time to the medical profession. In 1867 he was appointed director of the surgical section of the Ospedale Maggiore. In 1876 he was proposed to succeed Luigi Porta as professor of clinical surgery in Pavia.

From the 1850s onward, Rizzoli was a dominant figure in the medical circles of Bologna, covering the most prestigious positions as president of the local Accademia delle Scienze and, for twenty-two years (1854–76), of the Medical-Surgical Society. He was a member of various European and North American academies and societies, held several local political offices, and was nominated senator of the Italian Kingdom in 1879. He had a severe, solitary, and imperious personality, disciplined by his hard youth and by the sanitary misery that surrounded his work. Without a proper family, he donated all of his riches (about three million lire) to the provincial administration of Bologna to fulfill his dream of founding a large, clean and modern hospital, outside the city on the hillside, 'for the prevention and treatment of the deformations of the body'. Rizzoli died a few weeks after signing the purchase of the big building, which was inaugurated in 1896 and today is known as the Istituto Ortopedico Rizzoli.

Rizzoli was famous for the extraordinary quickness of his operations, an aspect that was of extreme importance in times without anesthesia or sterility. His main scientific merits concern orthopedics, especially osteoclasis. Around the mid-nineteenth century, orthopedics was still waiting to take off, and Rizzoli contributed by inventing a series of surgical instruments and apparatuses. His two most famous innovations concern the treatment of the ankylosis of the lower jaw, carried out for the first time on 15 May 1857, and his procedure for people that were unilaterally lame. On 24 April 1847 he improved and applied the osteoclast, recently invented by Bernhard Heine, on a nine-year-old girl with one leg three centimeters shorter than the other. Rizzoli carried out a subcutaneous fracture on the longer femur and then shortened and immobilized it in such a way that the fragments healed according to their longitudinal axis. Furthermore, he applied the osteoclast to straighten rachitic shinbones and to mobilize the angular ankylosis of knees and elbows. Other innovations involved the surgery of hernia, aneurysm, and calculus. He carried out subcutaneous operations of the Achilles tendon and, from 1862, opened the stomach in order to extirpate fibroid tumors.

Bibliography

Primary: 1869. *Collezione delle Memorie chirurgiche ed ostetriche* (Bologna) [French edn., 1872].

Secondary: Bernabeo, Raffaele A., 1981. 'Ricordo di Francesco Rizzoli (1809–1880) e di Vittorio Putti (1880–1940).' *Minerva ortopedica* 32: 485–488; Putti, Vittorio, 1939. 'Francesco Rizzoli.' *La Chirurgia degli Organi di Movimento* 25: 149–152.

Ariane Dröscher

ROBB, GEORGE DOUGLAS (b. Auckland, New Zealand, 29 April 1899; d. Auckland, 28 April 1974), *surgery, medical reform.*

Robb, the son of Agnes Rough, a school teacher, and John Robb, a timber company manager, was educated at Auckland Grammar School and Otago University, from which he graduated MB ChB in 1922. He became FRCS in 1926 after surgical training at the Middlesex Hospital, London. On his return to Auckland in 1929, he set himself up as a consultant without observing the convention of spending further time in general practice.

An interest in medical audit saw Robb appointed first registrar of the Auckland Hospital committee, which reported to the British Empire Cancer Campaign Society. In 1935 he fell foul of colleagues and board members alike because of his scathing critique of the hospital's clinical practices. Robb's forced departure from the hospital world coincided with a deterioration in health (his elder brother died of spinal TB in 1921, and Douglas was affected by recurring pulmonary illness from the early 1920s).

Obliged to withdraw from clinical work, Robb applied his intellect to health reform, stimulated by A. J. Cronin's 1937 novel *The Citadel.* In a series of publications, he examined the relationship between general practice, specialists, and hospital medicine; his proposed solutions included group practice, polyclinics, and a salaried state medical service—anathema to many New Zealand doctors. The jointly authored *A National Health Service* (1943), masterminded by Robb, paralleled a British study by the 'Under 45s'; this had been completed prior to the release of the 1942 Beveridge Report which outlined the future welfare state.

Reinstated by the Hospital Board after a seven-year absence, Robb joined the Green Lane Hospital Thoracic Surgery Unit. Five years later he established a Cardio-Surgical Clinic, following a six-month trip to Baltimore to study current practice. The unit flourished under his astute recruitment and leadership. Upon retiring in 1964, he noted that true success came when 'a man's successor and pupils not only equal him but surpass him'.

Robb was also a leader in medical education. A 1943 conference on medicine and surgery was the prelude to the Auckland Postgraduate Medical Committee. Robb, initially the Committee's secretary, soon became president, a position he retained until 1957. He also spearheaded the drive for a second New Zealand medical school, chairing the local Medical Education Committee from its inception in 1945. His efforts were rewarded nineteen years later when he received a telegram from his wife while he was visiting India: 'GOVERNMENT APPROVES AUCKLAND MEDICAL SCHOOL CONGRATULATIONS DARLING ALL WELL'.

Formal recognition came late in life. Robb was knighted in 1960 and served as Chancellor of the University of Auckland from 1961 to 1968 (having held the deputy's post since 1953). In 1961 he was elected President of the British Medical Association, which met in Auckland that year. His presidential address, on reducing inequalities of health in the Commonwealth, led the *British Medical Journal* to describe him as a 'medical statesman molding the medical services of New Zealand'.

In 1944 the American psychiatrist, Merrill Moore, described Robb as New Zealand's equivalent to 'what Osler once was in our country and England', and 'the greatest living authority and the most liberal and progressive thinker on [public health] in New Zealand if not in the entire British Commonwealth'. Following Robb's death in 1974, Sir Robert Aitken, an Otago contemporary, summed him up as 'the restless purveyor of new suggestions, the persistent dissenter and the passionate reformer'. Robb would have approved.

Bibliography

Primary: 1940. *Medicine and Health in New Zealand: A Retrospect and a Prospect* (Auckland); 1947. *Health Reform in New Zealand* (Christchurch); 1967. *Medical Odyssey* (Auckland).

Secondary: Roche, E. H., and A. H. G. Roche, 1983. *Green Lane Saga. Green Lane Hospital, Auckland: 1889–1982 and Its Development of Cardiology and Cardiothoracic and Vascular Surgery* (Auckland); Roche, E. H., 1978. *Continuing Medical Education in Auckland. The First 25 Years of the Auckland Postgraduate Medical Committee* (Auckland).

Derek A. Dow

ROBB, ISABEL ADAMS HAMPTON (b. Welland, Ontario, Canada, July 1860; d. Cleveland, Ohio, USA, 15 April 1910), *nursing.*

Hampton was the fourth of seven children reared by Samuel Hampton and Sarah Lay Hampton. Her parents emigrated from Scotland to Canada, where her father made his living running a tailor shop. Hampton attended school in Welland and at the Collegiate Institute in nearby St Catherine's. She earned a teaching certificate and taught in a district school in Merriton, Ontario. There she learned of the new Bellevue Hospital Training School for Nurses in New York City. She applied to the school, was accepted, and completed the two-year course in 1883.

For two years, she nursed English and American travelers at St Paul's House in Rome, Italy, traveling throughout Europe with a group of nurses from Bellevue. Standing an unusual five feet, ten inches tall, she combined striking good looks with intelligence, charm, and poise, attracting respect and attention.

In 1886 the philanthropic women directing the Illinois Training School in Chicago hired her as superintendent. She spent three years trying to improve the education of the pupil nurses, who, however, spent the majority of their time caring for patients at the Cook County Hospital. By 1889 she was ready to consider a more attractive and promising opportunity as superintendent at the new Johns Hopkins Hospital Training School for Nurses in Baltimore.

At Johns Hopkins, a carefully selected group of apprentices overseen by graduate nurses and the new superintendent worked in a modern hospital with high quality sanitary and technological capabilities. Hampton selected each pupil herself, placing emphasis on previous education, personal cultivation, and willingness to share in the welfare of the school. She also gave all the nursing instruction. Her essential balancing act, however, was to manage admissions and systematic education of the pupils without distracting from the care of patients in the hospital. The pupils were also the nursing staff; each worked ten-hour to twelve-hour days, making instruction somewhat incidental to hospital work. Still, both Hampton and the graduate nurses who taught them on the job fostered a sense of the importance of the work they were doing.

Hampton's sphere of influence expanded with the opportunity to organize the subsection on nursing at the International Congress of Charities, Correction, and Philanthropy held in Chicago during the World's Columbian Exposition in 1893. She brought together a group of international nursing leaders to explain the significance and problems of nursing reform before a large audience. An immediate result was the formation of the American Society of Superintendents of Training Schools for Nurses of the United States and Canada. Later, in 1899, a collaboration begun in 1893 led to the creation of the International Council of Nurses, the first international professional organization of women.

Isabel Hampton resigned in 1894 to marry Hunter Robb, MD. They moved to Cleveland, where he was professor of gynecology at Western Reserve University. They had two sons, Hampton and Phillip. But Isabel Hampton Robb continued her professional work by establishing the Nurses' Associated Alumnae of the United States and Canada (after 1911, the American Nurses Association), which pushed for legal status for nurses in all states. Hampton Robb served as the first president.

In 1910, while crossing the street in Cleveland, Hampton Robb was struck by a streetcar and killed instantly. She was buried in Burlington, New Jersey.

Bibliography

Primary: 1894. *Nursing: Its Principles and Practice* (Philadelphia); 1900. *Nursing Ethics: For Hospital and Private Use* (Cleveland).

Secondary: Connolly, Cynthia A., 1998. 'Hampton, Nutting and Rival Gospels at the Johns Hopkins Hospital and Training School for Nurses, 1889–1906.' *Image: Journal of Nursing Scholarship* 30: 23–29; James, Janet Wilson, 1979. 'Isabel Hampton and the Professionalization of Nursing in the 1890s.' in Vogel, Morris J., and Charles E. Rosenberg, eds., *The Therapeutic Revolution: Essays in the Social History of American Medicine* (Philadelphia) pp. 201–244; *DAMB*.

Joan E. Lynaugh

ROCK, JOHN CHARLES (b. Marlborough, Massachusetts, USA, 24 March 1890; d. Temple, New Hampshire, USA, 4 December 1984), *medicine, obstetrics, gynecology.*

Rock and his twin sister were the youngest of the five children of Frank Sylvester Rock, a successful businessman, and Ann Jane Murphy. Educated at Boston's High School of Commerce (1909), he was fired successively from jobs in Guatemala and Rhode Island before deciding on a medical career. Graduation from Harvard (1915) was followed by residencies at Massachusetts General Hospital, Boston Lying-in Hospital, and the Free Hospital for Women. Thereafter, he established a practice in obstetrics and gynecology, became an obstetrics assistant (later professor) at Harvard Medical School (1922), and founded an infertility clinic at the Free Hospital (1924). A devout Roman Catholic, his marriage to Anna (Nan) Thorndike (1925) was conducted by Boston's Cardinal William O'Connell; the marriage produced five children.

Although Rock believed sex to be fundamental to love and marriage, he supported Catholic teaching that its purpose was procreation. Later, his stance against maternal ill health and family poverty caused by continuous pregnancies led him to promote marital contraception. His was the only Catholic signature among sixteen Boston physicians on a petition (1931) urging repeal of the Massachusetts (Comstock) anti-birth control laws. During the Cold War, he perceived a link between overpopulation, communism, and a threat to world peace. When Pope Pius XII sanctioned the rhythm method of birth control, Rock opened the first rhythm clinic in the United States at the Free Hospital (1936). Much of his practice, however, was devoted to solving infertility problems, for which he established the Reproductive Study Center (1956). He and Arthur Tremain Hertig made a unique collection of embryos (1938–52) from women undergoing hysterectomy, representing the first seventeen days of gestation. He experimented on artificial insemination techniques, freezing and storing sperm, and, with Miriam Menkin, reported the first in vitro fertilization of a human egg (1944).

In the 1940s Rock experimented with progesterone and estrogen to induce false pregnancy in infertile women, about 16 percent of whom became pregnant after stopping treatment: the 'Rock rebound'. Since these hormones prevented ovulation, he realized that they could also be used for contraception. His work drew the attention of Gregory Pincus and Min-Cheuh Chang, themselves developing a contraceptive pill with a grant in 1951 from the Planned Parenthood Federation of America. Rock and Pincus combined hormone trials on infertile women with investigations into contraception with volunteers in 1953, after which Rock, supported by Margaret Sanger, Katherine McCormick, and medical colleagues, conducted the pill's first clinical trials in 1954, in areas including New York, Mexico, Puerto Rico, Japan, and India. Sanger, a lapsed Catholic, considered Rock a useful ally in gaining the pill's acceptance. He saw it as a 'natural', 'harmless', morally permissible variant of the rhythm method. 'The steroid compounds are the first physiologic means of contraception . . . they prevent reproduction by modifying the time sequences in the body's own functions . . .' (1963, pp. 100–101). When the pill was marketed for menstrual disorders and prevention of miscarriage (1957), Rock was encouraged by Pope Pius XII's endorsement in 1958 of its therapeutic benefits. Following its launch as a contraceptive (Enovid, 1960), Rock published his views in *The Time Has Come: A Catholic Doctor's Proposals to End the Battle over Birth Control* (1963).

The ensuing controversy thrust him into the international spotlight, although he remained steadfast to 'his' Church despite being labeled a 'moral rapist' by the Family Life Bureau of Cleveland Catholic diocese and threatened with excommunication. He was bitterly disappointed, as were other Catholics, when Pope Paul VI issued the encyclical *Humanae Vitae* (1968), condemning the pill and 'artificial' birth control methods. *Humanae Vitae* is considered to be a reply to issues raised by Rock's book. That year, Harvard closed his clinic following the Free Hospital's merger with other obstetric units. Rock sold his practice (1969) and retreated to New Hampshire with a small research grant from Searle, manufacturers of Enovid. Later, he stopped attending church. By the end of the 1960s, 8–10 million American women were using the pill.

Bibliography

Primary: 1940. (with Fleck, Stephen, and Elizabeth F. Snedeker) 'The Contraceptive Safe Period: A Clinical Study.' *New England Journal of Medicine* 223: 1005–1009; 1943. 'Medical and Biological Aspects of Contraception: The Scientific Case against Rigid Legal Restrictions on Medical Birth Control Advice.' *Clinics* 1: 1601–1602; 1944. 'In Vitro Fertilization and Cleavage of Human Ovarian Eggs.' *Science* 100: 105–107; 1951. (with Tietze, C., and S. R. Poliakoff) 'The Clinical Effectiveness of the Rhythm Method of Contraception.' *Fertility and Sterility* 2(5): 444–450; 1963. *The Time Has Come: A Catholic Doctor's Proposals to End the Battle over Birth Control* (London).

Secondary: Marks, Lara V., 2001. *Sexual Chemistry: A History of the Contraceptive Pill* (New Haven and London); McLaughlin, Loretta, 1982. *The Pill, John Rock, and the Church: The Biography of a Revolution* (Boston).

Carole Reeves

RODRÍGUEZ LAFORA, GONZALO (b. Madrid, Spain, 25 July 1886; d. Madrid, 28 December 1971), *neurology, psychiatry.*

Lafora was the son of an infantry colonel and the grandson of a renowned lawyer who would eventually become a Member of Parliament and Senator of the Kingdom. In 1900 Lafora began his studies of medicine in Madrid, and was a student of Santiago Ramón y Cajal and Federico Olóriz, among others.

Granted a pension by the Board of Advanced Studies and Scientific Research, he traveled to Germany to study the anatomy of the nervous system, first in Berlin's La Charité Psychiatric Clinic, and later in Munich with Emil Kraepelin and Alois Alzheimer. It was then, late in 1909, that he received a proposal from his friend and mentor, Nicolás Achúcarro, to substitute for him as pathologist at the Government Hospital for the Insane in Washington, D.C., USA.

Lafora's stay in Washington, from May 1910 to September 1912, is particularly significant in his life's path and scientific career, since it was then that he made his earliest, yet most decisive contribution—his description in 1911 of intracytoplasmic bodies within ganglion cells in the nervous system of patients with a particular, so-called myoclonic type of epilepsy (Lafora's disease).

Lafora returned to Madrid in October 1912, where he joined the Laboratory of Experimental Nervous System Physiology, which Cajal himself founded for him within his Institute. In 1914 he was appointed vice-secretary of Patronato Nacional de Subnormales [National Agency for the Mentally Disabled].

Lafora became a reference point for a relevant group of colleagues and disciples who made up a significant core of activity, a renewed 'school of Madrid', that would ultimately be dubbed by historiography 'the *Archivos de Neurobiología* generation', in reference to the scientific journal that Lafora founded in 1920.

Only three months after the proclamation of the Second Republic, the Decree of 3 July 1931 was promulgated. This Decree, the text of which had been drafted by Lafora, Sacristán, and Escalas, regulated admissions and discharges of patients in psychiatric institutions, but also favored the implementation of a new 'Healthcare Model' that no longer considered mental hospitals the only sites available for treatment, and which underscored the importance of prophylactic aspects. In 1933 Lafora passed a competitive examination for the position of head physician of '2nd Ward for demented women' at the Provincial Poor Law Hospital, and was appointed a permanent member of the National Academy of Medicine.

Once the civil war broke out, by mid-1938 Lafora decided to leave Spain. He obtained military permission and moved to France, where he stayed for a few months before crossing the Atlantic to settle in Mexico for nine years. Shortly after his arrival in Mexico he had his medical degree ratified, commenced medical practice, and undertook intellectual and scientific activities; together with his widely-recognized prestige, this won him great renown not only in medical spheres, but also in the diverse environments of Mexican society.

Lafora decided to return to Madrid in 1947. He immediately joined the Cajal Institute, but it was not until 1950 that he was pardoned and reinstated to his former position as department head of the Provincial Hospital. He retired in 1955 at the age of seventy; however, he kept his private clinic and continued to attend scientific lectures and meetings. In 1961 he was appointed honorary president of the Congress of Neuropathology held in Munich, in international recognition of a lifetime devoted to this discipline.

Bibliography

Primary: 1911. 'Ueber das Vorkommen amyloider Köperchen im Inner der Gangliensellen; zugleich ein Beitrag zum Studium der amyloiden Substanz in Nervensystem.' *Virchows Archiv* 205: 295–303; 1917. *Los niños mentalmente anormales* (Madrid).

Secondary: Huertas, Rafael, 2002. *Los médicos de la mente. De la neurología al psicoanálisis (Lafora-Vallejo-Garma)* (Madrid); Moya, Gregorio, 1986. *Gonzalo R. Lafora. Medicina y cultura en una España en crisis* (Madrid); Valenciano, Luis, 1977. *El doctor Lafora y su época* (Madrid).

Rafael Huertas

RÖSSLIN, EUCHARIUS (THE ELDER) (b. Waldkirch ?, Germany, *c.* 1465–1470; d. Frankfurt am Main, Germany, 1526), *obstetrics, pediatrics.*

Rösslin's fame rests almost exclusively on a single book. His *Der Swangeren frawen und hebammen Rosegarten* was one of the most successful and popular obstetrical and pediatric textbooks in early modern Western medicine. About Rösslin's origin and life, little is known. By all appearances he was identical with a pharmacist by the name of Eucharius Rösslin who was accepted into the merchants' guild of Freiburg in southwest Germany in 1493. A pharmacist by the same name continues to appear in various local documents, worked also as a scribe, and acquired citizen rights in 1502. From 1504 this pharmacist is no longer mentioned. But now various documents mention a physician, a 'medicus', by the same name: Eucharius Rösslin. In view of the rare first name, we can assume that it was one and the same person; but other possibilities remain, such as a father-son relationship. How and where the physician Eucharius Rösslin received his medical training is not known, but others (and he himself) referred to him as 'doctor', which suggests that he had obtained an academic degree. From 1506 until about 1511, he worked as a town physician in Frankfurt am Main. During this period he treated Duchess Katharina of Braunschweig and Lüneburg, to whom he later dedicated his *Rosengarten*. He then seems to have moved to Worms, where he wrote the preface to his *Rosengarten*. In 1517 he moved back to Frankfurt to work again as a town physician, an office in which his homonymous son followed him after his death.

The success of Rösslin's *Rosengarten* is, at first glance, somewhat surprising. In terms of content, the book offered virtually nothing new; it was a mere compilation. The parts on pregnancy, birth, and childbed are largely borrowed from the *Gynaecea* of Moschion (or Mustio) which was, in turn, based on the work, *On the diseases of women*, by the Greek physician, Soranus. It was probably also out of a manuscript of the Moschion text that Rösslin took the famous illustrations of the different positions of the child in the maternal womb. The pediatric parts, in turn, are based largely on the section about diseases of the newborn in Bartholomäus Metlinger's *Kinderbüchlein*. To both parts a Latin-German glossary was added.

The way in which Rösslin put these texts together, however, was new and seems to have been responsible, to a large degree, for *Rosengarten*'s success. Rösslin created a comprehensive textbook dealing systematically with the various medical problems that midwives might face when they took care of women before, during, and after birth, or when they treated their newborn children. The book included a fairly detailed account of the various drugs to which midwives could resort.

Repeatedly revised and published under changing titles, *Rosengarten* served as the leading German vernacular textbook on midwifery for a long time, and enjoyed great success abroad, as well. More than a hundred editions, revisions and translations are known. Rösslin's son, known also for his herbal, came out with a new edition, entitled *Ehstandsarzneybuch*, in 1526. Adam Lonicerus, in 1562, published another revised German text entitled *Hebammenbüchlein*, which went, in turn, through almost a dozen editions. Walther Ryff, in 1545, presented his *Frawen Rosengarten* with at least another five editions. Translations helped disseminate the work all over Europe. It was probably Rösslin's son who produced a Latin translation, *De partu hominis*, in 1532. A French edition appeared in 1536. The 1540 English translation, *The byrth of mankynde*, was followed by at least fourteen more English editions.

Bibliography

Primary: 1513. *Der Swangern frawen und hebammen rosegarten* (Hagenau); 1536. *De partu hominis, et quae circa ipsum accidunt libellus* (Venice); 1997–98. 'The pregnant women's and midwives' rose garden' (English trans. by Plassmann, Sybille) in Hess, H. H., ed., *Gynaecia Mustionis* Vol. 2 (Frankfurt am Main) pp. 104–166.

Secondary: Kruse, Britta-Juliane, 1994. 'Neufund einer handschriftlichen Vorstufe von Eucharius Rößlins Der schwangeren Frauen und Hebammen Rosengarten und des Frauenbüchleins Pseudo-Ortolfs.' *Sudhoffs Archiv* 78: 220–236; Klein, Gustav, 1909–10. 'Zur Bio- und Bibliographie Rößlins und seines Rosengartens.' *Archiv für Geschichte der Medizin* 3: 304–334; Ingerslev, E., 1909.

Rösslin's 'Rosegarten': Its relation to the past (the Muscio manuscripts and Soranos), particularly with regard to podalic version (rprt. from *Journal of Obstetrics and Gynaecology of the British Empire*, Jan.–Feb. 1909) (London); Baas, Karl, 1907. 'Eucharius Rößlins Lebensgang.' *Archiv für Geschichte der Medizin* 1: 429–441.

Michael Stolberg

ROGERS, LEONARD

(b. Helston, Cornwall, England, 18 January 1868; d. Truro, Cornwall, England, 16 September 1962), *tropical medicine.*

Rogers was the seventh son of Naval Captain Henry Rogers and Jane Mary Enys. He attended St Mary's Hospital Medical School, London (1888), graduating MB, BS (University of London, 1892). A strong Christian faith and early flair for pathology and bacteriology directed Rogers toward the Indian Medical Service (IMS) and a research career in tropical medicine. After training at the Army Medical School Netley, developing his pathology skills under Almroth Wright, he sailed for India (1893).

Like all new recruits, he started work for the military branch of the IMS. In 1896 he was seconded to investigate an outbreak of kala-azar (visceral leishmaniasis) in Assam. His results were largely incorrect, but he would return to kala-azar later, successfully culturing the newly discovered Leishman-Donovani parasite to its flagellate stage (1904).

In 1900 he transferred to the civil branch of the IMS and acted as professor of pathology at the medical college in Calcutta, assuming the chair formally in 1906. Rogers remained here for the remainder of his Indian career. It provided the base for his long-term goals of improving the clinical, pathological knowledge of the major diseases in India. He worked on a wide variety of fevers and bowel diseases. He hoped his work would aid the differential diagnosis of fevers and dysenteries, where diagnostic laboratory equipment was limited. He supplemented his clinical work at the Medical College Hospital by cycling early in the morning to other hospitals, taking shorthand (self-taught) notes on cases he observed in life and at postmortem. His energy and determination to collect and record this large amount of clinical material increased the robustness of his basic statistical analyses of the data.

Rogers was always keen to make his research therapeutically useful. His introduction of hypertonic saline solution in the rehydration treatment of cholera ('Rogers Fluid') was based on careful examination of the ion balance in the body. After identifying *Entamoeba histolytica* as the cause of amoebic dysentery, he advocated aseptic aspiration of liver abscesses (a common sequel of amebiasis) rather than open drainage. Although it was quickly superseded by Brahmachari's drug, Rogers introduced tartar emetic against kala-azar (1912). He also researched the native use of chaulmoogra oil as a treatment for leprosy (1916). He considered it a partial cure: it was able to arrest symptoms if applied early, and, therefore, it constituted something to encourage the infected to come forward, rather than hiding away where they might pose a source of infection to those living in close contact. This idea went to drive his postretirement founding of the British Empire Leprosy Relief Association (1923) now LEPRA.

In 1910 Rogers began to raise funds for the Calcutta School of Tropical Medicine and the Carmichael Hospital for Tropical Diseases. Plans for the hospital were drawn up on honeymoon in 1914 with his wife, Una Elsie North, a nursing sister. (There were three sons.) Emulating the schools of tropical medicine in the UK, Rogers hoped to prevent the need for British IMS officers returning home for specialist education and to promote research among all races of the service. The outbreak of war delayed the opening of these institutions, and Rogers retired from India (1920), leaving Sir John Megaw as the first director and professor of tropical medicine.

Rogers served on the India Office's medical board (1922–8) and as its president (1928–31). He also maintained his interest in data analysis, using their meteorological data to predict epidemics, e.g., cholera. Knighted (1914) and elected FRS (1916), Rogers was twice nominated for a Nobel Prize, but the diversity of his career and achievements made it difficult to single out a particular piece of work necessary for Nobel success.

Bibliography

Primary: 1908. *Fevers in the Tropics* (Oxford); 1911. *Cholera and Its Treatment* (Oxford); 1921. *Bowel Diseases in the Tropics* (Oxford); 1925. (with Muir, Edwin) *Leprosy* (Bristol); 1930. (with Megaw, John) *Tropical Medicine* (London); 1950. *Happy Toil: Fifty-Five Years of Tropical Medicine* (London).

Secondary: Gould, T., 2005. *Don't Fence Me In. From Curse to Cure Leprosy in Modern Times* (London); Power, Helen, 1996. 'The Calcutta School of Tropical Medicine.' *Medical History* 40: 197–214; *Oxford DNB.*

Helen Bynum

ROKITANSKY, CARL VON

(b. Königgrätz [Hradec Králové], Bohemia [now Czech Republic], 19 February 1804; d. Vienna, Austria, 23 July 1878), *pathology.*

Rokitansky was the son of an imperial Habsburgian district administrator. He went to school in Königgrätz and, from 1818, studied philosophy at the University of Prague. Between 1822 and 1828, he studied medicine in Prague and then Vienna, where he received his MD (1828) and worked as assistant to Johann Wagner (1800–32), professor of pathological anatomy, between 1828 and 1832. After Wagner's death in 1832, Rokitansky administrated the chair of pathological anatomy temporarily, and became curator of the pathological museum. In 1834 he became assistant professor (Extraordinarius) and prosector of the General Hospital in Vienna (Wiener Allgemeines Krankenhaus) and, in 1844, regular professor (Ordinarius) of pathological anatomy.

Thereafter, Rokitansky achieved leading positions in the medical and scientific administration in Vienna. In 1848 he became a member of the Viennese Academy of Sciences (Wiener Akademie der Wissenschaften) and would serve as its president from 1869 to 1878. In 1850 he was named chairman of the Society of Viennese Physicians (Gesellschaft der Ärzte in Wien) and, in 1863, court advisor for medical affairs (Hofrat und Ministerialreferent für die Medizin). Rokitansky, who in 1870 also became a member of the Paris Academy of Sciences, retired in 1875.

Rokitansky is regarded as the founder of the so-called Second Viennese School, in which pathological anatomy had a key position. Based on the Paris School, where autopsies became a routine measure of hospital medicine, Rokitansky institutionalized the correlation of clinical findings in the living patient with postmortem findings in the deceased one by establishing the cooperation of clinician and pathologist in medical practice. Rokitansky autopsied thousands of corpses, and considered also the chemical analysis of material. He enriched special pathology through his discovery of many separate results in different fields of morbid anatomy, which he published in his handbook of pathology (*Handbuch der pathologischen Anatomie*, 1842–46). He categorized diseases according to anatomical lesions.

Rokitansky's efforts to correlate clinical symptoms and postmortem findings, and his idea to develop a specific disease system, led him to postulate a hematohumoral theory of different dyscrasias of the blood, which he took to be responsible for specific diseases. He found the origins of altered morphological structures in changed conditions of the blood plasma. Lesions were caused by an imbalance of plasma proteins. This theory was based on contemporary concepts of the pathology of humors, e.g., that of the Paris physician Gabriel Andral (1797–1876). The chemical analysis of material and the performance of experiments helped Rokitansky to further develop his ideas, which he published in the first volume of his handbook.

Rokitansky's theory was fashionable at the time. Although it rested basically on the analysis of morphological substrate, it was heavily criticized by the Berlin pathologist, Rudolf Virchow (1821–1902). Virchow was a keen advocate of solidist pathology, and especially hostile to any 'systems' which were not well reasoned. Criticism caused Rokitansky to abandon his ideas, and to omit his theory in a new edition of his handbook (1855–61).

Although Virchow would decisively influence the further uptake of morbid anatomy in the second half of the nineteenth century, Rokitansky was one of the founding fathers of modern scientific pathology. He promoted morphological thinking and, above all, the firm and institutionalized cooperation of clinician and pathologist. Rokitansky, who also improved medical education, bolstered the reputation of Viennese medicine with his work, and had a long impact on medicine through his students.

Bibliography

Primary: 1842–46. *Handbuch der pathologischen Anatomie* 3 vols. (Vienna) (English edn., 4 vols., 1849–54); 1960. (Lesky, Erna, ed.) *Selbstbiographie und Antrittsrede* (Vienna).

Secondary: Miciotto, Robert Joseph, 1979. *Carl Rokitansky: Nineteenth-Century Pathologist and Leader of the New Vienna School* (Ann Arbor, MI); Miciotto, Robert Joseph, 1978. 'Carl Rokitansky: A Reassessment of the Hematohumoral Theory of Disease.' *Bulletin of the History of Medicine* 52: 183–199; Lesky, Erna, 1965. *Die Wiener Medizinische Schule im 19. Jahrhundert* (Graz and Cologne) (English edn., 1976).

Cay-Ruediger Pruell

ROLFINCK, WERNER (b. Hamburg, Germany, 15 November 1599; d. Jena, Germany, 6 May 1673), *anatomy, chemistry.*

Rolfinck was the son of a grammar school teacher. From 1616 to 1618, he studied medicine at Wittenberg under Daniel Sennert. He continued his studies at Leiden and Padua. A pupil of Adrian van den Spiegel, he graduated MD in Padua in 1625. In 1628 he declined a professorship there. Shortly afterwards, in 1629, he was called to Jena to teach—first anatomy, then surgery, later botany and, finally, chemistry. He played a key role in introducing the study of anatomy and chemistry to German universities. While at Jena he set up an anatomy theater, a botanical garden, and chemistry laboratories, all based on the Paduan model. The chemical laboratory was established in 1638. In that same year he took charge of teaching chemistry (director exercitii chymia), a position which became a professorship in 1641. The university of Jena was thus among the first to recognize the importance of a course in chemistry for future physicians.

Rolfinck was one of the pioneers in this rather new field. He did experimental research on various chemical substances such as iron, tin, silver, gold, antimony, copper, and mercury, studying their effects on the human body. He was, however, opposed to alchemy, which he considered as superstition. In the preface to his multi-volume study entitled *Chemia in artis formam redacta*, he stated that this work was not about transmutation, but dealt with 'the resolution of mixtures for the benefit of human health'. Rolfinck was therefore a representative of a movement away from alchemy into chemistry, away from magic into the realm of science. He also wrote a book on 'chemical nonentities'—i.e., on unnatural products that cannot be achieved by chemical operations, such as oils from precious stones. He vehemently opposed the homunculus of Paracelsus, debunking the myth of creating creatures with a human appearance. Rolfinck considered this popular notion to be ridiculous, and did not think any better of the claim that gold could be generated in the human body, as in the episode reported in 1593 of a Silesian boy who grew a gold tooth.

Rolfinck played a decisive role in the reformation of the Jena medical school—by introducing chemistry into the syllabus, by organizing botanical excursions, and by building the first anatomical theater. Nonetheless, he was still grounded in traditional medical thinking. He wrote, for example, a commentary on Hippocrates and on al-Rāzī. All the same, he was the first German professor to support Harvey's theory of the circulation of the blood, discussing this theory in one of his lectures as early as 1632.

Rolfinck taught anatomy, too. He was the first to demonstrate the locations of cataracts in the lens of the eye. As his lectures on anatomy involved dissection of criminals sentenced to death, Rolfinck became a controversial figure outside the university. His name became proverbial in the German language, used to describe the state of being subjected to dissection (rolfincken), although Rolfinck was certainly not among the most prolific anatomists of his time.

Rolfinck also had a private medical practice in Jena. He was six times rector of the University of Jena, and supervised 104 doctoral candidates.

Bibliography

Primary: 1655. *Epitome methodi cognoscendi & curandi particulares corporis affectus, secundum ordinem Abubetri Rhazae ad Regem Mansorem libronono, Hippocraticis, Paracelsicis [et] Harveanis principiis* (Jena); 1656. *Dissertationes anatomicae methodo synthetica exaratae* (Nuremberg); 1661. *Chimia: in artis formam redacta* (Jena); 1662. *Commentarius in Hippocratis primum libri primi aphorismum* (Jena); 1664. *Ordo et methodus generationi dicatarum partium, per anatomen cognoscendi fabricam* (Jena); 1670. *Non-ens chymicum* (Jena); 1670. *De vegetabilibus, plantis, suffruticibus, fructibus, arboribus in genere libri duo* (Jena).

Secondary: Pagel, Julius, 1962. 'Rolfinck, Werner.' *Biographisches Lexikon der hervorragenden Ärzte* (3rd edn., vol. 4) (Berlin) pp. 861–862; Chemnitius, Fritz, 1929. *Die Chemie in Jena von Rolfinck bis Knorr (1629– 1921)* (Jena); *DSB*.

Robert Jütte

ROSÉN VON ROSENSTEIN, NILS   (b. probably in Sexdrega, Västergötland, Sweden, 11 February 1706; d. Uppsala, Sweden, 16 July, 1773), *anatomy, medical education, pediatrics, preventive medicine.*

Rosén was the second child of the Reverend Erik Rosenius and his wife, Anna Wekander. His father ran a private school where Rosén was taught until he was twelve. After studies at the gymnasium of Gothenburg, he matriculated at the University of Lund in 1723, intending to study theology. His interests, however, soon turned toward medicine. In 1725 he made a decisive move to Stockholm, as tutor for a family with close connections to important physicians and surgeons in the capital. While he was there, he attended lectures in experimental physics, translated French and German literature, and kept up to date with current ideas in medicine, philosophy, and science. In 1728 he became an adjunct to the Faculty of Medicine at the University of Uppsala, on the condition that he travel to universities abroad for practical medical training, and to acquire the doctor's degree which it was not possible to obtain in Sweden at the time. His journey, which lasted nearly three years, took him to Germany, Switzerland, France, and the Netherlands, where he finally received his degree.

After his return in 1731, Rosén remained in Uppsala. He published an anatomical textbook in Swedish, *Compendium anatomicum* (1736–38), and was appointed professor of medicine in 1740. After Carl Linnaeus received the other chair of the Faculty, Rosén's responsibilities included anatomy, physiology, pathology, therapeutics, and chemistry, as well as directorship of the University Hospital. As a professor in anatomy, he conducted public demonstrations of the human body in the anatomical theater, in addition to dissecting examinations on animal and human corpses for the students. Rosén reformed the University Hospital, where he lectured and performed bedside teaching. He resigned in 1756, leaving his professorship to his son-in-law, and lived mostly in Stockholm as a practitioner and physician to the Royal family.

Rosén belonged to the iatromechanical school, and was influenced by the medical system of Herman Boerhaave, whose theories reached Sweden in the early eighteenth century. In his 1746 book, *Tal, om en Opartisk och Förnuftig Medici förnämsta Göromål* [The most important tasks of an impartial and rational physician], Rosén supported a mechanistic approach to medicine firmly grounded in anatomy.

Rosén's best known and most influential book was *Underrättelser om Barnsjukdomar och deras Botemedel* [The diseases of children and their remedies] (1764), in which he stressed general care, feeding, and simple hygiene, with many references to contemporary literature. The work was based on a series of articles published in the almanacs of the Royal Swedish Academy of Sciences, written to promote a better understanding of the needs of children—an urgent task since data collected on a national basis by the newly established Bureau of Statistics had shown a high mortality rate for infants and small children. In 1764 the Academy published the articles as a separate volume, the first modern textbook of pediatrics, which was soon translated into German (1766), Dutch (1768), English (1776), and French (1778).

Rosén also championed the use of variolation against smallpox, and he was one of the first Swedish physicians to use quinine as a treatment for malaria. He was a member of the Academy of Sciences, and he carried on a large correspondence with colleagues in Sweden and abroad, among whom should be mentioned Albrecht von Haller.

Bibliography

Primary: 1736–38. *Compendium anatomicum, eller En kort beskrifning om de delar, af hwilka hela menniskians kropp består* 2 vols. (Uppsala); 1746. *Tal, om en Opartisk och Förnuftig Medici förnämsta Göromål* (Stockholm); 1764. Underrättelser om Barnsjukdomar och deras Bote-medel (Stockholm).

Secondary: Vahlquist, Bo, 2004. 'Nils Rosén von Rosenstein and his textbook on paediatrics' in Rosén von Rosenstein, Nicholas, *The Diseases of Children and Their Remedies* [First reprinting of the 1776 English translation] (Uppsala) pp. 15–36; Nyström, Eva, 1999. 'Rosén von Rosenstein, Nils' in *SBL* 30 (Stockholm) pp. 425–433; Wallgren, Arvid, 1964. 'Nils Rosén von Rosenstein, a Short Biography' in Vahlquist, Bo, and Arvid Wallgren, eds., *Nils Rosén von Rosenstein and His Textbook on Paediatrics*, Supplement 156 of *Acta Paediatrica* (Uppsala) pp. 11–26.

Eva Nyström

ROSENBACH, OTTOMAR (b. Krappitz, Silesia, Prussia (now Poland), 4 January 1851; d. Berlin, Germany, 20 March 1907), *medicine*.

The son of a physician, Rosenbach was born in Krappitz (now Krapkowice), a town on the banks of the river Odra in Silesia, then a province of Prussia. He attended the gymnasium in neighboring Ratibor (Racibórz). After graduating, he studied medicine at the university of the Silesian capital, Breslau (Wrocław) and later in Berlin, where he came under the influence of his uncle, the renowned clinician Ludwig Traube (1818–78). Rosenbach served as a volunteer in the 1870–71 Franco-Prussian war, and participated in the siege of Paris. He received his doctorate in 1873. From 1874 to 1877, he worked as an assistant at the medical clinic at Jena University under Wilhelm Olivier Leube (1842–1922) and Carl Wilhelm Nothnagel (1841–1905), the latter a leading representative of the Vienna School of internal medicine. In 1877 he took a position at the Allerheiligen Hospital Breslau where, initially influenced by Julius Cohnheim's (1839–84) experimental approach, he became interested in pathological problems. In 1878 he obtained his Habilitation at the University of Breslau, with a study on artificially induced valvular heart defects (*Ueber artifizielle Herzklappenfehler*), which prepared the ground for later work on the function and pathology of the heart. In 1887 he was appointed physician in chief of the medical ward of the Allerheiligen Hospital, and in 1888 associate professor at the university. As he was Jewish, Rosenbach was not eligible for a full professorship. In 1893 he resigned from his hospital appointment, and in 1896 from his teaching position, in order to move to Berlin and dedicate his time exclusively to research and writing. He lived and worked in the capital until his untimely death in 1907.

Rosenbach was a prolific writer who published widely on issues in pathology and physiology, and especially on clinical problems. His bibliography lists more than 300 items, including a number of textbooks. Various tests, symptoms, and diseases carry his name, but much of his work was rather theoretical. He published on epistemological questions, and worked on an organismic theory of life, which contemporaries characterized as Naturphilosophie. Furthermore, Rosenbach left his mark as a critic of an important development in modern medicine, the shift away from the bedside toward the laboratory. He challenged what he saw as an uncritical reliance among physicians on specialist subjects, and practices such as radiology or bacteriology. Rosenbach was an ardent critic of Robert Koch in the tuberculin controversy. He was skeptical about the promises of bacteriology, doubting not only its value for clinical diagnoses, but also whether the new specialism contributed much to a better understanding of disease etiology. Instead, Rosenbach embraced a concept of functional diagnosis, based on technologies that could be used by generalist clinicians to monitor the functions of the human body under controlled conditions. In his view, clinical science should deal with 'insufficiencies', or failures of the body's organ systems, and he challenged the notion that the presence of localized lesions or isolated strains of pathological microbes was sufficient to identify a patient as ill. Equally, not every deviation from the norm was necessarily pathological, he argued, and generalists were better placed than specialists to make this distinction. He also assigned an important role to psychotherapy. His position toward bacteriology was especially responsible for Rosenbach's relative marginality in the final years of his life. However, he had a number of devoted followers, and his writings were popular with a vocal group of holistic physicians in the interwar period.

Bibliography

Primary: 1891. *Grundlagen, Aufgaben und Grenzen der Therapie* (Vienna and Leipzig); 1897. *Energetik und Medizin* (Vienna and Leipzig); 1899. *Grundriß und Pathologie der Herzkrankheiten* (Berlin and Vienna); 1903. *Arzt contra Bacteriologe* (Berlin) [English trans., 1904]; 1907. *Heilkunde und Spezialistentum* (Munich).

Secondary: Faber, Knud, 1930. *Nosography: The Evolution of Clinical Medicine in Modern Times* (New York); Hönigswald, R., 1910. 'Rosenbach, Ottomar.' *Biografisches Jahrbuch u. Deutscher Nekrolog*, Vol. 13, p. 510.

Carsten Timmermann

ROSS, RONALD (b. Almora, India, 15 May 1857; d. Putney, London, England, 16 September 1932), *malariology*.

Ross was the eldest of ten children of Captain (later General Sir) C. C. G. Ross of the Indian Army and Matilda Charlotte Ross (née Elderton). Ross was sent to England for his schooling and was educated at Springhill, near Southampton, where he developed a love of outdoor pursuits, mathematics, and the arts. Despite his early interests, his father urged him to join the IMS and, to this end, he entered St Bartholomew's Hospital, London (1874). He was a mediocre student and did not pass the LSA examination until his second attempt.

After working as a ship's surgeon and attending the Army Medical College, Ross left for Madras in 1881, after which he followed the army to a variety of stations in southern India, Burma, and the Andaman Islands. His duties were light and he had ample time to pursue his interest in sports, mathematics, and literature. On returning to England on furlough in 1888, Ross took a diploma in public health and studied bacteriology, marking the start of a lifelong interest in preventive medicine. In London, Ross also met and married Rosa Bloxam, who accompanied her husband back to India, where they had two of their four children. After serving with the army in Burma, Ross was appointed surgeon in Bangalore, southern India, where he became interested in malaria. He also continued with his literary endeavors, writing a novel and some poems, which were later published.

Ross's interest in malaria developed further when he met Patrick Manson (1844–1922) in London (1894). Manson demonstrated the existence of the malaria parasite (which Ross had earlier doubted) and told him of his belief that the mosquito was involved in its transmission. On returning to India, Ross began to test this hypothesis. He corresponded frequently with Manson, often expressing his frustrations with the lack of time and facilities he had for research. However, on 20 August 1897 ('Malaria Day'), Ross made an important breakthrough and announced that he had transmitted the parasite from human blood into a species of mosquito.

Transfer to a nonmalarious area interrupted Ross's research, but, at Manson's request, he was given six months' special duties in Calcutta, where he continued his research into malaria using birds rather than human patients. In February 1898, he proved that the transmission of malaria occurred through the bite of an infected mosquito, and, in July, he showed that mosquitoes could themselves become infected by biting infected birds. The complete cycle of transmission had thus been elucidated.

In 1899 Ross returned to England, becoming a lecturer at the new Liverpool School of Tropical Medicine. He thought deeply about the epidemiology of malaria and made innovative use of his knowledge in mathematics. He also set out his ideas on how to combat malaria using mosquito brigades, which aimed to destroy adult insects and larvae. Ross was now convinced that public health was essential to civilization and that the prevention of epidemic diseases, particularly malaria, was vital to economic development.

From Liverpool, Ross organized a number of malaria expeditions to West Africa, and he gave advice on malaria prevention in other parts of the British Empire. The failure of experimental mosquito control at the military station of Mian Mir, in the Punjab, was a major setback, but mosquito control remained an important element of malaria prevention. During World War I, when Ross was appointed as a consultant on malaria to the British army, he used his position to argue for mosquito control instead of reliance on quinine prophylaxis.

From the early 1900s, Ross was engaged in a bitter dispute over priority with the Italian parasitologist Giovanni Battista Grassi (1854–1925), whose team had demonstrated the malaria cycle in human beings, and their rivalry became intense after Ross alone was awarded the Nobel Prize in medicine or physiology (1902). The controversy revealed the unpleasant side of Ross's personality, yet he was a stalwart defender of those whom he believed to have been wronged, including the Russian-born Jew Waldemar Haffkine (1860–1930), who had been unjustifiably dismissed by the government of India.

Ross left Liverpool for London in 1912, where he was appointed consultant physician to King's College Hospital. In his later years, much of Ross's formidable energy was dissipated in continuing disputes with Grassi and in trying to establish his reputation as a mathematician. Despite his Nobel Prize, he died feeling that his contribution had been insufficiently recognized, especially financially.

Bibliography

Primary: 1910. *The Prevention of Malaria* (London); 1923. *Memoirs* (London).

Secondary: Power, Helen, 1999. *Tropical Medicine in the Twentieth Century: A History of the Liverpool School, 1898–1990* (London); Bynum, W. F., and C. Overy, eds., 1998. *The Beast in the Mosquito: The Correspondence of Ronald Ross and Patrick Manson* (Amsterdam and Atlanta); Nye, M. E., and M. E. Gibson, 1997. *Ronald Ross: Malariologist and Polymath* (London); *DSB*; *Oxford DNB*.

Mark Harrison

ROTHSCHILD, HENRI DE   (b. Paris, France, 26 July 1872; d. near Lausanne, Switzerland, 10 October 1947), *pediatrics, medical philanthropy.*

Rothschild was the son of James-Edouard and Theresa, a Frankfurt Rothschild. Henri was the quintessential Parisian, prominent man-about-town, bibliophile and art collector, playwright, and, above all, for many years an important figure in French medicine. Under the Teutonic discipline of his widowed mother, Rothschild took his medical degree at the Paris Faculty of Medicine (1898). A steady parade of top doctors to the family residence, both for Rothschild and his mother, along with family support of a hospital in Berck-sur-Mer, ensured that the young student would be well connected in high medical circles. His mentors were Georges Dieulafoy, Pierre Budin, Paul Poirier, and Alfred Fournier. Though he did not succeed in passing the patron-controlled intern examination for the Paris hospitals, it hardly mattered except for the damage to his tender ego. His early training and publications were in what came to be called pediatrics, with a specialty in infant feeding. Rothschild soon made his mark in medicine by supporting research and publications, and by supporting and building clinics and hospitals. His work in pediatrics received praise and awards from the medical establishment.

The Rothschilds have a distinguished history of hospital building in London, Frankfurt, Vienna, and especially

Paris. Henri was a remarkable institution builder. He began in 1895 by opening a small Consultation spéciale de nourrissons on the property of the hospital built by his great grandfather (James) in east Paris. The 'Consultation' soon became a polyclinic, and its success led him to build a new hospital in northwest Paris in order to provide the latest in medical and surgical care for babies, children, and adults of the eighteenth arrondissement. In a twenty-year period (1903–24), more than 2,600 patients were hospitalized, with 1,681 of them undergoing major surgery. More than 220,000 people received free consultations with free medicines. Many of these consultations were nursing mothers and their babies. Free sterilized milk and layettes were also distributed. During World War I the Rothschild hospitals were militarized. Rothschild and his wife (Mathilde) spent much of the war at the front, both in medical roles. The war provided a fertile, ghastly theater for Rothschild to continue his work on serious burns, a new affliction of industrializing societies.

He was a fervent Pastorian, though he appreciated the clinical acumen of the anti-Pastorian Michel Peter. His work on infant feeding, and his medical teaching and practice, were firmly rooted in germ theory. His hospital was the center of considerable medical research and teaching, with an emphasis on the latest equipment and techniques. There was an excellent library with many foreign journals, mostly German. Top specialists gave lectures and courses. With collaborators, Rothschild himself pursued work in endocrinology and venereal disease; he introduced Ehrlich's '606' treatment for syphilis. He promoted radium therapy for cancer patients by his heavy financial support of several institutions, including the Institut du Radium (La Fondation Curie). After the death of Mathilde in 1926, Henri rebuilt his hospital (La Fondation Mathilde-Henri de Rothschild) to make it into a true surgical hospital, chiefly for the poor of northwest Paris. Vichy rewarded him with loss of citizenship and seizure of his property. He spent the war years in Portugal.

Bibliography

Primary: 1898. *L'Allaitement mixte et l'allaitement artificielle* (Paris); 1902. *L'Oeuvre philanthopique du lait (Paris)*; 1919. *Traité des brûlures. Etude clinique et thérapeutique* (Paris); 1929. *Exposé des travaux scientifiques du docteur Henri de Rothschild* (Paris); 1933–36. *Croisière autour de mes souvenirs* 2 vols. (Paris).

Secondary: Ferguson, Niall, 1998. *The World's Banker: The History of the House of Rothschild* (London).

Harry W. Paul

ROUSSY, GUSTAVE SAMUEL (b. Vevey, Switzerland, 24 November 1874; d. Paris, France, 30 September 1948), *oncology.*

Roussy was an emblematic figure of the French Third Republic: reform-minded, founder of the Cancer Institute before becoming rector of the University of Paris, and an ally of left-wing politicians with ties to Léon Blum, Prime Minister of the 'Front Populaire' (1936).

Roussy was born in Switzerland to a family that shared ownership of the Nestlé Company. He studied medicine in Geneva, where he received his degree in 1906, then did his hospital internship in Paris. He was trained in the French school of clinical medicine, but with interest in the nervous system and endocrinology, Roussy did not see anatomo-pathology solely as a descriptive science, but rather as a dynamic approach to biology. As a result, in 1913 he went to the Paul Brousse Hospital in the Parisian suburb of Villejuif to study cancer, at that time a relatively neglected disease. After World War I he became involved in the experimental study of cancer, first the etiology of the disease, and then the mechanisms of defense of the organism against cancer. Roussy studied diverse carcinogenic substances and the problem of metastasis, from which he concluded that cancer was a disturbance of cell activity. He was also involved in prevention, and participated in the organization of regional anticancer centers created by government minister Paul Strauss.

His cancer service at Paul Brousse Hospital became the 'Research Institute for Cancer Treatment' of the Faculté de Médecine in Paris in ceremonies presided over by the President of the Republic in 1934. Thanks to support from the Communist city council of Villejuif, as well as the Rockefeller Foundation and the French government, this institute served both hospital and research functions, and housed a 600-watt high-penetration radiotherapy apparatus, next to laboratories of anatamo-pathology, biochemistry, physical chemistry, and experimental medicine. As a result, beginning in the 1930s Roussy introduced at Paul Brousse Hospital one of the first full-time hospital practices in France, a first step on the path which eventually made the hospital a modern 'healing factory', according to historian Patrice Pinell. Paradoxically, this made hospitals—institutions founded for a charitable purpose—the only places with the technical capacity necessary for modern medicine.

When Roussy was named dean of the Faculté de Médecine in 1933, he tried to modernize the teaching of medicine. In collaboration with André Mayer, chair of experimental medicine at the Collège de France, Roussy attempted to introduce the science of biology into the curriculum, changing the 'PCN' certificate (physics, chemistry, natural sciences) into 'PCB'. 'It is necessary', he argued, 'to give priority to the sciences (like biology) that have real educational value for the beginning year [of medical study].' Likewise, he proposed a rationalization of the 'Agrégation de médecine', the examinations that determined professors of the Faculté, by reducing the number of medical specialties from twenty-four to fifteen.

But Roussy collided with the conservatism of the Paris hospitals and the corporatism of the medical establishment, and he was unsuccessful in his project (financed by the Rockefeller Foundation) to integrate the Paris hospitals and the medical school into one organization, along the North American model. Nonetheless, thanks to his connections to the leaders of the Popular Front, Roussy was named to head the Section of Experimental Medicine at the new Centre National de la Recherche Scientifique (CNRS), and was made rector of the University of Paris. In this capacity in 1937, he laid the cornerstone of the new medical school building on Rue des Saints Pére in the 6th arrondissement of Paris. Several months after France's surrender to the Germans, and following demonstrations by Paris students against the Occupation in November 1940, Roussy was fired by the Vichy government. He was reinstated as rector after the Liberation.

He ended his life on 30 September 1948 following accusations of fiscal fraud in a minor affair by the Christian-democrat Minister Robert Schumann. Roussy's reputation was subsequently rehabilitated, and the French government decided to honor him by naming the cancer institute at Villejuif after him. Today, at the gates of Paris leading to Roussy's workplace, a traveler cannot fail to notice the immense buildings of the Institut Gustave Roussy.

Bibliography

Primary: 1920. (with Desmarets, E. E.). *À propos d'une mission scientifique aux Etats-Unis. L'enseignement médical aux États-Unis, The National Board of Medical Examiners* (Paris); 1924. *L'état actuel du problème du cancer* (Paris); 1935 (with Huguenin, R., and Ngo Quoc Queyn). *Les tumeurs noires de la peau* (Paris); 1942. (with Leroux, R., and C. Oberling). *Précis d'anatomo-pathologique* (Paris).

Secondary: Pinell, Patrice, 1992. *Naissance d'un fléau, Histoire de la lutte contre le cancer en France, 1890–1940* (Paris).

Jean-François Picard

ROUX, (PIERRE PAUL) EMILE   (b. Confolens, France, 17 December, 1853; d. Paris, France, 3 November 1933), *bacteriology, immunology.*

Roux was the most famous Pastorian, a term coined in 1895 by a medical journalist in reference to the dedicated group of scientists working under Louis Pasteur's leadership. Roux was the son of Jean Roux, head of a college, and Martha Pintaud, from the petite bourgeoisie. Orphaned at nine, he was educated at Aurillac and Clermont-Ferrand, where he obtained his baccalauréat, began medical studies, and met his future mentor, the chemist Emile Duclaux. Roux chose the military medical school in Paris, which charged no tuition, and he won a hospital internship in 1873. He displayed both his dedication to science, and his spirit of opposition to hierarchy, by declining to finish his medical thesis on rabies in the allotted time (he did not complete it until 1883). He was dismissed from the army in 1877.

At that difficult stage, lacking a medical degree, Roux met Duclaux again, who recommended him to Pasteur. Hired as an assistant to inoculate animals, the rebellious Roux progressively integrated himself into Pasteur's research team that was studying bacteria and immunity. The collaboration culminated in two famous episodes. The first involved Roux's contribution to the anthrax vaccine trials at the Pouilly le Fort farm near Paris, in 1881. Roux was able to produce an effective vaccine against anthrax by adding bichromate, which impeded spore formation, to the attenuated vaccine.

The second episode concerned rabies. Roux was the central figure in the process leading to the manufacture of a vaccine. He introduced the intracranial inoculation of rabid brains in animals to facilitate standardization of virulent products with a fixed incubation time, and then decreased the virulence level of infectious spinal cords by exposing them to progressive desiccation. This time of intense work was also a period of tension between pupil and master. Roux disagreed with what he perceived to be the premature initial trial of the vaccine in 1885 on young Joseph Meister, the victim of extensive bites by a rabid dog. Pasteur's broad success, however, led to the foundation of the Pasteur Institute in 1888.

Roux's last important scientific work was the one for which he received several nominations without winning a Nobel Prize. With Alexandre Yersin, he demonstrated in 1889 that a virulent poison, a toxin, produced by the bacillus discovered by Klebs and Loeffler and circulated by blood, was responsible for the paralysis and necrotic swelling and obstruction of the throat in diphtheria, the infantile scourge. In 1891 he tested the curative effects of Emil Behring's antidiphtheric serum, developed in horses, on a population of hospitalized ill children whom he compared against a sample of untreated siblings in another hospital. The positive results, which Roux reported at the Budapest Congress in 1894, were hailed as the first effective treatment of diphtheria. Serotherapy entered medical practice and proved effective against many infectious diseases.

After Pasteur's death, Roux dedicated himself to the management of research at the Institute. Although he collaborated in 1905 with his friend Elie Mechnikov on the investigation of syphilis in monkeys, Roux gradually reduced his own scientific work. In 1904 he became the powerful director of the Pasteur Institute, a position he held for thirty years until his death. He met the double challenge of promoting research in the Paris motherhouse, as well as in the emerging network of Pasteur institutes in French colonies and foreign countries. He taught the 'grand cours', in which a whole generation of bacteriologists was trained.

In France, Roux enjoyed a unique position of prestige and expertise. He was a member of the Academy of Sciences and the Academy of Medicine. He sat on all committees dealing with hygiene, and acted as an expert for the approval of vaccines and preventive or curative seras. He lent all his authority to the dissemination of BCG (Calmette and Guérin's bacillus, a vaccine against tuberculosis), and he shared Albert Calmette's anxiety when, in 1929, the news of the Lubeck disaster broke. In this incident, 100 children died after vaccination with contaminated material.

Roux contributed to a great scientific adventure which transcended his personal stature. He concentrated his energy on the maintenance of a scientific family, which has been compared with a religious order, sharing intellectual goals and a style of laboratory practices. He faced his various tasks with limited finances and administrative staff. His inspired direction and ascetic behavior nurtured his legend as a scientific saint (although he seemed himself to have been an agnostic). In the end, however, he was sharply criticized by colleagues such as Charles Nicolle, who believed Roux's mismanagement had resulted in the relative decline of the Pasteur Institute prior to World War II.

Some early biographies provided clues to Roux's psychology. His niece suggested the importance of a variety of female companions for the eternal bachelor; Emile Lagrange depicted a man trapped by a legend which he had helped to create. No biography addresses all the aspects of this versatile man. Unfortunately, most of his huge correspondence is not yet available, and this lacuna deprives historians of the documentation necessary for a fresh reappraisal of Roux's impact on French and international public health. Roux was a passionate and original character, who carried the weight of a tradition that mixed archaism and modernity.

Bibliography

Primary: 1896. *L'oeuvre scientifique de Pasteur* (Paris); 1899. *Notice sur les travaux scientifiques d'Emile Roux* (Paris); Complete list of publications at http://www.pasteur.fr/infosci/biblio/bibliogr/roux.html

Secondary: Geison, Gerald L., 1990. 'Pasteur, Roux and Rabies, Scientific versus Clinical Mentalities.' *Journal of the History of Medicine and Allied Sciences* 45: 341–365; Lagrange, Emile, 1954. *Monsieur Roux* (Brussels); Cressac, Mary, 1950. *Le docteur Roux, mon oncle* (Paris).

Anne Marie Moulin

RUBIO GALI, FEDERICO (b. Puerto de Santa María, Cádiz, Spain, 30 August 1827; d. Madrid, Spain, 31 August 1902), *surgery.*

Rubio was born to a liberal family that experienced persecution by the absolutist regime of King Ferdinand VII until 1833. He studied medicine and surgery at the Royal College of Surgery in Cádiz (1842–50). Upon completion of studies he moved to Seville (1850), where he opened a private practice that provided him with a considerable income. In addition, he practiced surgery in operating rooms at public hospitals. During the two-year progressionist period (1854–56) he held several political offices in Seville, where he advocated for the inception of a democratic regime. In 1859, in view of the repression brought about by moderate liberals, he exiled himself to London, where he met the surgeon William Fergusson. A few months later he went to Paris, where he completed his surgical training with Alfred Velpeau and Auguste Nelaton.

Upon his return, Rubio introduced surgical techniques such as hysterectomy (1861) and ovariotomy (1863) to Spain, whereupon he wrote various papers. He also was one of the first Spanish surgeons to study and then use anesthesia. In 1870 he became a Doctor of Medicine at the School of Medicine and Surgery in Seville, to the founding of which he had contributed.

Rubio's political activity increased during the Revolutionary Sexennium (1868–74). He was a Member of Parliament and Senator for the Federal Republican Party, and was appointed ambassador of the Spanish Republic to Great Britain in June 1873, with the mission of gaining official recognition of the Republican regime from the British government. Following his failed mission and the fall of the Republic, he returned in 1874 to Madrid, where he gave up politics. From then on he devoted himself intensely to his professional work, which focused exclusively on surgery. His major accomplishments included the introduction of nephrectomy (1874) and laryngectomy (1878) to Spain.

His prestige and political relationships, which reached the Royal House, allowed him to found the Institute for Operative Therapeutics (1880) within the facilities of *Hospital de la Princesa* (Princess Hospital), an institution managed under the Poor Law. The Institute had fifty beds in three wards (children's, women's, and men's), as well as a dispensary, clinic, anatomy amphitheater, and pharmacy. The Institute was moved to a dedicated, specifically constructed building in 1897. The aim was to set up a teaching center for the clinical and doctrinal cultivation of medicosurgical specialties, and to provide Madrid with a hospital center specializing in high-level surgery. From 1899 the new center produced a house organ of scientific expression, the journal *Revista Iberoamericana de Ciencias Médicas*, which in addition to recording the Institute's activities, included papers on surgery. Rubio's work in the fields of medical teaching and healthcare was eventually completed with the creation within his Institute of Escuela de Enfermeras de Santa Isabel de Hungría—Spain's first school for nurses.

Near the end of his life Rubio wrote several works on social topics, wherein he expressed his organistic conception of society and the need to apply social therapeutics to ease social tensions. Rubio contributed to the development and modernization of nineteenth-century Spanish surgery by introducing into the country novel surgical techniques, and by training a new generation of surgeons at *Instituto de Terapéutica Operatoria*. This institution disappeared during the Spanish Civil War (1936–39).

Bibliography

Primary: 1868. *Apuntes de mi práctica sobre los tumores y quistes y el resultado de su tratamiento médico* (Madrid); 1878. *La ovariotomía* (Madrid); 1878. *Caries y stenose laríngea. Extirpación total de la laringe* (Madrid); 1890. *La Sociopatología* (Madrid).

Secondary: Carrillo Martos, Juan Luis, ed., 2003. *Medicina y sociedad en la España de la segunda mitad del siglo XIX: una aproximación a la obra de Federico Rubio y Gali* (Puerto de Santa María); Campos Marín, Ricardo, 2003. *Curar y gobernar. Medicina y liberalismo en la España del siglo XIX. Monlau, Rubio, Giné* (Madrid).

Ricardo Campos

RUBNER, MAX (b. Munich, Germany, 2 June 1854; d. Berlin, Germany, 27 April 1932), *hygiene, physiology.*

Rubner, son of Johann Nepomuk Rubner, a locksmith, and Barbara Duscher, studied medicine at the University of Munich from 1873 to 1877. He received his doctorate in 1878. His trailblazing medical dissertation, *Über die Ausnutzung einiger Nahrungsmittel im Darmkanal des Menschen*, was published in 1880.

After completing his medical studies, Rubner became an unpaid assistant at the physiological institute. Since the director, Carl Voit, was not interested in his novel approach to bioenergetics, Rubner spent a year at Carl Ludwig's physiological institute at Leipzig, where he conducted research on the physiology of blood circulation, the muscles, and digestion. In 1883 Rubner contended that the log of the metabolic rate would vary with the log of body mass in the same way that the log of surface area does, because heat is lost through the external surface of the animal. If the animal is to balance the loss of heat across its external surface, then it must increase heat production in proportion to the surface area. Thus, Rubner concluded, specific metabolic rate should decrease with size as the cube root of mass. In 1885 he proved by animal experiments that an increase in metabolic rate was evident soon after the ingestion of food, independent of other activities.

In 1885 Rubner was offered a chair in pharmacology in Munich. He declined, accepting instead a professorship in hygiene at the University of Marburg, where he taught until 1891. In his teaching he made a point that, in studying medicine, one had to learn how to 'include hygiene into one's observation'. While at Marburg he published on heat regulation, body surface, and the exchange of substances, although he constantly complained to the authorities about the working conditions in his laboratory. At Marburg he also constructed in 1889 the first accurate respiration calorimeter.

Two years later he succeeded Robert Koch in the chair of hygiene in Berlin, despite the fact that he was a former student of Koch's rival, Max Pettenkofer. A large new institute with a focus on hygiene was built for him in 1905. For his achievements in this field he received the Pettenkofer Prize. Rubner was one of the leading experts on hygiene in Germany at the time, publishing, for example, the *Lehrbuch der Hygiene* (1890), which ran into several editions, and editing the renowned journal, *Archiv für Hygiene and Bakteriologie* (from 1892).

However, Rubner was much more interested in his scientific work on physiology. In 1894 he demonstrated that the amount of energy produced by food used by the body is the same as the energy produced if the food is burned (after urea—an organic compound of carbon, nitrogen, oxygen, and hydrogen that the body does not consume in respiration—is removed). The energy consumption hypothesis (Gesetz des Energieverbrauchs) proposes that animals are born with a limited amount of some substance, potential energy, or physiological capacity, and that the faster they use it, the faster they will die. In 1908 Rubner discovered a relationship between metabolic rate, body size, and longevity. In brief, long-lived animal species are, on average, bigger, and spend fewer calories per gram of body mass than smaller, short-lived species.

In 1909 Rubner was offered the Berlin chair of physiology as successor to Theodor Wilhelm Engelmann. From 1910 to 1911 he was rector of the University of Berlin and cofounder of the Kaiser-Wilhelm-Institut für Arbeitsphysiologie. In 1913 he became director of this new institute. Rubner also served as permanent secretary of the Preussische Akademie der Wissenschaften. He was member of the scientific academies of Munich, Vienna, Oslo, Washington, D.C., Stockholm, and Uppsala. Today, many research institutes all over the world bear his name. His claim that the German people were suffering from nutritional problems due to the blockade maintained by the Allies after World War I made him a well-liked figure in conservative circles during the Weimar Republic.

Bibliography

Primary: 1883. 'Die Vertretungswerthe der hauptsächlichsten organischen Nahrungsstoffe im Thierkörper.' *Zeitschrift für Biologie* 19: 313–396; 1889. 'Ein Calorimeter für physiologische und hygienische Zwecke.' *Zeitschrift für Biologie* 25: 400–426; 1909. *Volksernährungsfragen* (Leipzig); 1911. 'Die Kalorimetrie' in Tigerstedt, Robert, ed., *Handbuch der physiologischen Methodik*, vol. 1 (Leipzig) pp. 150–228; 1913. *Die Ernährungsphysiologie der Hefezelle bei alkoholischer Gärung* (Leipzig); 1982. *The Laws of Energy Consumption in Nutrition*, with a biography of Max Rubner by Chambers, William H. (New York).

Secondary: Peer, Elizabeth, 1983. *Max Rubner. Forscher und Mensch. Biographie* (Wattens); *DSB.*

Robert Jütte

RUDBECK, OLAUS (OLOF), Sr (b. Västerås, Sweden, December 1630; d. Uppsala, Sweden, 17 September 1702), *anatomy.*

Rudbeck was the son of the bishop in Västerås, Johannes Rudbeckius, and his second wife, Magdalena née Hising.

After completing primary school in his hometown, Rudbeck commenced medical studies at Uppsala University in 1648. Early on, he began doing dissections of smaller animals, and after discovering a milk-like substance oozing from the subclavian vein of a freshly butchered calf, he became aware of the lymphatic channels. These had first been observed in 1622 by the Italian Gasparo Aselli and were at the center of the anatomist's interest. Rudbeck, who had already begun teaching anatomy, got an opportunity to demonstrate his findings to Queen Christina in the spring of 1652, but he did not make his discoveries public until the summer of 1653. In the fall of that year, he went to Holland on a scholarship from the queen, and stayed until August 1654. At the famous university in Leiden, he immediately drew attention to his insights, and his great manual skills were displayed at the anatomical demonstrations headed by Professor van Horne.

In his work *Nova exercitatio anatomica*, Rudbeck demonstrated the central parts of the lymphatic system, with the nourishing veins from the bowels through the thoracic duct to the subclavian vein. He also proved the existence of a string of lymphatic channels carrying transparent liquid in different organs in the body. Of particular relevance for the debates of his time was his demonstration that the lymphatic channels carried fluid from the liver to the thoracic duct, since it was believed that the liver transformed nourishment from the bowels into blood. Through this demonstration, Rudbeck aligned himself with Harvey in the debates on the circulatory system. He had skillfully disclosed the direction of the movement of lymph in the body, and drawn attention to the system of shutters that prevented the lymph from traveling in the wrong direction. His illustrations of the examined organs were excellent. Rudbeck did his research on what was a hot topic at the time, and he was one of the pioneers in this field, but it is difficult to trace the exact order of discoveries because of their rapid pace. The thoracic duct had (without Rudbeck's knowledge) been described just prior to Rudbeck's demonstration by the Frenchman, Jean Pecquet, and most of the vessels presented by Rudbeck had been published by the Dane, Thomas Bartholin, in his book *Vasa lymphatica* a few months before Rudbeck's own work was published. This led to a heated debate on priorities. In 1654 the Dutchman Sieboldus Hemsterhuis published a collection of treatises that had produced new results on the lymphatic tracts (*Messis aurea triennalis*), which included both Rudbeck's and Bartholin's reports. During the proofreading, Rudbeck discovered that Bartholin had introduced new material, and he succeeded in having included a letter to Bartholin accusing him of trying to steal the credit for the discoveries. Rudbeck then received a rather aggressive letter from Bartholin's student, Martin Bogdan, and a written feud ensued. Rudbeck later made a series of addenda to his report.

In 1660 Rudbeck was appointed professor of anatomy at the University of Uppsala. Later on, he had less time for anatomy, and devoted himself to other fields of study. He did build an anatomical theater, and he founded the university's first botanical garden to help the study of medicine. Working with materials from the garden and available literature, in 1679 he began to depict all the plants of the world in their natural size in the magnificent collection of prints, *Campus Elysii*. Only a few prints were printed before Rudbeck's death, and almost all the remaining unpublished ones were destroyed in a great fire in 1702, the year he died.

Rudbeck also practiced medicine, but few traces remain of this. It is known that he found use for his surgical skill at the birth of one of his sons. He was forced to remove an obstructing tumor from his wife, a procedure mistakenly called a caesarean section. That he considered it such a procedure can be seen from the name he gave his son—Johannes Caesar.

Bibliography

Primary: 1653. *Nova exercitatio anatomica*. (Västerås) (also found in Hemsterhuis, 1654) [English trans. Liljestrand, Göran, 1942. *Bulletin of the History of Medicine* 11: 304–339]; 1654. *Insidiae structae* (Leiden); Hemsterhuis, Sieboldus, 1654. *Messis aurea triennalis*. (Leiden) [2nd printing, Heidelberg, 1659]; 1657. *Ad Thomam Bartholinum epistola* (Uppsala).

Secondary: Lindroth, Sten, 1957. 'Harvey, Descartes and Young Oluas Rudbeck.' *Journal of the History of Medicine and Allied Sciences* 12: 209–219; *DSB*.

Gunnar Eriksson

RÜDIN, ERNST (b. St Gallen, Switzerland, 19 April 1874; d. Munich, Germany, 22 October 1952), *psychiatry, medical genetics.*

Rüdin was the son of Conrad Rüdin, teacher and businessman, and Dorothea, housewife. He studied medicine at the universities of Geneva, Naples, Heidelberg, Berlin, and Zurich. In 1899 he commenced his clinical work at the psychiatric hospital Burghölzli in Zurich; he later worked in Heidelberg, Basel, and Berlin. He took his MD in 1901 (Zurich). In 1905 he was among the founding members of the German Society for Racial Hygiene (Deutsche Gesellschaft für Rassenhygiene), and was also part of the editorial team of the journal, *Archiv für Rassen- und Gesellschaftsbiologie.*

From 1907 he worked as clinical resident at the department of psychiatry at the University of Munich under Emil Kraepelin. In 1909 he completed his Habilitation, and was appointed consultant at the same department. In 1917 he became head of the department of genealogy and demography (Genealogisch-Demographische Abteilung, GDA) at the newly established German Institute for Psychiatric Research (Deutsche Forschungsanstalt für Psychiatrie, DFA) in Munich. The GDA was the first institution worldwide exclusively devoted to research in psychiatric epidemiology and genetics. Together with the DFA, it was integrated into the prestigious Kaiser-Wilhelm-Society for the Advancement of Science in 1924. In 1925 Rüdin accepted appointment as professor and chair at the department of psychiatry at the University of Basel in Switzerland, but returned to the GDA in 1928 where he was offered a tripling of his budget. In 1930 Rüdin was appointed full professor of psychiatry at the University of Munich. From 1931 until the end of the Nazi regime in 1945, he acted as director of the entire DFA. From 1935 until 1945, he was also president of the Association of German Neurologists and Psychiatrists (Gesellschaft Deutscher Neurologen und Psychiater, GDNP).

Rüdin's book *Zur Entstehung und Vererbung der Dementia praecox* (1916) introduced the method of 'empirical prognosis of hereditary states' [empirische Erbprognose] and established him as the leading scholar in the field for the next two decades. At the same time, he continued his activities in the context of the eugenics movement, and in 1932 was elected president of the International Federation of Eugenic Organizations. After the Nazi takeover in 1933, Rüdin took on a leading position in the Expert Committee for Population and Race Policies associated with the Reich's Ministry of the Interior. He was one of three authors of the official commentary to the Law for the Prevention of Hereditary Diseased Offspring, a law that de facto allowed forced sterilization.

Rüdin joined the Nazi party in 1937. In 1940, in his position as president of the GDNP, he refused to join a coordinated protest against the systematic killing of psychiatric patients ('Euthanasie') organized by the regime. In 1942 he argued for the high priority of research into the criteria for selecting children of 'minor value' for 'elimination' within the context of the war effort of German psychiatry. From 1943 until 1945, he supported a related research program of Julius Deussen, a member of the GDA, carried out at the department of psychiatry, University of Heidelberg. A constitutive part of this program was the killing of research subjects to systematically correlate clinical with postmortem data. After the war, Rüdin lost his position, and was expatriated as a Swiss citizen.

Bibliography

Primary: 1911. 'Einige Wege und Ziele der Familienforschung, mit Rücksicht auf die Psychiatrie.' *Zeitschrift für die gesamte Neurologie und Psychiatrie* 7: 487–585; 1916. *Zur Vererbung und Neuentstehung der Dementia praecox* (Berlin); 1934. (Gütt, Arthur, Ernst Rüdin, and Falk Ruttke, eds., with commentary) *Gesetz zur Verhütung erbkranken Nachwuchses* (Munich).

Secondary: Ritter, Hans Jakob, and Volker, Roelcke, 2005. 'Psychiatric Genetics in Munich and Basel between 1925 and 1945: Programs, Practices, Cooperative Arrangements.' *OSIRIS* 20: 263–288; Roelcke, Volker, 2000. 'Psychiatrische Wissenschaft im Kontext nationalsozialistischer Politik und "Euthanasie". Zur Rolle von Ernst Rüdin und der Deutschen Forschungsanstalt für Psychiatrie' in Kaufmann, Doris, ed., *Die Kaiser-Wilhelm-Gesellschaft im Nationalsozialismus* (Göttingen) pp. 112–150.

Volker Roelcke

RUFUS OF EPHESUS (fl. *c.* late first century BCE to early first century), *medicine, anatomy.*

A 'Hippocratic' doctor, yet with a critical stance toward Hippocrates, Rufus was a remarkably independent figure, standing on his own in an age of school allegiances. He studied and practiced in Ephesus and lived for a long time in Alexandria. As he wrote in Greek and there is no indication that he ever set foot in Italy, the connection with Rome implicit in his name is a puzzle. His chronology is disputed. Suda placed Rufus 'under Trajan', yet a Rufus was also mentioned by Damocrates, who lived earlier, under Emperors Nero and Vespasian. There is scholarly disagreement between the two possible dates, but the argument for identifying Rufus with the character in Damocrates is weak, so Suda's later dating is probably to be preferred.

The list of his genuine works comprises ninety-six titles ranging over an enormous variety of subjects, such as *On the Naming of the Parts of the Human Body*, *A Physician's Questions*, *Living at Sea*, *On Kidney and Bladder Ailments*, *On Joints' Diseases*, *The Purchase of Slaves*, *Satyriasis and Spermatorrhoea*, and *Ointment for a Powerful Erection*. Some of these treatises were in verse, following the tradition of didactic medical poems that goes back to Nicander.

Rufus's most popular and original work was *A Physician's Questions of the Physician*—a questionnaire for the patient, designed to give his doctor the relevant diagnostic and therapeutic information through a reconstruction of the exact clinical environment. With its close examination of psychological factors, and its focus on modes of questioning, this work testified to a sense of responsibility to, and awareness of, the patient that was unique in ancient medical literature (Andorlini, 2004). Rufus was also famous for studies of diseases such as melancholia, which combined the richness and detail of clinical observations with extreme rigor, care, and lucidity in their evaluation. He was a physician of enormous breadth of knowledge and interests. His approach was sharp, cautious, objective, and, above all, precise. Precision is illustrated, for instance, by his work *On the Naming of the Parts of the Human Body*, a didactic introduction attempting to clarify the confused area of anatomical terminology by fixing the meaning of terms. This treatise also reflected the increasing tendency of physicians in Rufus's era to regard anatomy as a theoretical discipline, 'from the perspective of medical education' (Kudlien in *DSB*), rather than as an afterthought of surgical practice.

Rufus was a figure of considerable authority and prestige. In Byzantine medicine he was referred to as one of the 'quieting foursome of diseases', together with Hippocrates,

Galen, and Cheiron. He exerted a strong influence on the Western tradition through medieval authors who quoted him (e.g., Constantine the African). Most of the surviving Rufus material can be recovered from quotations and paraphrases in Oribasius and Aëtius, and from late Latin and Arabic translations. The Arabic tradition, in particular, is rich in quotations and analytical lists of works by Rufus.

Bibliography

Primary: 1933. (Morland, H., ed.) *De podagra* (Oslo); 1939. (Morland, H., ed.) *Oribasius Latinus* (Oslo); 1960. (Kowalski, G., ed.) *De corporis humani appelationibus.* Dissertation, University of Göttingen; 1962. (Gärtner, H., ed.) *Rufus von Ephesos. Die Fragen des Arztes an den Kranken* (Berlin); 1963. (Daremberg, C., and E. Ruelle, eds.) *Oeuvres de Rufus d'Ephèse* (Amsterdam); 1977. (Sideras, A., ed.) *De renum et vesicae morbis* (Berlin).

Secondary: Andorlini, I., 2004. *Medicina, medico e società nel mondo antico* (Florence) pp. 51–52, 102, 153, 231; Pormann, P., 1999. 'Paul of Aegina's Therapy of Children.' MPhil Dissertation, University of Oxford; Sideras, A., 1994. 'Rufus von Ephesos und sein Werk im Rahmen der antiken Medizin' in Temporini, H., and W. Haase, eds., *Aufstieg und Niedergang der römischen Welt* (1974–) (Berlin) II, 37.2: 1077–1253; 2036–2062; Sideras, A., 1971. *Textkritische Beiträge zur Schrift des Rufus von Ephesos 'De renum et vesicae morbis'* (Mainz and Wiesbaden); Flaschar, H., 1966. *Melancholie und Melancholiker in den medizinischen Theorien der Antike* (Berlin); Morland, H., 1932. *Die lateinischen Oribasiusübersetzungen* (Oslo); Ilberg, J., 1930. *Rufus von Ephesos. Ein griechischer Arzt in Trajanischer Zeit* (Leipzig); DSB.

Manuela Tecusan

RUSH, BENJAMIN (b. Byberry, Pennsylvania, USA, 4 January 1746; d. Philadelphia, Pennsylvania, USA, 19 April 1813), *medical education, medical ethics, medicine, mental health, psychiatry, public health, politics.*

Rush was born on a Pennsylvania plantation and was raised by his mother and stepfather after his father died when Rush was only six years old. Rush studied with his uncle, Samuel Finley, in Maryland, before going on for his undergraduate studies at the College of New Jersey (now Princeton University), completing his studies in 1760, including extensive study of then-contemporary Scottish moral philosophy. He apprenticed for five years to the Philadelphia physician, John Redman. Rush then traveled to Scotland, to undertake his medical studies at the University of Edinburgh and received his medical degree in 1768. After a brief tour of the European continent, he returned to Philadelphia in 1769 and embarked on a career that made him, some would say, the most accomplished physician in American history. Rush married Julia Stockton in 1776, with whom he had thirteen children.

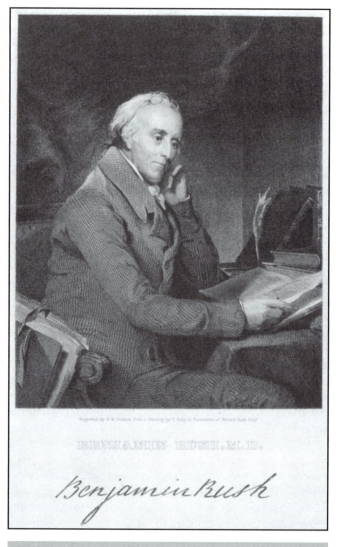

Benjamin Rush. Line engraving by R. W. Dodson after T. Sully. Iconographic Collection, Wellcome Library London.

American Patriot and Model Physician-Citizen

In only his twenties Rush became actively involved in politics, taking up causes such as the abolition of slavery, later serving as president of the Pennsylvania Society for the Abolition of Slavery. Upon his return to Philadelphia, Rush joined in the drive for the independence of the English colonies of North America. He published on the topic of colonial rights and played a leadership role in calling for independence from the crown in London. Rush is famous for his participation in the Continental Congress and as a signatory to the American Declaration of Independence for the colony of Pennsylvania in July 1776. He served as a military surgeon in the Pennsylvania navy and then in the revolutionary army from 1775 to 1778. He served in the convention that ratified the United States Constitution for the state of Pennsylvania in 1787. He capped his service to his country by becoming treasurer of the United States mint, a position that he held until his death in 1813. His long and distinguished public service makes him a role model of the conscientious physician-citizen and civic leader.

Medical and Liberal Arts Education

Rush had a long career in medical education, starting in 1769 as professor of chemistry at the Philadelphia medical college, the first medical school in the English North American colonies. He subsequently held faculty positions as professor of the theory and practice of medicine (from 1787) and professor of the institutes and practice of medicine (from 1791), serving in all three positions until his death. Rush brought to his teaching a dedication to Baconian scientific method that he learned as a medical student in Edinburgh in the 1760s. Rush also emphasized another Edinburgh theme: the scientific competence of physicians was the bedrock on which professional virtues and practice should be built. Rush emphasized scientific competence for the same reason his professors in Edinburgh did, to reform medicine into a profession worthy of the name and thus more than a mere occupation.

Rush also helped found Dickinson College in the Pennsylvania countryside. In doing so, he helped create a distinctively American institution of higher education, the freestanding liberal arts college that awarded only undergraduate degrees and did not include the graduate or professional schools of a university. These colleges were founded to educate the sons of the wealthy (American liberal arts colleges for women came in the nineteenth century) and to prepare them for leadership in civic and religious life. Upon completion of undergraduate studies in the liberal arts, students would go into business or to a university for professional study of law, medicine, or divinity. Rush thus helped create the pattern of the formal education of physicians in the United States that continues to this day.

Contributions to the Scientific and Learned Literature

Rush contributed to the scientific literature of medicine. His *Medical Inquiries and Observations*, published in several editions, ranged very widely. Topics included 'the natural history of medicine among the Indians of North-America'; the management of diseases, including bilious fever, cholera, consumption, parasitic worms, sore legs, dropsy, measles, yellow fever (extensively), and influenza; the clinical efficacy of various treatments, including blistering and bleeding for 'intermitting fevers', common salt to treat hemoptysis, arsenic to treat cancers, and inoculation to prevent smallpox; military medicine during the Revolutionary War; geriatrics; diseases of the brain, making him a forerunner of modern neuropsychiatry; and accounts of yellow fever during its several outbreaks in Philadelphia,

thus helping create the field of public health. He also wrote on moral philosophy and comparative physiology, again following the example of his Edinburgh professors.

Public Health

Rush distinguished himself within public health by helping found the Philadelphia dispensary and personally attending to scores of patients daily during the yellow fever epidemic of 1793 in Philadelphia. Whether physicians had an ethical obligation to remain with their patients in times of epidemics—risking health and life—was a matter of controversy in the history of Western medical ethics. Rush's example may well have influenced the writers of the *Code of Ethics* of 1847 of the American Medical Association, a provision of which makes it ethically obligatory for physicians to remain and care for their patients during epidemics.

Medical Ethics

At the medical school of the University of Edinburgh, Rush attended the clinical and medical ethics lectures of John Gregory (1724–73). Gregory based his medical ethics both on Baconian scientific method, as the basis for physicians' scientific and clinical competence, and on sympathy, a natural fellow feeling that motivated one to recognize the plight of the sick and to relieve the pain, distress, and suffering of their diseases and injuries. Like Gregory, Rush gave lectures on medical ethics for medical students before they undertook their clinical training in public hospitals for the care of the worthy, sick poor. Rush's published version of his medical ethics lectures were borrowed from the titles of Gregory's books on medical ethics, *Observations on the Duties of a Physician and the Methods of Improving Medicine*, to which Rush added the distinctive subtitle, *Accommodated to the Present State of Society and Manners in the United States*. The latter signaled his interest in topics that Gregory did not address, such as the size of the farm that a physician should seek to maintain, an important consideration at a time when most of the population of the United States was rural. Rush also took up topics that concerned Gregory, such as keeping medications simple so as to better study their effects and avoiding ostentation of dress or manners, since these were not true signs of competence in medicine and commitment to the well-being of patients, but indulgences of entrepreneurial self-interest. Gregory's medical ethics was secular in that it appealed to foundations in Baconian method and Scottish moral sense philosophy that were discoverable upon disciplined observation. Gregory defended physicians from the charge of atheism by arguing for deism in the evident design of an ordered natural world. Rush, in sharp contrast, gave his medical ethics a distinctively religious, indeed Christian, emphasis. In doing so, he created a distinctive theistic approach to medical ethics in the United States that lasted for the next two centuries. The introduction to the American Medical Association's *Code of Ethics*, for example, appeals explicitly to religion as one of its sources. In the twentieth century, both Roman Catholic and Protestant theologians and scholars made major contributions to medical ethics, and most of the nonphysician founding figures of bioethics in the United States were trained in theology or religious studies (Veatch, 2005). Both trends give evidence of Rush's lasting influence on the history of medical ethics in the United States.

Rush was a physician of considerable accomplishment in medicine, medical education, public health, and medical ethics. He was a leading colonial citizen and founder of the American republic and has been considered a worthy role model of the 'compleat physician' for doctors to emulate still.

Bibliography

Primary: 1789–98. *Medical Inquiries and Observations* (Philadelphia); 1798. *Essays, Literary, Moral, & Philosophical* (Philadelphia); 1811. *Sixteen Introductory Lectures to Courses of Lectures upon the Institutes and Practice of Medicine, with a Syllabus of the Latter* (Philadelphia); 1812. *Medical Inquiries and Observations upon the Diseases of the Mind* (Philadelphia); 1948. (Corner, George W., ed.) *The Autobiography of Benjamin Rush.* (Princeton).

Secondary: Veatch, Robert, 2005. *Disrupted Dialogue: Medical Ethics and the Collapse of Physician-Humanist Communication (1770–1980)* (New York); Brodsky, Alyn, 2004. *Benjamin Rush: Patriot and Physician* (New York); Burns, Chester, 1999. 'Setting the Stage: Moral Philosophy, Benjamin Rush, and Medical Ethics in the United States before 1846' in Baker, Robert, Arthur L. Caplan, Linda L. Emanuel, and Stephen R. Latham, eds., *The American Medical Ethics Revolution: How the AMA's Code of Ethics Has Transformed Physicians' Relationships to Patients, Professionals, and Society* (Baltimore) pp. 3–16; Haakonssen, Lisbeth, 1997. *Medicine and Morals in the Enlightenment: John Gregory, Thomas Percival and Benjamin Rush* (Amsterdam); Fox, Claire G., Gordon L. Miller, and Jacquelyn M. Miller, 1996. *Benjamin Rush, M.D. A Bibliographic Guide* (Westport, CT); Goodman, Nathan G., 1934. *Benjamin Rush Physician and Citizen 1746–1813* (Philadelphia); *DSB; DAMB.*

Laurence B. McCullough

IBN RUSHD, ABŪ L-WALĪD MUḤAMMAD IBN AḤMAD IBN MUḤAMMAD (aka AVERROES 'THE COMMENTATOR')   (b. Cordova, Spain, 1126; d. Marrakech, Morocco, 1198), *philosophy, jurisprudence, astronomy, medicine.*

Ibn Rushd was born into a family of prominent jurists of Cordova, in the south of Spain. He received a thorough education in Islamic law; he also studied the science of traditions, theology, astronomy, and medicine. Ibn Rushd studied medicine under Abū Jaʿfar Hārūn at-Tajālī, who also taught him Aristotelian philosophy, which probably influenced his interests in natural sciences and physics. Ibn Rushd adhered to the Almohad doctrines, and by 1153 he

had settled in Marrakech, the capital of the Almohad dynasty, where he spent a number of years. Toward 1168 he gained the favor of the caliph Abū Yaʿqūb Yūsuf (r. 1163–84). Ibn Rushd was introduced to him by the caliph's personal physician, the Andalusian philosopher and astronomer Ibn Ṭufayl (d. 1185). This period was the most fruitful time of Ibn Rushd's life in terms of scientific production and public activity. According to sources, the caliph complained of the obscurity of Aristotle's texts and asked Ibn Ṭufayl to make commentaries on them. Ibn Ṭufayl thought himself too old, so he asked Ibn Rushd to undertake the project. In 1169 Ibn Rushd was appointed *qāḍī* (judge) of Seville and, still holding the same position, he moved in 1171 to Cordova, although he continued to work on his writings throughout this period. In 1182 he was appointed chief *qāḍī* of Cordova. At the same time he was summoned to Marrakech to replace Ibn Ṭufayl as chief physician to the caliph Abū Yaʿqūb and kept this appointment under the caliph's son Abū Yūsuf Yaʿqūb al-Manṣūr (r. 1184–99), whose favor Ibn Rushd enjoyed for more than ten years. In 1195 their close relationship ended suddenly when the government in Al-Andalus prohibited philosophical studies and ordered the burning of philosophy books. Ibn Rushd was banished to Lucena, near Cordova, for two years and his doctrines anathematized. A few months before his death, he returned to Marrakech and was reinstated in the caliph's favor. Ibn Rushd died at the end of 1198, and three months later his corpse was brought back and buried in Cordova.

Although Ibn Rushd and his works had little influence in medieval Islam, his philosophical and medical ideas exerted a major impact in the Western Latin tradition. He was known as 'the Commentator': his commentaries on Aristotle's writings became part of them, and some of his doctrines formed a corpus under his name. As a physician, Ibn Rushd belongs to the sphere of such physician-philosophers as Ibn Sīnā, whose philosophical ideas Ibn Rushd criticized and corrected. His major work in medicine is the *Kitāb al-Kulliyāt fī ṭ-ṭibb* [Generalities of medicine], which is devoted to general principles of medicine, included challenging ideas regarding, for instance, the nature of fever, the nonexistence of female semen, and pharmacological issues that provided the Latin tradition with material for fruitful discussion. The book is divided into seven sections, which deal with anatomy, physiology, pathology, symptoms, drugs and foods, hygiene, and therapy. In contrast with the Galenic tradition, Ibn Rushd developed the anatomical discourse without reference to the physiological function of each bodily organ. Translated into Hebrew twice, *Kitāb al-Kulliyāt fī ṭ-ṭibb* was also translated into Latin by the Jew Bonacosa in 1255 under the title *Colliget*, first printed in Venice in 1482. Ibn Rushd also wrote a commentary on Ibn Sīnā's *Poem of Medicine*, translated into Hebrew prose in 1260, into Hebrew verse in 1261, and into Latin around 1280. Andrea Alpago, who also translated Ibn

Rushd's 'Treatise on Theriac', made a revised Latin translation. Particularly relevant to the Latin medical tradition were Ibn Rushd's *Talkhīs*, or paraphrases of Galen's works.

Bibliography

Primary: Forneas, J. M., and C. Álvarez de Morales, eds., 1987. *Kitāb al Kulliyāt* 2 vols. (Madrid) (El libro de las generalidades de la medicina [Kitāb al-Kulliyyāt *fi* l-*ṭibb*]/Abu-l-Walid Ibn Rusd (Averroes); traducción Vázquez de Benito, de María de la Concepción, y Camilo Álvarez Morales (Madrid) 2003.); Vázquez de Benito, C., ed., 1984. *Talkhisat Ibn Rushd ila Jalinus (Commentaria Averrois in Galenum)* (Madrid) ([Talhisat Ibn Rusd `alà Galinus] Obra médica/Averroes; traducción de Vázquez de Benito, Mª Concepción.—[S.l.]: Universidad de Córdoba, imp. 1998; La medicina de Averroes: comentarios a Galeno/Averroes; traducción de María Concepción Vázquez de Benito; introducción Cruz Hernández, Miguel. Colegio Universitario de Zamora, 1987.)

Secondary: García Ballester, L., 2002. 'La recepción del Colliget de Averroes en Montpellier (c. 1285) y su influencia en las polémicas sobre la naturaleza de la fiebre' in *Galen and Galenism* (Aldershot); Jacquart, D., 1996. 'The Influence of Arabic Medicine in the Medieval West' in Rashed, R., ed., *Encyclopedia of the History of Arabic Science* 3 vols. (London and New York) 3: 975–977; Jacquart, D., and F. Micheau, 1990. *La médicine arabe et l'occident médiéval* (Paris) pp. 142–145, 182–185; Renan, E., 1861. *Averroes et l'averroisme* (Paris); *DSB*.

Cristina Álvarez Millán

RUTGERS, JOHANNES (b. Hallum, the Netherlands, 24 August 1850; d. Heerenveen, the Netherlands, *c.* 3 August 1924), *contraception, sexology.*

Rutgers came from a family of Dutch Reformed clergymen and was a minister himself for a short time before he studied medicine and became a physician in Rotterdam in 1879. His first wife, Cornelia Everharda Thiens Abresch, died in 1884 after a long illness, brought on by childbed fever after the birth of their fourth child. Rutgers remarried, this time to the teacher and feminist Maria Wilhelmina Hendrika ('Mietje') Hoitsema. Together, they drifted into vegetarianism, radical politics, feminism, and socialism, although Rutgers never became a member of any socialist party. In 1892 he followed the example of Aletta Jacobs and started to provide contraception in his medical practice, although as a student he had opposed Neo-Malthusianism. He became active in the Dutch New Malthusian League (NMB), founded in 1881 after the British example of George Drysdale.

After 1900 Rutgers and his wife sat together on the board of the NMB. They brought about a reorientation of the NMB by reforming Neo-Malthusianism from a social gospel offering a solution to overpopulation and poverty by birth control, to concentrating instead on making low-cost contraceptive aid available all over the country. They managed to accomplish this by teaching lay women how to instruct other women about the use of the pessary. They also devoted themselves to lifting the legal ban on *abortus provocatus*. Because of the risk that illegal abortion would also be practiced by these so-called 'expert collaborators', there was strong opposition to this scheme among the few supporters of contraception in the Dutch medical profession, and among the old Neo-Malthusians. Although membership of the NMB rose, the social and intellectual isolation of the Dutch birth control movement increased. In the changing political climate in the Netherlands, where political parties along denominational lines became established at the center of political power, there was a serious threat that contraception would be forbidden. A 'League for the Struggle against Neo-Malthusianism' was formed in 1898. When in 1911 a law was passed to curb propaganda for contraception, no one in the Dutch parliament defended the practice of contraception on principle. Despite this general hostility, the prohibitive measures proved to have little effect.

Rutgers—who was editor of *Het Gelukkig Huisgezin* [the Happy Family]—continued his tireless efforts to spread knowledge on contraception and to teach the 'expert collaborators'. In 1915 Margaret Sanger was among the many women who stayed for some weeks in his household to pick up the routine. However, the idealistic attitude that had been typical of the NMB was gradually replaced by a more commercial spirit. When Rutgers left the NMB in 1919, there were no capable successors. The birth control movement in the Netherlands—to that moment the best organized in the world—entered a period of decline.

In his last years, Rutgers published extensively on sexual matters; he was the first author in the Netherlands to present a coherent theory of sexuality. He valued the satisfaction of the sexual drive as an aim in itself, and as a precondition for health and happiness, but was at the same time suspicious of yielding to lust. To cope with these conflicting considerations, he stressed the importance of self-control and hygiene in sexual behavior. The necessity to defend himself against accusations of immorality made him develop an exacting morality of his own. The roots of his outlook upon the world were an eclectic variety of socialism, anarchism, and social Darwinism. Rutgers combined a pessimistic view of life with a strong belief in progress. In many respects his philosophy was based on nineteenth-century utilitarian and materialist ideas. Rutgers committed suicide in 1924.

Bibliography

Primary: 1900. *Een Boek voor Jonge Vrouwen en Meisjes. Wenken voor het Geslachtsleven* (Amsterdam); 1905. *Rasverbetering en Bewuste Aantalsbeperking. Kritiek van het Malthusianisme en het Nieuw-Malthusianisme* (Rotterdam); 1916. *Het Geslachtsleven van den Man. Een Biologische Studie* (Almelo); 1940. *How to Attain and Practice the Ideal Sex Life: Ideal Sex and Love Relations for Every Married Man and Woman* (New York).

Secondary: Röling, H.Q. 1987. '*De Tragedie van het Geslachtsleven.*' *Dr. J. Rutgers (1850–1924) en de Nieuw-Maltusiaansche Bond (opgericht 1881)* (Amsterdam); Nabrink, G., 1978. *Seksuele Hervorming in Nederland* (Nijmegen).

Hugo Röling

RUYSCH, FREDERIK   (b. the Hague, the Netherlands, 28 March 1638; d. Amsterdam, the Netherlands, 22 February 1731), *anatomy, botany, obstetrics.*

Ruysch was a renowned anatomist whose fame lasted well into the nineteenth century. He owed his reputation to a preparation method that transformed anatomy from an unpleasant, grisly, activity into a widely admired art form. His technique enabled him to lay bare even the minutest parts of the body, making him a valuable guide on the early modern journeys of discovery through the human body. His preparations had wide appeal; visitors to Ruysch's anatomical collection marveled at his allegorical compositions. His embalmed bodies, adorned with lace, seemed not dead but merely asleep. One visitor, Russia's Tsar Peter the Great, was so astonished at the sight of a child's lifelike corpse that he knelt down to kiss it.

Ruysch, born into a family of clerks, first became an apothecary's apprentice. Keen to learn everything he could about plants, he began—while still an apprentice—to collect the flora of the area and such wonders of nature as shells, fossils, and insects. He soon turned to anatomy, however, experimenting with conservation methods that made use of alcohol. As soon as he had established himself as an apothecary, in 1661, he married Maria Post (1643–1720), the daughter of a famous architect, and went to Leiden to study medicine.

In Leiden he continued to develop his preservation techniques, which in turn facilitated further research. Anatomists working in the mid-seventeenth century continually encountered one apparently insurmountable obstacle: the rapid decay of corpses made systematic physiological research impossible. The great haste required to remain one step ahead of decomposition led to mistakes and misunderstandings. Another impediment was the fact that death altered the state of a body. After death, the arteries emptied, becoming almost invisible, so there was an urgent need for a method of preserving body parts and making previously invisible parts visible. Consequently, all manner of experiments were carried out, especially at Leiden University, by Ruysch and his fellow students Jan Swammerdam, Niels Stensen, and Reinier de Graaf. After graduation (1664) Ruysch persisted in developing better and more lasting methods of preservation. His successful injection techniques enabled him to demonstrate the occurrence of blood vessels in almost all the tissues of the body.

In 1666 the Amsterdam town council called upon Ruysch to reorganize the training of surgeons and midwives. To this end, and to finance his own anatomical research, he took on a number of medical and teaching posts, serving as professor of anatomy (1668), court physician (1672), accoucheur (1672), and professor of botany (1685). His success was envied by his rivals, and their jealousy led to conflicts that permeated Amsterdam's elite circles. Although power, money, and status were at stake, ideology also played a role in these controversies. Backed by several friends of Spinoza, Ruysch was cast in the role of champion of those seeking to explain the mysteries of the world in a rational way by providing answers based on their own insights, unencumbered by the dictates of tradition and authority.

Ruysch found theorizing a waste of time and placed little value on speculation, preferring to trust only his own eyes. In the early 1690s, having perfected his method of preparation, he felt confident enough to publish anatomical and surgical treatises based on his own observations, without the usual references to the classical medical literature. His observations impressed a number of prominent scientists, including Herman Boerhaave, who based much of his medical teaching on 'Ruyschian anatomy'.

Frederik Ruysch died in 1731, survived by three daughters, one of whom was the accomplished painter, Rachel Ruysch (1664–1750). He carried with him to the grave the secret of his preparation techniques, but his specimens have been preserved, thanks to Peter the Great. In 1717 Tsar Peter purchased Ruysch's entire collection and shipped it to St Petersburg, where Ruysch's anatomical specimens—a substantial part of which have survived for three centuries—still attract thousands of visitors each year.

Bibliography

Primary: 1737. *Opera omnia anatomica-medico-chirurgica* (Amsterdam); 1744. *Alle de ontleed-, genees- en heelkundige werken* (Amsterdam).

Secondary: Kooijmans, Luuc, 2004. *De doodskunstenaar. De anatomische lessen van Frederik Ruysch* (Amsterdam); *DSB*.

Luuc Kooijmans

RYLE, JOHN ALFRED   (b. Barnet, Middlesex, England, 12 December 1889; d. Pulborough, Sussex, England, 27 February 1950), *medicine, social medicine.*

Of a distinguished family (a grandfather and an uncle were bishops, a brother Waynflete professor of metaphysics at Oxford, and a son a Nobel prizewinner in physics), Ryle was the eldest son of a physician who later practiced in Brighton. With nine other children, however, his father could not afford to educate him at Oxford, sending him instead to Guy's Hospital Medical School, where he graduated in 1914. He joined the Royal Army Medical Corps almost immediately, spending four years in Flanders, where he undertook research into Weil's disease in the trenches.

Returning to Guy's Hospital as a registrar and becoming a consultant physician soon afterward, Ryle specialized in gastroenterology, devising a test meal and a gastric (Ryle's) tube much used in investigating peptic ulcer. Nevertheless, as someone who subsequently was in favor of nationalized medicine, he became increasingly unhappy with his large private practice in Wimpole Street, London, and in 1935 accepted the invitation to become Regius professor of physic at Cambridge. Conditions there, however, proved equally unattractive: there was no undergraduate school and his access to hospital beds was limited by the hostility of local consultants (who felt threatened by academia). Ryle was unhappy with the smugness of college life, whose members were unlikely to have sympathized with his work for Spanish Civil War relief and help for medical refugees. Thus, at the start of World War II, having failed to be elected as an independent member of parliament for Cambridge, he renounced his pacifist views and returned to Guy's Hospital as a consultant for the Emergency Medical Service, also helping treat patients injured in the bombing raids.

In 1942 Ryle accepted the offer of a newly created chair of social medicine at Oxford. He had long been disillusioned with the failure of clinical research based on laboratory studies to tackle the problems of clinical disease. Instead, in his view, as expressed well before in *The Natural History of Disease* (1936), the study of etiology needed to be expanded to recognize the patient's social environment and psychological history. Such a concept was much in vogue in the early 1940s with official bodies such as the Health Department and the RCP, being given practical expression with Lord Nuffield's funding of the Oxford chair. Until his early death from coronary disease, Ryle continued to speak and write about social medicine, with seventy-seven out of his lifelong total of 135 published papers devoted to the topic, as well as two of his five books, including the influential *Changing Disciplines* (1948). Nevertheless, although a few other chairs were established in the discipline (as well as a British journal), the Oxford Institute was closed after his death and the term 'social medicine' drifted into obscurity. In part, this was possibly because of the obscure language that some of the proponents of social medicine had used. Although the tall and handsome Ryle had enormous charisma and powers of persuasion, some practical implications of his philosophy were not always easy to perceive, and, with the newly emerging antibiotics and other powerful drugs, orthodox medicine was changing fast. Moreover, there were exciting discoveries in the related discipline of epidemiology, such as the statistically established links between lifestyle and disease (for example, smoking and lung cancer). Almost certainly, however, Ryle did have a profound and lasting influence on medical practice. Many of his lessons became subsumed, unacknowledged, into current thought, particularly in general practice; today's persistent emphasis on holism surely owes much to his work.

Bibliography

Primary: 1936. *The Natural History of Disease* (London) [2nd edn., 1948; reprint 1988, with an introduction by Shepherd, M. (London)]; 1948. *Changing Disciplines* (London) [reprint, 1994, with an introduction by Porter, D. (New Brunswick, NJ)].

Secondary: Porter, D., 1992. 'Changing Disciplines: John Ryle and the Making of Social Medicine in Britain in the 1940s.' *History of Science* 30: 137–164; *Oxford DNB.*

Stephen Lock